AIR & SURFACE TRANSPORT NURSES ASSOCIATION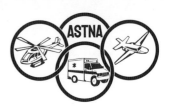

PATIENT TRANSPORT

MEDICAL CRITICAL CARE

AIR & SURFACE TRANSPORT NURSES ASSOCIATION

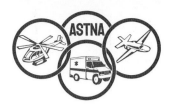

PATIENT TRANSPORT

MEDICAL CRITICAL CARE

Allen C. Wolfe Jr., MSN, CNS, APRN, CFRN, CCRN, CTRN, TCRN, CMTE, FAASTN

Senior Director of Education
Clinical Nurse Specialist
Life Link III
Minneapolis, Minnesota

Michael A. Frakes, APRN, FCCM, FAEN, FAASTN, FACHE

Chief Quality Officer and Director of Clinical Care
Boston MedFlight
Bedford, Massachusetts

B. Daniel Nayman, MBA, NRP, FP-C, CCP-C, CMTE

Vice President
Board of Directors
International College of Advanced Practice Paramedics
Washington, DC

Paramedic
Life Flight Duke University Hospital System
Durham, North Carolina

Product Manager
Patient Care
ZOLL Data Systems
Broomfield, Colorado

ELSEVIER

Elsevier
3251 Riverport Lane
St. Louis, Missouri 63043

Executive Content Strategist: Lee Henderson
Senior Content Development Specialist: Kristen Helm
Publishing Services Manager: Julie Eddy
Senior Project Manager: Joanna Souch
Design Direction: Margaret Reid

Printed in India

Last digit is the print number: 9   8   7   6   5   4   3   2   1

Working together to grow libraries in developing countries

www.elsevier.com • www.bookaid.org

This work is dedicated to the late Kelley Holdren, ASTNA President, flight nurse, wife, mother, colleague, and friend. We are inspired by her commitment to patient-centered care, education, and the transport community. She is missed every day.

Thanks to my mom for just being awesome and supportive! A huge shout-out and thanks to Mary Ann Melville, who was one of the first flight paramedics who trained me in Air Medical; she passed away this year. Thanks to my colleagues at Life Link III in Minnesota for their constant focus on providing great care for people on their worst days. Thanks to Ed Rupert and MedSTAR (DC) and Rob Hamilton for my start in this industry. An international thanks to my big supporters in Italy who invite me out to speak often and take great care of me in their country. Michele Masotto, Fabrizio Lorenzoni, Gianfranco Magi, and Isabella Garancini, you are amazing.

Allen C. Wolfe Jr., MSN, CNS, APRN, CFRN, CCRN, CTRN, TCRN, CMTE, FAASTN

Thank you to the colleagues and mentors who continue to help me be a better transport nurse. I appreciate the work that ASTNA, Allen, and Danny put into this work, and the efforts of the multiprofessional team of collaborators who worked on this book. I am proud to be able to dedicate my part of this book to Malisa, Charlie, and Gabriele, who support and inspire me every day; to the late Ray and Agnes Frakes, who taught me the value of books and language; and to the late Dr. Suzanne Wedel, for her visions of excellence and collaboration.

Michael A. Frakes, APRN, FCCM, FAEN, FAASTN, FACHE

My work on this book is dedicated to my wife, Angie, and kids, Braydan and Amelia, for the love, support, and inspiration they give me. I want to thank Dr. Brent Myers, René Borghese, Dr. Donna York, Phil Ward, Chris Hall, Sue Hollowell, Jenn Killeen, Michael Bachman, David Bump, John Clark, Charlie Swearingen, Eric and Ashley Bauer, Sean Gibson, Dr. Aaron Byrd, and the many other colleagues and mentors I have had in my life who have believed in me and pushed me to achieve more than I ever could have otherwise. Thank you to the ASTNA board, Allen Wolfe, and Michael Frakes for allowing me to work on this project with them, and to the I-CAPP board for allowing me to represent the organization on this project. To my Mom, Dad, and sisters (Trish, Rebecca, Kelli, and my late sister Jaime) for always believing in me. It has been an honor to work with each of the authors, reviewers, and collaborators on this project and to have a small part in creating content that will improve the knowledge of clinicians and the lives of patients for years to come.

B. Daniel Nayman, MBA, NRP, FP-C, CCP-C, CMTE

Contributors

Janna Baker-Rogers, MD, MS
Assistant Professor
Department of Medicine
West Virginia University School of Medicine
Morgantown, West Virginia

Francesca Baruffi, MD
Resident Physician
Department of Emergency Medicine
West Virginia University School of Medicine
Morgantown, West Virginia

Chad Bowman, MSN, RN, CFRN, CCRN, NR-P
Assistant Nurse Manager
Lifeline Critical Care Transport Team
Johns Hopkins Hospital
Baltimore, Maryland
Director of Transport Operations
Johns Hopkins Special Pathogen Center
Johns Hopkins Hospital
Baltimore, Maryland

Shellie A. Brandt, MSN, RN, NP, AANP
Nurse Practitioner
Department of Emergency Medicine
Children's Mercy Hospital
Kansas City, Missouri

Sarah Brock, BSN, BA, BES, CFRN, TCRN, CEN
Flight Nurse
Clinical
Life Link III
Marshfield, Wisconsin
Registered Nurse
Emergency
Marshfield Medical Center
Marshfield, Wisconsin

Ashley M. Chitty, BSN, RN, CFRN, CPEN, CEN
Registered Nurse
Flight Nurse
Life Link III
Anoka, Minnesota

Sahil Dayal, BA, BS, MD
Resident Physician
Emergency Medicine
West Virginia University School of Medicine
Morgantown, West Virginia

Jamie R. Eastman, BSN, RN, NRP, CCRN-A, CCRN-P, CCRN-N, CFRN, FP-C, CEN, TCRN, C-NPT, C-ELBW, CMTE
Pediatric Staff Educator, Critical Care Transport Nurse-Paramedic
Boston MedFlight
Bedford, Massachusetts
Critical Care Nurse
United States Army Reserve
Bedford, Massachusetts

Tonya I. Elliott, MSN, RN, CCTC, CHFN
Program Development Specialist
Medstar, Washington Hospital Center
Washington, DC

Vahe Ender, NRP, FP-C
Clinical Project Manager
Clinical Division
Boston MedFlight
Bedford, Massachusetts

Shane Farmer, MHA, NREMTP, FP-C
Senior Vice President
Medical Flight Operations
CSI Aviation
Kileen, Texas

Jade B. Flinn, MSN, RN, CCRN, CNRN
Director of Operations
Department of Medicine, Special Pathogens Center, Biocontainment Unit
Johns Hopkins Hospital
Baltimore, Maryland

Michael A. Frakes, APRN, FCCM, FAEN, FAASTN, FACHE
Chief Quality Officer and Director of Clinical Care
Boston MedFlight
Bedford, Massachusetts

Michael D. Gooch, DNP, APRN, CCP, ACNP-BC, FNP-BC, ENP-C, CFRN, CTRN, CEN, TCRN, NRP, FAASTN, FAANP
Flight-Emergency Nurse Practitioner
LifeFlight
Vanderbilt University Medical Center
Nashville, Tennessee
Assistant Professor
Acute and Chronic Care Community
Vanderbilt University School of Nursing
Nashville, Tennessee
Faculty
Middle Tennessee School of Anesthesia
Madison, Tennessee

Christian Greengrass, BSN, RN, EMT-P, CCRN, CFRN, CTRN, FP-C
Flight Nurse and Paramedic
Air Clinical Division
CareFlite
Grand Prairie, Texas

Francis Guyette, MD, MS, MPH
Professor of Emergency Medicine
Emergency Medicine
University of Pittsburgh
Pittsburgh, Pennsylvania
Medical Director
STAT MedEvac
Center for Emergency Medicine
West Mifflin, Pennsylvania

Joseph Hill, APRN, MSN, FNP-C, CFRN, CMTE
Nurse Practitioner
Family Practice
Sterling Health
Mt. Sterling, Kentucky
Clinical Director II
Air Methods
Midwest Region
Englewood, Colorado

Hunter Hix, BSN, RN, CCRN, TCRN, CNRN, CEN, CFRN
Flight Nurse
Medevac
Northern Colorado Medical Center
Greeley, Colorado

Kyle Hurst, MD, FACEP, EMS Physician
Assistant Professor
Emergency Medicine
West Virginia University School of Medicine
Morgantown, West Virginia
Director of Emergency Services
United Hospital Center
Bridgeport, West Virginia

Marion L. Jones, RN, MSN, CFRN, CMTE
Quality and Education Manager
Medical Operations
STAT MedEvac
West Mifflin, Pennsylvania

Bradley Arthur Kuch, MHA, RRT-NPS, NREMT, CMTE, FAARC
Director, Medical Operations
STAT MedEvac
Center of Emergency Medicine
Pittsburgh, Pennsylvania

Roger L. Layell, AAS, FP-C, CCP-C, C-NPT, CCEMT-P, NRP
Flight Paramedic
MedCenter Air
Atrium Health
Charlotte, North Carolina

Lorie J. Ledford, MSN, RN, CCRN, CEN, CPEN, TCRN, CFRN, CTRN
Bedford, Flight Nurse
Native Air 8
Air Methods Corporation
Greenwood Village, Colorado
Adjunct Faculty
Nursing
Estrella Mountain Community College
Goodyear, Arizona

Kayla S. Lynch, RN-BSN, CFRN, CCRN, PHN, NREMT-B
Director of Nursing Education and Interprofessional Development
Department of Education and Professional Development
MedStar Transport/MedStar Health
Washingon, DC

P.S. Martin, MD, FACEP, FAEMS
Associate Professor
Emergency Medicine
West Virginia University School of Medicine
Morgantown, West Virginia
West Virginia Office of EMS State Medical Director
Department of Health
Charleston, West Virginia

B. Daniel Nayman, MBA, NRP, FP-C, CCP-C, CMTE
Vice President
Board of Directors
International College of Advanced Practice Paramedics
Washington, DC
Paramedic
Life Flight Duke University Hospital System
Durham, North Carolina
Product Manager
Patient Care
ZOLL Data Systems
Broomfield, Colorado

Sandra Nixon, BA, MD
Resident Physician
Emergency Medicine
West Virginia University
Morgantown, West Virginia

Emily A. Ollmann, MS, MD
Emergency Medicine Resident
Emergency Department
West Virginia University
Morgantown, West Virginia

James Scheidler, MD, FACEP
Assistant Professor
Emergency Medicine
West Virginia University School of Medicine
Morgantown, West Virginia

Jessica Schmoyer Rispoli, DNP, FNP-C, RN, CMTE, CFRN, CEN, PHRN, EMTP
Flight Nurse, Base Lead
EastCare
ECU Health
Greenville, North Carolina

Michael Shukis, MD
Assistant Professor
Department of Emergency medicine
West Virginia University School of Medicine
Morgantown, West Virginia

Charles F. Swearingen, BS, NRP, FP-C
Flight Paramedic
Helicopter Transport
University of Mississippi Medical Center
Jackson, Mississippi
Owner/Educator
MeduPros.com
Brandon, Mississippi

Leslie C. Sweet, BSN, RN
Senior Principal, Medical Affairs, Medical Sciences, Publication Specialist
MCS Medical Affairs, Medical Sciences
Medtronic
Minneapolis, Minnesota

Allison Tadros, MD
Professor
Emergency Medicine
West Virginia University
Morgantown, West Virginia

Brooke Turner, BSN, RN, CCRN, CEN, CFRN, CMTE
Flight Nurse, Regional Clinical Manager
Clinical
Life Link III
Shoreview, Minnesota

John vonRosenberg, PhD, FP-C
Flight Paramedic
East Care
ECU Health
Edenton, North Carolina

Allen C. Wolfe Jr., MSN, CNS, APRN, CFRN, CCRN, CTRN, TCRN, CMTE, FAASTN
Senior Director of Education
Clinical Nurse Specialist
Life Link III
Minneapolis, Minnesota

Reviewers

Janna Baker-Rogers, MD, MS
West Virginia University School of Medicine
Morgantown, West Virginia

Francesa Baruffi, MD
West Virginia University School of Medicine
Morgantown, West Virginia

Paul Boackle, BSN, RN, CCRN, CEN, CFRN, CPEN, NPT-C, EMT
University of Mississippi AirCare
Jackson, Mississippi

Theresa Bowden, MSN, RN
Washington State University
Life Flight Network
Spokane, Washington

Cherish Brodbeck, MSN, FNP-BC, RNC-OB, LP, CMTE
Kite Flight Specialty Transport
Covenant Children's Hospital
Lubbock, Texas

Joshua Chan, BA, NRP, FP-C, CCP-C
Glacial Ridge Health System
Glenwood, Minnesota

Sahil Dayal, BA, BS, MD
West Virginia University School of Medicine
Morgantown, West Virginia

Michael W. Dexter, MSN, RN, CCRN, CEN, CFRN, CPEN, CTRN, TCRN, EMT
Board of Certification for Emergency Nursing
Chicago, Illinois

David Fifer, MS, NRP, WP-C, FAWM
Eastern Kentucky University
Richmond, Kentucky;
Kentucky Board of Emergency Medical Services
Lexington, Kentucky

Michael D. Gooch, APRN, CCP, ACNP-BC, FNP-BC, ENP-BC, ENP-C, CEN, CFRN, CTRN, TCRN, NRP
Vanderbilt University School of Nursing
Nashville, Tennessee

Cindy Goodrich, MS, RN, CFRN, CCRN
Airlift Northwest
University of Washington
Seattle, Washington

Robert L. Grabowski, DNP, MBA, APRN-CNP, AGACNP-BC, CPNP-AC, CEN, CCRN, CFRN, CMTE, EMT-P
Metro Life Flight
The MetroHealth System
Cleveland, Ohio

Russell Haight, MBA, BSN, RN, PHN, CFRN, CCRN-CMC, EMT-P
Stanford Life Flight
Palo Alto, California

Ray Hummel, MSN, RN, AGACNP-BC, CFRN, TCRN
UCLA School of Nursing
Los Angeles, California;
Memorial Care Long Beach Medical Center
Long Beach, California

Kyle Hurst, MD, FACEP, EMS Physician
West Virginia University School of Medicine
Morgantown, West Virginia;
United Hospital Center
Bridgeport, West Virginia

Ryan Kerr, CFRN, CEN, FP-C
Air Methods
Albuquerque, New Mexico

Frederick (Bud) Lavin, BSN, CFRN, RCIS, NREMT-P
Robert Wood Johnson Barnabas Health Life Flight
Robert Wood Johnson University Hospital
New Brunswick, New Jersey

Leslie Lewis, DNP, APRN, CPNP-AC, CCRN, C-NPT, CPEN, CPN, EMT-LP, FP-C, CCP-C
UT Southwestern/Children's Health
Dallas, Texas

P.S. Martin, MD, FACEP, FAEMS
West Virginia University School of Medicine
Morgantown, West Virginia

Conner McDonald, MD
West Virginia University School of Medicine
Morgantown, West Virginia

Lee McMurray, CFRN, CEN, FP-C, BSN, MSN
Stanford Life Flight
Palo Alto, California

Michael Moscone, BSN, RN, CEN
Penn Medicine
University of Pennsylvania Health System
Philadelphia, Pennsylvania

Sandra Nixon, BA, MD
West Virginia University School of Medicine
Morgantown, West Virginia

Emily A. Ollmann, MS, MD
West Virginia University School of Medicine
Morgantown, West Virginia

Katherine E. Riedel, RN, CCRN, C-NPT, CEN
Air Methods
Durham, North Carolina

Paul Rigby, BSN, RN, BS, CCRN, CFRN, EMTP, CCEMTP, CMTE
West Michigan Air Care
Kalamazoo, Michigan

Kandi (Karen) Sagehorn, BSN, CFRN, CMTE
Air Methods
Omaha, Nebraska

James Scheidler, MD, FACEP
West Virginia University School of Medicine
Morgantown, West Virginia

Michael Shukis, MD
West Virginia University School of Medicine
Morgantown, West Virginia

Allison Tadros, MD
West Virginia University School of Medicine
Morgantown, West Virginia

Foreword

The members of the Air & Surface Transport Nurses Association (ASTNA) Education and Publications committees, along with the Board of Directors, recognize that the aspects of critical care transport medicine can be overwhelming. Because of this, we introduce you to this first edition of *Patient Transport: Medical Critical Care*. This book has been written to serve as a comprehensive guide for transport professionals taking care of complex medical patients in a unique environment. Our goal is to bridge the gap between hospital-based critical care and the unique challenges faced every day when transporting these patients.

The realm of patient transport medicine is intricate and demanding, necessitating a unique blend of clinical expertise, swift decision-making, and an understanding of the logistical and environmental factors that can affect patient outcomes. Throughout this text, you will find detailed information on a variety of medical topics written by experts in the medical transport field.

As president of the Air & Surface Transport Nurses Association (ASTNA), I would like to extend my gratitude to all the contributors and reviewers who have made this publication possible. I am honored to have been a support person for this endeavor.

Sue Hollowell, BSN, RN, CFRN, FP-C, CMTE
President, ASTNA
Regional Clinical Educator, Air Methods

Preface

Critical care transport requires a precise and collaborative approach, which is why this book, supported by the Air & Surface Transport Nurses Association (ASTNA) and the International College of Advanced Practice Paramedics (I-CAPP), serves as an essential resource for transport clinicians. This text focuses on medical critical care transport. It covers foundational principles, research, and emerging practices tailored to patient care in air and ground transport. Every chapter is written to provide a clear and thorough understanding of critical care transport.

For the authors, reviewers, and editors who put in long hours to put this together, we appreciate your devotion to providing your expertise to the industry. Thanks for your dedication!

Allen C. Wolfe Jr., MSN, CNS, APRN, CFRN, CCRN, CTRN, TCRN, CMTE, FAASTN
Michael A. Frakes, APRN, FCCM, FAEN, FAASTN, FACHE
B. Daniel Nayman, MBA, NRP, FP-C, CCP-C, CMTE

Acknowledgments

We extend our deepest gratitude to everyone who contributed to *Patient Transport: Medical Critical Care*. This book reflects the collective expertise and dedication of transport professionals across multiple disciplines. From pilots and communication specialists to flight nurses and paramedics, their insights and experience helped shape the content, ensuring that it remains practical and relevant to the realities of critical care transport. Without their contributions and commitment to high-quality patient care, this book would not have been possible.

A special thank you is also due to our collaborators and supporters who believed in this vision from the start. Your encouragement and trust made the process smoother and more rewarding. To the team at Elsevier, Sarah Loiero, Nikole Good, and the ASTNA Board of Directors, your support is greatly appreciated. We hope this book will serve as a valuable resource, inspiring continued growth and collaboration in the field of patient transport. Together, we can continue striving to deliver the best care possible for those who need it most.

Allen C. Wolfe Jr., MSN, CNS, APRN, CFRN,
CCRN, CTRN, TCRN, CMTE, FAASTN
Michael A. Frakes APRN, FCCM, FAEN, FAASTN, FACHE
B. Daniel Nayman, MBA, NRP, FP-C, CCP-C, CMTE

Contents

1

Hematologic System

JESSICA SCHMOYER RISPOLI

COMPETENCIES

1. State the components of the hematologic system and their function.
2. Describe the clotting cascade intrinsic and extrinsic pathways.
3. List reversal agents for coagulopathies.
4. Describe common blood disorders.
5. Describe blood compatibility and transfusion requirements.

Introduction

The hematologic system is a complex and vital system that performs many essential functions. Transport clinicians should be able to interpret complete blood counts (CBC) and understand the effects of the coagulation cascade which guide their decision to implement different treatment modalities for patients with specific blood disorders or who require transfusion therapy. This chapter is intended to help the critical care transport clinician understand the vital role the hematologic (circulatory) system provides for organ and cellular survival by supplying important nutrients and eliminating toxins from the body. Knowledge of these coagulation disorders and the transfusion standards are key to effectively care for critical care patients.

Brief Anatomy and Physiology Overview

The hematologic system is composed of blood and bone marrow. Blood is a connective tissue that circulates throughout the body and consists of platelets, red blood cells (RBCs), plasma, clotting factors, and white blood cells (WBCs). RBCs, WBCs, and platelets make up about 45% of blood, while plasma and extracellular fluid make up the other 55%. The average adult has a volume of about 5–6 L of blood, which makes up around 7% to 8% of a human's total body weight.[1]

Red Blood Cells

RBCs, or erythrocytes, transport oxygen throughout the body due to the protein called hemoglobin. RBCs have no nuclei, which allows them to change shape. An average RBC has a lifespan of about 120 days (Fig. 1.1).[1] RBC production relies on the hormone erythropoietin, which is produced by the kidneys. Therefore, patients with chronic kidney disease are often anemic due to their decreased erythropoietin production.

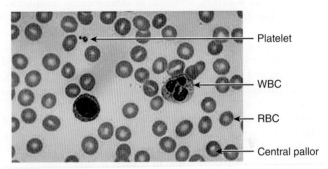

• **Fig. 1.1** Blood smear under a microscope. (From Navya KT, Prasad K, Singh BMK. Analysis of red blood cells from peripheral blood smear images for anemia detection: a methodological review. *Med Biol Eng Comput*. 2022;60(9):2446. Figure 1.)

White Blood Cells

WBCs, or leukocytes, make up 1% of blood volume. Produced by the bone marrow, neutrophils are the most common WBCs, totaling 55%–65% of the WBC count. Neutrophils act as the initial defense against foreign substances, bacteria, and fungi.[1] Eosinophils account for 1%–3% of WBCs and are noted to be elevated in both parasitic infections and allergic reactions.[1] Basophils account for even less than eosinophils and are involved with allergic reactions. The clotting cascade and the immune system have an indirect relationship. As the immune system is activated by toxins or infections and injury, a coagulation response occurs. Endotoxin triggers the formation of tissue factor initiating coagulation, downregulates anticoagulant mechanisms including the protein C pathway and heparin-like proteoglycans, and upregulates plasminogen activator inhibitor.[2] Therefore, a slight increase in WBC count may be expected in injured patients.

Lymphocytes are important for immunity in humans, as they may be stored for years in the blood and lymph system.[1] Lymphocytes include B cells, T cells, and natural killer cells, which will be discussed in a later chapter (see Chapter 5).

Platelets

Platelets are essential for forming the platelet plug, which controls bleeding once a vessel wall sustains an injury. Platelets also have no nucleus and circulate for about 8–9 days if they are unused. Platelets are produced each day from the bone marrow. In addition to the regulation of hemostasis, platelets have also been shown to play an important role in innate immunity.

Plasma

Plasma is a liquid composed of water (90%), proteins (6.5%–8%), and molecular substances (2%).[1] Plasma acts as a transport medium for the body, delivering nutrients while also collecting waste products to take to organs that will excrete them. Plasma proteins include albumin, fibrinogen, and globulins. Fibrinogen only comprises 7% of plasma proteins, but it plays a large role in blood clotting.[1]

Laboratory Values

The CBC, or complete blood count, is a blood test that is highly useful in the clinical setting as it can indicate dyscrasias or disorders such as anemia, infection, leukemia, or other medical conditions.[1] Normal values are shown in Table 1.1.

Hemoglobin, or Hgb, is the protein responsible for carrying oxygen. Normal hemoglobin levels for adult males are 14–17 g/dL and for adult females are 12–15 g/dL.[3] Hemoglobin is decreased in anemias and increased (polycythemia) in different disorders, such as chronic hypoxia, high-altitude living, and people who smoke.[1]

Hematocrit, or Hct, is the percentage of RBCs per whole blood volume. A normal hematocrit in relation to the hemoglobin should be three times the hemoglobin value. A normal hematocrit in adult males is 42%–52% and in females is 36%–48%.[3]

The CBC also contains platelet levels, mean corpuscular volume (MCV), mean corpuscular hemoglobin concentration (MCHC), mean corpuscular hemoglobin (MCH), red cell distribution width (RDW), and the neutrophil, lymphocyte, monocyte, eosinophil, and basophil counts. Normal values can be seen in Table 1.1. The MCV is the average size of the RBCs in the blood sample. Low MCV is seen in microcytic anemias, whereas elevated MCV is seen in macrocytic anemias. The MCHC indicates the average color of a red blood cell. A decreased value is found in certain anemias. The MCH is another, but indirect, measure of the red blood cell color. RDW shows the variations in the size of the RBCs which can be elevated in certain anemias and blood loss.[1]

Hemostasis

Hemostasis refers to the processes involved to stop bleeding which occurs in five stages and two different phases. Hemostasis comes from "hem-" meaning "blood" and "-stasis" meaning "to stop." After an intrinsic or extrinsic injury or insult, the first stage, or *vessel spasm*, occurs, which reduces blood flow by constricting the blood vessel.[1] This is the start of primary hemostasis. Intrinsic is defined as an insult from within such as a toxin in the bloodstream launching the clotting cascade or an extrinsic pathway which is an external penetration of the skin barrier.

TABLE 1.1   **Normal CBC and Coagulation Values**

Complete Blood Count (CBC)		
Red Blood Cells		
Red blood cell count	Male:	4.5–6 million/mm³
	Female:	4.0–5.5 million/mm³
Hemoglobin (Hgb)	Male:	14–17 g/dL
	Female:	12–15 g/dL
Hematocrit (Hct)	Male:	42%–52%
	Female:	36%–48%
Mean corpuscular volume (MCV)	80–100 μm³	
Mean corpuscular hemoglobin concentration (MCHC)	30–36 g/dL	
Red cell distribution width (RDW)	12%–15%	
White Blood Cells		
White blood cell count	4–10 ×10³/μL	
Neutrophils	40%–60% (of white blood cells)	
Lymphocytes	20%–40% (of white blood cells)	
Monocytes	2%–8% (of white blood cells)	
Eosinophils	1%–4% (of white blood cells)	
Basophils	0.5%–1% (of white blood cells)	
Bands (immature neutrophils)	0%–3% (of white blood cells)	
Platelets		
Platelet count	150–400 ×10³/mm³	
Coagulation		
Prothrombin time (PT)	10–13 seconds	
International normalized ratio (INR)	<1	
Activated partial thromboplastin time (aPTT)	22–34 seconds	

Following vessel spasm, the second stage is the formation of an unstable *platelet plug*.[1] In this stage the platelets are activated and aggregate and adhere to the vessel wall. Glycoprotein receptors are exposed on the platelets' outer surfaces.[1] One of the glycoproteins is GPIIb/IIIa, which is responsible for binding fibrinogen and bridging platelets together. This is where GPIIb/IIIa inhibitor drugs (abciximab [Reopro], eptifibatide [Integrillin], tirofiban [Aggrastat]) impact platelet adhesion, which is used in acute coronary syndrome or after percutaneous coronary intervention (PCI).[3] Platelet adhesion also relies on a protein called von Willebrand factor (vWF). Platelet receptors bind to vWF at the site of the endothelial injury.[1] After adhesion, platelet aggregation occurs. Adenosine diphosphate (ADP) is produced by platelets' mitochondria and enzyme systems and enzymes that synthesize thromboxane

A$_2$ (TXA$_2$), which are both essential to the enlargement of the platelet aggregate and the creation of the primary plug.[1] Clopidogrel (Plavix) and other similar medications (ticagrelor, ticlopidine, and prasugrel) inhibit the adenosine diphosphate (ADP) pathway by blocking the ADP receptor, preventing platelet aggregation.[3] Clopidogrel is commonly used during acute coronary syndrome (including myocardial infarction), stroke, and MI prevention.[3] Aspirin (ASA) inhibits platelet aggregation by inhibiting TXA$_2$ synthesis. ASA binds to platelets for the life of the platelet. Therefore, daily ASA allows for any platelets produced in the bone marrow to be covered to prevent aggregation.

The platelet plug is stabilized once the coagulation cascade, or clotting cascade, begins and starts the third stage and second phases of hemostasis.[1] This is the process involving the conversion of fibrinogen into fibrin. Fibrin is then able to form the clot by facilitating the adhesion of other blood components and platelets together.[1] The coagulation cascade requires the activation of numerous clotting factors, a majority of which are synthesized in the liver. These clotting factors are labeled with Roman numerals, and once they become activated are followed by the letter "a." For coagulation to occur there are three pathways: extrinsic, intrinsic, and common (Fig. 1.2).

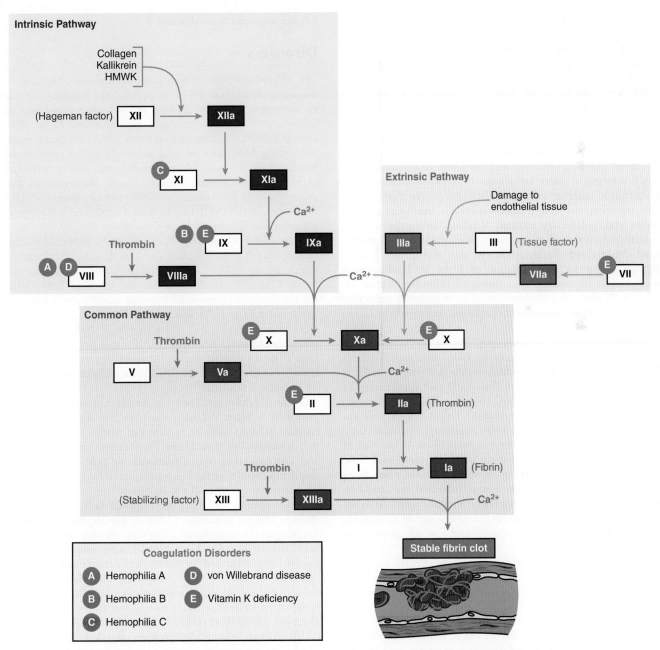

• **Fig. 1.2** Coagulation cascade. Series of steps in response to bleeding caused by tissue injury. Each step activates the next and ultimately produces a blood clot. Coagulation disorders can either cause excessive or inadequate clotting. Deficiency in >1 clotting factor can exist. (Modified from Tarantino C. Coagulation cascade: What it is, steps, and more. *Osmosis (from Elsevier)*. Updated 2023. https://www.osmosis.org/answers/coagulation-cascade.)

The *extrinsic pathway* begins at the initial endothelial injury, exposing tissue factor III. Factor III then binds with calcium (factor IV) and factor VIIa, which leads to the activation of factor X. Vitamin K is essential in this step as it helps activate factor VII.[4]

The *intrinsic pathway* starts when factor XII (Hageman factor) is activated by exposure to high molecular weight kininogen (HMWK), kallikrein, and collagen. Factor XI becomes activated by factor XIIa.[4] The intrinsic pathway heavily relies on calcium. Calcium and factor XIa then activate factor IX. Factor VIII is activated by factor IIa (thrombin). Calcium, combined with factor IXa and factor VIIIa, activate factor X.[4]

The *common pathway* starts after the activation of factor X from either previous pathway.[4] Calcium, factor Xa, and factor Va bind together and form a prothrombinase complex.[4] This complex then activates factor II (prothrombin) into factor IIa (thrombin). Factor I (fibrinogen) is then cleaved by thrombin into factor Ia (fibrin).[4] Thrombin then cleaves factor XIII into its activated form, XIIIa, which binds with calcium to develop fibrin crosslinks and clot stabilization.[4]

Multiple medications are utilized for coagulation prevention by impacting different parts of the coagulation cascade. Warfarin (Coumadin) is an oral medication that stops the activation of vitamin K and reduces the synthesis of the coagulation factors in the liver that are dependent on vitamin K.[3] This results in an impact on both the extrinsic and common coagulation pathways.[3] Warfarin is used for venous thromboembolism (VTE) prevention in patients with atrial fibrillation, atrial flutter, heart valve replacements, and thromboembolism treatment such as strokes and pulmonary emboli. Warfarin treatment requires frequent monitoring of the patient's prothrombin time/International Normalized Ratio (PT/INR) for therapeutic levels.[3] Heparin suppresses the formation of fibrin by binding with antithrombin III causing inactivation of thrombin, factor Xa, and IXa. Heparin is commonly used in myocardial infarction treatment and thromboembolism treatment and prophylaxis, but it is administered intravenously (IV) or subcutaneously (SC). Low-molecular-weight heparins only impact the activation of factor X and are given subcutaneously. Direct oral anticoagulants (DOACs) are oral medications broken into two categories: direct thrombin inhibitors (dabigatran [Pradaxa]) and direct factor Xa inhibitors (rivaroxaban [Xarelto], apixaban [Eliquis], edoxaban [Savaysa], and betrixaban [Bevyxxa]).[5] DOACs were first approved in 2010 and have become exceedingly popular since frequent INR monitoring is not necessary, there is less risk of intracranial hemorrhage[6] and there are fewer drug and food interactions than with warfarin. Reversing DOACs has been a challenge, but more reversal agents have become available. The most common anticoagulant reversal agent is prothrombin complex concentrate (PCC, KCentra).[6] PCC supplies factors II, VII, IX, X, and proteins C and S which all promote coagulation.[6]

The fourth stage of hemostasis is *clot retraction*.[1] The actin and myosin in platelets contract, resulting in the fibrin strands being pulled closer to the platelets, and serum is squeezed from the clot.[1] The clot then shrinks.

The last stage of hemostasis is *clot dissolution* or *lysis*. This stage is imperative as it allows for blood flow to be restored and the start of permanent tissue repair.[1] *Fibrinolysis* is the term used for the process of how a clot dissolves. Plasminogen is converted to plasmin which begins to digest the fibrin strands, fibrinogen, factor V, factor VIII, prothrombin, and factor XII.[1] Plasmin is deactivated by α_2-plasmin inhibitor to prevent the action from occurring throughout the circulation.[1] There are two plasminogen activators, including tissue-type plasminogen activator and urokinase-type plasminogen activator and they are released as a response to a variety of stimuli.[1]

Tissue plasminogen activators (alteplase, tenecteplase, and reteplase) are commonly used for the treatment of myocardial infarctions, acute ischemic strokes, massive pulmonary emboli, and peripheral arterial occlusions.[3] Alteplase (commonly referred to as tPA) binds to the fibrin in a clot and promotes the conversion of plasminogen to plasmin.[3] Tenecteplase (commonly referred to as TNKase) is very similar but has three differences that make it more fibrin-specific and aid in a longer half-life.[3] There is some off-label use of TNK in ischemic stroke, however at the time of publishing many studies are in process but the FDA has not approved it for this use.[7,8]

Disorders

Von Willebrand disease is a fairly common hereditary bleeding disorder, occurring in about 1% of the population.[3] It is most commonly an autosomal dominant disorder and is broken down into three subtypes with varying severity and manifestations.[9] In the disorder there is a defect or deficiency in the von Willebrand factor, resulting in bleeding. Most cases are mild and may manifest as spontaneous bleeding from the nose, GI tract, mouth, excessive menstrual flow, or bleeding with a normal platelet count. These patients should avoid ASA and nonsteroidal anti-inflammatory drugs (NSAIDs).[9] Desmopressin (DDAVP) may be used if implicated as it triggers the release of von Willebrand factor from storage.[3]

Hemophilia A and B are both genetically inherited disorders. Hemophilia A is an X-linked recessive disorder that most commonly affects males.[1,3] In hemophilia A there is a defect in the factor VIII gene, resulting in varying levels of factor VIII in the circulation.[3] Hemophilia B occurs when there is a mutation in the factor IX gene.[3] Severe hemophilia is noted in childhood as there is spontaneous and severe bleeding.[1] Patients with hemophilia should avoid ASA and NSAIDs that impair platelet function.[1,3] Factor concentrate replacement therapy can be given at home or in the hospital[3] and should be initiated before interfacility transfers if possible.[10]

Factor V Leiden, also known as activated protein C resistance, is caused by a factor V Leiden mutation that makes the factor Va resistant to being inhibited by activated protein C.[1] It is an autosomal dominant, inherited disease. These patients are hypercoagulable and can have deep vein thrombosis or pulmonary embolism.[3] Approximately 5% of the US population of European descent have a heterozygous presence of this mutation.[3]

Some clotting disorders are acquired rather than inherited. *Antiphospholipid syndrome* (APS) is an autoimmune disorder resulting in thrombophilia.[3] Most patients have recurrent thrombotic events, but 1% have a rapid progression with multiple organs being impacted by small-vessel occlusions.[3] APS is more common in females, and multiple fetal demise is a common feature of the disorder.[1] Antiphospholipid antibodies are present in up to 5% of healthy young people, but APS only develops in a small portion of these people.[3]

Thrombocytopenia, or a low platelet count (less than 150,000/mL, can occur from a variety of reasons including destruction, loss, and decreased production.[1] It can be triggered by diverse etiologies including viruses, drugs, or idiopathic reasons. *Heparin-induced thrombocytopenia* (HIT) occurs when components of the clotting cascade are activated inappropriately, and venous and arterial clotting occurs.[3] These patients develop antibodies that fight against the heparin-platelet factor 4 complex.[1,3] Platelet counts decrease because they are bound and used in both large and small clots.[3] Patients with HIT will need anticoagulation other than heparin and warfarin as they are at increased risk for thrombosis.[3] *Drug-induced immune thrombocytopenia* has been linked to over 200 medications caused by decreased platelet production or increased platelet destruction.[3] It often occurs 5–14 days after the start of medication, and platelet counts often improve after cessation of the drug.[3] *Immune thrombocytopenia* (ITP) may be classified into two categories – primary and secondary – and is an acquired syndrome leading to increased platelet destruction.[1,3,9] The primary classification was also formerly known as idiopathic thrombocytopenic purpura, and the secondary classification occurs when it has been associated with other conditions such as autoimmune disease or infections.[1] A petechial rash is a common presenting symptom (Fig. 1.3).[11] In severe cases with life-threatening bleeding, corticosteroids, immunoglobulin, and platelet transfusions should be initiated.[3]

Disseminated intravascular coagulation (DIC) occurs when there is widespread activation of the coagulation system. Clotting factors and platelets get consumed and there are resultant small vessel thrombi.[3] DIC is associated with a variety of conditions including, but not limited to, pregnancy, trauma, infection, cancers, and transfusion reactions.[1,3] Hyperfibrinolysis and major bleeding complications can occur. The most common laboratory abnormality is thrombocytopenia, with other laboratory abnormalities including decreased fibrinogen level, prolonged PT, and elevated D-dimer and fibrin degradation products.[3] The most important part of treatment in DIC is eliminating the causative problem.[3] Blood product transfusions may be necessary when there is active bleeding, yet VTE prophylaxis is recommended if major bleeding is not present.[3]

Anemias

In critical care transport, clinicians are exposed to many patients with anemia, resulting in a patient having decreased capacity to bind and transport oxygen in their blood.[9] Anemia is defined as a

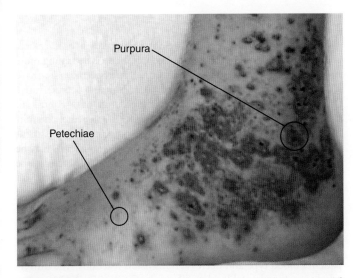

• **Fig. 1.3** Petechia and purpura. (From Santistevan J. What's that rash? An approach to dangerous rashes based on morphology. *emDocs*. http://www.emdocs.net/9009-2/. July 18, 2016.)

hemoglobin level of less than 13 g/dL in males or 12 g/dL in females according to the World Health Organization (WHO).[12] *Acute anemias* occur usually from direct blood loss but can also result from hemolysis.[12] Emergent conditions that can cause acute anemia include, but are not limited to, GI hemorrhaging, ruptured aneurysms, DIC, ruptured ectopic pregnancies, traumatic injuries to organs or blood vessels, or hemolytic reactions.[12] Signs and symptoms of significant blood loss include altered mental status, hypotension or postural hypotension, tachycardia, clammy or cool skin, although healthy individuals can usually tolerate a blood loss of 20% of their blood volume before these symptoms start to occur.[12]

Chronic anemias involve a more gradual decline in RBCs and have a variety of causes. *Iron deficiency* anemia is the most common anemia worldwide and is characterized by small and pale RBCs or microcytic and hypochromic.[9] These patients will have decreased MCV and MCHC values in their CBC and may complain of fatigue, weakness, dizziness, or pica (craving ice or other non-nutritional items).[9] Patients with severe anemias may have heart murmurs, tachycardia, or heart failure.[13]

Cyanocobalamin deficiency anemia, or *vitamin B_{12}* anemia, is caused by a deficiency in vitamin B_{12}. Vitamin B_{12} is essential for DNA synthesis and red blood cell maturation as well as the health of neurons.[13] It is found in food originating from animals, so patients with vegan or vegetarian diets may have a dietary deficiency of vitamin B_{12}. Outside of vegan diets, an autoimmune disorder known as pernicious anemia can occur where there is an inability to absorb vitamin B_{12} in the gastrointestinal tract.[9] Patients who have had gastric bypass also have malabsorption.[9] Vitamin B_{12} anemia is a macrocytic anemia characterized by large RBCs, so the MCV will be elevated. With a prolonged deficiency, demyelination can occur in the spinal cord, resulting in neurologic symptoms including paresthesia in the hands and feet or ataxia.[9]

Folic acid deficiency anemia is another macrocytic anemia, meaning is it characterized by large RBCs (elevated MCV).[13] The folate deficiency causes a problem in DNA synthesis and maturation of RBCs, similar to vitamin B_{12} deficiency.[1] Unlike vitamin B_{12} deficiency, folic acid deficiency anemia does not manifest any neurological symptoms, and the most common cause is of dietary origin. Dietary folate requirements are much higher in pregnancy, and deficiency has been linked to neural tube defects[1] and behavioral problems in offspring.[9]

Sickle cell disease (SCD) encompasses a wide range of disorders including sickle cell trait, where people have one gene mutation (heterozygous) and remain usually asymptomatic,[9] to fully manifested severe disease with homozygous gene mutation.[8,13] Sickle cell disorders are hemolytic anemias that involve vaso-occlusive episodes and often premature death.[9] About 4.5% of the world's population are at least carriers of the sickle cell gene.[3] Sickle cell is an inherited, autosomal recessive disease where there is an abnormal hemoglobin, hemoglobin (HbS).[1] HbS may become sickled when deoxygenated, which can lead to blood vessel occlusions and hemolytic anemia (Fig. 1.4).[14] Patients with a high percentage of hemoglobin molecules that are HbS have increased severity of their symptoms, however, many patients with sickle cell trait are asymptomatic.[1,14] Diagnosis is usually determined at birth, as most newborns are screened in the United States.[1,13] Life-threatening complications for patients with sickle cell disease include acute chest syndrome, stroke (ischemic and hemorrhagic), sepsis, and aplastic crisis.[3] Acute chest syndrome is the presence as a new infiltrate noted on chest x-ray, with an additional symptom including fever, tachypnea, wheezing, cough, or pain, usually

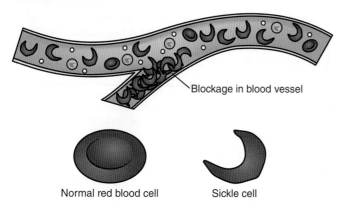

Blockage in blood vessel

Normal red blood cell   Sickle cell

• **Fig. 1.4** Sickle cell versus normal red blood cell. (From Ohio State University Comprehensive Cancer Center. Sickle cell anemia. Updated 2023. https://cancer.osu.edu/for-patients-and-caregivers/learn-about-cancers-and-treatments/cancers-conditions-and-treatment/benign-blood-diseases/sickle-cell-anemia.)

occurring within 3 days of hospitalization for a pain crisis.[3] Acute chest syndrome is the leading cause of death for SCD deaths in the United States.[3] SCD patients are also at increased risk for infarctions of multiple organs including the spleen, heart, and brain.[3] Treatment should be focused on pain management, hydration, and treatment of the cause of the crisis, and oxygen should be provided if hypoxemia is present.[3]

As with SCD, *thalassemias* can cause a wide range of microcytic and hemolytic anemia and are hereditary.[3] In thalassemia diseases there is a defect in the synthesis of the globin chains, causing a deficiency in the production of regular RBCs.[3] Beta (β)-thalassemia occurs when the defect is in the beta-globin gene and alpha (α)-thalassemia occurs when there is a defect with the alpha-globin gene.[3] Thalassemia is noted to occur in people from Asia, the Mediterranean, the Middle East, and North Africa.[13] β-thalassemia major, also referred to as Cooley's anemia, is a severe disease where patients require lifelong treatment and frequent blood transfusions.[3]

Acquired hemolytic anemias destroy RBCs before their usual lifespan.[1] These patients usually present with similar symptoms as in other anemias, including fatigue, dizziness, chest pain, new heart murmur, and tachycardias.[3] Acquired hemolytic anemias are considered autoimmune, alloimmune, or drug-induced.[3] Around 100 drugs are known to cause hemolytic anemia, but the incidence is rare.[3] Drugs most commonly linked to hemolysis include cephalosporins, chemotherapies, NSAIDs, penicillins, and other miscellaneous medications.[3] Blood transfusions can also cause hemolytic reactions, which will be discussed later in this chapter.

Aplastic anemia is caused by a disorder of bone marrow stem cells and subsequently can cause a decline in RBCs, WBCs, and platelets causing pancytopenia.[1,9] Aplastic anemia can occur at any age and can have a very acute onset or be more insidious.[1] It can be acquired, but more commonly occurs from medications, viral illnesses including hepatitis and Epstein–Barr, chemotherapies/radiation, chemicals, and pregnancy.[9] Future avoidance of the known causative agent is essential, and some patients may receive stem cell replacement, immunosuppressive therapies, and antibiotics as needed for infection.[1,9]

Anemias of chronic disease cause a shortened red blood cell life and a deficiency in the production of RBCs.[1] Chronic disease anemias are most commonly caused by chronic infections, autoimmune disorders, inflammatory bowel diseases, or chronic kidney disease.[1] Chronic renal failure patients tend to have anemia based on their deficiency of erythropoietin.[1]

In comparison to anemias, *polycythemia*, or erythrocytosis, is recognized as abnormally high hemoglobin and hematocrit, known as an RBC mass.[1,9,15] The largest risk with these patients is thromboembolic events, as their blood is hyperviscous.[15] Polycythemia vera is a subtype that is a myeloproliferative, acquired disorder with a male predisposition.[1,5] Common treatment is phlebotomy, which often occurs weekly where around 500 mL of blood is removed.[15] Secondary polycythemia results from hypoxia, which occurs in those living in higher altitudes, smoking, and chronic heart and lung disease.[1] Treating the causative problem is essential for secondary polycythemia.[15]

Blood Types and Transfusions

ABO Compatibility

In the critical care transport industry, it is fairly common to administer blood products or care for patients who have received recent transfusions. There are four main ABO blood groups. A patient's blood type depends on if the patient has red cell antigens, A and/or B, resulting in blood types A, B, AB, and O.[1] If someone has neither antigen, they are an O blood type. There are also Rh types, indicating whether or not someone has the D antigen or protein.[1] If the D antigen is present then the patient is RhD positive (i.e. A+ blood type), whereas if they do not have the D antigen, they are RhD negative (i.e. A− blood type).[1] RhD antibodies develop from exposure, which occurs most commonly in pregnancy or blood transfusions. These antibodies usually take weeks to be produced, resulting in possibly a mild reaction.[1] Subsequent exposure to these antigens may result in a severe reaction. RhD-negative pregnant patients should receive Rho(D) immune globulin (RhoGAM is a common brand) at around 28 weeks of pregnancy, and then within 72 hours of giving birth if the baby is Rh positive.[16] Rho(D) immune globulin is utilized to prevent the Rh sensitization from occurring, which will prevent blood from developing antibodies that will attack future exposure to RhD-positive blood, including fetuses in subsequent pregnancies causing spontaneous abortion or miscarriage.[16]

Blood Products

Whole blood is ideal in the acutely hemorrhaging patient as it replaces all blood products needed that the patient lost and is becoming more frequently used in the prehospital setting.[3] *Packed red blood cells* (PRBCs) are commonly transfused and contain a preservative containing citrate. Many facilities use the cutoff of 7–8 g/dL of hemoglobin to decide on transfusing PRBCs.[3] In an acutely hemorrhaging patient, transfusion should be based on physical assessment and estimated blood loss since the drop in hemoglobin levels may be delayed.[3] It is estimated that one unit of PRBCs will increase the adult patient's hemoglobin by about 1 g/dL.[3]

The administration of blood products does not come without risks, which is why consent should be obtained before administration. An IV line must be established without other medications and a piggyback line of normal saline. Prior to administration patients should have a Type and Crossmatch completed to assess the patient's blood type and decrease transfusion reactions. The universal donor for these blood products is O negative.[3] O-negative donors are difficult to find, as they are one of the least common blood types.[3] Due to availability, some critical care air and ground

EMS services are carrying O-positive whole blood for in-the-field resuscitation.[17] For patients with a uterus of childbearing age, some caution should be considered with administering RhD-positive blood products, as the patient could be RhD negative. Although fetal demise due to RhD-positive infusions in an RhD-negative patient is low at around 0.3%,[17] caution should still be advised in administering RhD-positive blood products to this patient population. Receiving facilities should be notified of the type of blood products administered in the prehospital environment to ascertain the appropriate blood type of the patient and administered Rho(D) immune globulin as appropriate if the patient is RhD negative.[17] Another important consideration in blood transfusions is hypocalcemia, as calcium binds to the citrate preservative in transfusions.[3] Calcium replenishment should be considered with subsequent blood transfusions.[3]

Platelet transfusions are indicated in patients with severe decreased platelet levels to prevent bleeding, or they may be transfused in a patient already having active bleeding. One unit (pack) should increase a patient's platelet level to around 50,000/mm,[4] so values should be checked after transfusion and then at the 24-hour mark.[3] If the platelet levels are not rising as expected, this may indicate other issues such as increased platelet destruction or platelet consumption from active bleeding.[3]

Fresh-frozen plasma (FFP) or *liquid plasma* may be transfused in patients with coagulation deficiencies, warfarin over coagulation, DIC, and massive transfusions.[3] In contrast to PRBCs and whole blood, the universal donor for FFP is blood type AB. FFP is not likely to reverse any anticoagulation caused by dabigatran or the DOACs[3] which were discussed earlier in this chapter.

Cryoprecipitate is another blood product, which is composed from plasma and includes fibronectin, factor XIII, fibrinogen, factor VIII, and von Willebrand factor.[3] It may be administered to bleeding patients, from severe liver disease, DIC, and dilutional coagulopathies.[3] Cryoprecipitate is made from FFP which is frozen and repeatedly thawed in a laboratory to produce a source of concentrated clotting factors. The volume of cryoprecipitate is smaller than and more concentrated than FFP. Cryoprecipitate is also being used for patients with post-fibrinolytic administration hemorrhaging, such as the ischemic stroke patient who has hemorrhagic conversion after tPA.[18] Before cryoprecipitate is given, fibrinogen levels are completed.[18]

Up to 20% of transfusions may have *transfusion reactions* occur,[3] although most reactions are minor. If a transfusion reaction is expected, the very first step is *stopping the transfusion*.[3] The blood bank should also be notified as soon as possible.

Transport Considerations

Critical care transport clinicians are responsible for both continuing blood product infusions from referring facilities during interfacility transfers and initiating blood product infusions based on their protocols or guidelines if their service carries blood products. Blood products are infused using tubing with filters to prevent particulates from being administered.[19] Normal saline is the only compatible fluid that can run with blood products and is often used to prime blood tubing.[19] Infusion rates for blood products vary based on the patient's clinical status. Massive transfusion involves infusing multiple blood products, often simultaneously, as quickly as possible as these patients are actively hemorrhaging at a life-threatening rate. Blood product transfusions in nonemergent settings are often started at a slow rate for the first 15 minutes to assess for transfusion reactions.[19] Utilizing a blood warmer is highly recommended to prevent hypothermia,[20] which is part of the trauma diamond of death.[21]

Although not previously discussed in this chapter, tranexamic acid, or TXA, is an antifibrinolytic medication that is commonly administered in situations of blood loss such as surgery, gynecological or obstetrical hemorrhage, or trauma.[3] It prevents the degrading of fibrin and cleavage of plasmin.[3] TXA has been found to decrease mortality rates, especially if given within 3 hours of injury, with the most benefit noted in the first hour.[3]

Unfortunately, there is limited available data to prove or disprove the theory that there is a delay in a drop in hemoglobin in acute blood loss. When agencies have blood available to them, this lack of data reinforces the concept of treating the patient rather than just numbers. The understanding of the coagulation cascade as well as what and how medications impact the cascade can aid in the transport clinicians' understanding and knowledge of treatments available.

This chapter will assist in providing the building blocks for the understanding of the hematologic system, its components, and current therapies for treating these conditions.

References

1. Porth C, Matfin G. *Pathophysiology*: *Concepts of Altered Health States*. 8th ed. Philadelphia: Wolters Kluwer Health | Lipincott Williams & Wilkins; 2009.
2. Esmon CT, Xu J, Lupu F. Innate immunity and coagulation. *J Thromb Haemost*. 2011;9(Suppl 1):182–188. doi: 10.1111/j.1538-7836.2011.04323.x
3. Tintinalli JE. *Tintinalli's Emergency Medicine*: A Comprehensive Study Guide. 8th ed. New York: McGraw-Hill Education; 2016.
4. Tarantino C. Coagulation cascade: What it is, steps, and more. *Osmosis*. Updated 2023. Available at: https://www.osmosis.org/answers/coagulation-cascade.
5. Chen A, Stecker E, Warden BA. Direct oral anticoagulant use: a practical guide to common clinical challenges. *J Am Heart Assoc*. 2020; 9(13):1–18.
6. Milling TJ, Pollack CV. A review of guidelines on anticoagulation reversal across different clinical scenarios—is there a general consensus? *Am J Emerg Med*. 2020; 38(9):1890–1903.
7. Katsanos AH, Psychogios K, Turc G. Off-label use of tenecteplase for the treatment of acute ischemic stroke: a systematic review and meta-analysis. *JAMA Network Open*. 2022;5(3):e224506.
8. Gerschenfeld G, Liegey JS, Laborne FX, et al. Treatment times, functional outcome, and hemorrhage rates after switching to tenecteplase for stroke thrombolysis: insights from the TETRIS registry. *Eur Stroke J*. 2022;7(4):358–364.
9. Goldman L, Schafer AI. *Goldman's Cecil Medicine*. 24th ed. Philadelphia: Saunders Elsevier; 2012.
10. Pollack AN, eds. *Critical Care Transport*. 2nd ed. Massachusetts: Jones & Bartlett Learning; 2018.
11. Santistevan J. What's that rash? An approach to dangerous rashes based on morphology. *emDocs*. Available at:http://www.emdocs.net/9009-2/. July 18, 2016.
12. Alder L, Tambe A. Acute anemia. In: StatPearls [Internet]. Treasure Island, FL: StatPearls Publishing; update July 18, 2022. Available at: https://www.ncbi.nlm.nih.gov/books/NBK537232/.
13. Leik MT. *Family Nurse Practitioner Certification*: Intensive Review. New York: Springer; 2014.

14. Ohio State University Comprehensive Cancer Center. Sickle cell anemia. Updated 2023. Available at: https://cancer.osu.edu/for-patients-and-caregivers/learn-about-cancers-and-treatments/cancers-conditions-and-treatment/benign-blood-diseases/sickle-cell-anemia.

15. Pillal AA, Fazal S, Mukkamalla SK, Babiker HM. Polycythemia. In: StatPearls [Internet]. Treasure Island, FL: StatPearls Publishing; update November 17, 2022. Available at: https://www.ncbi.nlm.nih.gov/books/NBK526081/.

16. American College of Nurse-Midwives. Rh-negative blood type and pregnancy. *J Midwifery Womens Hlth*. 2013;58(6):725–726.

17. Yazer MH, Gorospe J, Cap AP. Mixed feelings about mixed-field agglutination: a pathway for managing females of childbearing potential of unknown RHD-type who are transfused with RhD-positive and RhD-negative red blood cells during emergency hemorrhage resuscitation. *J AABB Transfusion*. 2021;61(S1):S326–S332.

18. Yaghi S, Willey JZ, Cucchiara B, et al. Treatment and outcome of hemorrhagic transformation after intravenous alteplase in acute ischemic stroke: a scientific statement for healthcare professionals from the American Heart Association/American Stroke Association. *American Stroke Association*. 2017;48:e343-e361.

19. Lotterman S, Sharma S. Blood transfusion. In: StatPearls [Internet]. Treasure Island, FL: StatPearls Publishing; update June 25, 2022. Available at: https://www.ncbi.nlm.nih.gov/books/NBK499824/.

20. Poder TG, Nonkani WG, Leponkouo ET. Blood warming and hemolysis: a systematic review with meta-analysis. *Transfusion Med Rev*. 2015;29(3):172–180.

21. Wray JP, Bridwell RE, Schauer SG, et al. The diamond of death: hypocalcemia in trauma and resuscitation. *Am J Emerg Med*. 2021; 41:104–109.

2

Vascular System

SHANE FARMER

COMPETENCIES

1. Describe the definitions of hypertension, aortic dissection, abdominal aortic aneurysm, peripheral vascular disease, and deep vein thrombosis.
2. Describe the anatomy and pathophysiology involved in commonly encountered vascular emergencies in the transport environment.
3. Identify the causes of vascular emergencies.
4. Understand treatment and management goals of vascular emergencies in the transport environment.

Introduction

While the topic of the vascular system and associated emergencies is quite broad, this chapter will focus on providing an overview of the anatomy, pathophysiology, causes, and treatment of emergencies specifically related to the central and peripheral vascular system, and not attempt to cover subcategories of the vascular system, such as neurovascular emergencies, which are covered in detail in Chapter 7, or cardiovascular emergencies, which are described in Chapter 8.

Emergencies involving the central and peripheral vasculature are frequently life-threatening, and associated mortality rates are often high.[1] The critical care transport provider must be able to provide a thorough assessment to identify the potential for such emergencies and provide rapid intervention to these patients when necessary. In this chapter, we will review the most common vascular emergencies critical care transport providers are likely to encounter, summarize their pathophysiology, and primary and secondary causes, and provide treatment guidance based on the latest research and evidence.

Hypertension

Definition

Hypertension is a chronic elevation of blood pressure that, over time, causes end-organ damage and results in increased morbidity and mortality. Blood pressure (BP) is the product of cardiac output and systemic vascular resistance. Patients with arterial hypertension may have an increase in cardiac output (CO), an increase in systemic vascular resistance (SVR), or both. In general practice, the level of blood pressure above which treatment of hypertension is indicated is now set at 140/90 mmHg. "Severe" hypertension, also sometimes classified as urgent or emergent, is typically recognized to be systolic blood pressure >180 mmHg and/or diastolic blood pressure >120 mmHg (Table 2.1).[2]

TABLE 2.1	Stages of Hypertension (Joint National Committee VI Guideline)	
Stages	Systolic BP (mmHg)	Diastolic BP (mmHg)
Optimal	<120	<80
Normal	120–129	80–84
High normal	130–139	85–89
Hypertension	>140	>90
Severe	>180	>120

Modified from Foëx P, Sear J. Hypertension: pathophysiology and treatment. *Cont Educ Anaesth Crit Care Pain*. 2004;4(3):73.

Pathophysiology

Systolic blood pressure (SBP) reflects the blood pressure when the heart is contracted, or in systole, and diastolic blood pressure (DBP) reflects the blood pressure during relaxation, or diastole. Hypertension can be diagnosed when either systolic pressure, diastolic pressure, or both are raised.

Blood pressure is determined by the CO balanced against SVR. The process of maintaining blood pressure involves numerous physiological mechanisms. These include arterial baroreceptors, the renin-angiotensin-aldosterone system (RAAS), atrial natriuretic peptide, endothelins, and mineralocorticoid and glucocorticoid steroids. These complex systems work together to manage the degree of vasodilatation or vasoconstriction within the systemic circulation and the retention or excretion of sodium and water. The balancing act of these systems works in concert to maintain an adequate circulating blood volume.[2]

Long-term control of blood pressure occurs via the renal–body fluid feedback system. This system involves pressure natriuresis (the increase in sodium and water excretion by the kidney). Impaired pressure natriuresis can result from impaired renal function, altered activation of hormones that regulate salt and water excretion by the kidney (such as those in the RAAS), or excessive activation of the sympathetic nervous system.[3,4]

Dysfunction in any of these processes can lead to the development of hypertension. This may be through increased cardiac output, increased systemic vascular resistance, or both (Fig. 2.1).[3,4]

Causes

The risk factors for developing hypertension include[4]:
- Increasing age (50% of the population aged over 60 years have hypertension)
- Ethnicity (hypertension is more prevalent in patients of Black African or Caribbean descent)
- Obesity
- Physical inactivity
- Stress
- Diabetes
- Chronic kidney disease
- Excessive salt consumption
- Excessive alcohol consumption
- Sleep apnea

There is no specific cause of hypertension found for most (>95%) patients with high blood pressure, and this is often referred to as primary or essential hypertension.[2] The secondary causes identified in the remaining 5% of cases are extensive and include:
- Medicines
  - Corticosteroids
  - Sympathomimetics
  - Non-steroidal anti-inflammatory drugs (NSAIDs)
  - Oral contraceptives
- Renovascular disease
- Primary hyperaldosteronism
- Pheochromocytoma
- Coarctation of the aorta
- Cushing's syndrome

Most hypertensive emergencies occur in patients already diagnosed with chronic hypertension. Noncompliance with antihypertensive medications and the use of sympathomimetics are two of the more common causes of hypertensive emergencies.[4]

Acute Treatment

At the time of publication of this text, the medications of choice typically seen in the transport environment for hypertensive crisis include labetalol and nicardipine.[5,6] When treating a hypertensive emergency with acute pulmonary edema the medications of choice are intravenous (IV) nitroglycerin, clevidipine, or nitroprusside. Beta-blockers are contraindicated in the treatment of acute pulmonary edema.[5] The medications of choice in treating patients with a hypertensive emergency and acute renal failure are clevidipine,

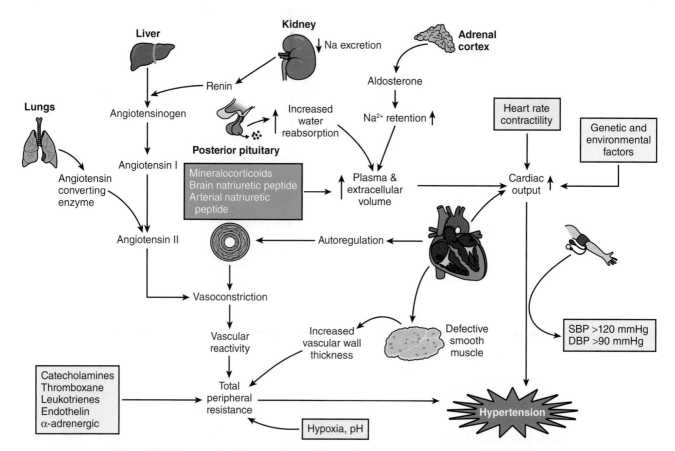

• **Fig. 2.1** How hypertension develops. (Modified from Adua E. Decoding the mechanism of hypertension through multiomics profiling. *J Hum Hypertens.* 2022; 37:255. Creative Commons licence: http://creativecommons.org/licenses/by/4.0/.)

fenoldopam, and nicardipine.[6] Providers should follow their program protocols or physician orders for medications and dosing.

Acute Blood Pressure Management

The target blood pressure is less than 140/90 mmHg in patients with acute myocardial infarction or unstable angina pectoris who are hemodynamically stable. In hypertensive emergencies, except for acute aortic dissection, blood pressure should not be rapidly lowered. Goal therapy includes a 10%–20% reduction of mean arterial pressure (MAP) in the first hour, and then 5%–15% further over the next 23 hours. This usually results in an acute target of <180/<120 in the first hour, then <160/<110 over the next 23 hours.

Aortic Dissection

Definition

Aortic dissection is defined as the separation of the layers within the aortic wall. Tears in the intimal layer result in the formation of a false lumen that allows blood to flow behind the intimal layer of the vessel and subsequent propagation of dissection (proximally or distally) secondary to blood entering the intima–media space.

Pathophysiology

The aortic wall consists of three layers: the intima, media, and adventitia (Fig. 2.2). Constant exposure to high pulsatile pressure and shear stress leads to a weakening of the aortic wall resulting in an intimal tear. Following this tear, blood flows into the intima–media space and creates a false lumen. Most of these tears take place in the ascending aorta, usually in the right lateral wall where the greatest shear force on the aorta occurs. In an aortic dissection, the true lumen is lined by the intima whereas the false lumen is within the media. In most cases, the true lumen is smaller than the false lumen. Over time, the blood flowing through the false lumen leads to the development of an aneurysm with the potential for rupture.[7,8]

Classification

There are two primary classification systems for aortic dissections (Fig. 2.3)[9]:
- DeBakey
- Stanford

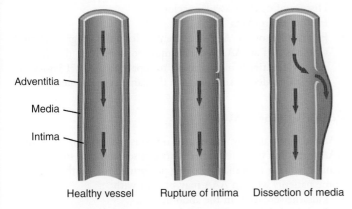

Adventitia
Media
Intima

Healthy vessel   Rupture of intima   Dissection of media

• **Fig. 2.2** Aortic dissection is where blood enters the vessel wall via a tear in the tunica intima. (Copyright © Shutterstock.com.)

The DeBakey classification uses a three-type model (Types I, II, IIIa, IIIb) to describe the aortic dissection by location and extent. In contrast, the Stanford classification uses a two-type model (Type A and B). DeBakey Type I and Type II, and Stanford Type A involve the ascending aorta, whereas Debakey Type IIIa and Type IIIb, as well as Stanford Type B are limited to the descending aorta.

Causes

- Chronic hypertension
- An abrupt, transient, severe increase in blood pressure
- Consumption of sympathomimetic agents such as cocaine, ecstasy, or energy drinks
- Inflammatory or infectious diseases that cause vasculitis (e.g., syphilis)
- Aortic instrumentation or surgery
- Genetic conditions including Marfan syndrome
- Atherosclerosis
- Pre-existing aortic aneurysm
- Pregnancy and delivery (risk compounded in pregnant women with connective tissue disorders)

Patient Presentation

The pain of an aortic dissection is often sudden in onset, reaches maximal severity quickly, and can feel "tearing" in nature. Patients often present with tearing chest pain that radiates to the back. Classically cited physical findings, such as a discrepancy of blood pressure in the upper extremities, a pulse deficit, or the presence of a diastolic murmur, should increase suspicion of an aortic dissection. Additionally, the presence of chest pain with any neurological finding, the combination of chest and abdominal pain, or chest pain accompanied by limb weakness or paresthesia should alert the clinician to the possibility of aortic dissection. Syncope (due to arrhythmias, myocardial infarction (MI), or an increased vagal tone) and hypertension are both very common findings in aortic dissection. A difference of more than 20 mmHg in blood pressure between the arms should raise suspicion of dissection.[10] Other features include:
- Wide pulse pressure
- Diastolic murmur
- Muffled heart sounds (suggesting cardiac tamponade)
- Syncope
- Altered mental status
- Loss of peripheral pulses
- Horner syndrome (stroke-like symptoms, specifically: decreased pupil size, a drooping eyelid, and decreased sweating on the affected side of the face)[11]

Acute Treatment

Acute management of the aortic dissection should be focused on reducing pressure within the vessel and limiting the volume of blood being ejected into the false lumen created by the dissection. Rapid and immediate reduction of blood pressure within 5–10 minutes is needed for patients with acute aortic dissection. The target blood pressure goal in these patients is a systolic blood pressure below 120 mmHg.[10] Due to the pain encountered with an aortic dissection, pain management through the use of opioid analgesic medications can assist with managing the pain and subsequently reduce catecholamine-mediated hypertension. Beta-blockers, such as IV esmolol, should be used to

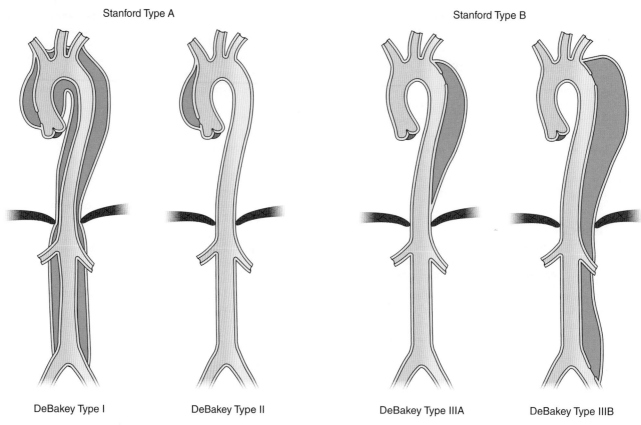

Stanford Type A

Stanford Type B

DeBakey Type I   DeBakey Type II   DeBakey Type IIIA   DeBakey Type IIIB

• **Fig. 2.3** DeBakey and Stanford classification of aortic dissection. (Modified from Conrad MF, Cambria RP. Aortic dissections. In: Cronenwett JL, Johnston KW, eds. *Rutherford's Vascular Surgery*. 8th ed. Philadelphia: Elsevier; 2014:2169–2188.)

manage contractile force and heart rate. If the blood pressure remains elevated after beta-blockade, a vasodilator such as IV nitroglycerin or nitroprusside should be considered.

Abdominal Aortic Aneurysm

Definition

An aortic aneurysm is a swelling, weakened area in the wall of the aorta. Once formed, an aneurysm will gradually increase in size and get progressively weaker.

Pathophysiology

An abdominal aortic aneurysm (AAA) is a dilation in which the aortic diameter is ≥3.0 cm. If untreated, the aortic wall continues to become weaker and unable to withstand the forces of the luminal blood pressure.[12] This force results in progressive dilatation (Fig. 2.4). This dilatation can result in a rupture and is associated with a mortality rate of up to 80%.[13]

Aortic aneurysms can develop in both the thoracic and abdominal aorta, however the abdomen is the most common location. AAAs can be further categorized into supra-renal if they involve the origins of the renal arteries, para-visceral aneurysms if they involve the visceral arteries, or infra-renal if they begin lower than the renal arteries. The majority of AAAs are infra-renal in nature.[14]

Causes

It is not always clear why an AAA occurs, but there are associated risk factors. These factors can include:
• Men age 66 years and older
• Women age 70 years and older
Both of the above age groups typically have one or more compounding risks present as well:
• Hypertension
• Chronic obstructive pulmonary disease (COPD)
• Hyperlipidemia
• Cardiovascular disease
• History of cerebrovascular accident
• History of smoking
• Familial history of AAA.[15] Patients with a first-degree relative who has had an AAA are 12 times more likely to develop an AAA. Of patients in treatment to repair an AAA, 15%–25% have a first-degree relative with the same type of aneurysm.[16]

Patient Presentation

AAAs do not usually cause any obvious symptoms. Typically, AAAs are often only discovered during a screening or found incidentally during tests that are being performed for another reason. Some patients with an AAA may present with[17]:
• Pulsatile sensation in the abdomen
• Persistent abdominal discomfort
• Persistent lower back pain

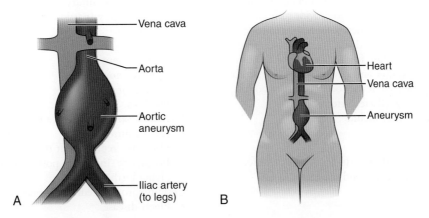

• **Fig. 2.4** Anatomy of abdominal aortic aneurysm. **A,** Aorta with large abdominal aneurysm. **B,** Location of the aorta in the abdomen. Leaking or rupture causes pain in the abdomen, back, and flank. (From Abdominal pain. In: Higgins T, Auerbach PS, Arastu AS, eds. *Medicine for the Outdoors: The Essential Guide to First Aid and Medical Emergencies.* 7th ed. Elsevier; 2024.)

If a AAA ruptures, associated symptoms may include:
- Sudden and severe pain in the lower back or abdomen
- Lightheadedness
- Pale skin
- Diaphoresis
- Tachycardia
- Shortness of breath
- Syncope[18,19]

Acute Treatment

Initial management for a ruptured AAA aims to correct hypovolemia and includes starting two large-bore IVs and initiating IV crystalloid fluids and blood products. Do not wait for a crossmatch if the patient is in shock, give uncrossmatched blood. If available, a mass transfusion protocol (MTP) should be activated. In addition to fluid and blood product resuscitation, consider permissive hypotension, reversal of anticoagulation, and airway management.[17] Timely transfer to a facility with operating room capabilities should be at the forefront of your treatment plan.[18,20,21]

Small asymptomatic AAAs that are not expanding quickly are usually left alone and watched for changes in size, most often by ultrasound examination of the abdomen every 6 months. The definitive treatment for an abdominal aneurysm may include surgical repair, removal of the aneurysm, or insertion of a metal mesh coil stent to support the blood vessel and prevent rupture.[18,20–22]

Acute Blood Pressure Management

In AAA rupture the goal SBP should be 90–100 mmHg.[22] Blood pressure higher may cause clot dislodgement and increase bleeding. Vasopressors should be a last resort in any treatment plan. Permissive hypotension guidelines should be initiated where available.[14]

Peripheral Vascular Disease

Definition

Peripheral vascular disease (PVD) refers to any disease or disorder of the circulatory system outside of the heart and brain. The term can include any disorder that affects blood vessels.

Pathophysiology

Peripheral vascular disease (PVD), also known as peripheral artery disease (PAD), is insufficient tissue perfusion caused by atherosclerosis.[23] Plaque (made of fat, cholesterol, and other substances) forms gradually inside vessel walls and slowly narrows the available space for blood flow. Many of these plaque deposits are hard on the outside and soft on the inside. The hard surface can crack or tear, allowing plaque to congregate in the area. Blood clots can form around the plaque, making the artery even narrower. This narrowing and subsequent lack of blood flow cause damage and eventually tissue death in the areas below the blockage. This most often occurs in the toes and feet.[24]

Causes

- Blood clots
- Diabetes
- Inflammation of the arteries or arteritis
- Infection
- Structural defects
- Injury
  Risk factors for peripheral vascular disease include[23]:
- Age over 50
- Male
- Postmenopausal women
- Heart disease
- Family history
- Coronary artery disease
- Diabetes
- Hyperlipidemia
- Hypertension
- Obesity
- Smoking or tobacco use[25]

Patient Presentation

About 50% of people with PVD are symptom-free.[26] For those presenting with symptoms, the most common is leg cramping that occurs with exercise and is relieved by rest (intermittent claudication). In an active state, the vasculature is unable to provide sufficient oxygen and nutrients to support aerobic metabolism, thus causing the musculature to suffer from hypoxia and forcing anaerobic metabolism; at rest, however, the vasculature feeding peripheral muscles is able to provide sufficient blood flow and oxygen to support aerobic metabolism, thus resolving the pain. It may occur in one or both legs depending on the location of the affected artery.

Other symptoms of PVD may include:
- Changes in the skin
  - Temperature
  - Appearance: thin, brittle, shiny skin on the legs and feet
- Weak peripheral pulses in the legs and the feet
- Gangrenous tissue
- Hair loss on legs
- Impotence
- Wounds that will not or are slow to heal over pressure points, such as heels or ankles
- Pain at rest, commonly in the toes and at night while lying flat
- Reddish-blue discoloration of the extremities
- Restricted mobility
- Thickened, opaque toenails[26]

Acute Treatment

Acute limb ischemia (ALI) from PVD is somewhat rare but it is a true medical emergency requiring rapid diagnosis and intervention to prevent limb loss. Emergent treatment typically consists of antiplatelet and anticoagulant therapy. Unfractionated heparin may be immediately administered to prevent the proximal and distal progression of secondary thrombosis to the site of occlusion (Fig. 2.5).[26]

Deep Vein Thrombosis

Definition

Deep vein thrombosis (DVT) is a medical condition that occurs when a blood clot forms in a deep vein. These clots usually develop in the lower leg, thigh, or pelvis, but they can also occur in the arm.

Pathophysiology

The following are the main pathophysiological mechanisms involved in DVT and are also known as Virchow's triad:
- Damage to the vessel wall
- Blood flow turbulence
- Hypercoagulability[27]

Thrombosis is the protective mechanism that prevents the loss of blood and seals off damaged blood vessels. The triggers of venous thrombosis are frequently multifactorial and each aspect of Virchow's triad[28] contributes in varying degrees in each patient. All result in early thrombus interaction with the endothelium.[28] This then stimulates local cytokine production and causes leukocyte adhesion to the endothelium, both of which promote venous thrombosis. Depending on the relative balance between the coagulation and thrombolytic pathways, thrombus propagation occurs. DVT occurs most often in the lower limb below the knee and starts at low-flow sites, such as the soleal sinuses, behind venous valve pockets.[29]

Causes

Common causes of DVT are:
- Injury to a vein, often caused by:
  - Fractures

- Severe muscle injury
- Major surgery (particularly involving the abdomen, pelvis, hip, or legs)
- Slow blood flow, often caused by:
  - Confinement to bed
  - Limited movement
  - Sitting for a long time
  - Paralysis
- Increased estrogen, often caused by:
  - Birth control pills
  - Hormone replacement therapy
  - Pregnancy (including post-partum of up to 3 months after giving birth)
- Certain chronic medical illnesses
  - Heart disease
  - Lung disease
  - Inflammatory bowel disease
- Other factors that increase the risk of DVT include:
  - Previous DVT or pulmonary embolism (PE)
  - Family history of DVT or PE
  - Obesity
- A catheter located in a central vein
- Genetic clotting disorders

Patient Presentation

Some of the most common symptoms of DVT that occur in the affected part of the body are:
- Swelling (70% of patients)
- Pain (50% of patients)
- Tenderness
- Redness of the skin
- Warmth in the affected area
- Limb edema (may be unilateral or bilateral if the thrombus is extending to pelvic veins)

Complications

Patients suffering from DVT are at risk for pulmonary embolism (PE), but may experience a PE without any symptoms of a DVT. PE, the most serious complication of DVT, happens when a part of the clot breaks off and travels through the bloodstream to the lungs, causing a blockage and the inability to oxygenate. Pulmonary embolisms are responsible for approximately 100,000 to 200,000 deaths in the United States each year.[30] Signs and symptoms of PE can include:
- Dyspnea
- Hemoptysis
- Tachycardia
- Arrhythmias
- Chest pain, which usually worsens with a deep breath or coughing
- Hypotension
- Dizziness[31]

Acute Treatment

The supportive care for hypoxemia and hemodynamic instability should be instituted. Anticoagulation is the mainstay for the treatment of acute pulmonary embolism.

Anticoagulants should be used as a first line of treatment. Most patients will receive a heparin bolus. A heparin drip may then be initiated to a maximum dose. Use caution and be mindful of anticoagulant use in patients with a high risk of bleeding.[30,32]

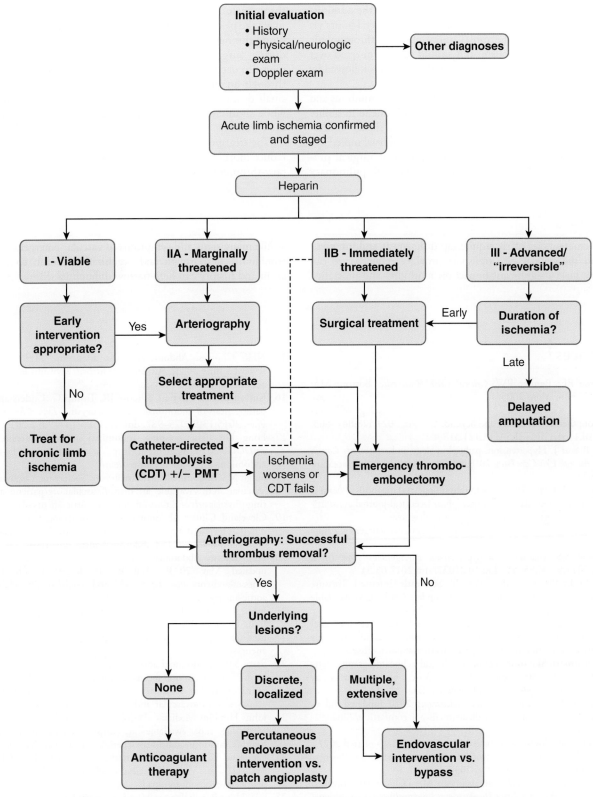

• **Fig. 2.5** Treatment algorithm for acute limb ischemia separated by Rutherford degree of ischemia. Rutherford class IIB ischemia is classically treated with surgical revascularization, but with the development of advanced endovascular techniques, catheter-directed therapy (CDT) or pharmacomechanical thrombolysis (PMT) may be the treatment option of choice for some surgeons. This is depicted with a dashed line. (From Go CC, Avgerinos ED, Chaer RA. Thrombolysis in acute limb ischemia. In: *Complications in Endovascular Surgery: Peri-Procedural Prevention and Treatment.* Elsevier; 2022. Figure 31.1.)

Systemic thrombolysis may also be facilitated by the administration of tissue plasminogen activator (tPA) over several hours via IV. Alteplase (rt-PA) is the most commonly used thrombolytic agent in pulmonary embolism. tPA should be administered over 2 hours, or may be administered as a smaller IV bolus followed by an infusion over 2 hours.[32,33]

Fibrinolytic therapy counteracts or stabilizes the thrombosis and is an option in the treatment of patients with PE due to its ability to rapidly dissolve thromboembolic clots. However, the use of fibrinolytic therapy in the treatment of PE is a controversial topic.[29]

More tertiary care may include nonsurgical or surgical pulmonary thrombectomy. Nonsurgical or medical pulmonary thrombectomy is more common, but surgical thrombectomy may take place with patients who cannot receive thrombolysis or blood thinners. It involves the manual removal of the blood clot during surgical intervention. Catheter-directed thrombolysis may also occur in patients with large clots. A catheter is inserted through an incision in the leg or neck using fluoroscopy and small doses of thrombolytics are applied directly into the clot while simultaneously using ultrasound waves to help break up the thrombus.

The treatment of DVT aims to prevent pulmonary embolism, reduce morbidity, and prevent or minimize the risk of developing post-thrombotic syndrome.[29]

Summary

Vascular emergencies often require rapid diagnosis and intervention from the critical care transport provider. Timely care can frequently have a significant impact on morbidity and mortality. While many signs and symptoms of vascular emergencies may be ambiguous, a thorough and organized approach to a physical exam and history can help narrow differential diagnoses.

References

1. Bledsoe BE, Benner RW. *Critical Care Paramedic*. Boston, MA: Pearson Education; 2005.

2. Harrison DG, Coffman TM, Wilcox CS. Pathophysiology of hypertension: the Mosiac theory and beyond. *Circ Res*. 2021;128:847–863. doi: 10.1161/CIRCRESAHA.121.318082

3. Foëx P, Sear J. Hypertension: pathophysiology and treatment. *Contin Educ Anaesth Crit Care Pain*. 2018;4(3):71–75. doi: 10.1093/bjaceaccp/mkh020

4. Williams H. Hypertension: pathophysiology and diagnosis. *Pharm J*. 2015, Feb 11. Available at: https://pharmaceutical-journal.com/article/ld/hypertension-pathophysiology-and-diagnosis.

5. Breu AC, Axon RN. Acute treatment of hypertensive urgency. *J Hosp Med*. 2018;13(12):860–862.

6. Aronow WS. Treatment of hypertensive emergencies. *Ann Transl Med*. 2017;5(S1):S5–S5. doi: 10.21037/atm.2017.03.34

7. Levy D, Le JK. Aortic dissection. In: StatPearls [Internet]. Treasure Island, FL: StatPearls Publishing; 2020 [update April 2023]. Available at: https://www.ncbi.nlm.nih.gov/books/NBK441963/.

8. TeachMe Surgery. Aortic dissection is where blood enters the vessel wall via a tear in the tunica intima. n.d. [update Dec 2022]. Available at: https://teachmesurgery.com/vascular/arterial/aortic-dissection/.

9. Hagen-Ansert SL. Introduction to clinical echocardiography: left-sided valvular heart disease. In: Hagen-Ansert SL, ed. *Textbook of Diagnostic Sonography*. 9th ed. Elsevier; 2023.

10. Mancini MC. Aortic dissection. *Medscape*; 2020 [updated Jul 6, 2022]. Available at: https://emedicine.medscape.com/article/2062452-overview.

11. Mayo Clinic. Horner syndrome. Mayo Clinic; 2018 [updated 2022]. Available at: https://www.mayoclinic.org/diseases-conditions/horner-syndrome/symptoms-causes/syc-20373547.

12. Mayo Clinic. Abdominal aortic aneurysm. Mayo Clinic; 2019 [updated 2023]. Available at: https://www.mayoclinic.org/diseases-conditions/abdominal-aortic-aneurysm/symptoms-causes/syc-20350688.

13. Avishay DM, Reimon JD. Abdominal aortic repair. In: StatPearls [Internet]. Treasure Island, FL: StatPearls Publishing; July 24, 2023 [update Jan 25, 2024]. Available at: https://www.ncbi.nlm.nih.gov/books/NBK554573/.

14. Kuivaniemi H, Ryer EJ, Elmore JR, Tromp G. Understanding the pathogenesis of abdominal aortic aneurysms. *Expert Rev Cardiovasc Ther*. 2015;13(9):975–987. doi: 10.1586/14779072.2015.1074861

15. NHS Choices. Abdominal aortic aneurysm. NHS; 2019 [last reviewed June 2023]. Available at: https://www.nhs.uk/conditions/abdominal-aortic-aneurysm/.

16. Kuivaniemi H, Ryer EJ, Elmore JR, Tromp G. Understanding the pathogenesis of abdominal aortic aneurysms. *Expert Rev Cardiovasc Ther*. 2015;13(9):975–987. doi: 10.1586/14779072.2015.1074861

17. Long DA. The crashing abdominal aortic aneurysm patient. *emDOCs*; 2019. Available at: http://www.emdocs.net/the-crashing-abdominal-aortic-aneurysm-patient/.

18. Singh MJ. Abdominal aortic aneurysm. Society for Vascular Surgery. Vascular; n.d. Available at: https://vascular.org/patients-and-referring-physicians/conditions/abdominal-aortic-aneurysm.

19. Cleveland Clinic. Abdominal aortic aneurysm. Cleveland Clinic; n.d. [last reviewed Aug 2023]. Available at: https://my.clevelandclinic.org/health/diseases/7153-abdominal-aortic-aneurysm.

20. NHS Inform. Abdominal aortic aneurysm. NHS Inform; 2019 [last updated May 2023]. Available at: https://www.nhsinform.scot/illnesses-and-conditions/heart-and-blood-vessels/conditions/abdominal-aortic-aneurysm.

21. Johns Hopkins Medicine. Abdominal aortic aneurysm: overview. John Hopkins Medicine; n.d. Available at: https://www.hopkins-medicine.org/health/conditions-and-diseases/abdominal-aortic-aneurysm.

22. Parsa MD. Abdominal aortic aneurysm. SAEM; n.d. Available at: https://www.saem.org/about-saem/academies-interest-groups-affiliates2/cdem/for-students/online-education/m4-curriculum/group-m4-cardiovascular/abdominal-aortic-aneurysm.

23. Johns Hopkins Medicine. Peripheral vascular disease. John Hopkins Medicine; n.d. Available at: https://www.hopkinsmedicine.org/health/conditions-and-diseases/peripheral-vascular-disease.

24. Cleveland Clinic. Peripheral arterial disease. Cleveland Clinic; n.d. Available at: https://my.clevelandclinic.org/health/diseases/17357-peripheral-artery-disease-pad.

25. GW Heart (Cardiology and Cardiac Surgery). Peripheral arterial disease (PAD). George Washington University Hospital; n.d. Available at: https://www.gwhospital.com/peripheral-arterial-disease-pad.

26. Obara H, Matsubara K, Kitagawa Y. Acute limb ischemia. *Ann Vasc Dis*. 2018;11(4):443–448. doi: 10.3400/avd.ra.18-00074

27. Centers for Disease Control and Prevention. What is venous thromboembolism? Centers for Disease Control and Prevention; 2018 [updated June 2023]. Available at: https://www.cdc.gov/ncbddd/dvt/facts.html.

28. Bagot CN, Arya R. Virchow and his triad: a question of attribution. *Br J Haematol*. 2008;143(2):180–190. doi: 10.1111/j.1365-2141.2008.07323.x

29. Aday AW, Beckman JA. Pulmonary embolism and unfractionated heparin: time to end the roller coaster ride. *Acad Emerg Med*. 2019;27(2):176–178. doi: 10.1111/acem.13871

30. Waheed SM, Hotwagner DT. Deep vein thrombosis (DVT). In: StatPearls [Internet]. Treasure Island, FL: StatPearls Publishing; 2018 [update Jan 2023]. Available at: https://www.ncbi.nlm.nih.gov/books/NBK507708/.

31. Yale Medicine. Pulmonary embolism. Yale Medicine. n.d. Available at: https://www.yalemedicine.org/conditions/pulmonary-embolism.

32. Root CW, Dudzinski DM, Zakhary B, Friedman OA, Sista AK, Horowitz JM. Multidisciplinary approach to the management of pulmonary embolism patients: the pulmonary embolism response team (PERT). *J Multidiscip Healthc*. 2018;11:187–195. doi: 10.2147/JMDH.S151196

33. Hughes RE, Tadi P, Bollu PC. TPA therapy. In: StatPearls [Internet]. Treasure Island, FL: StatPearls Publishing; 2019 [update Jul 2023]. Available at: https://www.ncbi.nlm.nih.gov/books/NBK482376/.

3

Renal Failure

HUNTER HIX AND B. DANIEL NAYMAN

COMPETENCIES

1. Understand the anatomy and structure of the kidneys.
2. Identify the function and pathophysiology of the renal system.
3. Recognize the two primary types of renal failure and their subcategories.
4. Understand treatment goals for renal failure patients and how to achieve them.

Pathophysiology of the Kidney

Gross Anatomy of the Kidney

The kidneys, located retroperitoneally on either side of the vertebral column against the posterior abdominal wall, filter blood, remove waste products, and maintain fluid and electrolyte balance in the body. Each kidney is approximately 10–12 cm in length, 5–7 cm in width, and 2–3 cm in thickness, and due to the location of the liver displacing the right kidney, it typically sits slightly lower than the left kidney.[1] The adrenal gland is located on the superior aspect of each kidney. A tough, fibrous connective tissue, the renal capsule, encapsulates the kidney, providing structural support and protection. Additionally, a layer of adipose tissue, known as perirenal fat, surrounds each kidney and works to cushion and protect them from traumatic forces.[2]

Each kidney is divided into two main regions. Different portions of the nephron and its functions can be found in both layers of the kidney. The renal cortex, where most filtration occurs, is the outermost layer, containing renal corpuscles and convoluted tubules. The renal medulla, situated deeper within the kidney, helps regulate fluid and sodium concentration. The medulla contains renal pyramids, conical-shaped structures responsible for urine formation. These pyramids converge at the renal papilla, from where urine is collected and transported through the minor calyces, major calyces, and eventually to the renal pelvis before leaving the kidney through the ureter.[1]

Renal Blood Flow

Renal blood flow is a crucial and highly regulated mechanism that ensures the kidneys receive an adequate supply of blood to maintain fluid and electrolyte balance and remove waste products from the bloodstream. The kidneys receive approximately 20%–25% of the cardiac output, making them one of the most highly perfused organs in the body.[3] Renal blood flow is primarily governed by the balance between vasoconstrictor and vasodilator mechanisms within the renal vasculature. The afferent arterioles that supply

blood to the glomerulus have alpha-adrenergic receptors, which respond to sympathetic stimulation by constricting the arterioles, reducing renal blood flow. On the other hand, prostaglandins, nitric oxide, and adenosine act as vasodilators in the kidney, promoting relaxation of the smooth muscle in the afferent arterioles and increasing blood flow to the glomerulus. Moreover, the renin-angiotensin-aldosterone system (RAAS) also plays a crucial role in regulating renal blood flow, particularly in response to changes in blood pressure and volume.[4]

Renal autoregulation is another essential mechanism that helps maintain a relatively constant renal blood flow and glomerular filtration rate (GFR) over a wide range of systemic blood pressures. This autoregulatory mechanism allows the kidneys to maintain their vital functions even during fluctuations in blood pressure. The two main components of renal autoregulation are the myogenic response and tubuloglomerular feedback. The myogenic response involves the contraction and relaxation of smooth muscle cells in the arterioles in response to changes in intravascular pressure, while tubuloglomerular feedback relies on the detection of sodium chloride concentration at the macula densa, leading to adjustments in afferent arteriolar resistance and ensuring stable renal blood flow and GFR.[4]

The Nephron

The nephron is the fundamental functional unit of the kidney, responsible for filtering blood and forming urine. Each kidney contains thousands of nephrons consisting of a renal corpuscle and a renal tubule. The renal corpuscle comprises the glomerulus, a network of capillaries surrounded by the Bowman's capsule. Blood entering the glomerulus is subjected to high pressure, allowing water, electrolytes, waste products, and small molecules to pass through the capillary walls into the Bowman's capsule, forming a fluid known as the filtrate.[5]

The filtrate then proceeds through the renal tubule, which consists of several segments, including the proximal convoluted tubule, the loop of Henle, and the distal convoluted tubule. As the filtrate moves through the proximal tubule, essential substances, such as glucose, are reabsorbed back into the bloodstream to be retained by the body. The majority of water reabsorption occurs in the loop of Henle, and the distal tubule is responsible for maintaining sodium levels by allowing sodium to be reabsorbed or continue through the tubule to be excreted.[5]

Glucose, water, sodium, potassium, and other reabsorbed items within the tubule are passed to the peritubular network to be sent back to the bloodstream, while waste products continue through the tubule to the collecting ducts for elimination. At the end of the collecting ducts, the filtrate becomes urine. It flows into the renal pelvis before being transported to the bladder for temporary storage and eventual excretion from the body through the urethra.

Glomerular Filtration Rate (GFR)

Glomerular filtration rate (GFR) is a critical clinical parameter used to assess kidney function and estimate the rate at which blood is filtered through the glomeruli of the nephrons. GFR is a crucial indicator of the kidney's ability to maintain homeostasis by filtering waste products, excess ions, and water from the bloodstream.

A normal GFR is essential for maintaining fluid and electrolyte balance, removing metabolic waste products, and preventing the accumulation of toxins in the body.[3]

GFR is typically measured in milliliters per minute of body surface area (mL/min/1.73 m^2) and is influenced by various factors, including blood pressure, renal blood flow, and the integrity of the glomerular filtration barrier. The glomerular filtration barrier comprises three layers: the endothelial cells lining the glomerular capillaries, the glomerular basement membrane, and the podocytes covering the outer surface of the capillaries. This barrier selectively allows certain substances to pass into the glomerular filtrate while preventing the passage of larger molecules, such as proteins and blood cells. The GFR is tightly regulated by intricate mechanisms, including the autoregulation of renal blood flow, the RAAS, and tubuloglomerular feedback, ensuring that GFR remains relatively constant under varying physiological conditions.[4]

Clinically, GFR is an essential tool for assessing kidney function and diagnosing renal diseases. A decrease in GFR may indicate reduced kidney function, and a persistently low GFR can be an early sign of chronic kidney disease (CKD). Conversely, an abnormally high GFR can be associated with certain medical conditions or medications. Estimation of GFR is commonly done using serum creatinine levels and equations like the Modification of Diet in Renal Disease (MDRD) equation or the Chronic Kidney Disease Epidemiology Collaboration (CKD-EPI) equation. GFR measurements are crucial in determining the severity of kidney dysfunction, guiding treatment decisions, and monitoring disease progression.[6] GFR reflects the efficiency of the kidneys in filtering blood and maintaining a balance in fluids, acid-base, and electrolytes. The clinical importance of GFR lies in its role as a diagnostic tool for kidney diseases and in guiding treatment strategies to preserve kidney function and improve patient outcomes.

Most GFR estimations (eGFR), however, have historically included race-specific adjustments due to physiological differences in African Americans, notably in creatinine production. These demographic-specific considerations have been addressed in the clinical setting by applying race-specific correction factors when using the MDRD or CKD-EPI formulas, in an effort to enhance

	TABLE 3.1	The Stages of Development of Chronic Kidney Disease

Stage	Description	Glomerular Filtration Rate (GFR) (mL/min/ 1.73 m^2)	Treatment Stage
1	Kidney function is normal	≥90	Observation, blood pressure control
2	Kidney damage is mild	60–89	Observation, blood pressure control and risk factors
3	Kidney damage is moderate	30–59	Observation, blood pressure control and risk factors
4	Kidney damage is severe	15–29	Planning for end-stage renal failure
5	Established kidney failure	≤15	Treatment choices

From Senan EM, Al-Adhaileh MH, Alsaade FW, et al. Diagnosis of chronic kidney disease using effective classification algorithms and recursive feature elimination techniques. *J Healthc Eng.* 2021;2021:1–10.

the accuracy of those GFR estimates by increasing the estimated GFR values which could otherwise underestimate kidney function in African Americans if unadjusted.[7] The inclusion of race as a modifier in GFR estimation, however, has sparked considerable debate. There is a legitimate concern that such race-based adjustments may reinforce racial biases and fail to consider individual physiological variability. Recent medical research and discussions advocate for a move towards more personalized GFR measurements that do not solely rely on racial categorization but include a variety of biological and environmental factors.[7] Recently the National Kidney Foundation (NKF) and the American Society of Nephrology (ASN) have developed new eGFR equations that incorporate both creatinine and cystatin C, but do not utilize race as a factor for calculating eGFR, and have recommended that these new equations be utilized by all labratories.[8] However, when utilizing these new equations that omit race for diagnosis it is important to note that utilizing both creatinine and cystatin C is more accurate than utilizing either creatinine or cystatin C individually.[9] While Table 3.1 describes the various stages of CKD based on eGFR values, it is important to note that the diagnosis of CKD may include factors other than a decreased GRF, including but not limited to albuminuria, urine sediment abnormalities, or structural abnormalities. Each of these factors, including decreased GFR, must be present for more than 3 months to be diagnostic of CKD.[10]

The Renin-Angiotensin-Aldosterone System (RAAS)

The renin-angiotensin-aldosterone system (RAAS) is a crucial hormonal pathway that regulates blood pressure, fluid balance, and electrolyte homeostasis. It plays a central role in maintaining cardiovascular function and ensuring adequate perfusion to vital organs, particularly the kidneys. The RAAS is activated in response to decreased blood flow or sodium concentration in the renal arteries. It triggers a response, leading to increased blood pressure and sodium retention.[11]

The initial response of the RAAS is the release of renin from the juxtaglomerular cells in the kidneys. Renin is an enzyme that acts on the precursor molecule angiotensinogen, primarily produced in the liver, to form angiotensin I. Angiotensin I is an inactive peptide that requires further enzymatic processing for its biological effects. This conversion occurs primarily in the lungs and other tissues with the help of the angiotensin-converting enzyme (ACE). ACE cleaves angiotensin I to form angiotensin II, the biologically active peptide responsible for most of the effects of the RAAS system.[12]

Angiotensin II acts on various receptors in the body, including the angiotensin II type 1 receptor (AT1) and the angiotensin II type 2 receptor (AT2). Stimulation of the AT1 receptor leads to vasoconstriction of blood vessels, increasing peripheral resistance and raising blood pressure. Additionally, angiotensin II promotes the secretion of aldosterone from the adrenal cortex. Aldosterone is a hormone that acts on the distal tubules and collecting ducts of the kidneys, enhancing sodium reabsorption and potassium excretion leading to increased water retention and expanded extracellular fluid volume. This mechanism contributes to the maintenance of blood pressure and electrolyte balance.[13]

The RAAS system plays a crucial role in the regulation of blood pressure and electrolyte balance in both normal physiological conditions and various disease states. Dysregulation of the RAAS can lead to hypertension, a condition characterized by persistently high blood pressure, and may contribute to other cardiovascular diseases. The RAAS system is a target for several antihypertensive medications, including ACE inhibitors and angiotensin receptor blockers (ARBs), which work by inhibiting the effects of angiotensin II and reducing blood pressure. Understanding the complex interplay of the RAAS system is vital for managing hypertension and related cardiovascular disorders and developing targeted therapies for these conditions.[14]

Hormones and Their Renal Interactions

The kidney plays a vital role in hormonal regulation, interacting with various hormones significantly affecting the body. In addition to the RAAS, the kidney synthesizes and activates important hormones that contribute to calcium homeostasis and red blood cell production.

One of the crucial hormonal functions of the kidneys is the production of the active form of vitamin D, known as calcitriol. The process for the kidneys to synthesize 1,25-dihydroxyvitamin D3 into calcitriol is regulated by parathyroid hormone (PTH). When blood calcium levels are low, the parathyroid glands release PTH, which stimulates the conversion of inactive vitamin D (cholecalciferol) from the skin or diet into its active form, calcitriol, within the kidney. Calcitriol plays a crucial role in calcium metabolism by promoting calcium absorption from the intestine and the reabsorption of calcium in the renal tubules. This ensures that adequate levels of calcium are maintained in the bloodstream to support various physiological processes, including bone health, neuromuscular function, and blood clotting.[15]

Furthermore, the kidney produces erythropoietin (EPO), a hormone essential for erythropoiesis or the production of red blood cells. EPO is primarily synthesized and released by specialized cells in the kidneys, known as interstitial fibroblasts, in response to low oxygen levels in the blood. When the kidney senses decreased oxygen levels (hypoxia), it upregulates the production of EPO, which

then travels to the bone marrow, stimulating the production and maturation of red blood cells. This process helps maintain sufficient oxygen-carrying capacity in the blood and ensures adequate tissue oxygenation. EPO is a critical hormone for individuals with chronic kidney disease (CKD) or other conditions causing anemia, as it is used therapeutically to manage anemia and improve patient outcomes.[16] Understanding these hormonal interactions and their implications in various physiological processes is crucial for comprehending kidney function and managing related disorders effectively.

Acute Renal Failure (ARF)

Acute renal failure, also known as acute kidney injury (AKI), is a sudden and often reversible decline in kidney function. It is characterized by a rapid decrease in GFR, resulting in the accumulation of waste products, electrolyte imbalances, and fluid retention. ARF can be caused by various factors, including reduced blood flow to the kidneys (*prerenal*), direct damage to the kidney tissue (*intrarenal*), or obstruction of the urinary tract (*postrenal*).[17]

The clinical presentation of acute renal failure may vary depending on the underlying cause and the severity of kidney impairment. Common symptoms include oliguria, defined as a urine output of less than 400 mL per day, fluid overload, electrolyte abnormalities, and uremia (elevated blood urea nitrogen (BUN) and creatinine levels). Patients with ARF may experience nausea, vomiting, fatigue, and confusion. In severe cases, complications such as metabolic acidosis, hyperkalemia, and pulmonary edema can develop, requiring prompt medical intervention. Diagnosing acute renal failure (ARF) involves a comprehensive approach that combines clinical evaluation, laboratory tests, and imaging studies to determine the cause, severity, and appropriate management of the condition. A crucial step in the diagnosis of ARF is obtaining a detailed medical history, including information on medications, recent illnesses, surgeries, and exposure to nephrotoxic agents. Physical examination may reveal signs of fluid overload, electrolyte imbalances, or underlying conditions contributing to ARF. Additionally, assessing urine output and analyzing the characteristics of urine, such as color, sediment, and specific gravity, can provide valuable insights into kidney function. Blood tests, including serum creatinine and BUN, are essential in evaluating kidney function and estimating GFR. Elevated levels of creatinine and BUN indicate impaired kidney function, whereas a decreased GFR suggests a reduction in renal filtration capacity. Electrolyte abnormalities, such as hyperkalemia or metabolic acidosis, may also be evident in laboratory findings.[17]

Imaging studies play a significant role in diagnosing ARF and identifying any structural abnormalities that could obstruct the urinary tract. Renal ultrasound is a noninvasive imaging modality used to assess kidney size, shape, and the presence of hydronephrosis or renal masses. Computed tomography (CT) scans, or magnetic resonance imaging (MRI) can provide detailed information about the kidneys' anatomy, blood flow, and any obstructive lesions. Early recognition and treatment are crucial to prevent further kidney damage and improve outcomes.[18]

Prerenal ARF

In cases of prerenal ARF, the lack of perfusion does not always mean low-volume states. For example, the patient may have sufficient volume status but reduced flow efficiency to the kidney, such as in cardiogenic or distributive shock cases. As discussed previously, the kidneys attempt to compensate for this using the RAAS. Prerenal injury treatment should focus on the cause of the renal failure. Fluids can be helpful to increase arterial pressure and therefore increase perfusion to the kidneys and the glomerulus. However, not all causes of prerenal injury will respond to fluids. Patients in cardiogenic shock, for example, may require inotropic support. The main treatment goal of prerenal failure is to identify the cause of the lack of sufficient flow and then correct that issue.

Intrarenal ARF

In intrarenal ARF, specific interventions depend on the cause, including discontinuation of nephrotoxic medications, treatment of infections, or addressing immune-mediated processes. One of the most common causes of intrarenal ARF is acute tubular necrosis (ATN). ATN can occur from ischemia, nephrotoxic drugs, sepsis, or rhabdomyolysis. It is important to note that ATN can result from prerenal causes such as hypoperfusion. Overall, the ATN leads to cell injury or death, which causes a cascade of inflammatory effects and further damages the kidneys.

Treatment is focused on the prevention of this complication in high-risk patients, such as patients with preexisting kidney disease, diabetes, and cardiac conditions such as heart failure. High-risk procedures like cardiac bypass can strain the kidneys and lead to acute tubular necrosis.[19] Patients that are admitted with sepsis, major burns, and other forms of shock have a high risk of developing ATN. These patients must be monitored continuously, ensuring proper fluid status, cessation of nephrotoxic medications such as nonsteroidal anti-inflammatory drugs (NSAIDs), and proper management of the disease process causing the ATN.

Rhabdomyolysis

Patients presenting with myoglobinuria secondary to rhabdomyolysis are at high risk for developing ATN and subsequently intrarenal ARF. The cause of rhabdomyolysis may be traumatic or atraumatic, but the underlying pathway that results in muscle injury, cellular destruction, and necrosis is the same in either case, direct injury to the myocyte.[20] Diagnosis of rhabdomyolysis is generally confirmed through serum creatine phosphokinase (CPK) of greater than 1000 UI/L, or 5 times upper normal limit. In addition to cellular destruction and the resulting release of intracellular proteins and ions into the extracellular space, the risk of ARF in these patients is compounded by acidosis, the generation of oxidative free radicals, and decreases of circulating fluid volume, as injured muscles have the capacity to aggregate up to 12 L of fluid within 48 hours of injury.[21]

The goal when treating these patients is to decrease myoglobin precipitation in the renal tubules, where increased concentrations are likely to cause an obstruction. This is achieved though aggressive fluid resuscitation with isotonic saline and alkalinization of the urine. Alkalinization of the urine is important, as the nephrotoxic effect of myoglobin in the tubules is mitigated in alkaline urine. The treatment goals for patients experiencing rhabdomyolysis are to maintain a urine output of 200 to 300 mL/h, a serum pH of 7.5 or less, and a urine pH of greater than 6.5. These goals should be pursued and maintained until the patient's CPK is below 5000 IU/L.[22] Throughout treatment, however, providers must closely monitor serum metabolic lab values, as both the cause of the injury, and the subsequent treatments provided, are likely to result in significant fluctuations of calcium, potassium, and sodium. The addition of glucose to isotonic fluid may prove beneficial to supplement caloric demand, as well as mitigate

hyperkalemia. The administration of calcium, however, should be avoided, as these patients frequently present with hypocalcemia in the initial stages of injury, but can quickly evolve to hypercalcemia as cellular destruction progresses. Through the application of rapid treatment to address the cause and aggressive fluid management to mitigate effects of rhabdomyolysis, significant renal damage can be avoided in these patients.

Comparing Prerenal and Intrarenal

Prerenal and intrarenal failure are two of the most common causes of acute renal failure and can coincide. It is helpful to understand different characteristics of the diagnosis criteria to help differentiate the two. The BUN to creatine ratio and fractional excretion of sodium are helpful tools in evaluating prerenal versus intrarenal renal failure. Urea is primally reabsorbed in the proximal tubule, while creatine is not, and the majority is filtered and excreted. The normal ratio of BUN (10–20 mg/dL in blood) to creatinine (0.7–1.2 mg/dL in blood) is anywhere from 10:1 to 20:1.[23] In this equation, the urea is the larger number and is mostly reabsorbed whereas most of the creatinine is secreted in the urine. Larger ratios (those greater than 15:1) indicate prerenal failure, whereas a ratio less than 15:1 would coincide with intrarenal failure or ATN.[23] This is because the tubules in prerenal failure tend to function appropriately, meaning they can still maintain reabsorption and filtration. However, the GFR tends to slow in the presence of hypoperfusion, allowing for more reabsorption of urea. Therefore the body reabsorbs more urea but filters the same amount of creatine, increasing the ratio.[23] With intrarenal failure, the tubules are not functioning properly, and the body does not absorb as much urea or filter as much creatine. The ratio lessens as the difference between the two numbers is closer. It is important to note that urea can also be increased in other states, such as increased protein intake, dehydration, liver disease, pregnancy, and advanced age.[23] Plasma creatine concentration can also be influenced by other disease processes, such as trauma or increased steroid use or production, as seen with Cushing's disease. Creatinine, however, has a more stable rate of production and, therefore, may serve better in the diagnosis of renal failure. The fractional excretion of sodium (FEna) compares the ratio of filtered sodium to excreted sodium. In prerenal, the value is less than 1%.[23] This is because the RAAS is activated in the prerenal portion of the renal system, and the body absorbs more sodium to help increase blood pressure, resulting in less sodium being filtered and excreted in the urine. In intrarenal injury, the tubules cannot reabsorb properly, and therefore the body excretes more urine, and the value is greater than 1%.[24] This diagnostic tool must be interpreted in the clinical setting to ensure its usefulness, as other clinical cases can cause percentages below and above. Overall, both tools can be helpful in investigating prerenal and intrarenal injury, and there are many circumstances where their values can be skewed.

Postrenal ARF

The causes of postrenal ARF arise from compression of the urinary tract, such as obstruction of the urethra from benign prostatic hyperplasia or a kidney stone obstructing the ureter or urethra. Both examples cause a backup of urine, which then causes increased pressure within the tubules. This increased pressure gradient eventually affects the GFR. A FEna of less than 1% can also be seen here, as the tubules start to lose function and more sodium is excreted into the urine. Though postrenal failure is not the most common form of renal failure, it can cause injury to the tubule and lead to negative function of the nephron and, ultimately, the kidney. Treatment may require the removal of obstructions through surgical or catheter-based procedures.

Management of ARF

As a significant clinical condition with various underlying causes, ARF requires a multidisciplinary approach involving nephrologists, critical care specialists, and other healthcare professionals.[25] Treatment is first aimed at life-threatening complications such as fluid overload, hyperkalemia, or metabolic acidosis. Treatment of those conditions will be discussed later in this chapter as it relates to transporting these acutely ill patients. Treatment should be focused on the kidneys and the disease process causing insult to the kidney and should not be limited to just one or the other. Fluid status should be examined and treated to ensure proper perfusion to the kidneys. Vasoactive agents can be used in the treatment of shock (i.e., cardiogenic and septic shock) to help with renal perfusion. Low-dose dopamine and diuretics such as furosemide have previously been accepted clinical practice in the treatment or attempted prevention of ARF; however, multiple studies have failed to prove the efficacy of either of these modalities.[26,27] In fact, there is growing evidence to suggest that diuretic use in ARF may actually increase mortality.[27]

The overall focus of management of acute renal failure needs to be on prevention in high-risk populations, cautious administration of nephrotoxic drugs, and optimizing fluid status, all while correcting the cause of the renal failure. Treatment is individualized for each patient based on the cause of the failure. Overall management of acute renal failure is focused on balanced fluid management. Correcting and treating life-threatening electrolyte imbalances such as hyperkalemia is imperative, as well as refraining from administering drugs that might further damage the kidney.[25] Most acute renal injuries will recover with supportive care.[28] The provider must focus on early recognition to determine the underlying cause and fix the problem swiftly. If this cause is not addressed, the kidneys will likely sustain permanent damage and progress to chronic renal failure.

Chronic Renal Failure

Chronic renal failure is the progressive loss of the function of the kidneys, specifically the nephron. Individuals with renal failure often lack signs and symptoms until a large amount of the kidney is injured. This is because the kidney has many systems in place to deal with decreased GFR that lead to overall increased filtration and absorption. It is not until late renal failure that elevated levels of urea, creatine, and acidosis are seen. The most common signs and symptoms seen with chronic renal failure are systemic hypertension and proteinuria. The reason for this is the kidneys adapt to the decreased GFR by stimulating the RAAS. One of the essential parts of this system is aldosterone. Increasing levels of aldosterone lead to increased glomerular pressure and systemic hypertension. The overall increase in pressure and damage to the kidneys results in increased inflammatory markers. These inflammatory markers lead to increased permeability at the glomerulus and result in increased protein in the urine.

There are many causes of chronic renal failure; however, some of the most common are hypertension, diabetes, and lupus.[23] Each of these disorders has a unique process in how it relates to overall kidney damage. Lupus, for instance, is an autoimmune disorder that forms immune complexes that damage the kidney. Regardless of the causative factor, chronic renal failure is the result of the nephrons increasing their GFR until exhaustion and renal failure signs and symptoms appear.

Renal Replacement Therapy

The use of renal replacement therapy (RRT) for acute patients in the hospital is common, and transport providers should be familiar with these treatments. Patients with severe AKI in the ICU usually require RRT in the form of intermittent hemodialysis (HD), peritoneal dialysis (PD), extended hemodialysis (slow low-efficiency dialysis; SLED), or continous renal replacement therapy (CRRT).[29] The primary renal system functions that RRT supplements or substitutes are fluid balance, electrolyte balance, acid-base balance, and excretion of drugs and by-products of metabolism such as nitrogen, urea, and creatinine.[27] Because of this, indications for RRT may include non-renal failure-related needs, such as sepsis, acidosis, and multiple organ dysfunction syndrome (MODS).[30]

Terminology

Before discussing the principles of RRT, it is important to understand the terminology and methods used for RRT.

Extracorporeal Circuit

The extracorporeal circuit (EC) is the method by which blood flow is routed outside the body. It consists of tubing that carries the blood to the filter (or hemofilter or dialyzer) from the vascular access catheter and from the filter back to the body via the access catheter again.[31]

Dialysate

Dialysate is an electrolyte solution that typically contains physiologically normal concentrations of extracellular electrolytes, except for potassium and bicarbonate. As the dialysate, or dialysis solution, passes by the non-blood side of the semipermeable membrane during dialysis, it attracts and absorbs waste products from the blood.[31]

Diffusion

Diffusion is the process by which solutes move across a semipermeable membrane from an area of higher concentration to an area of lower concentration. Diffusion occurs within the hemodialyzer or hemofilter, where solutes in the patient's blood, such as urea, creatinine, and electrolytes, diffuse across the membrane into the dialysate solution or replacement fluid.[32] This process helps to remove waste products and normalize electrolyte levels in the bloodstream.[33]

Convection

Convection is the process by which solutes and fluids are removed from the bloodstream by the movement of solvent (typically water) across a semipermeable membrane under pressure. In CRRT, convection occurs primarily during hemofiltration, where excess fluid is removed from the patient's blood by convective clearance through the hemofilter membrane. As blood passes through the hemofilter under pressure, water and solutes are filtered across the membrane into the replacement fluid, effectively reducing fluid overload and maintaining fluid balance in critically ill patients.[33]

Ultrafiltration

Ultrafiltration removes excess fluid from the bloodstream by creating a pressure gradient across a semipermeable membrane. In CRRT, ultrafiltration occurs concurrently with hemofiltration, where hydraulic pressure is applied to the blood side of the hemofilter to facilitate the movement of water and solutes across the membrane. Ultrafiltration helps to alleviate fluid overload, reduce pulmonary congestion, and improve hemodynamic stability in patients with acute kidney injury or renal dysfunction.[33]

Adsorption

Adsorption is the process by which solutes are removed from the bloodstream by adhering to the surface of an adsorbent material. Adsorption can play a role in removing certain middle molecular weight solutes and inflammatory mediators that may not be effectively cleared by conventional dialysis techniques.[33]

Vascular Access for RRT

Central venous catheters (CVC) are commonly used for short-term vascular access in RRT due to their large size and ease of insertion. The CVC can be placed in the internal jugular, subclavian, or femoral veins. Typically, dual-lumen catheters are preferred for CRRT, with one lumen used for blood withdrawal to the circuit, using a negative pressure pump, and the other for returning the filtered or dialyzed blood from the circuit to the patient.[31,32] Patients who are expected to receive hemodialysis over a longer period of time typically have vascular access achieved through arteriovenous fistulas or grafts. Arteriovenous fistulas connect an artery and a vein directly, whereas an arteriovenous graft achieves this connection through additional synthetic tubing.[34]

Types of RRT

Continuous renal replacement therapy is a generic term used to refer to any extracorporeal blood purification process that is intended to be utilized 24 hours a day. CRRT involves continuously removing solutes and fluids through a semipermeable membrane, allowing for gentle fluid and solute removal and maintaining hemodynamic stability in critically ill patients.[29] Some of the techniques used to deliver RRT are the following:

Continuous Veno-Venous Hemofiltration (CVVH)

This process utilizes a pump to move blood through a highly permeable membrane. The plasma that crosses the membrane contains all of the molecules to which the membrane is permeable, including many toxins and electrolytes. This ultrafiltration process uses convection to remove impurities and excess fluid.[34]

Continuous Veno-Venous Hemodialysis (CVVHD)

This technique utilizes diffusion to remove impurities from the plasma by pumping an electrolyte neutral fluid (dialysate) through the membrane in the opposite direction of blood flow, inducing the movement of electrolytes and toxins from a fluid with high concentrations (the plasma) to a fluid with lower concentrations (the dialysate), such that it can be discarded.[34]

Continuous Veno-Venous Hemodiafiltration (CVVHDF)

This method utilizes both convection and diffusion, essentially combining CVVH and CVVHD to achieve the removal of toxins and high levels of electrolytes from the plasma.[34]

Hemodialysis (HD)

Hemodialysis involves the extracorporeal removal of waste products and excess fluids from the bloodstream using a dialyzer.[35] Patients usually undergo HD sessions three times weekly in a dialysis center or hospital setting, lasting 3–5 hours each.[36] Rapid fluid removal during HD sessions can pose risks such as hypotension and disequilibrium syndrome.[37] Despite its efficacy, HD may not be suitable for patients with poor vascular access or those unable to travel to a dialysis center regularly.

Peritoneal Dialysis (PD)

Peritoneal dialysis utilizes the peritoneum as a semipermeable membrane for fluid and solute exchange. A peritoneal dialysis catheter is inserted into the abdominal cavity for infusion and drainage of dialysis fluid.[38] PD offers greater flexibility as it can be performed at home, either manually throughout the day (continuous ambulatory peritoneal dialysis; CAPD) or with the assistance of a machine overnight (automated peritoneal dialysis; APD).[39] While PD may have fewer cardiovascular complications and preserve residual renal function better than HD, it carries risks of peritonitis, catheter-related issues, and hernias.[39]

Anticoagulation

Anticoagulation helps maintain circuit patency and prolongs the lifespan of the hemofilter, as well as reduces the risk of emboli by inhibiting clot formation.[40] Some anticoagulants used are unfractionated heparin, low-molecular-weight heparin (LMWH), and regional citrate anticoagulation. Unfractionated heparin is a commonly used anticoagulant in CRRT. It is typically administered as a continuous infusion at a titrated dose to maintain the desired level of anticoagulation while minimizing the risk of bleeding complications.[41] LMWH, however, is not commonly used in CRRT, as there is a concern for systemic anticoagulation and an inherent lack of reliable predictors of bleeding and antithrombotic efficacy.[42] Regional citrate anticoagulation is an alternative anticoagulation strategy used in CRRT that involves the infusion of citrate solution into the pre-filter blood circuit to chelate ionized calcium, thereby inhibiting the coagulation cascade. Regional citrate anticoagulation requires careful monitoring of ionized calcium levels and adjustment of citrate infusion rates to prevent systemic hypocalcemia.[41]

Transporting Patients Receiving RRT

RRT in the transport world remains a rare occurrence. Some military teams, however, have demonstrated its use in extended critical care air transport.[43] The use of RRT in the transport environment could be beneficial for acid-base, metabolic, and precise volume control.[30] For transport teams that encounter patients receiving RRT, which may be paused for transport, it is critical to ensure strict monitoring of intake and output, anticoagulation status, and protection of any access lines to ensure they remain patent and undamaged.[42] Providers should be vigilant for signs of access-related complications for patients with HD access, such as thrombosis, infection, or malfunction. Regular assessment of the access site for signs of redness, swelling, tenderness, or impaired blood flow is imperative.[43] In the case of patients on PD, transport providers should be aware of potential complications such as peritonitis, catheter-related issues (e.g., leakage, obstruction), or hernias.[39] Close observation for signs of peritoneal infection, including abdominal pain, cloudy dialysate, fever, or systemic signs of infection, is essential. By remaining vigilant and informed about potential complications associated with HD and PD, transport providers can ensure prompt recognition and appropriate management, thereby optimizing the safety and well-being of patients during transport.

Diagnosis of Chronic Renal Failure

The diagnosis of chronic renal failure begins with evaluating patients that are high risk, such as patients with chronic hypertension and diabetes. These patients will often have azotemia, increased levels of urea and creatine in the plasma, as well as uremia, which is a proinflammatory state.[23] Providers may look at the albumin-to-creatine ratio. This will compare the levels of protein, more specifically albumin, and creatine, in the urine. Protein is usually not present in the urine due to the negative charge on the glomeruli and tightly constructed cell walls. With renal failure, albumin is not prevented from moving through the glomerulus and entering the tubules to be excreted as filtrate. In general, protein levels in the urine can be of great concern for renal failure. Azotemia and albuminuria are markers for decreased renal function and can lead the provider in determining the cause of renal failure. Imaging, such as CT, MRI, ultrasound, or a kidney biopsy, may be performed to further understand the cause of renal failure. One of the more common ways of classifying renal failure is using the five stages of kidney disease (Table 3.1).[44]

Signs and Symptoms of Chronic Renal Failure

The signs and symptoms of early chronic renal failure can be broad and vague, sometimes only manifesting as mild hypertension. However, as GFR declines, the kidneys lose their ability to secrete and absorb many important factors needed to maintain homeostasis in the body. The kidneys also lose their ability to secrete important hormones, which leads to some of the diseases that correlate with chronic renal failure. The most common labs that are drawn for the progression of renal failure are urea and creatine. As discussed previously, these plasma markers can be influenced by many other factors, and their role is not the most specific for renal disease. Some of the broader signs and symptoms are nausea, vomiting, and diarrhea, which are caused by increased levels of uremia in the blood. In addition to this, electrolyte abnormalities occur frequently, and metabolic acidosis can be seen as the disease progresses.[45]

Hyperkalemia can be seen when the patient no longer can sustain the excretion of potassium, and it builds up in the blood. This is usually maintained by increased GFR, as seen in early chronic renal failure, but falls over time. Patients that develop oliguria are at increased risk of hyperkalemia due to decreasing levels of potassium being excreted into the urine. It is important to note that patients with chronic renal failure can develop potassium adaptation, which leads to their cells being accustomed to the increased potassium levels as they gradually increase over time. Patients with chronic renal failure tend to develop hypocalcemia and hyperphosphatemia. This is due to decreased synthesis of activated vitamin D, which leads to less absorption of calcium in the GI tract. The phosphorous levels also increase due to decreased excretion, which further compounds the hypocalcemia. Overall, this imbalance increases parathyroid hormone, which can further decrease GFR.

Metabolic acidosis can occur due to decreased excretion of hydrogen and decreased absorption of bicarbonate, resulting in increased levels of chloride, decreased amounts of bicarbonate, and a non-ion gap metabolic acidosis. The patient can have cardiopulmonary effects such as pulmonary edema, hypertension, and possible heart failure. Many of these patients can have anemia due to low levels of erythropoietin, which is used to stimulate the production and maturity of red blood cells.

Additionally, some patients with chronic renal failure have been shown to have elevated levels of troponin.[46] The exact reason for this is not fully known. This elevation can make it difficult to diagnose patients with possible cardiac injury that also have chronic renal failure, as they tend to present together.

Overall, there are many signs and symptoms of chronic renal failure, and the progression of this disease will only increase them further.

Treatment of Chronic Renal Failure

Treatment of chronic renal failure starts with the cause, as it is usually secondary to another disease process that damages the kidney. For instance, optimal glucose management in diabetic patients may help limit kidney injury. Strict management of hypertension may also help with declining GFR. Changes in diet may alleviate some of the signs of renal failure; for example, a low-protein diet may help decrease creatinine levels. The patient may receive vitamin D supplements to treat hypocalcemia and products containing aluminum to decrease phosphorus levels. These patients need to ensure their intake and output are adequately managed, including intake of potassium and sodium. For patients that continue to have declining renal function, options such as hemodialysis or kidney transplant may need to be introduced. Treatment of chronic renal failure needs to be focused on reducing the cause of the failure and attempting to maintain a normal balance of the body's essential products and waste.

Renal Failure and Transport

Transport providers are called many times to transport patients with kidney failure that have many life-threatening signs and symptoms, such as metabolic acidosis, fluid overload, and hyperkalemia. For the remainder of this chapter, these life-threatening symptoms and treatment will be reviewed in further detail.

Metabolic Acidosis

The kidneys are an important buffering system and help in many ways to keep a normal pH within the body.[23] This is first seen in the proximal tubule. Sodium and hydrogen are exchanged, and hydrogen binds with bicarbonate to create carbonic acid. Carbonic acid is then catalyzed with carbonic anhydrase and becomes H_2O and CO_2.[23] Thus, the original hydrogen is reabsorbed as H_2O. The CO_2, however, diffuses back into the cell, where it can be expelled as CO_2 through respiration or again combine with H_2O to form carbonic acid. The carbonic acid dissociates to produce bicarbonate and hydrogen. The bicarbonate is reabsorbed, and the hydrogen starts the cycle over again.

With renal failure, metabolic acidosis is caused by both decreased bicarbonate absorption and secretion along with decreased ammonia secretion.[47] Hyperchloremia usually accompanies this acidosis due to chloride and bicarbonate being extracellular anions and the blood wanting to maintain this balance.[23] Metabolic acidosis can have harmful effects on the cardiovascular system, including cardiac dysfunction leading to arrhythmias.[48] The treatment of renal failure with accompanying metabolic acidosis can be difficult. Many providers have administered sodium bicarbonate to help alleviate some of the detrimental effects of metabolic acidosis. However, bicarbonate administration can lead to increased carbon dioxide levels and decreased calcium levels, both of which can have negative effects on the cardiovascular system. While bicarbonate has been used by many providers for severe acidosis (<7.1) in the treatment of cardiac arrest, there is no recent evidence to support its use and growing evidence indicating potential harm.[49]

These patients may develop Kussmaul respirations or deep labored respirations in response to the acidosis. The provider must be aware of this protective compensation and take it into consideration when determining the need for intubation. Intubation of these patients can be detrimental. If intubation is required, then the provider must ensure that the apneic time is limited.[50] Some providers will allow the patient to breathe spontaneously during intubation to decrease any apneic time.[50] The provider must ensure that they are allowing the patient to reach the required minute ventilation, as it is often a larger minute ventilation than normal. It can be helpful to evaluate the patient's ability to maintain homeostasis, given their current level of respiratory compensation, either through spontaneous respirations, or a set minute ventilation on a mechanical ventilator, using the Winters' formula. The Winters' formula states that expected PCO_2 is = $(1.5 \times HCO_3 + 8)$.[51] If the patient's actual PCO_2 is higher than the calculated value by two or more mmHg, more minute ventilation, or respiratory compensation, is needed. If the patient's actual PCO_2 is lower than the calculated value by two or more mmHg, the minute ventilation, or level of respiratory compensation, is too high.[51]

Depending on the ventilator mode being used, it may be beneficial to administer less sedation or utilize medications that do not depress the patient's respiratory drive, thereby allowing the patient to control their own rate and use the ventilator to support the patient's goal tidal volume or minute ventilation as needed.[50] If the patient is paralyzed and/or significantly sedated, it is up to the provider to ensure minute ventilation needs are met, and goal PCO_2 values are being achieved. It is helpful to remember here that the frequently monitored $ETCO_2$ values and blood-gas PCO_2 values are not 1:1. Depending on factors that may affect gas exchange at the alveolar level, $ETCO_2$ values may be falsely lower than blood-gas PCO_2 values; however, $ETCO_2$ values cannot be falsely higher than blood-gas PCO_2 values. That is to say, blood-gas PCO_2 values are always greater than or equal to $ETCO_2$ values. Many of the strategies for the treatment of patients with metabolic acidosis are still under research. The provider needs to focus on proper management of the cause of metabolic acidosis and support the patient.

Hyperkalemia

Hyperkalemia is the most common electrolyte disturbance associated with renal disease.[52] One of the reasons for hyperkalemia is the result of the kidney's inability to properly eliminate potassium, which is done primarily in the distal tubules.[53] In addition to this, hyperkalemia coincides with metabolic acidosis, due to potassium moving from the intracellular space to the extracellular space.[53] Potassium is primarily located intracellularly and is

needed for many cardiac, skeletal muscle, and nerve conductions.[23] The signs and symptoms of hyperkalemia may be related to how rapidly potassium increases more so than the actual amount of potassium.[23,54] This means that patients with chronic renal failure may adapt to higher levels of potassium and show no symptoms in the setting of hyperkalemia versus a patient that develops a rapid increase in potassium levels.[54,55] Some of the effects of potassium can be seen on the EKG, such as peaked T waves; however, as potassium increases, the ECG can show prolonged PR interval, widening QRS, and loss of p waves.[54] Ultimately, a sine wave pattern can be seen on ECG.[56]

One of the first treatments for this hyperkalemia is the administration of calcium, as calcium works to stabilize the resting membrane potential.[57] Calcium chloride is more irritating to the peripheral vasculature and may be best administered via central line.[54] When administering calcium, however, it is important to remember that, due to variations in bioavailability, it takes roughly 3 grams of calcium gluconate to equal the effectiveness of 1 gram of calcium chloride. Insulin has been shown to decrease extracellular potassium levels by activating the sodium-potassium pump, leading to an influx of potassium into the cell.[23] A dextrose solution should be administered concurrently with insulin when used for the management of hyperkalemia, to prevent hypoglycemia. The use of a short-acting beta agonist can help shift potassium back into the cell as well, and beta-2 agonists, such as albuterol, have been shown to effectively achieve this goal.[58] Management of hyperkalemia is multimodal, and the treatment must be goal-driven and evidence-based if it is to be effective in decreasing the detrimental effects of potassium.

Fluid Overload

Fluid overload is commonly found in patients with kidney failure. Diuretics are frequently utilized as one of the treatments for acutely ill patients with fluid overload secondary to renal insult.[59] It is important to recall, however, that there is a lack of evidence supporting the use of diuretics in renal failure patients and increasing evidence that their use may be harmful.[27] Ultimately, dialysis will help these patients and decrease the amount of fluid in the body. One of the lethal signs and symptoms of fluid overload is noncardiogenic pulmonary edema.[60] Pulmonary edema can cause shunt physiology, where blood from the right side of the heart is unable to pick up oxygen at the lungs as it returns to the left side.[61] A poor response to an increase in oxygen therapy is a typical feature of a shunt.[61] Hypercapnia is uncommon in shunt physiology but can be seen as the shunt worsens.[61] Positive-pressure ventilation should be utilized to help decrease the fraction of shunt and also recruit more alveoli.[62] Overall, the treatment of life-threatening symptoms of renal failure needs to be focused on addressing the problem and ensuring effective treatment.

Summary

Renal failure, both chronic and acute, has many causes and can present in many different ways. This disease is very common in acutely ill patients admitted to the hospital and is often the result of complications from a primary causative factor. For that reason, it is imperative for transport providers to better understand the renal system. Renal failure can be caused by a multitude of different disease processes and is a major cause of patient morbidity and mortality, and it is common during the career of a transport provider to care for patients with renal failure requiring transport to a higher level of care. Understanding the physiology and pathology of the renal system will help the provider to better treat and manage these patients.

References

1. Drake RL, Vogl AW, Mitchell AWM. *Gray's Anatomy for Students*. 4th ed. Philadelphia, PA: Elsevier; 2020.

2. Standring S, editor. *Gray's Anatomy: The Anatomical Basis of Clinical Practice*. 41st ed. Edinburgh: Elsevier; 2016.

3. Brenner BM. *Brenner & Rector's The Kidney*. 8th ed. Philadelphia, PA: Saunders Elsevier; 2007.

4. Guyton AC, Hall JE. *Textbook of Medical Physiology*. 13th ed. Philadelphia, PA: Saunders Elsevier; 2016.

5. Becker KL. *Principles and Practice of Endocrinology and Metabolism*. 4th ed. Philadelphia, PA: Lippincott Williams & Wilkins; 2001.

6. Levey AS, Coresh J, Greene T, et al. Using standardized serum creatinine values in the modification of diet in renal disease study equation for estimating glomerular filtration rate. *Ann Intern Med*. 2006;145(4):247–254. doi: 10.7326/0003-4819-145-4-200608150-00004

7. Delanaye P, Mariat C, Maillard N, Krzesinski JM, Cavalier E. Are the creatinine-based equations accurate to estimate glomerular filtration rate in African American populations? *Clin J Am Soc Nephrol*. 2011;6(4):906–912. doi: 10.2215/CJN.10931210

8. Delgado C, Baweja M, Crews DC, et al. A unifying approach for GFR estimation: Recommendations of the NKF-ASN Task Force on Reassessing the Inclusion of Race in Diagnosing Kidney Disease. *Am J Kidney Dis*. 2022;79(2):268–288. doi: 10.1053/j.ajkd.2021.08.003

9. Inker LA, Eneanya ND, Coresh J, et al. New creatinine- and cystatin C-based equations to estimate GFR without race. *N Engl J Med*. 2021;385(19):1737–1749. doi: 10.1056/NEJMoa2102953

10. National Kidney Foundation. *What is the Criteria for CKD?* Available at: https://www.kidney.org/professionals/explore-your-knowledge/what-is-the-criteria-for-ckd.

11. Schrier RW, Gottschalk CW. The mechanism of renin release. V. Factors affecting the release of renin. *J Clin Invest*. 1972;51(7):1950–1956. doi: 10.1172/JCI107017

12. Nussberger J, Brunner DB, Waeber B, Brunner HR. True versus immunoreactive angiotensin II in human plasma. *Hypertension*. 1985;7(5 Pt 2):II1–II6. doi: 10.1161/01.HYP.7.5_Part_2.II1

13. Carey RM, Siragy HM. The intrarenal renin-angiotensin system and diabetic nephropathy. *Trends Endocrinol Metab*. 2003;14(6):274–281. doi: 10.1016/s1043-2760(03)00111-4

14. Brenner BM, Cooper ME, de Zeeuw D, et al. RENAAL Study Investigators. Effects of losartan on renal and cardiovascular outcomes in patients with type 2 diabetes and nephropathy. *N Engl J Med*. 2001;345(12):861–869. doi: 10.1056/NEJMoa011161

15. Holick MF. Vitamin D deficiency. *N Engl J Med*. 2007;357(3):266–281. doi: 10.1056/NEJMra070553

16. Jelkmann W. Erythropoietin: structure, control of production, and function. *Physiol Rev*. 1992;72(2):449–489. doi: 10.1152/physrev.1992.72.2.449

17. Ronco C, Bellomo R, Kellum JA. Acute kidney injury. *Lancet*. 2019;394(10212):1949–1964. doi: 10.1016/S0140-6736(19)32563-2

18. Khwaja A. KDIGO clinical practice guidelines for acute kidney injury. *Nephron Clin Pract*. 2012;120(4):c179-c184. doi: 10.1159/000339789

19. Djordjević A. Acute kidney injury after open-heart surgery procedures. *Acta Clin Croat*. 2021;60(1):120–126. doi: 10.20471/acc.2021.60.01.17

20. Gupta A, Thorson P, Penmatsa KR, Gupta P. Rhabdomyolysis: revisited. *Ulster Med J*. 2021;90(2):61–69.

21. Gonzalez D. Crush syndrome. *Crit Care Med*. 2005;33(1):S34–S41. doi: 10.1097/01.CCM.0000151065.13564.6F

22. Stanley M, Chippa V, Aeddula NR, Quintanilla Rodriguez BS, Adigun R. Rhabdomyolysis. In: *StatPearls* [Internet]. Treasure Island, FL: StatPearls Publishing; 2023.

23. McCance K, Huether S. *Pathophysiology: The Biologic Basis for Disease in Adults and Children*. 8th ed. Elsevier; 2019.

24. Lima C, Macedo E. Urinary biochemistry in the diagnosis of acute kidney injury. *Disease Markers*. 2018;2018:1–7. doi: 10.1155/2018/4907024

25. Pannu N, James M, Hemmelgarn BR, Klarenbach S; Alberta Kidney Disease Network. Association between AKI, recovery of renal function, and long-term outcomes after hospital discharge. *Clin J Am Soc Nephrol*. 2013;8(2):194–202. doi: 10.2215/CJN.04660512

26. Bistola V, Arfaras-Melainis A, Polyzogopoulou E, Ikonomidis I, Parissis J. Inotropes in acute heart failure: from guidelines to practical use: therapeutic options and clinical practice. *Card Fail Rev*. 2019;5(3):133–139. doi: 10.15420/cfr.2019.11.2

27. Hegde A. Diuretics in acute kidney injury. *Indian J Crit Care Med*. 2014;24(S3):98–99. doi: 10.5005/jp-journals-10071-23406

28. Goyal A, Daneshpajouhnejad P, Hashmi MF, Bashir K. Acute kidney injury (acute renal failure). In: StatPearls [Internet]. Treasure Island, FL: StatPearls Publishing; 2020 [update Nov 2023]. Available at: https://www.ncbi.nlm.nih.gov/books/NBK441896.

29. Karkar A, Ronco C. Prescription of CRRT: a pathway to optimize therapy. *Ann Intensive Care*. 2020;10(1):32. doi: 10.1186/s13613-020-0648-y

30. Zhang J, Tian J, Sun H, et al. How does continuous renal replacement therapy affect septic acute kidney injury? *Blood Purif*. 2018;46(4):326–331. doi: 10.1159/000492026

31. Juncos LA, Chandrashekar K, Karakala N, Baldwin I. Vascular access, membranes and circuit for CRRT. *Semin Dial*. 2021;34(6):406–415. doi: 10.1111/sdi.12977

32. See EJ, Bellomo R. How I prescribe continuous renal replacement therapy. *Crit Care*. 2021;25(1):1. doi: 10.1186/s13054-020-03448-7

33. Claure-Del Granado R., Clark WR. Continuous renal replacement therapy principles. *Semin Dial*. 2021;34(6):398–405. doi: 10.1111/sdi.12967

34. Kallenbach JZ. *Review of Hemodialysis for Nurses and Dialysis Personnel*. 10th ed. Mosby; 2021.

35. Ronco C, Bellomo R, Kellum JA, Ricci Z. *Critical Care Nephrology e-book*. 3rd ed. Elsevier; 2017.

36. Ashby D, Borman N, Burton J, et al. Renal association clinical practice guideline on haemodialysis. *BMC Nephrol*. 2019;20(1):379. doi: 10.1186/s12882-019-1527-3

37. Tandukar S, Palevsky PM. Continuous renal replacement therapy. *Chest*. 2019;155(3):626–638. doi: 10.1016/j.chest.2018.09.004

38. Andreoli M, Totoli C. Peritoneal dialysis. *Rev Assoc Med Bras*. 2020;66(suppl 1):S37–S44. doi: 10.1590/1806-9282.66.s1.37

39. Oza-Gajera BP, Abdel-Aal AK, Almehmi A. Complications of percutaneous peritoneal dialysis catheter. *Semin Interv Radiol*. 2022;39(1):40–46. doi: 10.1055/s-0041-1741484

40. Abdosh K, Suliman I, Ahmed G. Complications of permanent vascular access in hemodialysis patients. *J Egypt Soc Nephrol Transplant*. 2020;20(3):157. doi: 10.4103/jesnt.jesnt_36_19

41. Li R, Gao X, Zhou T, Li Y, Wang J, Zhang P. Regional citrate versus heparin anticoagulation for continuous renal replacement therapy in critically ill patients: A meta-analysis of randomized controlled trials. *Ther Apher Dial*. 2022;26(6):1086–1097. doi: 10.1111/1744-9987.13850

42. Singh S. Anticoagulation during renal replacement therapy. *Indian J Crit Care Med*. 2015;24(suppl 3):112–116. doi: 10.5005/jp-journals-10071-23412

43. Dittman K, Pearson D. Crossing the pond: Transcontinental continuous renal replacement therapy in modern warfare. *Chest*. 2019;156(4):A167. doi: 10.1016/j.chest.2019.08.241

44. Senan EM, Al-Adhaileh MH, Alsaade FW, et al. Diagnosis of chronic kidney disease using effective classification algorithms and recursive feature elimination techniques. *J Healthc Eng*. 2021;2021:1–10. doi: 10.1155/2021/1004767

45. Kim HJ. Metabolic acidosis in chronic kidney disease: pathogenesis, clinical consequences, and treatment. *Electrolyte Blood Press*. 2021;19(2):29. doi: 10.5049/ebp.2021.19.2.29

46. Chesnaye NC, Szummer K, Bárány P, et al. Association between renal function and troponin T over time in stable chronic kidney disease patients. *J Am Heart Assoc*. 2019;8(21). doi: 10.1161/jaha.119.013091

47. Adamczak M, Masajtis-Zagajewska A, Mazanowska O, Madziarska K, Stompór T, Więcek A. Diagnosis and treatment of metabolic acidosis in patients with chronic kidney disease – position statement of the Working Group of the Polish Society of Nephrology. *Kidney Blood Press Res.* 2018;43(3):959–969. doi: 10.1159/000490475

48. Dhiman D, Mahajan S, Kumar S. Perioperative arrhythmias and metabolic status: an elephant in the room. *Ain-Shams J Anesthesiol.* 2022;14(1). doi: 10.1186/s42077-022-00228-z

49. Velissaris D, Karamouzos V, Pierrakos C, et al. Use of sodium bicarbonate in cardiac arrest: current guidelines and literature review. *J Clin Med Res.* 2016;8(4):277–283. doi: 10.14740/jocmr2456w

50. Capone J, Gluncic V, Lukic A, Candido KD. Physiologically difficult airway in the patient with severe hypotension and metabolic acidosis. *Case Rep Anesthesiol.* 2020;2020:1-4. doi: 10.1155/2020/8821827

51. Burger M, Schaller DJ. Metabolic acidosis. In: StatPearls [Internet]. Treasure Island, FL: StatPearls Publishing; 2019 [update July 2023]. Available at: https://www.ncbi.nlm.nih.gov/books/NBK482146/.

52. Bianchi S, Aucella F, De Nicola L, Genovesi S, Paoletti E, Regolisti G. Management of hyperkalemia in patients with kidney disease: a position paper endorsed by the Italian Society of Nephrology. *J Nephrol.* 2019;32(4):499–516. doi: 10.1007/s40620-019-00617-y

53. Hunter RW, Bailey MA. Hyperkalemia: pathophysiology, risk factors and consequences. *Nephrol Dial Transplant.* 2019;34(Suppl 3): iii2–iii11. doi: 10.1093/ndt/gfz206

54. Bianchi S, Aucella F, De Nicola L, Genovesi S, Paoletti E, Regolisti G. Management of hyperkalemia in patients with kidney disease: a position paper endorsed by the Italian Society of Nephrology. *J Nephrol.* 2019;32(4):499–516. doi: 10.1007/s40620-019-00617-y

55. Morales E, Cravedi P, Manrique J. Management of chronic hyperkalemia in patients with chronic kidney disease: an old problem with news options. *Front Med.* 2021;8. doi: 10.3389/fmed.2021.653634

56. Loubser J, Pinto Bronislawski L, Fonarov I, Casadesus D. Sine-wave electrocardiogram rhythm in a patient on haemodialysis presenting with severe weakness and hyperkalaemia. *BMJ Case Rep.* 2023;16(3):e255007. doi: 10.1136/bcr-2023-255007

57. Yamanoglu A, Celebi Yamanoglu N. The effect of calcium gluconate in the treatment of hyperkalemia. *Turk J Emerg Med.* 2022;22(2):75. doi: 10.4103/2452-2473.34281213

58. Hollander-Rodriguez JC, Calvert JF. Hyperkalemia. *Am Fam Phys.* 2006;73(2):283–290.

59. Novak JE, Ellison DH. Diuretics in states of volume overload: Core Curriculum 2022. *Am J Kidney Dis.* 2022;80(2):264–276. doi: 10.1053/j.ajkd.2021.09.029

60. Farha N, Munguti C. A dramatic presentation of pulmonary edema due to renal failure. *Kansas J Med.* 2020;13:56–57.

61. Sarkar M, Niranjan N, Banyal P. Mechanisms of hypoxemia. *Lung India.* 2017;34(1):47. doi: 10.4103/0970-2113.197116

62. Çoruh B, Luks AM. Positive end-expiratory pressure. when more may not be better. *Ann ATS.* 2014;11(8):1327–1331. doi: 10.1513/annalsats.201404-151cc

4

Psychiatric Disorders

SARAH BROCK

COMPETENCIES

1. Recognize the most common psychiatric illnesses in transport medicine, and identify each specific patient's needs.
2. Effectively communicate and anticipate the needs of patients in transport considering their unique presentations.
3. Understand and mitigate the risks associated with transporting a patient with psychiatric illness.
4. Effectively manage both overdose and suicide attempt.

Almost 5 million people visit the emergency department each year with a primary complaint stemming directly from a mental health diagnosis.[1] In 2020, 1 in 5 adults sought mental health treatment during the previous 12 months.[2] And in 2021, overdose-related deaths were 15% higher than just the year prior.[3] For every 100,000 people in the United States, 14 will end their life this year, not to mention the many more who will attempt. Over 2 million Americans receive social security benefits with the primary reason being mood or psychiatric disorder.[4]

These numbers are quite staggering. The mental health stigma may have improved, but a harsh reality remains. We are unequipped to care for both the volume and variety of mental health disorders in society today. As a transport provider, you will encounter other professionals, partners, and patients living with a mental health disorder, and undoubtedly many others who are undiagnosed. Perhaps you also function under the weight of a mental health diagnosis.

In this chapter, we will briefly discuss the most common mental health illnesses present in the United States and identify ways to improve the care we provide them. Focus will then turn to life-threatening situations, highlighting transport considerations, and recognizing potential medical mimics. Finally, we will conclude with Trauma Informed Care, and learn how to prevent unintentionally rooting a deeper mental health crisis within our patient(s) as we care for them.

Depression

The World Health Organization (WHO) estimates that up to 5% of the world population is clinically depressed. Depression is also the leading cause of disability worldwide. In the United States, heightened awareness and a nationwide push to destigmatize mental health have empowered individuals to speak up and reach out for assistance. Despite this, 75% of low to middle income individuals will receive no treatment. And of these people who are not treated, the greatest number are elderly.[5]

Depression knows no demographic. Between 2016 and 2019, 4.4% of children aged 3–17 were diagnosed with depression in the United States. In 2020, the NIH broke down the statistics and found that depression is highest among White women aged 18–25. However, depression is also quite high in other ethnicities and ages, as well as in men.

Depression is a very serious mood disorder marked by persistent sadness that encroaches on daily activities. It affects not only how a person thinks, but also how they feel, respond to their environment, and engage in normal activity. To be clinically diagnosed with depression, symptoms must be present for a minimum of 2 weeks and represent a change from previous functioning. The symptoms present must include a loss of interest in almost all activities, plus psychomotor changes, fatigue, or suicidal ideation. The full list of symptoms can be found in the *Diagnostic and Statistical Manual of Mental Disorders*, Fifth Edition (DSM-5).[6]

Depression is further delineated into five primary categories. These categories include Major Depression, Dysthymia, Perinatal Depression, Seasonal Affective Disorder, and Depression with Psychosis.[7] It is also a symptom within Bipolar Disorder, Disruptive Mood Dysregulation Disorder in children, and Premenstrual Dysphoric Disorder. Depression's span across so many disorders has led to a large number of people living with chronically depressive symptoms.

Medications and/or psychotherapy offer a patient some control over their depression. The most common class of medications used are selective serotonin reuptake inhibitors (SSRI), which increase the serotonin available in the brain. Some of the more common medications in this class include citalopram, sertraline and fluoxetine. Other antidepressants including tricyclics, tetracyclics, and monoamine oxidase inhibitors (MAOI) are also widely used today.[8] These other classes of medications are not typically first line in treatment, but also work by altering the levels of neurotransmitters in the brain, including, but not exclusively, serotonin. The side effect profile is similar in all classes with the most common including headache, drowsiness, dizziness, and sleep problems.

Providers should be alert to signs pointing to a patient experiencing depression, which include obvious lack of self-care, apathy, flat affect, pessimism, and helplessness. This is not an all-inclusive list, but these are the more easily recognizable given the limited time providers are able to spend with each patient. Depression looks slightly different across the lifespan. It is especially important to recognize depressive symptoms in elderly patients. They are the most at-risk subgroup of the population, as well as the most underdiagnosed. Geriatric patients spend the majority of their short appointments discussing chronic physical health conditions. The more subtle mental health disorders are often overlooked. The older generation are also more stoic and less forthcoming about depressive symptoms. Providers may also believe that a dismal outlook is a natural occurrence as patients near the end of life, and not recognize it as treatable.

Studies have demonstrated patients with depression report decreased satisfaction with their health care when compared to nondepressed patients, which leads to worse outcomes.[9] Further studies are needed to pinpoint the reason for the disparity, but a few philosophies attempt to explain this phenomenon. One is that depressed patients hold a negative world view and often do not advocate for themselves. Doctors may also find depressed patients more challenging to work with due to their persistent negativity. Effective communication is paramount in health care, but it is especially important when caring for depressed individuals.

Some of the easiest ways to support a depressed patient are by being compassionate and showing empathy. Acknowledge and accept their feelings without trying to rationalize a positive outlook. Attempt to meet each patient in their own mood and refrain from attempting to change their outlook. Attempting to change their attitude can further the feelings of "not being good enough." A flat affect can make it difficult to ascertain the complexity of their current situation; allow the patient ample time to speak and be comfortable with periods of silence.[10]

As a provider treating patients with depression, we must have a heightened level of suspicion for suicidal ideation and overdose attempt in any patient who is not managing their depression well. We will revisit this in depth later in the chapter.

We often see other medical conditions arise in patients who are depressed; lack of self-care starts a downward spiral to noncompliance. Many patients with depression are apathetic and have a dismal outlook. It may be difficult to rise from bed each morning. This can perpetuate not taking medications, attending medical appointments, or complying with suggestions from providers. The recommendations to exercise, eat well, and attend therapy are neglected when their mood is dark and motivation minimal. This in turn fuels exacerbations of chronic health problems. For example, a patient with end-stage congestive heart failure may struggle with worsening fatigue and shortness of breath through disease progression. He lays in bed until noon and skips morning medications. He then sees the edema in his legs, which makes it even more difficult to ambulate well. He is bed-ridden and ends up with delivery food for dinner. The meal is laden with sodium and leaves him without proper nutrition. He returns to bed upset as his condition deteriorates and wakes up again the following day to face the same spiraling challenges.

Depression may not be the reason why we are called for transport, but we must take it into our considerations. Patients with depression are less likely to be forthcoming and attempt to hide their non-compliance. It will be up to you to recognize the compounding factors that are contributing to their current presentation and intervene as appropriate.

Anxiety

Anxiety is the most common mental health disorder affecting American adults, impacting 40 million people throughout the country. Anxiety is an umbrella term used in psychology; it covers a broad host of individual mental health disorders. The two common denominators linking all anxiety disorders are a sense of fear and apprehension. DSM-5 classifies each of the anxiety disorders by how often they occur and how debilitating each occurrence becomes.[6]

Anxiety can be wrongly diagnosed when a clinician does not exclude mimic medical conditions. The most common medical diagnoses wrongly attributed to essential anxiety include hyperthyroidism, chronic obstructive pulmonary disorder, arrhythmia, and transient ischemic attack.[11] Substance use and abuse can also cause transient anxiety, but again must also be considered separately from a true anxiety disorder. Common medications that cause anxious feelings are albuterol, caffeine, decongestants, and various illegal substances. True anxiety is rooted in neurotransmitter imbalances in the brain, not as a symptom of substance use. The two need to be considered separately.

Many medications useful in treating depression are also found to be helpful in treatment for anxiety.[12] Depression and anxiety are both caused by imbalance of serotonin and norepinephrine levels in the brain. These medications aim to help restore that balance. SSRIs are again commonly prescribed, as well as serotonin-norepinephrine reuptake inhibitors (SNRI). Both work in similar fashion, with the core difference being reduction of the reabsorption of norepinephrine with SNRIs versus pure serotonin effect. Tricyclic antidepressants (TCA) are also prescribed, but less commonly due to a larger side effect profile. Monoamine oxidase inhibitors (MAOI) are most effectively utilized in treating panic disorder and social phobia, but are also used second line for general anxiety. Side effects common to all these medications include dizziness, headache, sleep problems, and drowsiness.

Benzodiazepines are one class of drug that are used to treat anxiety but not depression alone. This class of medication encourages relaxation in small dosages and is useful for sedation in larger quantity. Some of the common transport medications included in this class are midazolam, diazepam, and lorazepam. When a patient tells you they use a "rescue medication," these are most commonly prescribed. Onset of action is quick and they alleviate both physical and emotional symptoms of anxiety. Benzodiazepines cause a release of gamma-aminobutyric acid (GABA) in the brain, which makes your nervous system less active. This helps promote calm by reducing heart rate and lowering blood pressure.

Beta-blockers can also be prescribed to prevent the body from being able to increase blood pressure and heart rate associated with an anxious state. These drugs work by reducing the effect of norepinephrine which blunts the fight or flight response. The most prescribed for this purpose are atenolol and propranolol.

Immediate signs that your patient may be experiencing anxiety are worry, restlessness, tremor, irritability, muscle tension, and difficulty concentrating. You may also notice diaphoresis, hyperventilation, self-reported feelings of being smothered or choked, palpitations, paresthesia, and dizziness. Though these symptoms can be attributable to generalized anxiety, they are also part of a normal physiological response to a stressful situation. Either way, these responses can be detrimental to promoting a healing environment, and a clinician should do everything in their power to limit actions that invoke anxiety.

On physical exam, you may find diaphoresis, tremors, elevated heart rate and blood pressure. It is especially important to rule out underlying medical causes for each of these presentations.

There are many medical mimics. Medication side effects, intense pain, stroke, heart attack, and hypoxia can all have the appearance of anxiety. Performing an electrocardiogram with full vital signs is a quick and noninvasive way to rule out life-threatening situations.

Again, overdose needs to be considered in association with poorly managed anxiety. Patients are often not overdosing in attempts to end their lives, but in response to dependence. This is true especially for benzodiazepines. For example, a patient may be instructed to take one alprazolam as needed for acute anxiety. Life has been particularly stressful, and they find themselves now using it numerous times daily. One pill no longer calms their emotions, and they begin using two pills. This begins a spiral of increasing tolerance leading to the potential overdose. Patients will also commonly turn to illegal methods of obtaining medication when their prescribed dose no longer has the same effect. This adds the risk of not trusting the strength or purity of the substance.

Communicating in a soft and slow tone of voice can help lessen immediate panic. Validate the patient's feelings and show sincere empathy. If possible, calm yourself, work at a slower pace, keep the lights lowered, and shut off unnecessary alarms to minimize noise. If you can keep the situation under control and be a grounding presence, this will also help the patient stay calm.

Narrating care as you complete it is beneficial with all patients, but especially when trying to dispel anxiety. Patients who do not have diagnosed anxiety can still experience it in our care given their situation. A medical crisis or trauma that precedes transport is already stressful but transport itself often fuels unease. Narration not only helps to dampen the patient's anxiety but can keep you calm as well in a stressful situation. There is often a sense of fear in patients unfamiliar with medical presence and describing each intervention before you proceed can provide clarity and counter unease.

When possible, provide patients with choices in their care. Even simple choices will help the patient maintain a sense of control. Powerlessness is an emotion that can trigger anxiety. Asking which arm they would like a blood pressure reading taken, or where the best spot would be for an intravenous line (IV) will help foster trust. Even by offering a closed decision, such as, "Would you like the IV in your right arm or left arm," can help regain a semblance of control.

In transport, we as providers need to be very aware of the surroundings for our own safety. Patients may unintentionally become unsafe. If anxiety becomes severe, patients may attempt to exit the vehicle. Your intervention to prevent this can inadvertently lead to aggression and have unintended consequences. Patients may attempt to rip off medical equipment and can potentially cause themselves great harm in the process. It is imperative to the safety of the crew and patient to have the foresight to intervene on any anxiety in transport. This will greatly reduce the chance of escalation to a dangerous level. Attending to the emotion prior to transport is much more easily accomplished than attempting intervention during transport and after continued escalation.

Eating Disorders

Eating disorders comprise a very complex list of illnesses within the DSM-5.[6] These unhealthy eating habits are more than a maladjusted relationship with food; they can have serious health consequences, even resulting in death.[13] Common illnesses in this category include anorexia, bulimia, binge eating, and rumination disorders. As a group, eating disorders affect approximately 5% of the United States population.[14]

Eating disorders commonly coexist with another psychiatric disorder. Bulimia and anorexia nervosa commonly occur in connection to obsessive compulsive disorder (OCD) or mood disorders. Pica (eating nonedible items) is often seen in patients diagnosed with autism or intellectual disability. Patients with eating disorders, who also have body image distortion, are not likely to admit their issues. As a provider, you may not be able to outwardly notice physical traits of a disorder. These patients are typically ambivalent or outright resistant towards treatment.

It is important to note that not all eating disorders are created equal. Though many have the same underlying emotional components, they are quite varied in presentation. As a provider meeting a patient for the very first time, it would be difficult to recognize an eating disorder unless it is severe. Patients can range between underweight to obese depending on the disorder. Some have no affliction with food quantity itself. Pica, for example, is the compulsion to eat items that have no nutrient value such as paint, chalk, soap, clay, etc. and often does not affect weight. Patients with bulimia nervosa are sometimes overweight due to the inability to completely purge the stomach of its contents.

The most successful treatment option for many eating disorders is cognitive behavioral therapy. Sessions can occur outpatient, but in serious cases inpatient hospitalization is required. Inpatient options are most regularly utilized in the treatment for anorexia, especially when the patient denies the disorder. Evidence suggests patients with bulimia benefit greatest from antidepressant medication. Medication, combined with cognitive therapy, has shown to decrease the urge to binge and vomit better than either alone.

Many medical concerns exist for these patients, but the most common is electrolyte imbalance. A potassium and/or sodium imbalance is common in any restrictive-type disorder. Chloride loss is common in bulimia. These electrolyte imbalances occur gradually over a long period of time, and patients typically tolerate the imbalance better than a patient with acute loss. However, serious consequences can still arise, including cerebral edema, shock, and cardiac arrhythmia. Other concerns include nausea, vomiting, hypothermia, confusion, irritability, and lethargy. Specifically in pica, the most urgent task is identifying what was ingested. Toxic items or those that cannot safely pass through the gastrointestinal tract require intervention. Treatment may include an antidote, activated charcoal, or surgical removal.

Patients with these disorders pose no greater threat to the transport provider than a standard medical transport. However, continued vigilance while anticipating and mitigating any potential concern is what will ultimately keep you as a provider safe.

Substance Abuse Disorders

Substance abuse and dependence were historically two separate mental health diagnoses. The DSM-5 has now condensed these into one category, headed substance use disorder (SUD), which umbrellas both the use and dependence. A separate diagnosis covers substance-induced disorders. This explains the onset of a mental health disorder secondary to the use of substances (i.e., substance-induced psychotic disorder).[6,15]

Diagnosis fits under four major categories consisting of 11 criteria. These criteria also determine how severe the disorder has become; the more that are met, the more severe the disorder.

Severe disorders are marked by greater than six criteria, including creating danger to self or others, tolerance, withdrawal, use in the context of mental or physical symptoms, and effects on daily activities. These criteria are fully listed in the DSM.[6]

There are currently 10 separate classes of drugs recognized in the DSM-5. They include inhalants, PCP, stimulants, hallucinogenics, sedatives, cocaine, amphetamine-type, cannabis, alcohol, and opioids.[6] To be diagnosed with a SUD, activation of the dopamine reward system is so intense that a person neglects other normal activities.[16] There are other substances outside this list that can become addictive and activate the dopaminergic pathway. These other addictions, such as gambling, are their own disorder.

Treatment for substance abuse can include a combination of medical therapies and behavioral counseling. Medications can include a controlled method to obtain the "high" with a weaning treatment. For example, a psychiatrist may prescribe methadone for opiate addiction. Methadone itself is an opiate, but by offering a prescription, the patient no longer needs to obtain the drug illegally. This therapy helps correct the negative behaviors associated with obtaining the drug. By reinforcing positive lifestyle change, the commitment to break the addiction is more often adhered to without relapse.

There are many indicators of a potential substance use disorder. As we had to rule out substance use prior to diagnosing anxiety, we also must rule out medical condition mimics here. Signs of substance abuse may be quite obvious or very subtle. Symptoms may include pupil dilation or retraction, bloodshot eyes, irritability, palpitations, a general unkempt appearance, runny nose, unusual odor on body or breath, anxiety, and agitation. However, to truly diagnose substance use, these signs must be noted over time, and encompass a lifestyle surrounding addiction.[15] Many of these symptoms are vague and subjective, and often are present in medical illness as well.

There is a long list of medical concerns that must be on your radar when transporting someone with known substance abuse. Toxicity, withdrawal, seizures, loss of airway control, and cardiac arrest or arrhythmia are the most common and severe. Build rapport with the patient. They are more likely to be forthcoming about what substance they are using if they trust that you are acting in their best interest and remain non-judgmental. Knowing what substance the patient is abusing will really help hone into what symptoms need to be watched most closely. Reminding the patient of HIPAA laws and your complete detachment from legal repercussions can also ease misgivings and establish trust.

Crew and patient safety are also paramount in this transport. Anyone under the influence of a substance is highly unpredictable. The transport team should have a low threshold for sedation and/or intubation. If the crew decides against more aggressive interventions, a plan to mitigate an escalating situation should be discussed and agreed upon prior to transport. A very quick intervention should be immediately available. This may be medication drawn up and prepared with an intramuscular needle for use, should the patient display signs of violence or agitation that is not redirectable. Again, this is for the safety of both the patient and crew due to the confined space of transport.

It is important to know your company's policy on the use and documentation of restraints. Restraints are employed for patient safety, but never as a punishment or out of convenience. Both physical and chemical restraints exist and each situation will differ to which is most appropriate. Restraints should be the least invasive form that is appropriate for the situation. In transport, intubating someone for crew or patient safety is the most invasive restraint we can utilize, but is often the one that is the most appropriate. Wrist restraints are an obvious form of restraint, but a video camera encroaches on privacy and is also a restraint. Providing midazolam to an escalating patient is also a restraint. Even strapping a backboard to an aware patient can be a restraint if they are of sound mind and tell you no.

Post-traumatic Stress Disorder

PTSD (post-traumatic stress disorder) is diagnosable in children and adults alike, though in children, symptoms often manifest quite differently. PTSD can result from an actual experience of a traumatic event, witnessing the event, learning of an event that affected a close family member or friend, or having repeated or extreme exposure to a traumatic event.[17] To be diagnosed with PTSD there are numerous criteria that must be met, and each of these criteria must persist for greater than one month.[6]

PTSD is not always immediately recognizable after an event and may have delayed expression. Full diagnostic assessment is postponed for more than 6 months in some cases. Though many individuals will have clear-cut symptoms of PTSD, many others will fail to meet all criteria. Even if not fully diagnosable, these patients' lives are negatively impacted by their experiences.

Up to 30% of patients with PTSD will develop dissociative coping mechanisms. Dissociation is classified into two categories, depersonalization and derealization.[18] In depersonalization, the patient will detach from the event and explain it as if they had been an outside observer. When describing their own emotions and physical experiences, they will do so as if the event were only a dream. Derealization expands this "dream-like" description of the event into the patient's entire life. They will say that the world they currently live in feels distant or distorted, or that they are viewing life through an out-of-body experience.

As with many psychiatric disorders, a combination therapy and medication regimen is used for treatment. Many patients describe PTSD as living with a pervasive depressed mood, punctuated by anxiety triggers. Therefore, management typically includes antidepressants (most commonly SSRIs), and fast acting "rescue" medications to treat panic. Some studies have also shown prazosin (Minipress) to be beneficial in the reduction or complete suppression of nightmares common in PTSD. Minipress works primarily by blocking alpha-1 receptors for norepinephrine in the brain. This lessens the body's ability to respond to increased arousal.

In transport, you may recognize these patients present in much the same manner as a depressed person. They regularly describe feelings of hopelessness and have a generally negative world view. Their demeanor may be dull and flat. Other signs that are more separated from singular depression are being easily startled, demonstrating hypervigilance, engaging in self-destructive behavior, or being irritable. Suicidal ideation and suicide attempts are also common in PTSD.

It may be difficult to recognize a patient experiencing symptoms of PTSD in the transport environment. If a patient is forthcoming about their diagnosis, ask them what triggers their experiences and what will help them feel the most comfortable. Prevent triggers as much as possible to minimize traumatic flashbacks or panic attack. For example, loud noises are often a trigger and cannot be completely avoided. You may minimize noise by turning off alarms and warning the patient if you know a loud noise is going to occur. Engaging the siren is a good example of a process that could be warned of beforehand.

Watch for any indication during transport of the patient experiencing a flashback or panic attack; intervene when possible. Benzodiazepines are useful both as preventative and even if a panic attack begins. However, if the patient has a history of addiction they may not wish to receive these medications. Managing panic or flashbacks can also be accomplished through distraction, redirection, or breathing techniques. As the provider, make every effort to encourage the use of these coping mechanisms first, using medical management only as necessary.

Attention Deficit Disorder

Attention deficit/hyperactivity disorder (ADHD), previously known as attention deficit disorder (ADD), is a common diagnosis for children, but also affects the adult population. Those affected adults comprise 4% of total diagnoses.[19] In the DSM-5, ADD is in fact a subtype of ADHD, which is further delineated into three separate subtypes, which we will detail now.

The most diagnosed form of ADHD is primarily inattentive type (formerly ADD). In adults, this manifests as forgetfulness, poor focus, and lack of organization. Whereas in children, this is most often seen as apathetic or "spacey" behavior. The same criteria must be met in both adults and children for diagnosis with primarily inattentive type ADHD.[20]

Hyperactive-impulsive type ADHD encompasses more of the "stereotypical" traits people have come to recognize. Children with this subtype are seen as bouncing off the walls, fidgeting, and interrupting. The reality is that only a small number of children and adults truly meet the criteria for this subtype. One caution to note is diagnosis in girls; hyperactivity is diagnosed in boys more often but misdiagnosed in girls as a mood disorder.

The third presentation of ADHD is a combined type. To carry this diagnosis, patients must demonstrate six symptoms from both hyperactive and inattentive subtypes. Patients will have difficulty with both impulsivity and hyperactivity, as well as distractibility and inattention. This is the most diagnosed subtype, with more than half of all diagnoses being in this group.

Medications include two modalities, stimulants and nonstimulants. It would seem counterintuitive to provide a stimulant for a patient with hyperactive symptoms, but in fact, patients report a 70%–80% reduction in symptoms with the use of methylphenidate or amphetamines.[19] Stimulants work by increasing dopamine in the brain, which is associated with increased attention and motivation. In a patient with ADHD, this creates a calming effect, as they are more readily able to focus. Nonstimulants include Strattera (atomoxetine), Intuniv (guanfacine), Kapvay (clonidine), and Qelbree (viloxazine, which are currently the only nonstimulant medications approved for the treatment of ADHD.[21] Nonstimulants are categorized into two classes: norepinephrine modulators and alpha agonists. Both increase levels of norepinephrine in the brain, just through different modalities.

Transporting an adult with ADHD will be uncommon, as typically adults are more able to control their impulsive behaviors. Our focus here will be on the management of children. All children in transport will have some level of apprehension. In children with ADHD, increased fidgeting, picking at equipment, and constant movement are common. This can make it difficult to complete the simplest of tasks, such as obtaining vital signs. A calm demeanor and reassuring speech pattern, along with distraction, can assist in regaining a child's focus and limiting their hyperactivity. If you transport as part of a team, having one person dedicated to distraction and engagement will make the transport more successful.

Safety measures are aimed at keeping the child from pulling at medical equipment or moving in a way that could cause further injury. If the child becomes frustrated there may be aggression, but these are typically dispelled through distraction and redirection.

Autism Spectrum Disorder

Autism spectrum disorder (ASD) is present in all racial, ethnic, and socioeconomic groups, but affects boys at four times the rate of girls. The Centers for Disease Control and Prevention (CDC) current estimate is that 1 in 36 children has an ASD.[22] ASD is considered both a neurological disorder and a developmental disorder, with symptoms appearing within the first two years of life. ASD is a "spectrum disorder" because of the wide variety and severity of symptoms it encompasses. Though it is not known what causes ASD, it is likely a combination of genetics and environment. Several known factors that increase the likelihood of being diagnosed include having a sibling with ASD, being born to older parents, having other genetic conditions, and having very low birth weight.[23]

Behaviors associated with ASD largely encompass communication and social interactions. Some behaviors are restrictive or repetitive in nature, such as becoming overly focused on a specific interest or repeating a phrase. For example, a child may become fixated on spinning objects and therefore spend a lot of time watching front-load washers at a local laundromat. This fixation will often expand as the child ages to include other "spinning" objects, such as watching helicopters land, or studying the spinning tires of passing traffic on roadways. These fixations are often pervasive enough to meet the criteria for an OCD sub-diagnosis as well.

Transporting an individual with ASD can become quite challenging, as they often do not tolerate changes to their routine. Increased stimulation above baseline can also pose a threat to the person's sense of calm and control. Allowing a parent or caregiver to accompany the patient on transport can be extremely beneficial, both in calming the patient, but also educating the providers on how to best approach him or her. Simple measures that limit stimulation are turning off sirens, minimizing vital sign measurements, minimizing excessive light, and keeping the environment as quiet as possible. Those with ASD also can have a heightened tactile awareness. If possible, try using a wrapped gauze instead of a band-aid on wounds, and refrain from touching them if not necessary. Ask the caregiver about comfort items that can be brought on the transport. It is also very important to be aware of unusual pain responses; singing or humming instead of a typical cry may be present. Narrating your care may be beneficial, or describing cares before you complete them. The patient may be unwilling to talk or may be nonverbal and unable to speak, but they can likely understand what you are saying and may be able to communicate in other ways, such as using a tablet or some other assistive device. Again, parents or other caregivers will be the best source for information about these patients.

Down Syndrome

Down syndrome is the most common chromosomal condition, affecting 1 of every 772 babies born in the United States. Down syndrome occurs when a developing fetus has an extra copy of chromosome 21. Though there is much information known about Down syndrome, there is no known cause for the actual chromosomal abnormality. The only factor that is known to increase the incidence of Down syndrome is higher maternal age.

As healthcare providers, we can expect to see a greater number of individuals with Down syndrome through the coming years. Diagnosis is expected to increase as people continue to wait longer to begin having families. The incidence of a child being born with Down syndrome to a 25-year-old woman is 1 in 1200, but by age 40, the incidence is 1 in 100. Advances in clinical treatments are also helping patients live longer. In 1910, the survival age in Down syndrome was 9; today 80% are expected to live past 60.[24]

Most people with Down syndrome have mild to moderate cognitive delay. Severe delay is also possible, but not common. Certain physical features are typically identifiable when the patient's history is unknown. Some of these include low muscle tone, a flat facial profile (especially across the bridge of the nose), almond shaped eyes with an upward slant, a tongue that tends to protrude from the mouth, and a shorter stature.

As in ASD, if it is possible to bring a caregiver or parent on the transport, this may limit anxiety and prevent outbursts. Be acutely aware that these patients have a very high pain tolerance. Don't take a report of "no pain" as a reason to not treat an obviously painful condition. For example, a patient with a broken arm may not answer if you ask about their pain and may not grimace or cry. This verbal report is not a reason to withhold pain medication. A broken arm is an obviously painful condition and treating it as such remains important despite the lack of typical signs.

Medically, there is an increased prevalence of certain repeatable conditions in people with Down syndrome. Hearing loss, sleep apnea, and eye diseases to name a few, but most notable and concerning are heart defects. The three most prevalent defects are atrioventricular septal defect, patent ductus arteriosus, and tetralogy of Fallot.[25] These are surgically repaired as an infant but can lead to other cardiovascular complications later in life, including myopathies and heart failure. Though the transport may have no tie to cardiology, having the awareness of such deficits can alert you to potential confounding influences on the current situation.

Schizophrenia

Schizophrenia is most often diagnosed between 16 and 30 years of age. An abnormal period of acute psychosis almost always predicates diagnosis. Symptoms of schizophrenia are divided into four categories: positive, negative, cognitive, and mood. Positive symptoms are those present which are not typical of the general population, such as delusions or hallucinations. Negative symptoms are those that are absent from typical behavior, such as a loss of ambition or decrease in range of emotion. Cognitive deficits negatively impact attention and communication, and also include memory deficits. Lastly, mood symptoms are emotions displayed that do not fit a given situation.

There are three subtypes of schizophrenia: psychotic, negative, and cognitive. In psychotic presentation, reality is distorted and there is a lost sense of being. Symptoms include hallucinations, delusions, difficulty organizing speech (known as "flight of ideas"), and abnormal repetitive body movements.[26] In the negative subtype, withdrawal, along with a complete and profound loss of interest in anything, are hallmark. The most severe cases can actually lead the person to completely stop moving or talking for periods of time, a condition known as catatonia. Finally, in the cognitive presentation, there is a decreased attention span, lack of concentration, and poor memory.

Historically, people have incorrectly confused schizophrenia and multiple personality disorder. Though the symptoms may appear similar outwardly, especially for the cognitive subtype, these are two very different illnesses. Dissociative identity disorder (DID) is the psychiatric diagnosis given to a person presenting with multiple personalities. DID is very rare, affecting only 0.01%–0.1% of the population. In contrast, schizophrenia is quite common; it is estimated that 1 in every 300 people carry a diagnosis of schizophrenia worldwide, and in the United States, the numbers are closer to 1 in every 100.[27]

People living with schizophrenia are at a 10% higher risk of dying prematurely than the rest of the population. Depressive symptoms and psychosis are thought to contribute to numerous factors leading to this risk. Schizophrenics are also more likely to have comorbid medical illness such as type II diabetes, heart disease, and obesity. Medical diagnoses are often fueled by a lack of self-care or a complete lack of understanding of how to care for themselves. Sadly, they also die by suicide at a much higher rate than the general population. This grave number is nearly 13%. Studies have also proven that they have twice the number of vehicular accidents per mile driven than the rest of population.[28] Again, these statistics point to the disorganized thinking process hallmark to schizophrenia.

Patients with schizophrenia can be quite unpredictable. During transport it is likely unnecessary to exercise extreme measures of restraint, such as intubation, but providers should remain vigilant to changing mood and behaviors. Subtle cues often precede unsafe behaviors. Any small increases in repetitive motions or anxious language can cue a provider into an impending disruption. The exact opposite is also true, especially in negative subtype; these patients may get progressively quieter and begin to become noncompliant or withdrawn in small ways prior to an outburst.

Hopefully you are now able to recognize a few common mental illnesses and are more confident in your communication with these patients. Now we will discuss medical emergencies related to mental health. These transports can be emotional and extremely challenging, making them potentially traumatic for both the patient and provider.

Delirium

Delirium is defined as a disturbance of consciousness with reduced ability to focus, sustain, or shift attention. "Excited delirium" was once the verbiage that dominated description of this behavior set, but terminology has since been unsupported.[29] The fall-out from this is two-fold. Delirium diagnosis was based largely on case studies with no medically defined parameters, and due to agitation, large quantities of sedation were used in this patient population. The larger doses of medications to control behavior sadly also increased fatalities in the field.

Most recently, the American College of Emergency Physicians has recognized the existence of hyperactive delirium syndrome (HDS).[29] HDS is diagnosed by the exhibition of aggression, agitation, and distress, accompanied by hyperthermia and high blood pressure. This state can be drug abuse facilitated. The drugs of abuse most associated with HDS are those capable of severely altering the dopaminergic pathway, the most studied of which is cocaine. Acute intoxication and the presence of other mental illness is also common.[30]

HSD has high mortality and many patients die prior to any contact with medical personnel. Numerous factors increase mortality, but the most significant are direct physical trauma and effects from high metabolic demand. Acute hyperthermia poses the greatest immediate threat to the patient. Profound hyperthermia creates high metabolism, which alters the blood–brain barrier, and contributes to protein malfunction and degradation.

In transportation, airway intervention and temperature management are paramount. Securing the patient's airway is important in anticipation of the large doses of medication that will be required for sedation secondary to the hypermetabolic state. Even if the decision is made to not intubate a patient with HSD, end-tidal carbon dioxide (ETCO$_2$) monitoring is a gold standard for all patients receiving sedatives or opioid medications.

Cardiovascular collapse is common. Patients exert themselves beyond normal physiological limits causing lactic acidosis. This lactic acid production, when combined with hyperthermia, creates rapid onset of rhabdomyolysis. Continued accumulation is normally mitigated through the respiratory drive. However, as the patient tires, or is intubated, this compensation stops, which can cause arrest within seconds. Aggressive hydration for the patient, ice packs to the groin and armpits, and administering sodium bicarbonate early have shown to decrease the incidence of cardiac collapse. A continued hypermetabolic state and hyperthermia create a growing acidotic shift, which contributes to the cardiac etymology. The body's response to catecholamines is blunted and reduces the effect of epinephrine during the peri-arrest state, therefore withholding epinephrine is prudent.

The safest way to transport these patients is intubated. However, it is important to recognize the fragile state they exist in and resuscitate them prior to the intubation to prevent cardiac arrest. However, due to the large volume of benzodiazepines used, and their aggressive, uncontrollable behavior, both the patient's safety and yours is at great risk if their airway is not managed.

Overdose

Overdose is a growing epidemic in the United States. In 2021, data indicate that more than 105,000 lives were lost due to overdose. The United States continues to lead the world in overdose death rates by an overwhelming number: each year, 320 lives per million are lost to overdose. The next closest country is Scotland, with 267 deaths from overdose per million.[31] Though there are numerous substances that may lead to overdose death, the overwhelming majority occur with opioids.

Opioids are highly addictive and come in many forms; natural and synthetic, prescription or illegally obtained. Fentanyl and its derivatives are thought to be a contributing factor in the increase of overdose-related deaths. Fentanyl is a synthetic opioid that is up to fifty times stronger than heroin to obtain a more potent high. Other drugs may be laced with fentanyl, unbeknownst to the user. Heroin itself is also more widely available in recent years. This larger supply leads to lower costs, and decreased cost often means use by a greater number of people. The increased supply availability also spurs greater variance to the product, which is another considerable factor in the increase in overdose deaths. Many deaths are accidental.

Patient care must go beyond the administration of naloxone for these persons, as first responder services, police, and even patients themselves, now carry naloxone. On arrival, our care immediately needs to fall back to the ABCs (airway, breathing, circulation, and so on). With all opioid overdoses, airway management and proper ventilation remain paramount. Once an airway is secured and the patient is being ventilated appropriately, other cares can commence. Remember that even if the patient received naloxone and is currently breathing spontaneously, many opioid medications

have a longer half-life than naloxone itself. This disparity can lead to re-sedation, and if an airway has not been secured, it can again become compromised. Re-dosing is falling out of favor as research shows that large doses of naloxone can increase its adverse effects, causing acute withdrawal syndrome. This perpetuates vomiting, agitation, and pulmonary edema, which itself can lead to death.[32]

A broad range of differential diagnoses must also be considered. Other medications can mimic opioid use. Alcohol, sedatives, hypnotics, and clonidine all can have similar effects, even within a therapeutic dose range. Respiratory depression can stem from numerous medical conditions and should not be assumed to be related to a toxicity or overdose unless other factors suggest it. Opioids are frequently taken in conjunction with a sympathomimetic, such as cocaine, which counteract one another. In this case, once naloxone is used, the patient may become combative, tachycardic, hypertensive, and diaphoretic. If the overdose is truly unknown, intubation may be the safest management strategy.

Many drugs have deleterious cardiac effects as well. An electrocardiogram (EKG) is a priority for ruling out arrhythmias associated with various overdoses. Abuse of loperamide, a common over-the-counter medication, is known to affect cardiac conduction causing QT segment prolongation and ventricular tachycardia. Methadone is known to cause torsades de pointes if abused.[32] In recent years, diphenhydramine (Benadryl) has been in the news as part of social media "challenges." Overdose from diphenhydramine can cause profound tachycardia and has resulted in some deaths in the teenage pediatric population.

Patients with a long-standing history of drug abuse can have patterns of old injury present in the EKG. Changes in an EKG may signal a deteriorating condition before a patient becomes symptomatic of their overdose.

Any unresponsive patient must be fully evaluated for trauma or medical etiology prior to making overdose assumptions. A provider can become conditioned to select patients who they encounter frequently. It is easy to become complacent and not finish a full medical exam, but this is how many life-threatening emergencies are missed. They may include hypoglycemia, stroke, electrolyte imbalances, trauma, hypothermia, and sepsis. There is value in following the ABCs and head-to-toe assessment in every situation, on every call.

Providers must remain aware of the factors that may threaten their safety. Any overdose situation indicates a high level of risk to providers. If the overdose was unintentional and the patient received naloxone, they may now be upset, combative, or in a lot of pain. Many patients addicted to narcotics first began the pathway to addiction by using prescribed narcotics for pain control, and perceived pain still exists. For the intentional overdose, providers should be aware of the continued desire to hurt oneself. The interrupted attempt may be repeated, or the patient may turn violent in anger over the situation. Be always prepared to intervene for safety of both the patient and the crew. Verbalize a plan with your crew and be prepared to execute it quickly if the situations warrants.

Suicide Attempt

Suicide is endemic. Currently, it is the 12th leading cause of death in the United States. In 2020, there were almost 46,000 deaths; this equates to 130 per day. Sadly, it is also estimated that 1.2 million attempts were made during this same time frame.[33]

It is a widely incorrect belief that patients who repeatedly attempt suicide are trying to bring attention to themselves and are not truly suicidal. It is difficult as a transport professional to remain empathetic towards these patients. However, data show that 10% of these patients will ultimately go on to succeed in committing suicide.[34] For this reason, every attempt needs to be considered potentially lethal.

EMS providers also have become a front-line gatekeeper for education and resources for these patients. They often are non-compliant with therapy and extended treatments, leaving their only healthcare contact as EMS. Knowing local resources, community outreach, and other government services may mean the difference between life and death for this population.

Many patients do attempt to seek help in managing their suicidal ideations. Unfortunately, a growing lack of providers has led to long wait times for establishing care. Lack of federal funding has also created bed shortages in psychiatric facilities. This same funding shortage has also limited community resources that were at one time available. Understandably, these challenges lead to discouragement, and many patients give up completely on accessing resources.

Transport professionals are also expected to be familiar with laws pertaining to psychiatric illness. Many statutes exist to protect these patients from themselves as they do not have insight into their illness. If any suicidal attempt is made, the patient no longer has the option to refuse care. Having law enforcement involved early is prudent practice; patients are often unaware they can be held against their will for evaluation per federal laws. This can cause behavioral escalation and put both patient and providers at risk.

Furthermore, as medical professionals, we are mandated reporters.

Trauma-Informed Care

Trauma affects everyone differently. Some people will develop PTSD, while others seem to have a resilient response to stress. Ultimately, most adults have experienced some degree of trauma in their lives. Trauma-informed care (TIC) seeks to create an environment that promotes healing and recovery without re-traumatization. TIC goes beyond the patient, seeking to protect other individuals, staff persons, and organizations involved in the care of patients as well.[35]

Re-traumatization can occur in many ways. Any situation that may resemble the initial traumatic assault, even if only symbolically, carries the risk for re-traumatization. This occurrence is typically unintentional. It can be as "obvious" as restraints, but also as discreet as a smell or noise. It may be impossible to know what will trigger a re-traumatization experience. Being educated on its possibility is prudent, and simple awareness and help prevent its occurrence.

TIC adheres to five principles, which have become the framework for how providers can reduce the likelihood of re-traumatization. These five principles are: safety, choice, collaboration, trustworthiness, and empowerment.[35] Safety is the foundation of TIC; both physically and emotionally. This is accomplished through a welcoming environment that is free of judgment, and where privacy is respected. Individuals should also maintain control, with a clear message about their rights when making choices. These choices will lead to decisions that empower the individual and build an environment for collaboration. Trustworthiness comes from task clarity, consistency, and boundary setting. This shows respect to all parties involved and should be maintained throughout the relationship. Finally, empowerment provides validation and an affirmative atmosphere.

Effective communication has been mentioned numerous times throughout this chapter. TIC's success is also rooted in good communication. Using the principles above as a guide, a safe and supportive environment is established between patient and caregiver. Situational safety is the undercurrent that helps prevent re-traumatization.

In summary, encountering psychiatric illness is unavoidable. As transport professionals, we are likely to encounter mental health concerns in our patients, team members, and community. It is imperative that we stay educated and empathetic to these situations and practice effective communication skills across all situations and with every transport.

References

1. Centers for Disease Control and Prevention. FastStats – Mental Health. CDC; September 6, 2022. Available at: https://www.cdc.gov/nchs/fastats/mental-health.htm.
2. Terlizzi EP, Norris T. *United States, 2020.* NCHS Data Brief, no. 419. Hyattsville, MD: National Center for Health Statistics; 2021.
3. Centers for Disease Control and Prevention. U.S. overdose deaths in 2021 increased half as much as in 2020 – but are still up 15%. CDC; May 11, 2022. Available at: https://www.cdc.gov/nchs/pressroom/nchs_press_releases/2022/202205.htm.
4. National Alliance on Mental Illness. *Supplement Security Income (SSI) and Social Security Disability Insurance (SSDI).* Available at: http://tinyurl.com/yr6mjkeh.
5. World Health Organization. Depression. World Health Organization Fact Sheet; September 13, 2021. Available at: https://www.who.int/news-room/fact-sheets/detail/depression.
6. American Psychiatric Association. *Diagnostic and Statistical Manual of Mental Disorders, Fifth Edition.* Arlington, VA: American Psychiatric Association; 2013. [Revised edition *DSM-5TR*, 2023.]
7. U.S. Department of Health and Human Services. *Depression.* National Institute of Mental Health; n.d. Available at: https://www.nimh.nih.gov/health/topics/depression.

8. U.S. National Library of Medicine. Commonly prescribed antidepressants and how they work, *NIH MedlinePlus Magazine.* MedlinePlus; n.d. Available at: https://magazine.medlineplus.gov/article/commonly-prescribed-antidepressants-and-how-they-work.
9. Haerizadeh M, Moise N, Chang BP, Edmondson D, Kronish IM. Depression and doctor–patient communication in the emergency department. *Gen Hosp Psychiatry.* 2016;42:49–53. doi: 10.1016/j.genhosppsych.2016.06.004
10. Bettencourt E. Dealing with depressed patients. Blog; n.d. Available at: https://blog.diversitynursing.com/blog/dealing-with-depressed-patients.
11. Locke AB, Kirst N, Shultz CG. Diagnosis and management of generalized anxiety disorder and panic disorder in adults. *Am Fam Phys.* 2015;91(9):617–624. Available at: https://www.aafp.org/pubs/afp/issues/2015/0501/p617.html.
12. Medical News Today. Everything you need to know about anxiety medications. Medical News Today; n.d. Available at: https://www.medicalnewstoday.com/articles/323666#side-effects.
13. Sells N. The 5 most common mental disorders. Blog. Davis Behavioral Health; January 30, 2020. Available at: https://www.dbhutah.org/the-5-most-common-mental-disorders/.
14. Guarda A. What are eating disorders? Psychiatry.org. American Psychiatric Association; March, 2021. Available at: https://psychiatry.org/patients-families/eating-disorders/what-are-eating-disorders.

15. Gateway Foundation. DSM-5 and addiction – understanding changes over time. Gateway Foundation; August 26, 2021. Available at: https://www.gatewayfoundation.org/addiction-blog/dsm-5-substance-use-disorder/.

16. Hartney E. DSM 5 criteria for substance use disorders. Verywell Mind; August 25, 2022 [updated April 7, 2023]. Available at: https://www.verywellmind.com/dsm-5-criteria-for-substance-use-disorders-21926.

17. Center for Substance Abuse Treatment (US). DSM-5 Diagnostic Criteria for PTSD. In: *Trauma-Informed Care in Behavioral Health Services.* TIP Series, No. 57: Chapter 3, Exhibit 1-3-4. Rockville, MD: Substance Abuse and Mental Health Services Administration (US); 2014. Available at: https://www.ncbi.nlm.nih.gov/books/NBK207191.

18. Center for Substance Abuse Treatment (US). Understanding the impact of trauma. In: *Trauma-Informed Care in Behavioral Health Services.* TIP Series, No. 57: Chapter 3. Rockville, MD: Substance Abuse and Mental Health Services Administration (US); 2014. Available at: https://www.ncbi.nlm.nih.gov/books/NBK207191.

19. Centers for Disease Control and Prevention. Treatment of ADHD. CDC. Available at: https://www.cdc.gov/ncbddd/adhd/treatment.html.

20. Russo A, ADDitude Editors. ADD vs. ADHD symptoms: 3 types of attention deficit disorder. *ADDitude*; July 11, 2022. Available at: http://tinyurl.com/522m6c9x.

21. U.S. Food and Drug Administration. Treating and dealing with ADHD. U.S. Food and Drug Administration Consumer Updates; August 8, 2023. Available at: https://www.fda.gov/consumers/consumer-updates/treating-and-dealing-adhd.

22. U.S. Department of Health and Human Services. Autism spectrum disorder. National Institute of Mental Health; n.d. Available at: https://www.nimh.nih.gov/health/topics/autism-spectrum-disorders-asd.

23. Centers for Disease Control and Prevention. Data & statistics on autism spectrum disorder. CDC; March 2, 2022. Available at: https://www.cdc.gov/ncbddd/autism/data.html.

24. National Down Syndrome Society (NDSS). About Down syndrome. n.d. Available at: https://ndss.org/about.

25. Global Down Syndrome Foundation. Congenital heart defects and Down sndrome: What parents should know. March 24, 2020. Available at: http://tinyurl.com/mud7cj8t.

26. U.S. Department of Health and Human Services. Schizophrenia. National Institute of Mental Health; n.d. Available at: https://www.nimh.nih.gov/health/topics/schizophrenia.

27. World Health Organization. Schizophrenia. World Health Organization Fact Sheet; n.d. Available at: https://www.who.int/newsroom/fact-sheets/detail/schizophrenia.

28. Treatment Advocacy Center. Schizophrenia Fact Sheet. Treatment Advocacy Center; n.d. Available at: http://tinyurl.com/ukvn7bdj.

29. Moran M. Board adopts position against diagnosis of 'excited delirium,' police use of ketamine. *Psychiatric News*; February 4, 2021. Available at: https://psychnews.psychiatryonline.org/doi/10.1176/appi.pn.2021.2.21.

30. Bornstein K, Montrief T, Parris MA. Excited delirium: Acute management in the ED setting. *Emerg Mgmt Resident*. April 8, 2019. Available at: https://www.emra.org/emresident/article/excited-delirium/.

31. Baumgartner JC, Gumas ED, Gunja MZ. Too many lives lost: comparing overdose mortality rates and policy solutions across high-income countries. Commonwealth Fund; May 19, 2022. Available at: http://tinyurl.com/37srkkuy.

32. Taxel S, Hagahmed M. Beyond naloxone: Providing comprehensive prehospital care to overdose patients in the midst of a public health crisis. *JEMS;EMS, Emergency Medical Services – Training, Paramedic, EMT News.* JEMS; January 1, 2018. Available at: https://www.jems.com/patient-care/beyond-naloxone-providing-comprehensive-prehospital-care-to-overdose-patients-in-the-midst-of-a-public-health-crisis/.

33. Centers for Disease Control and Prevention. Suicide data and statistics. CDC; June 28, 2022. Available at: https://www.cdc.gov/suicide/suicide-data-statistics.html.

34. Evans K, Geduld H, Stassen W. Attitudes of prehospital providers on transport decision-making in the management of patients with a suicide attempt refusing care: a survey based on the Mental Health Care Act of 2002. *S Afr J Psychiatr.* 2018;24:1156. doi: 10.4102/sajpsychiatry.v24i0.1156

35. Institute on Trauma and Trauma-Informed Care. *What is Trauma-Informed Care?* Buffalo Center for Social Research; March 31, 2022. Available at: https://socialwork.buffalo.edu/social-research/institutes-centers/institute-on-trauma-and-trauma-informed-care/what-is-trauma-informed-care.html.

5

Immunologic Disorders

CHRISTIAN GREENGRASS

COMPETENCIES

1. Define and demonstrate basic concepts and applications of epidemiologic data pertaining to immunologic conditions encountered in transport.
2. Perform a detailed pre-transport examination and evaluation of a patient with a suspected immunologic condition.
3. Identify the related signs, symptoms, and assessment findings associated with immunologic conditions encountered in the transport environment.
4. Identify and provide critical care interventions for immunologic conditions and related complications during transport.

Introduction

Immunology, or the study of the immune system and its related disease processes, is a complex physiologic topic that is necessary knowledge for the transport professional. The immune system is a complex system of cells, proteins, and mediators that make up innate and acquired immunity (Fig. 5.1)[1] to assist the body in "fighting off" infection. The immune system continuously adapts throughout our lives to provide protection against pathogens and illnesses. Immunologic conditions are unique because many of the various disease processes may affect almost any organ or tissue. Most importantly, immunologic disease may complicate any primary condition necessitating transport. For instance, a late-stage HIV patient requiring transport with the primary condition of bacterial pneumonia could easily advance to septic shock. Several of these complex immunologic conditions may be encountered by transport crews while in the transport environment.

HIV and AIDS

Acquired immunodeficiency syndrome (AIDS) is a chronic and life-threatening disease process caused by infection with the human immunodeficiency virus (HIV). According to the World Health Organization, an estimated 38.4 million people are living with the HIV virus at the end of 2021. In 2021, 650,000 people died from HIV complications with 1.5 million new patients contracting the virus.[2] The transport provider must be competent in understanding how this virus and related immunodeficiency syndrome affect the body and how to navigate the related complications that may be encountered in the transport environment.

Pathophysiology of HIV and AIDS

The etiology and mechanisms of HIV are well documented and studied. HIV is a bloodborne retrovirus from the *Retroviridae* family that is most frequently transmitted by sexual intercourse,

human breastmilk, and through shared intravenous drug paraphernalia. HIV infection is comprised of three distinct phases: acute HIV, chronic HIV, then AIDS. HIV is composed of two subtypes, known as HIV-1 and HIV-2. The most common type of HIV is HIV-1, which may be found all over the globe.[2] HIV-2 is almost exclusively found in the region of West Africa.[3] Upon transmission of HIV into a new host, the virus will bind to CD4 molecules on the surface of helper-T cells and begin to replicate utilizing the helper-T cells as a host. This process of replication causes the virus to spread throughout the body. In response, numerous white blood cells that function in a healthy immune system are destroyed, creating a state of immunodeficiency. Fig. 5.2[4] describes this process in more detail by visually displaying the cyclic pathogenicity of the HIV virus. Immunodeficiency exposes the body to opportunistic infections and complications. HIV is diagnosed by multiple serologic assays to determine the patient's viral load and confirming the CD4[+] T cell count.[2,3,5–8] The severity or stage of the HIV infection is determined by physical exam findings and the CD4[+] T cell count found in serologic lab collections.[7,8]

Assessment of the HIV/AIDS Patient

The assessment of a patient infected with HIV/AIDS in transport may prove to be a challenge due to multiple existing factors. Physical assessment findings will vary depending on the progression of the disease at the time of contact. In the acute stage, the patient may experience flu-like symptoms such as headache, fever and rashes that may persist for several weeks.[3,5–7] Chronic HIV infection, the second stage, is characterized by the lack of symptoms that were experienced in the acute phase. If untreated, the virus may remain dormant for 10 years or longer prior to progression into the final stage of infection which is AIDS. In later stages of the disease process, patients will begin to experience opportunistic infections such as oral yeast infections (thrush), viral infection such as shingles, or bacterial infections that lead to pneumonia and/or sepsis.[7,8]

Innate vs. adaptive immunity: A summary

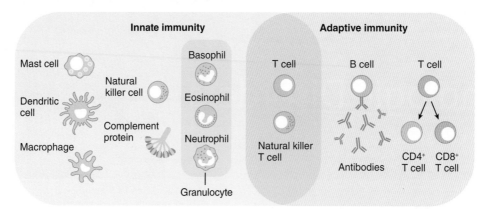

ATTRIBUTE	INNATE IMMUNITY	ADAPTIVE IMMUNITY
Response time	Fast: minutes or hours.	Slow: days.
Specificity	Specific only for molecular patterns that are generally associated with pathogens or foreign particles.	Highly specific. Can discriminate the molecular signatures of different pathogens and distinguish then from those of the body's own cells.
Major cell types	Macrophages, neutrophils, natural killer cells, dendritic cells, basophils, eosinophils.	T cells, B cells and other cells that help flag pathogens for destruction.
Key components	Antimicrobial peptides and proteins.	Antibodies: Molecules that latch onto pathogens and flag them for destruction.
Diversity and customization	Limited: Receptors only recognize patterns consistent with pathogens. No new receptors are made to adapt the immune response.	Highly diverse: Can be customized by genetic recombination to recognize a broad array of molecular targets.

• **Fig. 5.1** The different cells, characteristics and subtypes that comprise both the innate and adaptive immune system. (Modified from Landhuis E. Could the immune system be key to Alzheimer's disease? *Knowable Magazine*. Published 02.02.2021

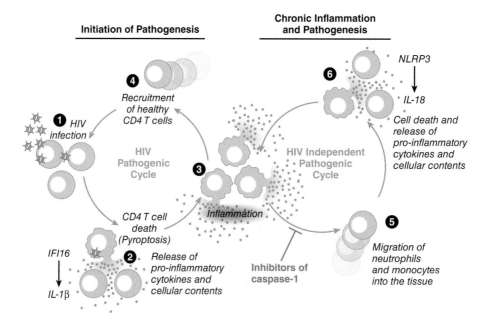

• **Fig. 5.2** The cycle of pathogenicity with infection of the HIV virus. (Modified from Doitsh G, Greene WC. Dissecting how CD4 T cells are lost during HIV infection. *Cell Host Microbe*. 2016;19(3):287. Figure 5.)

Treatment and Transport Considerations

Patients with HIV/AIDS requiring transport should have treatment pathways based upon the patient's specific presenting condition and etiologies. The transport provider should focus on the treatment of serious complications primarily related to opportunistic infections, multiorgan failure, respiratory failure, and cardiovascular collapse.[9] At this time, no cure exists for HIV infections, however, antiretroviral drugs (or ART) provide the most effective treatment for the patient infected with HIV.

Multisystem Inflammatory Syndrome (MIS) and SARS-CoV-2

In 2019, the world was introduced to the SARS-CoV-2 or COVID-19 virus that originated in Wuhan, China. The SARS-CoV-2 virus spread at an exponential rate around the world which led to the death and chronic disability of millions of people. In the transport environment, COVID-19 was proven to be difficult to manage due to overt pulmonary and hemodynamic dysfunction. The dysfunction was hypothesized to be related to systemic inflammatory response related to the infection. Over time cases grew in number which led to the identification of Multisystem Inflammatory Syndrome in children (MIS-C) and Multisystem Inflammatory Syndrome in adults (MIS-A). According to the Centers for Disease Control, as of 2022, the number of children diagnosed with MIS-C is roughly 9139, versus 221 of adult cases.[10,11]

Pathophysiology of Multisystem Inflammatory Syndrome (MIS)

The pathophysiology of MIS[12] with SARS-CoV-2 infections is not fully understood and is still under investigation. However, the syndrome is hypothesized to be secondary to an exaggerated (dysregulated) immune response, or cytokine release syndrome triggered by COVID-19 infection. Specifically, MIS affects organs of the gastrointestinal tract as well as the heart, eyes, lungs, kidneys, and the brain.[13] The release of inflammatory mediators such as cytokines leads to widespread inflammatory response. Cytokine release syndrome is described as an acute systemic inflammatory syndrome triggered by infection. Cytokines are small membrane-bound proteins released by cells to assist in cellular communication or signaling. The cellular communication leads to a broad range of physiologic effects based on the specific cytokine. In MIS related to SARS-CoV-2 infection, the related cytokine triggers the release with predominant effects originating from interleukin-6 (IL-6) and tumor necrosis factor-alpha (TNF-α). IL-6 and TNF-α are both pro-inflammatory cytokines secreted by T cells and dendritic cells. When these cytokines are released, they produce systemic clinical features ranging from mild generalized discomfort to neurologic dysfunction, or myocardial injury with manifestations similar to Kawasaki disease.[12,14]

Assessment of the MIS Patient

In the transport environment, assessment of MIS-C and MIS-A may prove to be difficult related to the collection of symptoms that may be presented. It is difficult to discern between severe COVID-19 cases and MIS-C/MIS-A due to the similar inflammatory response seen in both conditions. While most patients being transported for MIS have already been identified based on specific diagnostic criteria that will be confirmed by the sending facility, there are several markers differentiating COVID-19 from MIS that can be observed via diagnostic imaging. These differences are primarily noted in pulmonary findings: pulmonary edema, acute respiratory distress syndrome (ARDS) (possibly asymmetric), and bi-basal consolidation are more commonly associated with MIS; uni-/bilateral ground-glass opacities of the lower lobe and early-phase Halo sign are more commonly associated with COVID-19.[15–17] For MIS-C the following criteria have been identified by the Centers for Disease Prevention and Control (CDC) for the confirmation of diagnosis for MIS cases:

- Age: Less than 21 years old
- Temperature: 38.0°C or greater sustained for 24 hours or longer
- Labs: Presence of inflammation (such as elevated CRP, D-dimer, procalcitonin, LDH, etc.)
- Other: No alternative diagnosis plausible
- History: Positive for recent SARS-CoV-2 infection or exposure to confirmed COVID-19 case within 4 weeks prior to onset of MIS-C symptoms.[18]

When conducting a history of present illness assessment, a key difference is the noted duration of time between the initial SARS-CoV-2 infection and onset of MIS clinical manifestations. In most cases MIS may not begin until weeks after the initial diagnosis of a severe COVID-19 infection. Apart from the timeframe of onset, many of the manifestations remain the same between severe COVID-19 infection and that of MIS-C and MIS-A. In December of 2021, a meta-analysis was conducted among a total cohort of 2275 cases.[14] The results identified the stratification of clinical findings for MIS which included: Fever (100%), gastrointestinal (82%), abdominal pain (68%), cardiac symptoms (66%), respiratory symptoms (39%), and 28% of cases presented with neurologic manifestations.[19] A further breakdown of assessment findings is listed below by system affected:

- General: Skin rash, persistent fever
- Gastrointestinal: Diarrhea, abdominal pain, vomiting, GI bleeding
- Genitourinary/renal: Oliguria
- Neurologic: Headache, irritability, altered mental status, confusion, lethargy
- Cardiac: Hypotension, shock, acute heart failure
- Respiratory: Persistent cough, tachypnea, dyspnea[12]

After acquiring the history of present illness and related clinical data, monitoring the patient in transport for related complications is necessary for ensuring positive transport outcomes. Recommended ongoing assessment of the patient in transport includes the following measures:

- General: Temperature acquisition, note the presence of skin rash or mucosal lesions
- Cardiac: ECG monitoring, assessment of heart tones, 12-lead ECG, hemodynamic monitoring
- Neurologic: Ongoing assessment of mental status and alertness
- Genitourinary/renal: Intake and output (I/O), urinary output
- Respiratory: End-tidal CO_2 monitoring, auscultation of breath sounds
- Laboratory findings: Elevated BNP, elevated troponin, COVID-PCR positive, elevated lactate, ABG abnormalities secondary to shock state for severe cases.[12]

Treatment and Transport Considerations

Treatment in the transport environment for a known or suspected MIS diagnosis depends on the stability of the patient. In the hemodynamically stable patient, treatment is primarily supportive. Pharmacologic agents that may be administered by the transport provider for stable MIS patients include intravenous (IV) crystalloid fluids and antipyretics for fever. The provider must also continually assess for developing septic or cardiogenic shock state.[12,14] Patients with MIS who present with hemodynamic instability may require IV fluids, vasopressors, inotropic support agents and may be on a prophylactic anticoagulant infusion for transport. It is important for the transport provider to be aware of the inpatient care plan which may include IV immunoglobulin therapy (IVIg), corticosteroids and additional advanced cardiovascular and hemodynamic monitoring.[12,14]

Anaphylaxis

Anaphylaxis is a life-threatening allergic reaction, which in the transport environment is classically seen commonplace by both the air and ground transport professional. Anaphylaxis is most commonly triggered by foods, medication, or animal envenomation (bees, wasps etc.). Transport for patients with this condition typically requires immediate, lifesaving interventions or the continuation of ongoing lifesaving therapies such as vasopressors and placement of an advanced airway. Between 1.6% and 5.1% of the US population has experienced an anaphylactic episode, and the mortality is an estimated 1% of severe cases.[20] Mortality is typically related to drug-induced anaphylaxis.[20]

Pathophysiology of Anaphylaxis

The manifestation of anaphylaxis is comprised of cellular mediators and antibodies which contribute to its potentially lethal clinical picture. There are two types of anaphylactic reactions: immunologic and nonimmunologic. In the transport environment, the most common antibody to trigger an immunologic anaphylaxis reaction is IgE, or immunoglobulin E. IgE is most closely related to "classic" anaphylactic reaction presentation. Other mediators of anaphylaxis include immunoglobulin G or IgG, and immune complex/complement-mediated reactions. When a person is exposed to an allergen through contact, ingestion, or inhalation, the allergen will diffuse into tissues within close proximity of mast cells and basophils. Upon exposure to the allergen, the IgE antibodies will initiate cellular signaling to the mast cells and basophils which, in turn, lead to degranulation or "release" of its cellular contents. This degranulation or "release" refers to the release of mediators, enzymes, and cytokines such as histamine, tumor necrosis factor, or tryptase.[21] These mediators, enzymes, and cytokines will facilitate a chain reaction of events which directly cause the clinical manifestations seen in classic anaphylaxis. Fig. 5.3 shows this physiologic process starting from allergen exposure to the production of clinical manifestations.[21] Histamine is the predominant inflammatory mediator of immunologic IgE anaphylaxis. Histamine is unique in its physiology due to mast cells and basophils containing it within the cytoplasmic granules released with IgE-mediated anaphylactic reactions.[21] The effects seen with release of histamine into the tissues is created by the binding of histamine to the H_1 and H_2 receptors located in the vasculature, lungs, smooth muscle of the GI tract, central nervous system, and adrenal glands.

Assessment of the Anaphylactic Patient

A patient experiencing anaphylaxis in the transport environment presents on a spectrum based on the level of immunologic response

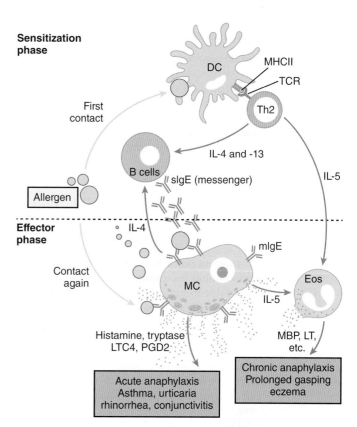

• **Fig 5.3** The cellular process of histamine degranulation during IgE mediated anaphylaxis response. (Modified from He S, Zhang H, Zeng X, et al. Mast cells and basophils are essential for allergies: mechanisms of allergic inflammation and a proposed procedure for diagnosis. *Acta Pharmacologica Sinica*. 2013;34:1271. Figure 1.)

to the exposed allergen. Anaphylaxis is a rapidly evolving process involving the pulmonary, integumentary, gastrointestinal, and cardiovascular systems.[22] When the transport provider is obtaining a history of present illness, the following assessment items are critical to obtain from the referring ground EMS crew, referring facility or from the patient as applicable prior to transport:

- Documented exposure source: Insect venom, food, and medication are the most common sources
- Interventions and medications provided prior to arrival
- Status of airway, presence of stridor
- Hemodynamic status with or without the presence of anaphylactic shock
- Integumentary assessment: Urticaria locations, angioedema severity and location

Physical assessment findings of anaphylaxis vary depending on the severity of the reaction, time of assessment after exposure, and type of allergen exposure. Clinical manifestations of anaphylaxis have been studied closely with a variable prevalence. Skin and mucosa symptoms comprise of 80%–90% of cases followed by bronchopulmonary (60%–70%), cardiac (40%–50%), gastrointestinal (40%–50%), and neurologic manifestations (<15%).[22] In the transport environment the following assessments and monitoring interventions should be considered:

- Airway/Respiratory: End-tidal CO_2, pulse oximetry, assessment of breath sounds, work of breathing, bronchospasm/bronchoconstriction and speech for evidence of stridor. Evidence of stridor is considered to be an ominous finding potentially requiring immediate lifesaving intervention.

- Cardiovascular: Increased capillary permeability, vasodilation with decreased SVR, coronary vessel dilation and/or constriction, positive atrial chronotropy, decreased diastolic blood pressure, hemodynamic monitoring with ABP/NIBP, and continuous ECG monitoring.
- Neurologic: Assessment of mental status
- Gastrointestinal/Genitourinary: Assess for complaints of nausea or gastrointestinal discomfort or pain.
- Integumentary: Location and spread of urticaria and angioedema. If localized edema or urticaria, consider using various methods of demarcation to monitor for spread.[22–24]

Treatment and Transport Considerations

In the transport environment, one should be prepared to perform the placement of an endotracheal tube in the case of respiratory failure secondary to angioedema or bronchospasm.[23] Surgical or needle cricothyrotomy should be considered in cases where the transport provider is unable to intubate or oxygenate the patient experiencing anaphylaxis.[23–25] First-line pharmacologic agents and related interventions, routes, and recommendations for the treatment of anaphylaxis in the transport environment include the following:

- Removal of the allergen with decontamination as needed. If HAZMAT in nature, appropriate PPE should be worn, and decontamination should be performed by qualified professionals prior to contacting the patient.
- Oxygen therapy: High-flow oxygen
- Epinephrine: Intramuscular is the first-line recommended route of administration. Subcutaneous route for the injection of epinephrine is no longer recommended for emergent cases of anaphylaxis.
- Intravenous access with administration of crystalloid fluids: 20–30 mL/kg for circulatory support.[22,25]

Secondary-line interventions and adjunctive therapies for anaphylaxis in the transport setting include the following agents[22,25]:

- Antihistamines: Diphenhydramine, famotidine
- Corticosteroids: Methylprednisolone
- Bronchodilators: Albuterol, terbutaline
- Vasopressors: Vasopressin

Additional therapies for anaphylaxis especially in the case of refractory hypotension in the inpatient setting include methylene blue and consultation for extracorporeal membrane oxygenation (ECMO).[24,25]

Angioedema

Angioedema is a localization of tissue swelling that is directly related to the movement of fluids from the intravascular space into the interstitial space (tissues). Typically, angioedema results in edema of the face, hands, feet, and mucosa of the lips and tongue.[26] In the transport environment, angioedema is a potentially life-threatening condition depending on the anatomic region affected. It must be treated promptly by the transport professional to prevent lethal complications.

Pathophysiology of Angioedema

Angioedema can be broken down into two subtypes: Mast cell mediated (histaminergic angioedema) and bradykinin mediated angioedema. The primary mechanisms for both subtypes are inflammation and extravasation of intravascular fluid into the surrounding interstitial tissue. The most observed angioedema in the transport environment is histaminergic angioedema which is caused by exposure to an allergen, such as certain foods or insect bites/stings. Upon exposure to the suspected allergen, the IgE mediated response triggers the degranulation of mast cells which release histamine. The histamine released then creates angioedema swelling of the tissues via increased capillary permeability and vasodilatation. This allows the extravasation of intravascular volume into the tissues. This can occur within a few minutes of exposure to the allergen. Bradykinin mediated angioedema presents with a different clinical picture. The most common bradykinin-related angioedema is angiotensin-converting enzyme (ACE) inhibitor induced angioedema, which takes usually over 24–36 hours with resolution of the symptoms occurring in 2–4 days.[26] However, in some cases, the time between the trigger and onset of symptoms may range from days to weeks or even years. Both bradykinin and histaminergic angioedema are caused by released granules contained within mast cells and basophils.

Assessment of Angioedema

In the transport environment, assessment of the patient experiencing angioedema should have a primary focus on determining airway patency with pre-planning for advanced airway management as necessary. When obtaining the history of present illness/report from the referring facility or ground EMS, the transport provider should assess the patient for recent use or prescription of ACE inhibitor medications, any known allergens, recent exposures to allergens, and history of any prior reactions. Timing of the onset of angioedema should also be assessed to possibly determine bradykinin versus histaminergic diagnosis. The following is a list of clinical manifestations differentiating between these two distinct types of angioedema. Keep note that many of the symptoms are similar with some key differences. In bradykinin-related angioedema, the angioedema is described as localized, erythematous but without the presence of urticaria, hypotension or bronchospasm. With histamine mediated angioedema, this is typically accompanied by the classic anaphylactic symptoms such as bronchospasm, urticaria, hypotension along with erythema that may be seen in bradykinin reactions. However, in both cases, the angioedema may develop in the larynx, which to the transport provider is a clinical emergency requiring prompt intervention to prevent asphyxiation. Other important assessments that should be performed in the transport environment include:

- Cardiovascular: Continuous ECG, blood pressure monitoring
- Respiratory: End-tidal CO_2, respiratory rate, respiratory effort, breath sounds, pulse oximetry
- Airway: Assess for presence of stridor, hoarseness, or voice changes
- Integumentary: Presence of urticaria and erythema. Skin with angioedema present will be taut and nearly firm to the touch.[27]

Treatment and Transport Considerations

In the transport environment, there are two important factors to consider as a primary priority to determine the appropriate treatment plan. It is initially necessary to determine whether or not the patient's airway is patent or if there is an anticipated clinical course with impending airway compromise. In the case of tongue or larynx angioedema, stridor, voice changes, or hoarseness the transport provider should consider an advanced airway. Minimal attempts should be made to perform laryngoscopy due to the potential worsening of edema with manipulation, especially for bradykinin mediated reactions.[28] In angioedema cases, cricothyrotomy or tracheostomy is needed in up to 50% of cases.[28] When preparing for intubation the transport provider should place the surgical airway kit in an easily accessible location. The second factor is the determination of which type of angioedema the patient is experiencing. Understanding how to differentiate between types of angioedema through a proper assessment is critical to ensure that effective treatments are given. In the case of histamine mediated angioedema (i.e., anaphylaxis), epinephrine, steroids, and antihistamines are critical life-saving parts of the treatment pathway.[27,28] However, in bradykinin mediated angioedema, the administration of epinephrine, steroids, and antihistamines are not proven to be effective.[27] The following is a list of medications commonly utilized for angioedema as organized by type of reaction.[27,28]

- Histamine mediated angioedema
  - Intramuscular (IM) epinephrine is the first-line agent for histamine-related angioedema and IV epinephrine. However, push doses may be used after multiple doses of IM epinephrine.
  - Corticosteroids such as methylprednisolone may be used as adjunctive therapy.
  - Antihistamines such as diphenhydramine for H_1-receptor antagonist effect may be used as an adjunctive therapy in combination with an H_2-receptor blocker such as loratadine, cetirizine, or fexofenadine.
- Bradykinin mediated angioedema[27,28]
  - In the prehospital environment pharmacologic treatment of bradykinin mediated angioedema such as with ACE inhibitor mediated angioedema is typically supportive. Many available targeted treatments for ACE inhibitor bradykinin mediated angioedema are still currently under investigation and require more study prior to field deployment.
  - The use of fresh-frozen plasma is currently under investigation but there is limited literature currently describing the use of FFP in these cases successfully.
  - The use of corticosteroids of these cases may be considered, but only to be used as an adjunctive therapy.

Systemic Lupus Erythematosus (SLE)

Systemic lupus erythematosus, SLE, is a serious chronic autoimmune condition that affects 20 to 150 people per 100,000 Americans annually. This population primarily comprises women between the ages of 15 and 44.[29] In the transport environment, this condition may present with the failure of critical organs secondary to the related inflammatory responses during exacerbations. Identification of SLE is challenging for providers to diagnose and predict prognosis due to the vast variability of clinical findings.

Pathophysiology of SLE

The etiology of SLE still remains mostly unknown. The specific key pathophysiologic features that occur are based on an autoimmune originated inflammatory response. It results in the destruction of tissues noted in multiple anatomic regions which commonly include the joints, skin, brain, vasculature, and kidneys. Most commonly, SLE presents with the age of onset between 16 and 55 and continues with the patient throughout their life with paroxysmal periods of "flare-ups" and periods of inflammatory remission.[29] The pathogenesis of this autoimmune disorder is mostly unknown but is suspected to be based on genetic or hormonal factors. Many of the clinical manifestations of SLE are related to the formation of antibodies which mediate inflammatory responses within the immune system of the patient. The inflammation and organ tissue damage is related to the immune response secondary to maladaptive responses from the B and T cells. The diagnosis of SLE is confirmed by a combination of clinical symptoms reported by the patient, laboratory tests, and tissue biopsy.[30] The antinuclear antibody test, or ANA test, is the primary method to confirm the diagnosis in conjunction to clinical assessment.

Assessment of the SLE Patient

Assessment of the patient with SLE is a challenge due to the constellation of clinical findings that may be observed. In the transport environment, assessment should be focused on the possible development of life-threatening conditions that require prompt treatment. Typically, whenever SLE is first diagnosed, the patient will present with constitutional symptoms such as fever, fatigue, mucocutaneous lesions, arthritis and arthralgia.[30] Severe complications of SLE could involve the renal, cardiovascular, pulmonary, hematological and neurologic system. These complications may be more highlighted in the presence of other etiologies. Renal complications including renal failure secondary to nephritis are among the most encountered (about 50% of cases).[31] In the early stages, assessment for renal complications includes the presence of protein in the urine. Then, lab studies may show an elevated blood urea nitrogen (BUN), elevated creatinine serum levels, and decreased glomerular filtration (GFR) levels. The patient may also experience oliguria and/or anuria. Pulmonary involvement of lupus may manifest as pleuritis, pleural effusion, acute reversible hypoxemia, pulmonary embolism, obstructive lung disease, and pulmonary hypertension.[32,33] In pulmonary manifestations, signs and symptoms of respiratory failure may be evident and ventilatory compliance may be diminished. Hematologic symptoms may include anemia and leukopenia. Neurologic complications manifest as headaches, seizures, aseptic meningitis infection, and related psychiatric conditions.[32] Cardiovascular symptoms include pericarditis, endocarditis, coagulopathy, and related thromboembolic complications such as myocardial infarction, CVA, and DVT.[32] Due to the immunosuppression, the transport provider should also assess for developing sepsis. Exacerbation of SLE can present with a characterized lupus skin rash on the face which covers the nose and maxillary regions. This rash presents in the shape of a butterfly.[34] General monitoring strategy should be focused on the patient-specific systemic complications and the transport provider's index of suspicion.

Treatment and Transport Considerations

The treatment of SLE in the transport environment is primarily based upon the patient-specific clinical presentation of their condition at the time of transport. Treatment of SLE complications may potentially include the following therapies based on etiology:[29,31,32,34]
- Renal manifestations: Cardiopulmonary support, blood pressure control, and transport to facility with dialysis capability in the case of renal failure.
- Neurologic manifestations: Pharmacologic seizure control, airway management, stroke care, and transport to primary or comprehensive stroke facility.
- Cardiac manifestations: Hemodynamic pharmacologic support, STEMI (ST-segment elevation myocardial infarction) care, transport to PCI center (percutaneous cornonary intervention) with related coronary thrombosis or STEMI.

- Pulmonary manifestations: Advanced airway management as needed, mechanical ventilation, corticosteroids, supportive care.

Definitive treatment of SLE is patient-specific and is focused on preventing exacerbations that lead to organ and tissue destruction from the related inflammatory response. Specific agents include corticosteroids such as IV prednisolone, hydroxychloroquine, and various immunosuppressant drugs.[29,31–33]

Sarcoidosis

Pathophysiology of Sarcoidosis

Sarcoidosis is a multisystem immunologic condition that affects an estimated 200,000 cases in the United States annually with 70% between the ages of 20 to 40 years.[35] Sarcoidosis presents with a largely unknown etiology or cause. However, exposure to environmental factors including certain molecular compounds such as beryllium, zirconium, aluminum, and other hazardous materials are strongly suspected to be the primary cause. During the 9/11 attacks at the World Trade Center, thousands of rescue workers were exposed to these deadly compounds during the collapse, rescue, and recovery operations. Afterwards, a cohort study was conducted which revealed an incidence of sarcoidosis to be 25 per 100,000 among those exposed at ground-zero.[36] The pathogenicity of this condition stems from T lymphocytes, granulomas, and phagocytes developing in the tissues of the patient which are known as "sarcoid granulomas." Sarcoid granulomas commonly form in the skin, eyes, lymph nodes and pulmonary tissue. The worst complication comes from the lymph node enlargement within the intrathoracic cavity (hilar adenopathy.) This causes pulmonary lesions and scarring from normally "elastic" pulmonary tissue which grows into pulmonary fibrosis.

Assessment of the Sarcoidosis Patient

Sarcoidosis presents with an arrangement of symptoms based on the organ system/tissues affected. For the transport provider, sarcoidosis may present with challenges in assessment based on the remarkable ability of sarcoidosis to affect any organ within the human body.[37] Patients with sarcoidosis frequently present with fatigue, weight loss, and fever.[38] These generalized symptoms are common and easily mistaken for other conditions similar to sarcoidosis such as hypothyroidism, depression, or severe inflammatory reaction.[38] As a distinguisher, early respiratory assessment may reveal a cough, intermittent dyspnea, chest pain or even chronic dyspnea with delayed diagnosis.[37] Late-stage symptoms include respiratory failure, hypoxemia, and pulmonary noncompliance from pulmonary fibrosis. One can also view chest radiographical imaging and CT revealing the presence of bilateral hilar lymphadenopathy which lead to the diagnosis of pulmonary fibrosis. The complication of pulmonary fibrosis is the primary contributor to 95% of the morbidity and mortality with sarcoidosis.[39] Other complications that may be observed with the sarcoidosis patient include cardiovascular (heart failure, thromboembolic disease, arrythmias, pulmonary hypertension), neurologic (depression, anxiety, neuropathy), and integumentary (sarcoidosis specific skin lesions).[26,37]

Treatment and Transport Considerations

Sarcoidosis requires a multidisciplinary plan due to the myriad of comorbid conditions that may develop secondary to the underlying inflammatory etiology.[37] In the transport environment, first-line agents such as corticosteroids, hydroxychloroquine, rituximab, and adrenocorticotropic hormone will be needed to provide immunosuppression. Otherwise, sarcoidosis is treated almost exclusively by supportive care. The transport provider should develop treatment plans for patients with sarcoidosis based on the severity/stage and system affected by the patient's disease process. One may need to provide administration of medications such as pulmonary dilator medications (beta-2 agonist medications), and corticosteroids. Due to the development of fibrosis, adequate ventilation is critical. Noncompliant pulmonary tissue may increase the incidence of complications when attempting to mechanically ventilate patients with sarcoidosis. Conclusively, the treatment of sarcoidosis in the transport environment is complex and nonstandardized. Development of preventative and curative therapies are still under investigation pending further research currently.

Organ Transplantation (Lung, Kidney, Heart, Lungs)

Organ transplantation is a relatively newer practice in medicine originating in 1954 with the successful transplant of a human kidney. Liver, pancreas, and heart tissue transplantations occurred during the 1960s.[40] In the transport environment, providers are expected to manage patients who require transplant and those who are a recipient of an organ transplant. Once a patient receives a transplanted organ, they require a dedicated regimen of immunosuppressive medications, lifestyle modifications, and other treatments. These treatments place the patient at a high risk for complications surrounding their prophylactically immunocompromised state. Transport professionals are expected to manage these complications appropriately and with competency to ensure positive patient outcomes.

Organ Transplant Physiology

Organ transplantation is a complex multisystem topic which involves multiple organ systems and mechanisms of physiology. In this section we will be discussing the pathophysiology of organ transplant and the related immunologic complications that may be observed in the transport environment. Transplantation is simply the movement of a tissue, cells, or organs from one subject to another, replacing a diseased tissue when other methods of repair are no longer feasible. However, this process is complicated due to the body's natural response to reject the transplantation. The recipient's immune system identifies the transplanted tissue as foreign, which triggers an immune response that will ultimately destroy the transplanted tissue and may result in the mortality of the recipient. Prior to the transplant procedure, the donor and recipient are matched based on hematologic tests and tissue typing. These tests assess the reactivity of recipient's serum when introduced to donor cells. *Graft versus host* is nomenclature commonly used to describe an organ rejection. However, graft versus host and rejection are not synonymous. Graft versus host describes a rare systemic immune response on the graft received which "attacks" the new host or the recipient of that transplant. Graft versus host can occur in any transplant but occurs most commonly in bone marrow transplant cases.

Assessment of the Organ Transplant Patient

Adequate assessment of the patient who has had an organ transplant must begin with a sufficient report. The provider must determine the length of time since the transplant, and the existence of any comorbidities or presence of concurrent illness. The focus should be the risk assessment of acute rejection, graft versus host disease, or any postoperative surgical complications. Organ transplant rejection may manifest acutely as flu-like symptoms, cardiac dysrhythmias, and fever. Other symptoms will be directly related to the organ received.[41] The transport provider should monitor organ-specific physical exam findings and related laboratory evidence. As an example, in a kidney transplant rejection, the patient would likely show oliguria, elevated creatinine, elevated BUN levels and other manifestations of renal failure.[41] The patient with graft versus host may present with painful maculopapular rash on the hands, feet, shoulders, and the nape of the neck.[42] Gastrointestinal symptoms may include diarrhea, abdominal pain, nausea, and vomiting. Hepatic clinical features of graft versus host disease may include elevated bilirubin levels, alkaline phosphatase levels, and ammonia levels.[42] Graft-versus-host rejection contains three distinct phases that may be potentially encountered in the transport environment: the hyperacute phase which presents with immediate onset, the acute phase which has an onset time of weeks to months, and the chronic phase which has an onset time of months to years. Other severe complications that may occur with an organ transplant include coagulopathy, infection/sepsis secondary to immunosuppressive therapies, respiratory failure, and hemorrhagic shock related to postoperative hemorrhage.

Treatment and Transport Considerations

The treatment pathway for patients with recent organ transplantation complications varies on the type of transplanted organ/tissue and the acuity of the complication. Regardless of compatibility, patients who are recipients of organ transplants will require exogenous pharmacologic immunosuppression agents to prevent rejection such as tacrolimus, cyclosporine, and steroids such as prednisone.[43] However, immunosuppressive drugs are noted to be nonspecific as to their spectrum of coverage, thus leaving the patients who require them to be susceptible to infection, sepsis, and unwanted side effects.[43] Acute rejection of an organ is treated with a multiple day course of IV methylprednisolone, supportive care, and consideration of retransplantation.[41]

The transplanted heart is not able to respond to drugs that act by blocking the parasympathetic system, such as atropine, because these connections were severed during the transplant. During the acute rejection period significant, symptomatic bradycardia can be managed with a temporary pacing, or alternatively, agents such as isoproterenol, theophylline, or terbutaline can be used to increase sinus rates while awaiting the return of normal sinus node function.[44,45] Isoproterenol is most commonly used for increasing heart rate in cardiac transplant recipients. Epinephrine may have exaggerated beta mimetic effects on the heart rate because the increase in blood pressure will not lead to a reflex slowing of the heart rate via the baroreceptor reflex (i.e., efferent vagus nerve).[44,45] Implanted mechanical pacemakers work normally in heart transplant recipients since the cardiac leads are placed directly into myocardium.[44,45]

In complications such as hemorrhagic shock, sepsis, or respiratory failure in the transport environment, treatment would include vasopressors, crystalloid fluids, blood products, broad spectrum antibiotics, advanced airway placement and mechanical ventilation as needed. The transporter should also consider the transfer destination. Many patients prefer the transplant center where the affected organ was implanted. The transport provider should reasonably make all efforts to ensure the patient is transported to their facility.

Stevens–Johnson Syndrome (SJS)/Toxic Epidermal Necrolysis (TEN)

Pathophysiology of SJS and TEN

Stevens–Johnson syndrome is classified as a rare and serious immunologic disorder which is distinguished by the severity of the clinical manifestations. Epidemiologic study reveals that Stevens–Johnson syndrome presents with 1 to 2 cases per million people per year with an overall global mortality rate between 10% and 30%.[46,47] Stevens–Johnson syndrome is a severe mucocutaneous reaction that is most commonly triggered by medications. Some of the most common medications that are known to potentially trigger this response include sulfa drugs, antibiotics, allopurinol, and lamotrigine.[48] A severe complication of SJS is toxic epidermal necrolysis or TEN.[49] TEN is characterized by an episode of extensive detachment and necrosis of the epidermal layer (>30% total body surface area [TBSA]) that is found in two or more distinct sites which may include genitalia, oral mucosa, and ocular mucosa. The mechanism for SJS/TEN is not entirely understood. It is argued that the triggering medication stimulates the immune system through major histocompatibility complex and T cell receptors. Upon receptor stimulation, cytotoxic T cells are produced which destroy dermal cells called keratinocytes. They stimulate other inflammatory-related mediators which promote further cellular destruction and detachment of the epidermal layer. This cellular process can cause partial- to full-thickness necrosis of the epidermal layer of the skin. Fig. 5.4 displays a young patient experiencing epidermal necrosis[49] that may be seen in severe cases.

Assessment of the SJS and TEN Patient

SJS and TEN are both rare and potentially severe life-threatening conditions which require careful assessment. In the transport environment, these cases will typically present with a confirmed diagnosis and need to transfer to a higher level of care. Upon receiving the patient, the transport provider should ask for confirmation of

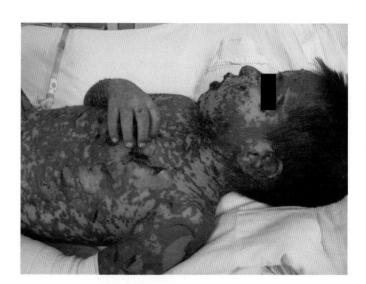

• **Fig. 5.4** A young patient afflicted with SJS exacerbation with TEN to the face, torso, and extremities. (From Romero-Tapia SJ, Cámara-Combaluzier HH, Baeza-Bacab MA, et al. Use of intravenous immunoglobulin for Stevens–Johnson syndrome and toxic epidermal necrolysis in children: Report of two cases secondary to anticonvulsants. *Allergol Immunopathol.* 2015;43(2):228. Figure 1.)

SJS/TEN diagnosis if available and a list of current medications with a lookout for potential triggering medications such as allopurinol, trimethoprim, aminopenicillins and cephalosporins.[48] Notably, patients with an immunocompromised diagnosis such as HIV, are at a 1000-fold higher incidence than the general population.[48] After acquiring a history of present illness, a prompt physical examination should be performed. The physical manifestations are integumentary which range from SJS (least severe) to TEN (most severe). In the early stages, patients present with scattered lesions, i.e., flat or raised pink appearance. The patients may also complain of fever, eye discomfort or stinging, and discomfort upon swallowing.[48] In the later stages, the lesions will worsen with blistering and peeling skin in a rash-like distribution on the body. After a few days the patient will typically begin manifesting the cutaneous symptoms on the trunk and face. This will also progress to involvement of the buccal, genital and/or ocular mucosa.[48] As the disease progresses from SJS to TEN, manifestations become more severe with systemic effects and greater percentage of body surface area detachment. TEN is a notably excruciatingly painful condition for most patients. It is necessary to continue assessing the pain levels to allow for proper treatment of pain. Other assessment items that should be collected in the transport of the SJS patient include the following:[48]

- Cardiovascular: Continuous ECG, blood pressure monitoring, hemodynamic pressures for assessing volume status such as CVP.
- Respiratory: Respiratory rate and depth, and pulse oximetry. End-tidal CO_2 monitoring is critical to deploy, especially with the use of higher dose opioids for analgesia.
- Integumentary: Note the size, spread, condition, color, and location of the SJS/TEN lesions.
- Genitourinary: Urinary output to assess fluid volume status related to fluid loss.

- Laboratory values: Electrolytes related to fluid loss, assessing for evidence of sepsis via inflammatory markers such as procalcitonin, lactate, and evidence of opportunistic infection such as elevated WBC and other related laboratory values.

Treatment and Transport Considerations

The initial treatment of a patient with SJS/TEN is the removal of the culprit drug that may have triggered the reaction. In many cases this should be performed by the sending facility prior to arrival of the transport team. The discontinuation of the culprit medication should be recorded in transport documentation. When treating and transporting a patient with SJS and TEN, regardless of the stage, they should be treated similarly to a burn patient.[46,50,51] The patient should be warmed by maintaining an ambient temperature of (31–32°C).[46,51] Intravenous fluids may be needed to maintain urinary output of 50–80 mL/hour.[48] The fluid of choice for SJS is 0.5% sodium chloride with 20 milliequivalents (mEq) of potassium due to the risk of hypophosphatemia and hypokalemia.[48] Analgesia is a critical intervention for SJS/TEN patients: transport providers are encouraged to provide with opioids as needed for acute pain.[52] The desired transport destination for this patient will be a burn center for comprehensive specialized care. A 15-burn multicenter in the United States conducted a study which concluded that SJS/TEN patients transported to a burn center within 7 days of disease onset showed significantly higher survival rates in comparison to cases admitted 7 days after disease onset (51.4% vs. 29.8%).[48] Currently, several therapies are being studied, however, there is no confirming data yet.[48] In years past, corticosteroids were popular treatments for SJS/TEN, however the data supporting this treatment definitively is not supportive.

Summary

In the transport environment immunologic etiologies that may be encountered by the transport professional are complex and commonly difficult to discern. In most cases, considerations of immunologic conditions are focused on identifying life-threats and the provision of supportive care. In the transport environment, curative interventions are typically not possible to provide. However, treatment of life-threatening complications related to or caused by the underlying immunologic condition may contribute to the positive outcomes of patients. The transport provider must have a comprehensive understanding of the underlying pathophysiology, common assessment findings, definitive treatment pathways and potential life-threatening complications to ensure patient safety.

References

1. Landhuis E. Could the immune system be key to Alzheimer's disease? BrainFacts.org. April 21, 2021. Available at: https://www.brainfacts.org/diseases-and-disorders/topic-center-alzheimers-and-dementia/2021/could-the-immune-system-be-key-to-alzheimers-disease-042121.
2. World Health Organization. Health Topics: HIV. World Health Organization. 2022. Available at: https://www.who.int/health-topics/hiv-aids#tab=tab_1.
3. Kapoor AK, Padival S. HIV-2. In: StatPearls [Internet]. Treasure Island, FL: StatPearls Publishing; 2022, Jan [update Sep 20, 2022]. Available at: https://www.ncbi.nlm.nih.gov/books/NBK572083/.
4. HIV pathogenesis. https://ars.els-cdn.com/content/image/1-s2.0-S1931312816300531-gr5_lrg.jpg.
5. Workowski KA, Bolan GA; Centers for Disease Control and Prevention. Sexually transmitted diseases treatment guidelines, 2015. *MMWR Recomm Rep.* 2015;64(RR-03):1–137 [published correction appears in *MMWR Recomm Rep.* 2015;64(33):924].
6. Cesarman E, Damania B, Krown SE, et al. Kaposi sarcoma. *Nat Rev Dis Primers.* 2019;5(1):9. doi: 10.1038/s41572-019-0060-9

7. Parekh BS, Ou CY, Fonjungo PN, et al. Diagnosis of human immunodeficiency virus infection. *Clin Microbiol Rev.* 2018;32(1): e00064-18. doi: 10.1128/CMR.00064-18
8. Mayo Clinic. HIV/AIDS. Available at: https://www.mayoclinic.org/diseases-conditions/hiv-aids/symptoms-causes/syc-20373524.
9. Wiewel MA, Huson MA, van Vught LA, et al. Impact of HIV infection on the presentation, outcome and host response in patients admitted to the intensive care unit with sepsis; a case control study. *Crit Care.* 2016;20(1):322. doi: 10.1186/s13054-016-1469-0
10. CDC. COVID Data Tracker. Centers for Disease Control and Prevention. Available at: https://covid.cdc.gov/covid-data-tracker/#mis-national-surveillance.
11. Mezochow G, Zlotoff D, Brenner L, Nestor J, Bebell LM. Multisystem inflammatory syndrome in adults (MIS-A) associated with COVID-19: a presentation of mixed shock. *Ann Intern Med Clinical Cases.* 2022;1(7). doi: 10.7326/aimcc.2021.0066
12. The Children's Hospital of Philadelphia. Multisystem inflammatory syndrome (MIS-C) clinical pathway – emergency, ICU and inpatient. Multisystem Inflammatory Syndrome (MIS-C) clinical pathway – emergency, ICU and inpatient. May 20, 2020. Available

at: https://www.chop.edu/clinical-pathway/multisystem-inflammatory-syndrome-mis-cclinical-pathway.

13. Mayo Clinic. Multisystem inflammatory syndromw in children (MIS-C) and COVID-19. Symptoms and causes. Available at: https://www.mayoclinic.org/diseases-conditions/mis-c-in-kids-covid-19/symptoms-causes/syc-20502550?p=1.

14. Children's Minnesota. Clinical Guideline: Suspected Multisystem Inflammatory Syndrome in children (MIS-C), possibly associated with COVID-19. September 2022. Available at: https://www.childrensmn.org/Departments/infectioncontrol/pdf/mis-c-clinical-guideline.pdf.

15. Ahmad F, Ahmed A, Rajendraprasad SS, et al. Multisystem inflammatory syndrome in adults: a rare sequela of SARS-CoV-2 infection. *Int J Infect Dis.* 2021;108:209–211. doi: 10.1016/j.ijid.2021.05.050

16. Yao Q, Waley L, Liou N. Adult presentation of multisystem inflammatory syndrome (MIS) associated with recent COVID-19 infection: lessons learnt in timely diagnosis and management. *BMJ Case Rep.* 2021;14(10):e243114. doi: 10.1136/bcr-2021-243114

17. Winant AJ, Blumfield E, Liszewski MC, et al. *Radiology: Cardiothoreacic Imaging.* 2020: 2(4). doi: 10.1148/ryct.2020200346

18. Feldstein LR, Tenforde MW, Friedman KG, et al. Characteristics and outcomes of US children and adolescents with multisystem inflammatory syndrome in children (MIS-C) compared with severe acute COVID-19. *JAMA.* 2021;325(11):1074–1087. doi: 10.1001/jama.2021.2091

19. Olivotto S, Basso E, Lavatelli R, et al. Acute encephalitis in pediatric multisystem inflammatory syndrome associated with COVID-19. *Eur J Paediatr Neurol.* 2021;34:84-90. doi: 10.1016/j.ejpn.2021.07.010

20. Turner PJ, Jerschow E, Umasunthar T, et al. Fatal anaphylaxis: mortality rate and risk factors. *J Allergy Clin Immunol Pract.* 2017;5(5):1169–1178. doi: 10.1016/j.jaip.2017.06.031

21. Shao-heng H, Hui-yun Z, Xiao-ning Z, Ping-chang Y. Mast cells and basophils are essential for allergies: mechanisms of allergic inflammation and a proposed procedure for diagnosis. *Acta Pharmacol Sinica.* 2013;34:1270–1283. doi: 10.1038/aps.2013.88

22. LoVerde D, Iweala OI, Eginli A, Krishnaswamy G. Anaphylaxis. *Chest.* 2018;153(2):528–543. doi: 10.1016/j.chest.2017.07.033

23. Li X, Ma Q, Yin J, et al. A clinical practice guideline for the emergency management of anaphylaxis (2020). *Front Pharmacol.* 2022;13:845689. doi: 10.3389/fphar.2022.845689

24. Nuñez-Borque E, Fernandez-Bravo S, Yuste-Montalvo A, Esteban V. Pathophysiologic, cellular, and molecular events of the vascular system in anaphylaxis. *Front Immunol.* 2022;13:836222. doi: 10.3389/fimmu.2022.836222

25. Whyte AF, Soar J, Dodd A, et al. Emergency treatment of anaphylaxis: concise clinical guidance. *Clin Med (Lond).* 2022;22(4):332–339. doi: 10.7861/clinmed.2022-0073

26. Tharayil AM, Chanda AH, Shiekh HA, et al. Life threatening angioedema in a patient on ACE inhibitor (ACEI) confined to the upper airway. *Qatar Med J.* 2014;2014(2):92–97. doi: 10.5339/qmj.2014.15

27. Long BJ, Koyfman A, Gottlieb M. Evaluation and management of angioedema in the emergency department. *West J Emerg Med.* 2019;20(4):587–600. doi: 10.5811/westjem.2019.5.42650

28. Pandian V, Zhen G, Stanley S, et al. Management of difficult airway among patients with oropharyngeal angioedema. *Laryngoscope.* 2019;129(6):1360–1367. doi: 10.1002/lary.27622

29. Centers for Disease Control and Prevention. Systemic lupus erythematosus (SLE). CDC. Available at: https://www.cdc.gov/lupus/facts/detailed.html#prevalence. July 5, 2022.

30. Alghareeb R, Hussain A, Maheshwari MV, Khalid N, Patel PD. Cardiovascular complications in systemic lupus erythematosus. *Cureus.* 2022;14(7):e26671. doi: 10.7759/cureus.26671

31. Almaani S, Meara A, Rovin BH. Update on lupus nephritis. *Clin J Am Soc Nephrol.* 2017;12(5):825–835. doi: 10.2215/CJN.05780616

32. Ameer MA, Chaudhry H, Mushtaq J, et al. An overview of systemic lupus erythematosus (SLE) pathogenesis, classification, and management. *Cureus.* 2022;14(10):e30330. doi: 10.7759/cureus.30330

33. Shin JI, Lee KH, Park S, et al. Systemic lupus erythematosus and lung involvement: a comprehensive review. *J Clin Med.* 2022;11(22):6714. doi: 10.3390/jcm11226714

34. Mayo Clinic. Lupus. October 21, 2022. Available at: https://www.mayoclinic.org/diseases-conditions/lupus/symptoms-causes/syc-20365789.

35. American Lung Association. Learn about sarcoidosis. November 17, 2022. Available at: https://www.lung.org/lung-health-diseases/lung-disease-lookup/sarcoidosis/learn-about-sarcoidosis.

36. Hena KM, Yip J, Jaber N, et al. Clinical course of sarcoidosis in World Trade Center-exposed firefighters. *Chest.* 2018;153(1):114–123. doi: 10.1016/j.chest.2017.10.014

37. Sève P, Pacheco Y, Durupt F, et al. Sarcoidosis: a clinical overview from symptoms to diagnosis. *Cells.* 2021;10(4):766. doi: 10.3390/cells10040766

38. Gerke AK. Treatment of sarcoidosis: a multidisciplinary approach. *Front Immunol.* 2020;11:545413. doi: 10.3389/fimmu.2020.545413

39. Gerke AK. Morbidity and mortality in sarcoidosis. *Curr Opin Pulm Med.* 2014;20(5):472-478. doi: 10.1097/MCP.0000000000000080

40. UNOS. History of transplantation. Available at: https://unos.org/transplant/history/.

41. Justiz Vaillant AA, Misra S, Fitzgerald BM. Acute transplantation rejection. In: StatPearls [Internet]. Treasure Island, FL: StatPearls Publishing; 2022 Jan [update Jul 8, 2022]. Available at: https://www.ncbi.nlm.nih.gov/books/NBK535410/.

42. Justiz Vaillant AA, Modi P, Mohammadi O. Graft versus host disease. In: StatPearls [Internet]. Treasure Island, FL: StatPearls Publishing; 2022 Jan [update Oct 10, 2022]. Available at: https://www.ncbi.nlm.nih.gov/books/NBK538235/.

43. Claeys E, Vermeire K. Immunosuppressive drugs in organ transplantation to prevent allograft rejection: mode of action and side effects. *J Immunol Sci.* 2019;3(4):14–21. doi: 10.29245/2578-3009/2019/4.1178

44. Costanzo MR, Dipchand A, Starling R, et al. International Society of Heart and Lung Transplantation Guidelines. The International Society of Heart and Lung Transplantation guidelines for the care of heart transplant recipients. *J Heart Lung Transplant.* 2010;29:914–956. doi: 10.1016/j.healun.2010.05.034

45. Open Anesthesia. Post-cardiac transplant patient. 6 March, 2015. Available at: https://www.openanesthesia.org/post-cardiac_transplant_patient/.

46. Medline Plus [Internet]. Genetics conditions. Stevens–Johnson syndrome/toxic epidermal necrolysis. Bethesda, MD: National Library of Medicine Medline. Jan 1, 2020. Available at: https://medlineplus.gov/genetics/condition/stevens-johnson-syndrome-toxic-epidermal-necrolysis/#frequency.

47. Watanabe T, Go H, Saigusa Y, et al. Mortality and risk factors on admission in toxic epidermal necrolysis: a cohort study of 59 patients. *Allergol Int.* 2021;70(2):229–234. doi: 10.1016/j.alit.2020.11.004

48. Harr T, French LE. Toxic epidermal necrolysis and Stevens–Johnson syndrome. *Orphanet J Rare Dis.* 2010;5:39. doi: 10.1186/1750-1172-5-39

49. Romero-Tapia SJ, Cámara-Combaluzier HH, Baeza-Bacab MA, et al. Use of intravenous immunoglobulin for Stevens–Johnson syndrome and toxic epidermal necrolysis in children: report of two cases secondary to anticonvulsants. *Allergol Immunopathol.* 2015;43(2):227–229. doi: 10.1016/j.aller.2013.12.008

50. Oakley AM, Krishnamurthy K. Stevens Johnson Syndrome. In: StatPearls [Internet]. Treasure Island, FL: StatPearls Publishing; 2022 Jan [update 2022, Aug 21]. Available at: https://www.ncbi.nlm.nih.gov/books/NBK459323/.

51. Kumar R, Das A, Das S. Management of Stevens–Johnson syndrome-toxic epidermal necrolysis: looking beyond guidelines! *Indian J Dermatol.* 2018;63(2):117–124. doi: 10.4103/ijd.IJD_583_17

52. Shanbhag SS, Chodosh J, Fathy C, et al. Multidisciplinary care in Stevens–Johnson syndrome. *Ther Adv Chronic Dis.* 2020;11:2040622319894469. doi: 10.1177/2040622319894469

6

Ethics and Wellness

JOHN VONROSENBERG

COMPETENCIES

1. List some of the benefits of an ethical approach to transport medicine.
2. Identify the components of a healthy lifestyle.
3. Describe how to integrate the components of a healthy lifestyle into the transport environment.
4. Identify causes of critical incident stress in the transport environment.
5. Discuss methods to manage critical incident stress in the transport environment.

Introduction

As a transport professional, you will be subjected to a variety of stressors and trauma throughout your career. Transport professionals are part of a unique branch of medicine that is utilized both in and out of the hospital settings, in collaboration with prehospital (EMS) teams and a variety of medical professionals. Transport professionals are often called to assist in management and resuscitation of some of the sickest, most complex, and most traumatically injured patients and are at the front line between members of the community and the trauma, sickness, and suffering of that community.[1]

The work of a transport professional is important to the worker and to the patients and to the communities we serve. It is important to perform at the highest possible level and remain ready to serve with dedication, humility, and intelligence. Transport professionals may feel an increased sense of purpose with the work that is completed and frequently develop a unique sense of family amongst those with whom we work side-by-side. This purpose empowers workers to persevere in the presence of difficult situations and provides support in times of need. The cost of a dramatically imbalanced work–life schedule takes the form of depression, anxiety, substance abuse, domestic strife, post-traumatic stress disorder (PTSD), and suicide.[2]

Exposure to chronic traumatic events influences the transport professional's perception of stressors and experience of strain. First responders are exposed to specific job stressors such as lack of social support, shift work, and unpredictable professional environments that generate emotional, physical, and cognitive strain.[3] Long-term exposure to professional stressors in ambulance personnel is correlated positively with anxiety, depression, burnout, and compassion fatigue.[4] Researchers found critical care healthcare workers had high rates of burnout that were correlated with variation of workload (84.1%), overload (76.8%), responsibility for people's lives (69.5%), and lack of perceived control (63.4%).[2] While we have historically suppressed sharing emotions and struggles related to the job of a transport profession, new strategies are emerging from the research to support an active pursuit of positive mental health, such as physical activity, peer support, and critical incident stress management (CISM).[5,6] In addition to celebrating the power of the work completed by healthcare workers, it is important to emphasize the value of positive mental and physical health.

First responders cultivate feelings of purpose through work, however a disproportionately high number of first responders experience psychological and emotional distress when compared to the general public.[7-9] First responders are exposed to chronic stressors that alter the appraisal and differentiation of stimuli and are also exposed to specific acutely traumatic events that cause sharp changes in their emotional, cognitive, and physical well-being.[10] Researchers found first responders reported increased strains following acutely traumatic incidents, such as the death of a pediatric patient, exposure to potentially harmful body fluids, and vehicle crashes, to name a few.[11] Acute stressors are high intensity, short duration situations that may lead to strain. The nature and frequency of exposure of first responders to traumatic events increased the risk of mental health consequences.[12] Attention has shifted over time to consider the impact of chronic stressors as well as acute stressors on first responders. Chronic stressors are often lower intensity, longer duration situations that are repeated over time. Chronic job stressors include time away from home and family, financial trouble, feeling unappreciated by management, inadequate resources, and lack of community.[13] Strain occurs when expectations exceed resources; there are a variety of stressors that lead to strains.[14] In addition to stressors that do not originate from the work environment, stressors of transport include hypoxia, barometric pressure changes, thermal changes, decreased humidity, vibration, noise, fatigue, and gravitational forces.

Stress in the transport environment can have positive effects. The way in which an individual perceives a stressor influences their emotional and physical response in either a positive or negative way. The term "positive stress" refers to a novel stimulus that is perceived as a challenge rather than a threat and leads to growth or development.[15] In these situations, the individual is more focused and aware of the surrounding environment with the intention of solving a problem.[15] The term "negative stress" refers to the individual feeling overwhelmed, frustrated, or defeated.[2] Stress then is neither inherently positive nor negative. The perception of the stressor and the individual response to it determines the emotions and behaviours for those who are involved.

Exposure to stressors can help one develop new skills needed to manage life-threatening situations, however a similar experience can be harmful if it is severe enough to become overwhelming or lead to a loss of control. According to cognitive appraisal theory, there is a two-stage mental process in which individuals consider the stress generated by undertaking a task and the resources required to accomplish the goals of the task.[16] The appraisal of the situation moderates the relationships between the environment and emotion and either amplifies or controls the response to the stimulus (Fig. 6.1).

Physical or emotional tension are very often signs of stress. They may be the reaction to a situation that causes anxiety or feelings of being threatened. Symptoms of stress are included in Box 6.1.

When individuals develop healthy methods of managing stress, the negative effects can be managed with less detrimental long-term effects. Without balance, stressors become overwhelming, and the exhaustion phase may become the norm rather than the anomaly.[17] Having a healthy lifestyle and seeking support from appropriate sources act as mitigating factors to professional stressors. This chapter will outline sources of mental, emotional, and physical stress for the transport provider and strategies for managing that stress.

Ethics

An individual's ethics drive much of their decision-making, including the setting of priorities and the decision to persevere in the presence of difficulties or not.[18] Ethics refers to well-founded standards of right and wrong that prescribe what humans ought to do, usually in terms of rights, obligations, benefits to society, fairness, or specific virtues.[19] Ethics become increasingly important when

> • BOX 6.1   **Symptoms of Stress**
>
> Common reactions to a stressful event include the following:
> - Disbelief and shock
> - Tension and irritability
> - Fear and anxiety about the future
> - Difficulty making decisions
> - Being numb to one's feelings
> - Loss of interest in normal activities
> - Loss of appetite
> - Nightmares and recurring thoughts about the event
> - Anger
> - Increased use of alcohol and drugs
> - Sadness and other symptoms of depression
> - Feeling powerless
> - Crying
> - Sleep problems
> - Headaches, back pains, and stomach problems
> - Trouble concentrating

the answer to a question is not immediately clear or obvious. As a result, ethics have the potential to impact safety, compliance, and patient advocacy. Ethics are especially impactful on the concept of risk through avoidance behavior and failure to act.[20] As a result, the choices and consequences of ethical dilemmas may result in low self-esteem, job dissatisfaction, poor productivity, moral distress, burnout, disengagement, and low retention.

Moral Philosophy

Moral philosophy describes the process by which an individual determines if an action is "good" or "bad".[21] There are a number of moral philosophies, including utilitarianism and deontology, however an in-depth discussion of the various philosophies is beyond the scope of this chapter. It is important for the transport provider to be aware of their own moral philosophy so that they can appropriately advocate for their patient and minimize any potential tension between personal belief and legal standard.

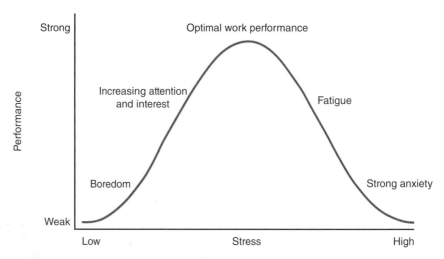

• **Fig. 6.1** Yerkes–Dodson curve. (Modified from Iglesias CA, Muñoz S. An agent based simulation system for analyzing stress regulation policies at the workplace. *J Comput Sci.* 2021;101326. Figure 1; and Yerkes RM, Dodson JD. The relation of strength of stimulus to rapidity of habit-formation. *J Comp Neurol Psych.* 1908;18:459–482.)

Some of the principles that factor into the ethical decision-making of the transport professional include nonmaleficence, beneficence, autonomy, justice, veracity, accountability, fidelity, and negligence.[22] Nonmaleficence follows the mantra of "first, do no harm", whereas beneficence is acting in a way that benefits others. Autonomy is the respect of others' decision-making, and justice is the equitable distribution of benefits. While the terms "ethical" and "legal" are not synonymous, many of the principles overlap. Table 6.1 outlines the definitions and examples of some of these ethical principles.

Moral Distress

Moral distress occurs when our actions are at odds with what we believe to be right; this inconsistency is both a precursor to and consequence of burnout.[23] Burnout, which is characterized by emotional exhaustion, cynicism, and reduced personal accomplishment, has been linked to poorer quality of care and decreased patient safety.[24] The inability to act in accord with individual and professional ethical values due to institutional constraints has been linked with moral distress and often leads to symptoms of PTSD and burnout.[25] As a transport professional, it is important to investigate options for places of employment and make a choice that – at least in part – enables providers to act according to their professional values. Furthermore, it is important for the transport professional to select a place of employment that has professional values that closely match their own.

It is appropriate to remain aware of the unintended consequences of having to perform interventions that may cause moral distress in ourselves and our team members. For example, the expectation of providing care in a futile resuscitation or managing multiple peri-mortem patients on a mass casualty incident may generate feelings of moral distress.[23] Other common triggers of moral distress include end-of-life care, inadequate staffing, value conflicts, and challenging team dynamics. Moral distress is the link between ethics and wellness; it is the responsibility of each transport professional to find ways to cope with personal feelings and support colleagues. Transport professionals can advocate for issues that impact their patients as a practical method of managing moral distress and can encourage their agency to adopt educational materials for the development of professional skills and best practices for wellness checklists and evaluation of organizational stressors.[25] Taking steps to support patients, team members, and ourselves empowers rather than distresses the individual.[26] The transport professional should pursue practical methods of decreasing moral distress in addition to other moderating factors such as resilience, mindfulness, and physical activity.

Moral Courage

Courage can be divided into two categories of critical moments – the courage to act and the courage to be.[27] Moral courage is the ability to use inner principles to do what is good for others.[28] Moral courage is influenced by previous work experience, individual traits, values, knowledge, maturity, and personal experience.[29] The concept of moral courage is often used synonymously with the ability to manage ambiguity and endure hardship.[30]

Moral courage is based on three foundational attributes: perseverance, resilience, and authenticity.[22] These qualities develop over the course of a lifetime and are sharpened by previous exposure to difficult situations. Perseverance refers to grit and self-confidence, resilience refers to bravery and mental strength, and authenticity refers to self-awareness and self-regulation. Moral courage is described as the energizing catalyst for choosing growth over safety needs and allowing one to effectively act under conditions of danger, fear, and risk.[31]

TABLE 6.1	Ethical Principles
Term	**Definition**
Nonmaleficence	The duty to do no harm. This is often the basis of ethical standards in health care and includes the consideration of the benefit of an intervention weighed against any potential harm that can be caused, such as the performance of chest compressions in cardiopulmonary resuscitation.
Beneficence	The concept of doing good and acting in the best interest of the patient.
Autonomy	Self-determination and the right to make one's own decisions. The patient has the right to consent or decline a particular treatment, including consent for transport to another facility.
Justice	Fairness and treating people equally. The transport professional may be called upon to provide care to someone who has done something that is discordant with their personal beliefs, including robbery, assault, murder, or other acts. It is important that the transport professional treat the individual with the same level of care independent of any allegations or background bias.
Veracity	Telling the truth. Veracity most commonly comes up when mistakes are made. If there is a mistake in medication administration or a negative patient reaction following an intervention, it is important that the transport professional communicate the actual events rather than an adapted or altered version of what happened.
Accountability	The ability and willingness to assume responsibility for one's actions and to accept the consequences of one's behavior.
Fidelity	To be faithful to agreements and responsibilities one has undertaken. This may mean following up with a promise provided to the patient, such as "I will be right here beside you the entire trip" or "Let me know if your pain increases and we will try to manage it."
Negligence	To fail to perform a legal duty.

Data from Marquis BL, Huston CJ. *Leadership Roles and Management Functions in Nursing Theory and Application.* 10th ed. Wolters Kluwer, 2021; and Blai, KK, Hayes JS. *Professional Nursing Practice Concepts and Perspectives.* 7th ed. Pearson Education; 2016.

Wellness

Wellness has been correlated with improved performance, job satisfaction, and job retention while poor mental health has been correlated with depression, substance abuse, marital distress, anxiety, PTSD, suicide, compassion fatigue, and burnout. In addition to the individual and personal cost of poor mental health, burnout has been associated with increased medical mistakes and increased risk of litigation.[32] Decreased well-being in first responders decreased safety of the professionals and resulted in increased medical mistakes and increased distraction while on shift.[12] Burnout was the result of high job demands and low job resources.[13] Burnout decreased performance of employees and increased turnover rates.[13]

Ways to Mitigate Stress

Hormones such as serotonin, dopamine, oxytocin, and phenylethylamine are often considered "happy hormones" because they ease the imbalance in neurological activity associated with stress and restore a positive emotional state.[33] An active lifestyle, a healthy diet, and a life full of love are each components for enjoying adequate happy hormone levels. Sometimes, taking small breaks from the tedium of daily life to appreciate small things can have a significant impact on the positive influence of hormones on emotion regulation. For example, a few minutes of petting a dog prompts a release of a number of positive hormonal changes in humans, with numerous studies having shown that dogs can help lower blood pressure.[33] In addition to participating in gentle demonstrations of compassion and companionship, participating in mindfulness, yoga, breathing techniques, coloring or drawing, listening to music, or writing in a journal may increase the number of hormones that generate feelings of happiness, enjoyment, or contentment.

Diet

A balanced diet is important to help counteract the effects of stress and to help maintain a healthy body.[34] While it may seem convenient to snack on pre-packaged foods that are high in fats, salts, and sugars, these ingredients provide short-term relief of hunger with only minimal long-term benefit.[35] A supply of healthy alternatives are often readily available, such as granola or high-protein bars, and may be helpful to avoid temptation. Enjoying small treats, such as sweet snacks, has been proven to be more effective in establishing overall healthy habits when compared to cutting out treats altogether.[36] Moderation and realistic goals are key ingredients in adherence to positive and sustainable behaviors.

Caffeine is a strong stimulant that can increase focus and wakefulness in the short term but is known to produce a stress reaction on the body with chronic use. The secretion of adrenaline results in nervous tension, irritability, and insomnia. If used, caffeine is best consumed before lunch and with a balanced meal. Energy drinks in particular have high amounts of caffeine, sugar, and other physiologically stimulating ingredients that have very little nutritious value.[37] Additionally, excessive amounts of caffeine may lead to or exacerbate tachydysrhythmias, the sensation of anxiety, or decreased sleep quality. Chronic consumption of energy drinks, including the sugar-free options, has been correlated with insulin resistance, increased triglycerides, increased blood pressure, endothelial dysfunction, increased white fat tissue, and other signs of metabolic syndrome.[37] Alternatives to caffeine, such as herbal teas, are acceptable and often healthier.[34]

Other drinks and foods, such as alcohol and fatty foods, may provide temporary positive feelings but stimulate the secretion of adrenaline and the depression of the immune system.[35] Alcohol, as an example, may be consumed as part of a transport professional's social behavior, however it is important to understand the limitations and risks of excessive alcohol consumption. One drink a day was associated with lower risk of hypertension, myocardial infarction, and stroke.[38] More than one alcoholic drink in a day transitions any potential benefit to a very different outcome. Individuals who consume more than one alcoholic drink per day have an increased risk of heart disease, stroke, liver disease, and all-cause mortality.[39] Additionally, alcohol consumptions is associated with increased risk-taking behavior, impaired judgment, domestic strife, and feelings of depression.[40]

Whole grains promote the production of serotonin in the body, which increases a sense of well-being. Yellow, green, and leafy vegetables are rich in vitamins and minerals, help boost the production of serotonin, and increase functioning of the immune system. The ideal food that will provide lasting energy is one rich in protein, fiber, and complex carbohydrates. Some of the best options for snacks or smart choices for a lunchtime meal that will keep your energy up are shown in Box 6.2.

Exercise

Exercise mitigates stress in several ways. Exercising releases endorphins that chemically make an individual feel better. Exercise also stops the production of the chemicals that are produced during the fight-or-flight phase of stress.[41] Exercise does not have to be extremely strenuous or take a long period of time. Any movement that engages the cardiovascular and musculoskeletal system produces positive effects.[35] Walking during a break or using the stairs can accomplish exercise. There are many ways to generate the benefits of strength training and aerobic workouts, such as yoga, martial arts, power lifting, swimming, cycling, running, and many others.

There are some public service departments that encourage employees to exercise while on shift and some that even take a resource out of service to provide the opportunity for physical fitness. In the absence of these options, there are still exercises that the transport professional can do while on shift without monopolizing large sections of time or becoming physically exhausted. Basic body weight exercises like squats and push-ups can be done repeatedly throughout the day in small numbers, and isometric exercises such as "wall sits" and planking may take 30 to 60 seconds at a time and can be repeated to an individual's comfort level.[42] Yoga has been shown to benefit individuals, not only in a

---

• BOX 6.2 **Foods That Boost Energy**

- One ounce of almonds
- Air-popped popcorn
- Two tablespoons of peanut butter
- Salmon
- Bananas
- Kale
- Oatmeal
- Pistachios
- Hummus
- Six ounces low-fat Greek yogurt

physical sense through increased strength, balance, and flexibility, but also through more purposeful mindful activities.[43] Higher intensity movement will burn more calories and build more muscle but can be distracting while at work.

Physical movement improves muscular tone and cardiovascular health; exercise has also been correlated with improved mental health. The different options of activity – resistance training, aerobic activity, flexibility, etc. – have a variety of benefits for the physical body. Professionals who participated in some type of physical activity had lower levels of depression and burnout than those who did not participate in physical activity.[44] The transport provider should take advantage of the opportunity to participate in physical activity both on shift and away from work in hopes of prolonging productive years of life and improving general wellness.

Laughter

Laughter has been found to be an effective stress management tool.[45] Laughter allows for the release of endorphins that produce feelings of euphoria and relaxation. Laughter has been proven to benefit both neuroendocrine and cardiac systems and has shown improved clinical courses for chronically and acutely ill individuals.[46] Watching a funny movie, visiting a comedy club, or joking with friends can help relieve stress through humor.

Verbalization of Feelings

Individuals often keep feelings of stress internalized for fear of showing weakness or loss of control.[47] When sharing feelings that involve stress, individuals should not minimize their feelings or the feelings of others. Transport professionals should share their concerns with others but must also be willing to seek professional help if these feelings begin to jeopardize their sense of well-being.

Even if the transport professional is not ready or willing to share feelings verbally, emotions can be expressed through nonverbal coping mechanisms, such as drawing, coloring, singing, playing a musical instrument, gardening, or journaling. It is important to allow time and space for the release of emotional pressure, which can look very different depending on the particular individual.

Sleep

Although inadequate sleep periods may not solely produce stress among transport professionals, sleep deprivation is associated with increased risk for accident and injury.[48–50] Disruption in circadian rhythm and shortened sleep cycles have been found to increase stress and increase the risk for injury and accident in transport professionals. Human beings are naturally disposed to a diurnal cycle of wake and sleep in which the night-time hours are spent sleeping and the day-time hours are wakeful.[51] There is some debate over how much sleep an adult requires for optimal performance, however disruption of sleep negatively impacts mental acuity and physical coordination.[51] Shift work, such as 24-hour shifts, 12-hour shifts, and working night shift all disturb the normal cycle of wake and sleep and thus can negatively impact the overall health of the transport provider. Transport providers who work shift work got progressively more sleep episodes both on and off shift but those episodes of sleep were progressively shorter year after year.[52] Sleep duration may be interrupted by noises, lights, or the inability to fully relax due to an awareness of the impending or possible call to duty while on shift.

Transport professionals can minimize the effects of shift work by minimizing secondary jobs, maintaining a consistent sleep pattern when not on duty, and avoiding activities that can disrupt sleep patterns (such as alcohol, caffeine, and exposure to electronic screens before sleep). Establishing specific times and locations for sleep when not on shift can also improve the quality of sleep. Sleeping in bed (rather napping or resting on a couch), in a bedroom with the lights off and other stimulation kept to a minimum can mimic the diurnal cycle and positively influence the amount of rest a transport provider gets while not on shift.[52] Additional environmental factors that can affect the quality of sleep are the temperature of the room, the amount of light, and ambient noise pollution.[53]

Resiliency Training

Resiliency refers to a personal trait that allows the individual to persevere through adversity and overcome obstacles.[54] Resiliency can be enhanced through training regimens and encouragement of natural ability.[6] The term resilience is often used within the context of exposure to stressors and the expectation of continued performance in the presence of stressors. Resilience does not imply the absence of a stressor, but rather the individual's ability to respond to the stressor in a productive way. Dispositional moderators of job stressors include self-efficacy, resilience, conscientiousness, negative affectivity, and emotional stability.[55] Individual dispositional differences have been found to influence both individuals' appraisals of job stressors as well as their reactivity to those job stressors.[56] In other words, certain skills and characteristics – such as resiliency – can change the way the transport provider experiences the stressors of the job and improve their overall wellness. Exposures to stressors in the transport professional work environment is inevitable, so it is imperative that providers develop methods to support their mental health.

As data increasingly support a preventative approach to psychological first aid (PFA) and resiliency training, more programs are supporting a "teach first" approach to mental health and wellness alongside reactive support platforms such as peer support programs and Critical Incident Stress Management (CISM) teams. Foundational training in PFA includes awareness of stress responses, stress and crisis mitigation techniques, alongside local resource awareness.

Mindfulness

Mindfulness is a technique of self-awareness practice based on Buddhist meditation that impacts resilience and manifests as a metacognitive monitoring of thought.[57] Mindfulness incorporates a number of specific qualities, such as being aware of a stimulus without feeling the need to respond to the stimulus. Mindfulness as a trait acts as a moderator of the relationships between fear, frustration, and burnout.[58,59] Mindfulness Based Resiliency Training (MBRT) moderates the relationship between work overload and burnout.[5] MBRT also acts as a moderator of the relationships between interpersonal conflict and fear, interpersonal conflict and frustration, and work overload and burnout.[5,60,61] Controlled breathing techniques, such as box breathing, and yoga, are two examples of physical activities that may facilitate mindfulness.

Critical Incident Stress Management (CISM)

Critical incident stress (CIS) can occur with one specific incident or situation or may accumulate over time with exposure to chronic stressors. Critical incidents usually involve a perceived threat to a person physically or the physical health of others.

Critical Incident Stress Management (CISM) is an interventional protocol designed to help manage the trauma associated with public service professions such as law enforcement, emergency services, and military. CISM is highly structured and requires specific standardized training for individuals involved in the processes after a major event. The seven components to CISM are pre-incident education, individual crisis or peer support, demobilization, defusing, debriefing, family support, and referral services. Grief and loss sessions are included when deaths are involved. These sessions are intended to help those involved to work through the grief process and deal with the sense of loss involved in the critical incident.

Not every individual requires CISM following every event. CISM is intended to be a cultural shift towards support and encouragement of individuals rather than only emergent responses to acutely traumatic events.[62] If done well, CISM prepares the transport provider for challenging calls before they even happen and educates them on the resources that are available for support when additional help is needed. CISM is based on the idea of crisis intervention, group psychotherapy, community psychology, and peer support.[62] If a transport provider is not ready to participate in a debriefing event, it is important to allow that individual space and time rather than force them into a situation in which re-living the traumatic events only adds to their discomfort.

Half of fire fighters who were surveyed preferred not to have a debrief session and that those who participated in debriefing sessions had significantly higher levels of secondary stress than those who did not participate.[63] These findings illustrate the importance of an individual approach rather than a mandated course of therapies as well as the importance of pre-incident preparation and peer support. There is significant overlap between CISM and more general ideas of wellness – strategies such as appropriate sleep, nutritious diet, physical activity, and encouragement of social support have been shown to be more impactful on developing provider resilience than debriefing sessions following events.[64] Perhaps the most important lessons from CISM are: (1) provide individual support for each member of the team and (2) begin preparation well before any incident actually occurs.

Summary

Transport providers act as an advocate for their patients; practicing wellness enables the provider to be an advocate for themselves. The transport provider is often self-motivated and accustomed to achieving a goal by overcoming ever-changing obstacles. While we care for our patients, it is important to care for ourselves as well. Small steps on a day-to-day basis may help lead to a long, healthy life and rewarding career.

References

1. Callaghan EL, Lam L, Cant R, Moss C. Compassion satisfaction and compassion fatigue in Australian emergency nurses: a descriptive cross-sectional study. *Int Emerg Nurs.* 2020;48:100785. doi: 10.1016/j.ienj.2019.06.008

2. Elshaer NSM, Moustafa MSA, Aiad MW, Ramadan MIE. Job stress and burnout syndrome among critical care healthcare workers. *Alex J Med.* 2018;54(3):273–277. doi: 10.1016/j.ajme.2017.06.004

3. Greinacher A, Derezza-Greeven C, Herzog W, Nikendei C. Secondary traumatization in first responders: a systematic review. *Eur J Psychotraumatol.* 2019;10(1):1562840. doi: 10.1080/20008198.2018.1562840

4. Petrie K, Milligan-Saville J, Gayed A, et al. Prevalence of PTSD and common mental disorders amongst ambulance personnel: a systematic review and meta-analysis. *Soc Psychiatry Psychiatr Epidemiol.* 2018;53(9):897–909. doi: 10.1007/s00127-018-1539-5

5. Kaplan JB, Bergman AL, Christopher M, Bowen S, Hunsinger M. Role of resilience in mindfulness training for first responders. *Mindfulness.* 2017;8(5):1373-1380. doi: 10.1007/s12671-017-0713-2

6. Thompson J, Drew JM. Warr;or21: a 21-day program to enhance first responder resilience and mental health. *Front Psychol.* 2020;11:2078. doi: 10.3389/fpsyg.2020.02078

7. Martin CE, Tran JK, Buser SJ. Correlates of suicidality in firefighter/EMS personnel. *J Affect Disord.* 2017;208:177–183. doi: 10.1016/j.jad.2016.08.078

8. McIntosh WL, Spies E, Stone DM, Lokey CN, Trudeau ART, Bartholow B. Suicide rates by occupational group—17 states, 2012. *MMWR Morb Mortal Wkly Rep.* 2016;65(25):641–645. doi: 10.15585/mmwr.mm6525a1

9. Barber E, Newland C, Young A, Rose M. Data suggests ways to reduce the impact of critical stress on EMTs and paramedics. *JEMS.* 2015;40(10). Available at: www.https://www.jems.com/special-topics/survey-reveals-alarming-rates-of-ems-provider-stress-and-thoughts-of-suicide/.

10. Scherer KR, Moors A. The emotion process: event appraisal and component differentiation. *Annu Rev Psychol.* 2019;70:719–745. doi: 10.1146/annurev-psych-122216-011854

11. Arble EP, Arnetz BB. CH 12: Evidence-based practices to enhance first responder well-being and performance. In: Bowers CA, Beidel DC, Marks MR, eds. *Mental Health Intervention and Treatment of First Responders and Emergency Workers* (pp. 205–229). Hershey, PA: IGI Global; 2020:205–229.

12. Jones S, Nagel C, McSweeney J, Curran G. Prevalence and correlates of psychiatric symptoms among first responders in a Southern State. *Arch Psychiatr Nurs.* 2018;32(6):828–835. doi: 10.1016/j.apnu.2018.06.007

13. Demerouti E, Bakker AB, Nachreiner F, Schaufeli WB. The job demands-resources model of burnout. *J Appl Psychol.* 2001;86(3):499. doi: 10.1037/00219010863499

14. McFarlane AC, Williamson P, Barton CA. The impact of traumatic stressors in civilian occupational settings. *J Public Health Policy.* 2009;30(3):311–327. doi: 10.1057/jphp.2009.21

15. Arble E, Arnetz BB. A model of first-responder coping: an approach/avoidance bifurcation. *Stress Health.* 2017;33(3):223–232. doi: 10.1002/smi.2692

16. Folkman S, Lazarus RS, Dunkel-Schetter C, DeLongis A, Gruen RJ. Dynamics of a stressful encounter: cognitive appraisal, coping, and encounter outcomes. *J Pers Soc Psychol.* 1986;50(5):992. doi: 10.1037/0022-3514.50.5.992

17. Kaye B, Jordan-Evans S. *Love'em or Lose'em.* San Francisco, CA: Berrett-Koehler; 1999.

18. Sanford K. The ethical leader. *Nurs Adm Q.* 2006;30(1):5–10.

19. Velasquez KR. When buying milk, do you care about the cow? Developing and validating a measure of focus on ethical considerations. Doctoral dissertation, The Florida State University; 2019. Available at: http://purl.flvc: fsu/fd/2019_Spring_Velasquez_fsu_0071N_15101.

20. Edmonson C. Moral courage and the nurse leader. *Online J Issues Nurs.* 2010;15(3):5. doi: 10.3912/OJIN.Vol15No03Man05

21. Buchanan A. Justice: a philosophical review. In: Shelp EE, ed. *Justice and Health Care Policy* (pp. 3–21). Dordrecht: Kluwer; 1981.

22. Merriman K. Leadership and perseverance. In: Marques AJ, Dhiman BS, eds. *Leadership Today*: Practices for Personal and Professional Performance (pp. 335–350). Cham, Switzerland: Springer; 2017.

23. Hlubocky FJ, Taylor LP, Marron JM, et al. A call to action: ethics committee roundtable recommendations for addressing burnout and moral distress in oncology. *J Oncol Pract*. 2020;16(4):191–199. doi: 10.1200/JOP.19.00806

24. Panagioti M, Geraghty K, Johnson J, et al. Association between physician burnout and patient safety, professionalism, and patient satisfaction: a systematic review and meta-analysis. *JAMA Intern Med*. 2018;178(10):1317–1331. doi: 10.1001/jamainternmed.2018.3713

25. Dzeng E, Wachter RM. Ethics in conflict: moral distress as a root cause of burnout. *J Gen Intern Med*. 2020;35(2):409–411. doi: 10.1007/s11606-019-05505-6

26. Wocial LD. Resilience as an incomplete strategy for coping with moral distress in critical care nurses. *Crit Care Nurse*. 2020;40(6):62–66. doi: 10.4037/ccn2020873

27. Harbour M, Kisfalvi V. In the eye of the beholder: an exploration of managerial courage. *J Bus Ethics*. 2014;119(4):493–515. doi: 10.1007/s10551-013-1835-7

28. Sekerka LE, Bagozzi RP. Moral courage in the workplace: moving to and from the desire and decision to act. *Bus Ethics: Eur Rev*. 2007;16(2):132–146. doi: 10.1111/j.1467–8608.2007.00484.x

29. Murray JS. Moral courage in healthcare: acting ethically even in the presence of risk. *Online J Issues Nurs (OJIN)*. 2010;15:2. doi: 10.3912/OJIN.Vol15No03Man02

30. Kidder R. *Moral Courage*. New York, NY: W. Morrow; 2005.

31. Goud NH. Courage: its nature and development. *J Humanist Couns Educ Dev*. 2005;44(1):102–116. doi: 10.1002/j.2164-490X.2005.tb00060.x

32. Hamilton S, Tran V, Jamieson J. Compassion fatigue in emergency medicine: the cost of caring. *Emerg Med Australas*. 2016;28(1):100–103. doi: 10.1111/1742-6723.12533

33. Hasin D, Pampori ZA, Aarif O, Bulbul KH, Sheikh AA, Bhat IA. Happy hormones and their significance in animals and man. *Int J Vet Sci Animal Husbandry*. 2018;3(5):100–103.

34. Marx W, Lane M, Hockey M, et al. Diet and depression: Exploring the biological mechanisms of action. *Mol Psychiatry*. 2021;26(1):134–150. doi: 10.1038/s41380-020-00925-x

35. Johnson TD. Address your stress, for a healthier life. *Nations Health*. 2008;38(3):24.

36. Ersche KD, Ward LH, Lim TV, et al. Impulsivity and compulsivity are differentially associated with automaticity and routine on the Creature of Habit Scale. *Pers Individ Dif*. 2019;150:109493. doi: 10.1016/j.paid.2019.07.003

37. Graneri LT, Mamo JC, D'Alonzo Z, Lam V, Takechi R. Chronic intake of energy drinks and their sugar free substitution similarly promotes metabolic syndrome. *Nutrients*. 2021;13(4):1202. doi: 10.3390/nu13041202

38. Mostofsky E, Chahal HS, Mukamal KJ, Rimm EB, Mittleman MA. Alcohol and immediate risk of cardiovascular events: a systematic review and dose–response meta-analysis. *Circulation*. 2016;133(10):979–987. doi: 10.1161/CIRCULATIONAHA.115.019743

39. Brennan SE, McDonald S, Page MJ, et al. Long-term effects of alcohol consumption on cognitive function: a systematic review and dose-response analysis of evidence published between 2007 and 2018. *Syst Rev*. 2020;9(1):1–39. doi: 10.1186/s13643-019-1220-4

40. Mukamal KJ, Stampfer MJ, Rimm EB. Genetic instrumental variable analysis: time to call mendelian randomization what it is. The example of alcohol and cardiovascular disease. *Eur J Epidemiol*. 2020;35:93–97. doi: 10.1007/s10654-019-00578-3

41. Sahakian A, Frishman WH. Humor and the cardiovascular system. *Altern Ther Health Med*. 2007;13(4):56–58.

42. Anderson GS, Di Nota PM, Groll D, Carleton RN. Peer support and crisis-focused psychological interventions designed to mitigate post-traumatic stress injuries among public safety and frontline healthcare personnel: a systematic review. *Int J Environ Res Public Health*. 2020;17(20):7645. doi: 10.3390/ijerph17207645

43. Gothe NP, Khan I, Hayes J, Erlenbach E, Damoiseaux JS. Yoga effects on brain health: a systematic review of the current literature. *Brain Plasticity*. 2019;5(1):105–122. doi: 10.3233/BPL-190084

44. Ochentel O, Humphrey C, Pfeifer K. Efficacy of exercise therapy in persons with burnout. A systematic review and meta-analysis. *J Sports Sci Med*. 2018;17(3):475.

45. North C, Wraa C. Stress: Taming Your Shadow 2000. Critical Care Transport Medicine Conference. 2000

46. Nollet M, Wisden W, Franks NP. Sleep deprivation and stress: a reciprocal relationship. *Interface Focus*. 2020;10(3):20190092. doi: 10.1098/rsfs.2019.0092

47. Cavanaugh MA, Boswell WR, Roehling MV, Boudreau JW. An empirical examination of self-reported work stress among US managers. *J Appl Psychol*. 2000;85(1):65. doi: 10.1037//0021-9010.85.1.65

48. Frakes MA, Kelly JG. Shift length and on-duty rest patterns in rotor-wing air medical programs. *Air Med J*. 2004;23(6):34–39.

49. Frakes MA, Kelly JG. Off-duty preparation for overnight work in rotor wing air medical programs. *Air Med J*. 2005;24(5):215–217.

50. Frakes MA, Kelly JG. Sleep debt and outside employment patterns in helicopter air medical staff working 24-hour shifts. *Air Med J*. 2007;26(1):45–49.

51. Lee CH, Sibley CG. Sleep duration and psychological well-being among New Zealanders. *Sleep Health*. 2019;5(6):606–614. doi: 10.1016/j.sleh.2019.06.008.

52. Betson JR, Kirkcaldie MT, Zosky GR, Ross RM. Transition to shift work: sleep patterns, activity levels, and physiological health of early-career paramedics. *Sleep Health*. 2022;8(5):514–520.

53. Miyama G, Fukumoto M, Kamegaya R, Hitosugi M. Risk factors for collisions and near-miss incidents caused by drowsy bus drivers. *Int J Environ Res Public Health*. 2020;17(12):4370. doi: 10.3390/ijerph17124370

54. Tabibnia G, Radecki D. Resilience training that can change the brain. *Consult Psychol J*. 2018;70(1):59. doi: 10.1037/cpb0000100

55. Sonnentag S. The recovery paradox: portraying the complex interplay between job stressors, lack of recovery, and poor well-being. *Res Organ Behav*. 2018;38:169-185. doi: 10.1016/j.riob.2018.11.002

56. Kilby CJ, Sherman KA, Wuthrich V. Towards understanding inter-individual differences in stressor appraisals: a systematic review. *Pers Individ Dif*. 2018;135:92-100. doi: 10.1016/j.paid.2018.07.001

57. Clarkson M, Heads G, Hodgson D, Probst H. Does the intervention of mindfulness reduce levels of burnout and compassion fatigue and increase resilience in pre-registration students? A pilot study. *Radiography*. 2019;25(1):4–9. doi: 10.1016/j.radi.2018.08.003

58. Vonderlin R, Biermann M, Bohus M, Lyssenko L. Mindfulness-based programs in the workplace: a meta-analysis of randomized controlled trials. *Mindfulness*. 2020;11(7):579–1598. doi: 10.1007/s12671-020-01328-3

59. McGee SL, Höltge J, Maercker A, Thoma MV. Sense of coherence and stress-related resilience: investigating the mediating and moderating mechanisms in the development of resilience following stress or adversity. *Front Psychiatry*. 2018;9:378. doi: 10.3389/fpsyt.2018.00378

60. Chiesa A, Serretti A. Mindfulness-based stress reduction for stress management in healthy people: a review and meta-analysis. *J Altern Complement Med*. 2009;15(5):593–600. doi: 10.1089/=acm.2008.0495

61. Guendelman S, Medeiros S, Rampes H. Mindfulness and emotion regulation: insights from neurobiological, psychological, and clinical studies. *Front Psychol*. 2017;8:220. doi: 10.3389/fpsyg.2017.00220

62. Mitchell J. Critical Incident Stress Debriefing (CISD). Available at: https://corpslakes.erdc.dren.mil/employees/cism/pdfs/Debriefing.pdf.

63. Sarabia-Cobo C, Pérez V, de Lorena P, et al. Burnout, compassion fatigue and psychological flexibility among geriatric nurses: a multi-center study in Spain. *Int J Environ Res Public Health*. 2021;18(14):7560. doi: 10.3390/ijerph18147560

64. Caldas MP, Ostermeier K, Cooper D. When helping hurts: COVID-19 critical incident involvement and resource depletion in health care workers. *J Appl Psychol*. 2021;106(1):29. doi: 10.1037/apl0000850

7

Neurologic Emergencies

LORIE J. LEDFORD

COMPETENCIES

1. Describe essential nervous system anatomy and physiology.
2. Apply physiologic principles of the nervous system to perform a rapid, focused neurologic patient assessment.
3. Initiate therapeutic interventions to manage neurologic emergencies throughout patient transport.

Introduction

Neurologic disorders present a high risk for significant morbidity and mortality. The effects on the patient's quality of life may be devastating. Without rapid recognition and intervention, neurologic disorders can be deadly. The transport team is fundamental in reducing morbidity and mortality by managing neurologic conditions while rapidly transporting the patient for definitive care.

Neurologic Anatomy and Physiology

Cellular Structure

The cellular structure of the central nervous system (CNS) is composed of neurons. Neurons are composed of a cell body with a nucleus, one or more dendrites, and a single axon. The dendrites receive the incoming messages to the cell and the axon sends out its messages. The neuronal cells are not in direct physical contact with each other. Neurotransmitters such as acetylcholine, dopamine, and serotonin carry the signal from cell to cell across the synaptic cleft. The signal can stimulate or inhibit the required function such as movement of an arm, hormone secretion or elicit a sneeze. The axon in the peripheral nervous system is covered with a myelin sheath. This myelin sheath is a lipoprotein layer that is interrupted at intervals by nodes of Ranvier. This complex permits rapid nerve conduction as the impulse jumps from node to node like taking the stairs two steps at a time. Nerves without a myelin sheath conduct the impulse much slower, taking the steps one at a time.[1-3]

Brain

The brain weighs approximately three pounds in the average adult. In a resting state, cerebral blood flow (CBF) is 50 mL blood per 100 g tissue per minute or about 15% of cardiac output. The brain consumes 20% of the body's oxygen and 25% of the body's glucose. It does not have the capability to store oxygen or glucose and is thus reliant on a steady blood supply. Autoregulation ensures adequate CBF with a mean arterial pressure (MAP) ranging from as low as 50 mmHg to as high as 150 mmHg. However, an insult to the brain interferes with these autoregulation capabilities.[1-3]

Knowledge of the functions of the brain's lobes can help determine the area of the brain affected by certain pathological conditions (Table 7.1). It is important to be mindful that awareness is the responsibility of the cerebral hemispheres. Dysfunction of the cerebral hemispheres will result in alterations of cognition ranging from mild confusion to complete absence of interaction with their environment.[1-3]

TABLE 7.1	Functions of the Brain Lobes
Lobe	Functions
Frontal	Intellect: problem-solving, planning Behavior/Affect Personality Working memory Concentration Judgment Initiation Inhibition Expressive language
Temporal	Hearing Receptive language Short-term memory Object recognition
Parietal	Touch, pain, temperature, position perception Body awareness Sensory interpretation: taste, hearing, sight, touch, and smell
Occipital	Vision interpretation
Cerebellum	Balance Coordination

The brain is protected by the skull, meninges, and cerebral spinal fluid (CSF). The skull has a capacity for approximately 1500 mL of content in an adult. In a healthy individual, this 1500 mL consists of 80% brain, 10% blood, and 10% cerebral spinal fluid (CSF). Under normal conditions, this balance of components maintains an intracranial pressure (ICP) of 5–15 mmHg (7–20 cmH$_2$O). The Monro–Kellie doctrine states the sum of these products must remain constant. If one component increases in volume, another must decrease, or intracranial pressure will elevate (Fig. 7.1). As intercranial pressure rises, brain tissues begin to get squeezed resulting in hypoperfusion. Unabated rising ICP will lead to shifting of brain tissues and ultimately cerebral herniation.[1-3]

The hypothalamus and the structures of the brain stem connect at the base of the cerebrum and transition into the spinal cord. The brain stem and hypothalamus regulate the many functions necessary to maintain homeostasis: body temperature, hunger, thirst, heart rate, respiration, vascular tone, hormone release, and circadian rhythms, to name a few. One notable network located in the brain stem is the reticular activating system (RAS). The RAS is responsible for arousal on the continuum from sleep to fully alert. Damage to both the RAS (alertness) and the cerebral hemispheres (awareness) results in a coma. Alertness without awareness is termed a persistently vegetative or a minimally responsive state. Awareness without alertness results in a phenomenon known as locked-in syndrome.

Blood–Brain Barrier

The capillaries in the brain form tight junctions creating the blood–brain barrier (BBB). The BBB protects the brain from toxins entering its delicate structures. Oxygen and glucose readily cross the BBB while other substances are held back. Insult to the brain can alter the BBB exposing the brain to substances that are irritating or toxic to its delicate tissues.[1,2]

Cerebral Blood Flow

Arterial cerebral blood flow is supplied bilaterally by the internal carotid arteries (that supply the anterior brain) and the vertebral arteries (that supply the posterior brain). The internal carotid arteries branch into the anterior cerebral artery and continue to form the middle cerebral artery. The vertebral arteries fuse together and form the basilar artery. These vessels in addition to the anterior and posterior communicating arteries round out the Circle of Willis. The Circle of Willis protects the brain by assuring continued blood flow in the event of a vessel blockage. However, a complete and functional Circle of Willis is present in only about 20% of individuals. Disruptions of blood flow to an area of the brain can cause loss of function secondary to hypoxia. Patients experiencing this will present with predictable symptoms representing the affected area[1-3] (see Table 7.5).

Cerebral blood flow is controlled by vasoconstriction and vasodilation of the cerebral arteries in response to the metabolic and oxygenation needs of the brain. Hypoxia and hypercapnia elicit vasodilatation which increases CBF. Fever, seizures, agitation, and pain cause an increase in cerebral oxygen demand; in response to this, autoregulation will initiate vasodilatation. Conversely, low $PaCO_2$ (hypocapnia) causes cerebral vasoconstriction. Hypothermia and sedation decrease cerebral oxygen demand; in response to this, autoregulation will initiate vasoconstriction[1-3] (Fig. 7.2).

Venous blood from the brain includes the superficial veins and the deep veins. The superficial veins are primarily the dural venous sinuses which flow along the midline of the brain and ultimately drain into the jugular veins. The deep vein system is composed of veins inside the structures of the brain. These vessels ultimately form into the confluence of sinuses and drain into the jugular vein.[1-3]

Cerebrospinal Fluid

Cerebrospinal fluid is predominately produced by the choroid plexus found on the lining of the lateral ventricles. Approximately 500 mL of CSF is produced daily in adults with roughly 150 mL circulating at any one time. CSF circulates through the four cerebral ventricles and around the spinal cord. CSF allows the brain and spinal cord to "float" in their space cushioning them from impact. CSF functions to provide nourishment and remove waste for the health of the CNS. Most of the CSF is reabsorbed by the arachnoid villi in the subarachnoid space. Blockage of the subarachnoid villi will inhibit reabsorption and can lead to hydrocephalus.[1-3]

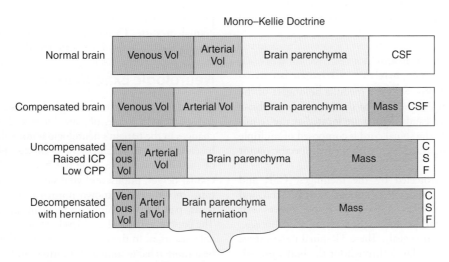

• **Fig. 7.1** Monro–Kellie doctrine. (Modified from Siddiqui E, Qazi GI. Role of dexamethasone in meningitis. In: Wireko-Brobby G, ed. *Meningitis*. InTech; 2012. Creative Commons license: https://creativecommons.org/licenses/by/3.0/.)

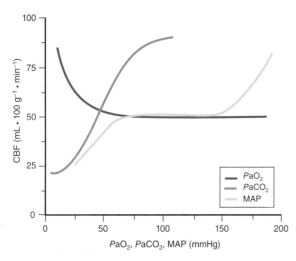

• **Fig. 7.2** Changes in cerebral blood flow (CBF) caused by independent alterations in $PaCO_2$, PaO_2, and mean arterial pressure (MAP). (From Miller RD, ed. *Miller's Anesthesia*. 8th ed. Philadelphia, PA: Saunders; 2015.)

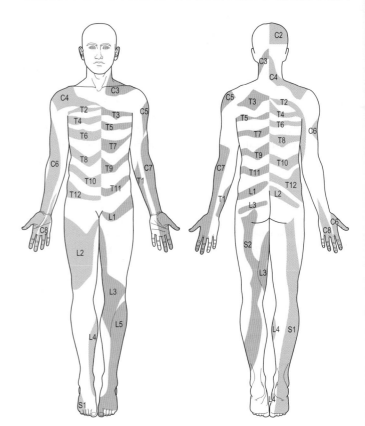

• **Fig. 7.3** Evidence-based dermatome map. (Reproduced from Lee MW, McPhee RW, Stringer MD. An evidence-based approach to human dermatomes. *Clin Anat*. 2008;21(5):363–373 Copyright © 2008 Wiley-Liss, Inc.)

Intracranial Pressure and Cerebral Perfusion Pressure

The Monro–Kellie doctrine mentioned earlier describes the pressure/volume gradient within the confines of the rigid skull. With all three parts (brain, blood, and CSF) in proper pro portion the pressure within the skull, known as the intracranial pressure (ICP), is 5–15 mmHg (7–20 cm H_2O). ICP above 20 mmHg is unfavorable and an ICP above 50 mmHg requires immediate attention to prevent herniation and brain death.[1,3]

Monitoring the ICP will not only portend shifting and potential herniation of the brain tissues, but also provides a means to monitor cerebral blood flow. Cerebral blood flow is driven by the cerebral perfusion pressure (CPP). CPP is determined by the following equation: MAP – ICP = CPP. The exact CPP required to maintain adequate cerebral oxygenation is not known and is likely to be patient-specific. Current guidelines recommend a minimum CPP of 60–70 mmHg. An elevation in ICP or a decreased MAP reduces the CPP indicating cerebral hypoperfusion and probable cerebral hypoxia.[1,3]

Spinal Cord

The spinal cord is continuous with the medulla oblongata of the brain stem and terminates at the level of the L1 or L2 vertebrae. The conus medullaris and cauda equina are located at the termination of the spinal cord. The spinal cord is composed of multiple ascending and descending tracts each with its own specific motor or sensory function.[2,3]

The spinal cord is protected by the meninges, CSF, and 33 vertebrae (7 cervical, 12 thoracic, 5 lumbar, 5 fused sacral, and 4 coccygeal). Thirty-one bilateral pairs of spinal nerves exit through the intravertebral foramina (8 cervical, 12 thoracic, 5 lumbar, 5 sacral, and 1 coccygeal). These 31 spinal nerves serve as the motor and sensory highway throughout the body, providing CNS communication to the PNS. Each nerve root provides enervation to a specific, unchanging, area of the body. Familiarity with dermatome distribution assists in the diagnosis of patients

with disease or injury of the spinal cord (Fig. 7.3). Symptoms will follow a predictable pattern of dermatome distribution.[2,3]

Cranial Nerves

There are 12 paired cranial nerves. In contrast to the peripheral nerves which are responsible for a specific area of the body, the cranial nerves are responsible for a specific function such as vision or eye movement. Cranial nerves I and II originate from the cerebral hemispheres, the other 10 originate from the brain stem. This placement makes the cranial nerves vulnerable to increased intracranial pressure. Cranial nerves are responsible for many of the criteria used to assess for neurologic disorders and brain death.[1–3]

Neurologic Examination

A rapid, yet thorough neurologic exam is essential prior to patient transport, both to identify alterations and to set a baseline. Subtle changes in the patient's neurologic status will go unnoticed if a solid baseline is not established. The exam should include an assessment of the Glasgow Coma Scale (GCS), mental status, motor/sensory, cranial nerves, pupils, and vital signs. A brief history of the symptoms including last known normal (LKN), temporality of symptoms, past medical history and medications should be obtained. The patient with an altered level of consciousness may not be a reliable historian. In these instances, family, friends, or bystanders may be a more reliable source of information.[1,3]

If rapid sequence intubation with sedation and paralytics is being considered, it is prudent to complete an abbreviated neurological exam or the ability to do so will be lost.

Glasgow Coma Scale

The GCS is undoubtedly the most familiar component of the neurologic exam (Table 7.2). It provides a score between 3 and 15 that is readily communicated and recognized by healthcare providers indicating the patient's level of consciousness. Each of the three components, eyes, verbal, and motor, are scored separately and the *best* performance is scored. The eye and verbal components are straightforward. The motor component is a little more challenging. A patient who can follow simple commands such as showing two fingers, giving a thumbs up, or making a fist scores a 6. The patient who does not follow commands should be stimulated with noxious stimuli to assess for impaired motor function.[1,3]

The stimuli need to be central in nature, such as trapezius squeeze, pressure on the corner of the jaw, glabellar pressure, and finally the sternal rub. Localization occurs when the patient moves away from the stimuli and attempts to remove the stimuli (i.e., reaches up to push the examiner's hand away). Withdrawal is the simple act of moving away from the stimuli. Decorticate (flexive) posturing occurs when there is an unnatural flexion of the arms and extension of the legs. Decerebrate (extensive) posturing is forced extension of the arms and legs. Often the decorticate gesture of bringing the arms up onto the chest is misinterpreted as the purposeful movement of reaching for the endotracheal tube. Flexed, fisted hands will be seen with decorticate posturing. Open-handed reaching is seen with purposeful movement. The application of nail bed pressure to perform a motor/sensory exam is useful to confirm the patient can move all four extremities. However, peripheral painful stimuli can elicit spinal reflexes, which can be active in a brain-dead patient and are not reliable for the GCS.[1,3]

Proposed changes to the GCS (GCS-40 or GCS-P) to include pupillary response have not been widely adopted at this time and may cause inconsistencies in reporting changes in patient condition as the numbers do not equate to the standard GCS.

The Full Outline of Unresponsiveness (FOUR) score may also be used to assess the level of consciousness (Table 7.3). It removes the verbal response component of the GCS and adds components for brain stem reflexes and respirations. A FOUR score has been shown to have superior predictability in determining in-hospital mortality, but its use in identifying clinical deterioration is still uncertain.[1,3–5]

Mental Status Exam

The information necessary to complete a brief mental status exam can often be gleaned from the patient's responses during initial patient contact. Components of the mental status exams include awake, oriented to person, place, time, and events, ability to appropriately answer questions, self-awareness, conversational and cooperative. It may not always be possible to differentiate the patient who is intentionally being inappropriate from one whose behavior is a symptom of neurologic dysfunction. Always err on the side of caution. Manage the patient as having a suspected neurologic insult until proven otherwise. Alterations in the level of consciousness is the first sign of an abnormality in the brain and needs to be examined thoroughly.[1,3]

TABLE 7.2	Glasgow Coma Scale	
Best eye response	Spontaneously opens	4
	Opens to speech	3
	Opens to pain	2
	No response	1
Best verbal response	Oriented	5
	Confused	4
	Inappropriate words	3
	Indecipherable sounds	2
	No response	1
Best motor response	Follows commands	6
	Localizes pain	5
	Withdrawal	4
	Abnormal flexion	3
	Abnormal extension	2
	No response	1
Total score		3–15

Modified from Royal College of Physicians and Surgeons of Glasgow. The Glasgow Structured Approach to Assessment of the Glasgow Coma Scale. https://www.glasgowcomascale.org/.

TABLE 7.3	Full Outline of Unresponsiveness (FOUR) Score			
Points	Eye Response	Motor Response	Brain Stem Reflexes	Respirations
4	Eyelids open, tracking or blinking to command	Thumbs up, fist or peace sign	Pupil and corneal reflexes present	Not intubated, regular breathing pattern
3	Eyelids open but pupils not tracking	Localize pain	One pupil wide and fixed	Not intubated, Cheyne–Stokes breathing pattern
2	Eyelids closed but open to loud voice	Flexion response to pain	Pupil OR corneal reflexes absent	Not intubated, irregular breathing
1	Eyelids closed but open to pain	Extension response to pain	Pupil AND corneal reflexes absent	Breathes above ventilator rate
0	Eyelids remain closed to pain	No response to pain or generalized myoclonus status	Pupil, corneal and cough reflexes absent	Breathes at ventilator rate or apneic

From Wijdicks EF, Bamlet WR, Maramattom BV, et al: Validation of a new coma scale: The FOUR score. *Ann Neurol.* 2005;58(4):585–593.

Motor/Sensory Exam

In the transport environment, the motor/sensory exam is brief. It includes assessing the ability to move each extremity, evaluating the strength between the left and the right side, and assessing for numbness, tingling, or loss of sensation. The presence of weakness or sensory deficit requires further investigation to discover the extent of impairment. Be alert for focal or lateralized deficits; they provide important diagnostic information. A patient whose entire leg is numb may have a spinal cord process developing. While a patient who has segmental numbness of the leg is more likely to have a spinal nerve dysfunction.[1,3]

Pupillary Response and Cranial Nerves

The cranial nerves (CN) originate on either the cerebral cortex (I and II) or the brain stem (III through XII). CN III, responsible for pupillary dilatation and constriction, sits directly above the tentorium. As ICP rises, CN III will be the first to show dysfunction as it gets squeezed against the tentorium. Pupillary changes are the second sign of increased ICP (altered level of consciousness being the first).[1,3]

CN III, IV, and VI control eye movement. CN VII is responsible for the facial droop seen in cerebral vascular accidents (CVA). Table 7.4 describes the cranial nerve assessment. Many CN assessments are readily apparent from interacting with the patient, such as facial droop, and may not require a targeted assessment. In the transport environment, the CN assessment should be guided by the individual patient complaint. Rarely are all 12 assessed.

Vital Signs

Vital signs are commonly overlooked as part of the neurologic assessment. The CNS is the "captain of the ship" controlling homeostasis and bodily functions, including vital signs.

Hypotension is rarely neurologic in origin except in neurogenic shock. The provider should look for other causes of hypotension. Heart rate, rhythm, the force of contraction, respiratory rate, depth and rhythm, vasoconstriction and vasodilatation, and body temperature are just a few of the functions of the CNS. Impaired brain stem function may reveal itself in vital sign changes.[1,3]

Neurogenic fever is caused by pressure on the hypothalamus. Core body temperatures can rise as high as 40°C to 41°C (104°F to 105°F). An elevated body temperature increases cerebral oxygen demand increasing the risk of cerebral hypoxia. An infectious source needs to be considered. Antibiotics are not indicated if an infectious source is not discovered. Tylenol has little effect on a neurogenic fever. Active cooling measures are required, such as a cooling blanket.[1,3]

Cushing's Triad

Cushing's triad is a constellation of symptoms consisting of bradycardia, hypertension with widening pulse pressure, and irregular respiratory patterns. This pattern of symptoms is an indication of pressure on the brain stem and pending cerebral herniation. The triad is a very late sign, usually observed in the moments preceding herniation. Immediate intervention to reduce ICP is necessary to prevent brain death.[1,3]

Management of Neurologic Emergencies

Increased Intracranial Pressure

Increased intracranial pressure occurs when there is an increase in the volume of one intracerebral component without a compensatory decrease in another component. Causes of increased ICP include mass lesions of the brain (hematoma, tumors, abscesses, etc.), cerebral edema, increased cerebral blood flow, and increased CSF.[1,3]

Increased cerebral blood flow occurs from increased arterial flow, decreased venous flow, or both. Primary hypertension is the most common cause of increased arterial flow. Stimulant use such as methamphetamine can cause a rapid spike in cerebral arterial flow. Conversely, reduced venous flow leads to cerebral vasocongestion.

Increased CSF volume, regardless of the cause, leads to hydrocephalus. Management of hydrocephalus requires the removal of

TABLE 7.4	Cranial Nerve Assessment		
Cranial Nerve	**Function**		**Testing**
I Olfactory	Smell		Identify familiar odors
II Optic	Vision		Visual acuity and visual fields
III Oculomotor IV Trochlear VI Abducens	Eye movement and pupil constriction		Full range of ocular movement and pupil size, shape and equality. Presence of diplopia
V Trigeminal	Facial sensation and mastication		Facial sensation, corneal reflex, clench teeth, chew
VII Facial	Facial motor, taste, salivary and lacrimal glands		Facial symmetry, corneal reflex (along with CN V), taste
VIII Auditory/Acoustic (Vestibular cochlear)	Hearing and equilibrium		Hearing acuity, presence of vertigo, nystagmus, imbalance of gait. Doll's eye test
IX Glossopharyngeal X Vagus	Posterior tongue, soft palate and pharynx sensation. Swallowing. Carotid bodies control blood pressure, heart rate, and respirations		Gag reflex, ability to swallow. Dysphonia.
XI Spinal accessory	Trapezius and head movement		Ability to shrug shoulders, ability to turn and lift the head
XII Hypoglossal	Tongue muscles		Ability to protrude tongue, move tongue side to side. Dysarthria

CSF. This can be accomplished with an external ventricular drain (EVD), lumbar puncture, lumbar drain, or a ventricular–peritoneal shunt. Extreme caution is required with a lumbar drain in the setting of elevated ICP. Elevating the patient's head with a lumbar drain open to drain can cause abrupt herniation from gravitational forces. In a patient with a ventricular–peritoneal shunt, signs and symptoms including altered level of consciousness, nausea, and vomiting can indicate a shunt failure requiring prompt treatment to avoid herniation.[3]

Treatment of a mass lesion varies depending upon the type of lesion. An abscess requires antibiotics. Epidural and subdural hematomas may require surgical evacuation. Arteriovenous malformation and aneurysms may be managed with embolization. Surgically, aneurysms can be clipped or coiled. Emergent management of a brain tumor includes the use of a steroid such as decadron to reduce vasogenic edema surrounding the tumor. Finally, cerebral edema from an ischemic stroke, cardiac arrest, and other causes is treated by the general principles of managing increased ICP (Box 7.1).[1,3,6,7]

The goal of managing increased ICP is to prevent herniation and to restore/maintain cerebral blood flow. Cerebral perfusion pressure (CPP) is the primary determinate of CBF. The formula to calculate the CPP is CPP = MAP – ICP. Current recommendations are to maintain a CPP between 60 and 70 mmHg. Follow the general principles of ICP management to maintain adequate CPP.

In the air transport environment, pneumocephalus can rapidly become a mass lesion. Pneumocephalus occurs when the cranial vault is penetrated either traumatically or therapeutically (basilar skull fracture, EVD, or craniotomy). According to Boyle's law of gas, the air in the cranial vault will expand as altitude increases. If the patient's neurologic status deteriorates while ascending during transport, then altitude adjustments should be made. On fixed-wing transport, request the pilot to pressurize the cabin to sea level (or altitude of origination).[8]

Intracranial pressure monitoring devices are inserted to obtain a direct measurement of the intercranial pressure. Subdural or epidural catheters, intraparenchymal wires or a subarachnoid bolt can provide an ICP measurement but have no capacity to treat increased ICP. The external ventricular drain is placed into one of the lateral ventricles. The EVD not only measures ICP but can be instrumental in decreasing ICP by draining small quantities of CSF when needed (Fig. 7.4) (Box 7.2).

Hyperosmolar Therapy

Two substances are used for hyperosmolar therapy for treatment of increased intracranial pressure – mannitol and hypertonic saline (HTS). There is no clear recommendation for use of one over the other. Mannitol is an osmotic diuretic. By creating an osmotic gradient across the BBB, CSF and brain water are drawn into the vascular space. There is a transient rise in CBF due to a decrease in blood viscosity. Results should be seen within 15–30 minutes and last from 2 to 6 hours. An indwelling catheter is suggested as a large quantity of urine output is expected. Mannitol is bolus

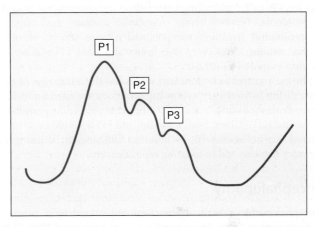

• **Fig. 7.4** Intracranial pressure waveform. Elevation of P2 indicates decreased brain compliance. P1 = percussion wave; P2 = tidal wave; P3 = dicrotic notch.

• BOX 7.1 General Management Principles of Increased ICP

- Elevate the head of the bed at least 30 degrees but no more than 45 degrees
- Maintain head in the midline position
- Remove circumferential devices around the neck (ETT holders, trach ties) but assure tube is secure
- Reduce external stimuli
- Administer pain and sedation medications
- Avoid activities that increase intrathoracic pressure (coughing, gagging, vagal maneuvers)
- Administer hyperosmolar therapy (bolus doses)
- Maintain blood glucose 140–180 mg/dL
- Treat fever with cooling devices
- Do not administer dextrose solutions
- Monitor ICP using an external ventricular drain, fiberoptic sensor or other device
- Drain CSF to maintain ICP ≤15 mmHg or as ordered
- Administer vasopressors as needed to maintain adequate MAP to sustain CPP ≥70 mmHg
- Target end-tidal carbon dioxide ($ETCO_2$) and $PaCO_2$ of 35–40 mmHg
- Hyperventilation for a short period is indicated to reduce herniation risk in acutely elevated ICP
- Avoid daily weaning trials with elevated ICP

For abbreviations, see text.

Data from Varghese R, Chakrabarty J, Menon G. Nursing management of adults with severe traumatic brain injury: a narrative review. *Indian J Crit Care Med.* 2017;21(10):684–697; and Zrelak PA, Eigsti J, Fetzick A, et al. Evidence-based review: nursing care of adults with severe traumatic brain injury. *American Association of Neuroscience Nurses.* Originally published 2009, revised May 2019. https://aann.org/uploads/Publications/CPGs/AANN20_sTBI_EBR.pdf.

• BOX 7.2 External Ventricular Drain Management

- The pressure line is primed with preservative-free saline to remove all air.
- The pressure line is connected to the EVD, and the transducer is connected to the monitor.
- The pressure transducer is levelled, and the drainage system zeroed at the foramen of Monro approximately located at the tragus of the ear.
- Raise the drainage system to 15 mmHg or the ordered drainage level. The transduced ICP waveform fluctuates with arterial blood flow.
- The drainage system must be turned off to drain prior to patient repositioning and movement. If the drain falls below the head with an open drain, rapid release of CSF may precipitate herniation.
- The pressure transducer is releveled and zeroed after every patient movement.
- The EVD system is a closed system. Do not flush, aspirate or empty the drain.
- Document the quality of the ICP waveform, quantity and quality of CSF drained.
- If possible, print a segment of the ICP waveform and post with the chart.

Data from American Association of Neuroscience Nurses. Care of the patient undergoing intracranial pressure monitoring/external ventricular drainage or lumbar drainage, 2014. https://aann.org/uploads/Membership/SFG/neurotrauma/2015/EVD_Poster.pdf; Liu X, Griffith M, Jang HJ, et al. Intracranial pressure monitoring via external ventricular drain: are we waiting long enough before recording the real value? *J Neurosci Nurs.* 2020;52(1):37–42.

dosed. Continuous dosing can lead to rebound increases in ICP. Visually inspect the mannitol solution for crystals prior to administration and use a 0.22-micron in-line filter for infusion.[1,3,6,7,9]

A minute amount of mannitol may cross the blood–brain barrier, which carries the risk of rebound cerebral edema, pulling fluid from the vascular space into the brain. Other considerations when using mannitol include excessive diuresis leading to acute kidney injury and hypotension. The resulting increase in serum osmolarity can lead to fluid overload exacerbating heart failure and/or causing pulmonary edema. Monitor the serum osmolarity and electrolytes. Replace electrolytes as needed. Hold mannitol if the serum osmolarity exceeds 320 mOsm/kg.

Hypertonic saline is believed to decrease ICP by osmotic effects. The onset of HTS is 15–30 minutes and lasts 4–6 hours. The Neurocritical Care Society recommends bolus dosing as there is insufficient evidence to recommend continuous infusion. HTS does not cross the BBB, eliminating the risk of rebound increased ICP as seen with mannitol. Reduced blood viscosity transiently increases CBF.[1,3,6,7,9]

HTS increases intravascular volume thus avoiding hypotension but has a risk of exacerbating heart failure and potentiating pulmonary edema. Hypernatremia, metabolic acidosis, and osmotic demyelination syndrome are potential adverse effects. Monitor serum sodium levels every 4–6 hours and hold HTS if serum sodium exceeds 160 mEq/L.

In the transport environment, HTS has the advantage of not crystalizing in your medication bag and does not need an in-line filter. Both medications are safe to be administered in peripheral intravenous (IV) lines. Both mannitol and HTS should be administered as a bolus over 10–15 minutes. Utilizing an IV pump or pressure bag may aid in assuring rapid delivery.

Encephalopathy

Encephalopathy is brain dysfunction not caused by a primary neurological disease. The causative factors are varied (Box 7.3). Delirium is one type of encephalopathy. Rapid identification and intervention are crucial to improving patient outcome.

Neurologic symptoms can range from mildly impaired cognition to deep coma. Information from the history of the present illness (HPI), past medical history, medications, and available diagnostic tests can assist the clinician in determining the cause of encephalopathy. Once the causative factor is determined, the transport clinician initiates treatment to manage encephalopathy.[1]

• BOX 7.3 Causes of Encephalopathy

- Hypoxia
- Hypercapnia
- Endocrine disorders: glucose imbalance, thyroid disorders, adrenal disorders
- Electrolyte disturbances: sodium, potassium, magnesium
- Temperature extremes: hypothermia, hyperthermia
- Hypertensive crisis
- Drugs, toxins, alcohol
- Drug and alcohol withdrawal
- Sepsis
- Organ failure: renal, hepatic
- Post-ictal state
- Nutritional deficiencies

Data from Hartjes TM, ed. *AACN Core Curriculum for Progressive and Critical Care Nursing*, 8th ed. Elsevier; 2023.

Ischemic Stroke

Every year, there are nearly 800,000 strokes in the United States. Stroke is the fifth leading cause of death in the United States (stroke fell from fourth place when COVID-19 took third place on the list). Stroke is a major cause of disability with a huge burden on patient quality of life and healthcare costs. Hypertension, diabetes mellitus, and cardiac disease are the leading modifiable risk factors for stroke. Ischemic stroke accounts for approximately 85% of all strokes. Emboli or thrombus blocks the blood flow in a cerebral vessel causing hypoxia and death of the brain tissue. An occluded vessel will produce predictable symptoms that are useful in identifying the vessel involved[1–3,7,10–12] (Table 7.5).

The FAST exam is commonly used for stroke education to the public, and is most predictive of the signs and symptoms of a stroke affecting the anterior circulation. BEFAST is a modified version of the FAST exam that adds balance and eye evaluations, which is beneficial when assessing for signs and symptoms of a stroke affecting the posterior circulation. The Cincinnati Stroke Scale or Los Angeles Prehospital Stroke Scale are highly predictive of a large vessel occlusion. The National Institutes of Health Stroke Scale (NIHSS) has been shown to have high reliability and validity in assessing and quantifying neurologic deficits during acute ischemic stroke. A proper stroke scale is used to rapidly assess for stroke prior to initiating transport.

Treatment of acute ischemic stroke, after the ABCs are assured, focuses on minimizing time to reperfusion. It is imperative to identify the time the patient was last known to be normal (LKN) – not the time the symptoms were first noticed. Family may report

---

TABLE 7.5 Acute Ischemic Stroke Symptoms by Occluded Vessel

Vessel	Symptoms of Ischemia/Infarct
Vertebral artery	Dizziness Nystagmus Dysphagia Facial Pain Ataxia Clumsiness
Anterior inferior cerebellar artery	Vertigo Nausea Vomiting Tinnitus Nystagmus
Anterior cerebral artery	Contralateral paralysis and sensory loss of foot and leg Impaired gait Loss of willpower Flat affect Perseveration
Posterior cerebral artery	Memory impairment Visual deficits Homonymous hemianopsia Color blindness Loss of depth perception Inability to recognize objects
Middle cerebral artery	Hemiplegia: face and arm > leg Sensory impairment Homonymous hemianopsia Global aphasia if dominant hemisphere

the symptoms started at 7 a.m. because they were first noticed upon waking. However, the patient was last seen normal at 10 p.m. the night before. There is no way to predict when the occlusion occurred for a "wake-up" stroke. Administration of thrombolytics outside the window of opportunity can have catastrophic effects. Thrombolytics may be administered up to 3 hours after symptom onset and up to 4.5 hours for select patients. Currently, alteplase is the sole thrombolytic with FDA approval for use in ischemic stroke. Tenecteplase is being used off-label for thrombolysis in ischemic stroke. In addition, patients may be eligible for embolectomy up to 24 hours after symptom onset.

The goal for thrombolytic administration is within 60 minutes of arrival at a stroke center. However, each minute of delay is costing the patient's brain cells. The sooner thrombolytics are administered the better the outcome. If the patient is within the administration window, they are given thrombolytics without regard to their eligibility for embolectomy.

Once a stroke is suspected, the transport clinician's responsibility is to rapidly transport the patient to a primary stroke center, thrombectomy-capable stoke center, or a comprehensive stroke center. The American Stroke Association has established best practices for prehospital providers, which can be reviewed in *Guidelines for the Early Management of Patients With Acute Ischemic Stroke: 2019 Update to the 2018 Guidelines for the Early Management of Acute Ischemic Stroke: A Guideline for Healthcare Professionals From the American Heart Association/American Stroke Association.*[12] Notable aspects of the *Guidelines* for prehospital providers include:

- Assess ABCs (airway, breathing, circulation)
- Do not treat high blood pressure (unless patient-specific order received)
- Ensure cardiac monitoring
- Administer oxygen as needed to maintain $SpO_2 \geq 94\%$
- Obtain blood glucose, treat if >60 mg/dL
- Initiate IV access, two 18G if possible
- Do not administer excessive IV fluids
- Do not administer glucose-containing IV fluids
- Maintain patient absolute NPO (nil by mouth)
- Determine last known normal
- Document medical history and medications
- Obtain family member/bystander contact information
- Initiate rapid transport to closest appropriate stroke center
- Notify receiving facility of incoming stroke patient

Air transport can be dispatched to transport a patient from a primary stroke center to a thrombectomy-capable center while a thrombolytic is infusing. Verify the dosing with the sending facility. DO NOT interrupt the infusion to facilitate patient movement. Upon completion of the infusion, infuse 50 mL of normal saline at the same rate the thrombolytic was infusing to flush the remaining dose from the line. Vital signs are required at least every 15 minutes during the infusion and for 2 hours post-infusion. Best practice dictates an NIHSS assessment every 15 minutes during infusion and for 2 hours post-infusion. Aircraft configuration may make completing an NIHSS difficult. Conduct the most complete neurologic exam possible with a heightened awareness for improvement or deterioration of the patient's symptoms. If deterioration is noted, stop the thrombolytic infusion, and assume the patient has converted to a hemorrhagic stroke. In addition to neurologic changes, symptoms of a hemorrhagic conversion include headache, nausea, and vomiting.

Hemorrhagic Stroke

Hemorrhagic strokes account for the remaining 15% of strokes, which encompasses aneurysm rupture, arteriovenous malformations (AVM) rupture, and intracerebral vessel hemorrhage (ICH). Aneurysms most often rupture in the subarachnoid space causing a subarachnoid hemorrhage (SAH). Bleeding into the brain will cause a sudden onset of symptoms which may include severe headache, nausea, vomiting, and altered level of consciousness from mild impairment to coma. Symptoms of increased intracranial pressure may rapidly develop.[1,3,13]

In the transport environment, a hemorrhagic stroke can be suspected based on symptoms but cannot be confirmed. Once the ABCs are assured, management is focused on limiting further bleeding, reducing intracranial pressure, and reversing anticoagulation if applicable. The American Stroke Association has issued guidelines for the management of hemorrhagic stroke (Box 7.4) and anticoagulant reversal (Table 7.6). Neurology and/or medical control should be consulted before initiating anticoagulant reversal. It is imperative the patient be rapidly transported to the closest facility with neurosurgical capability for definitive care.

Seizure

Seizure is caused by the excessive, dyssynchronous electrical activity within the brain. Epilepsy is just one cause of seizures. Hypoglycemia, traumatic brain injury, tumors, stroke, alcohol withdrawal, hyponatremia, encephalitis, and anoxic brain injury can also cause seizures. Seizure classifications include tonic-clonic, myoclonic, partial, focal, absence, and febrile. Non-convulsive seizures (NCS) present with altered consciousness without motor activity. Status epilepticus is defined as seizure activity lasting longer than 5 minutes, or repeated seizures without return to baseline. It is important to get a detailed description of the seizure activity witnessed by others. Non-medical providers use the word seizure to describe a variety of physical movements, many of which are not seizure activity. For example, the brief nodding of the head and eyes rolling back that precedes syncope is mistakenly described as a seizure.[1-3,14]

Seizures increase cerebral metabolic demand leading to increased CBF. Prolonged seizures can cause hypoglycemia, hyperthermia, cerebral edema, rhabdomyolysis, orthopedic injuries, and death.

During a seizure, the initial priorities are to maintain adequate oxygenation and to prevent patient injury, followed by intervention to stop the seizure. Intravenous lorazepam, midazolam, diazepam, or phenobarbital are recommended as first-line treatment for active seizure. If the patient has no IV access, IM versed should be administered

---

> **BOX 7.4** **Management of Intracranial Hemorrhage**

- Anticoagulant reversal
- Smooth and sustained reduction in blood pressure. Reduce systolic BP to 130–150 mmHg range. Reduction below 130 mmHg may be harmful
- Recombinant factor VII and tranexamic acid have not shown to improve outcome. Maintain nil by mouth
- Monitor blood glucose. Avoid hypoglycemia (<80 mg/dL) and hyperglycemia (<180 mg/dL)
- Maintain normothermia. Manage fever with acetaminophen. Prophylactic seizure medication is not recommended
- Treat seizure activity promptly
- Administer bolus dosing hyperosmolar therapy to reduce increased ICP
- External ventricular drain monitoring of ICP with CSF drainage is recommended for reduction in ICP
- Do not use dextrose-containing IV fluids

From Greenberg SM, Ziai WC, Cordonnier C, et al. Guideline for the management of patients with spontaneous intracerebral hemorrhage: A guideline from the American Heart Association/American Stroke Association. *Stroke.* 2022;53:e.282–e361.

TABLE 7.6	Recommendations for Anticoagulant Reversal in Intracerebral Hemorrhage
Anticoagulant	**Management**
Vitamin K agonist (VKA)	Stop VKA administration INR ≥2.0, 4 factor prothrombin complex concentrate (PCC) is recommended over fresh-frozen plasma (FFP) INR 1.3 to 1.9 PCC is suggested if rapid reversal is required Vitamin K administration after PCC to prevent rebound
Direct Factor Xa inhibitor	Andexanet alpha 4 factor PCC or activated PCC (aPCC)
Dabigatran	Idarucizumab If idarucizumab is unavailable, PCC or aPCC may be considered
Unfractionated heparin	Protamine
Low molecular weight heparin	Protamine

Data from Greenberg SM, Ziai WC, Cordonnier C, et al. 2022 Guideline for the management of patients with spontaneous intracerebral hemorrhage: A guideline from the American Heart Association/American Stroke Association. *Stroke.* 2022;53:e.282–e361.

rather than wait for IV access. Respiratory depression is a primary concern with large doses of benzodiazepines, however, one study showed more respiratory depression in patients receiving a placebo vs. benzodiazepine, indicating the seizure activity itself is a bigger threat to respiratory drive.[1–3,14]

Second-line therapy with an anticonvulsant should be given if seizure activity lasts longer than 20 minutes. Although the results have not yet been published, in the Established Status Epilepticus Treatment Trial, preliminary data suggest there is no superiority of fosphenytoin, valproic acid, or levetiracetam in aborting status epilepticus.[15] The second-line medication should be completed within 20 minutes. If the seizure continues (40 minutes total duration) a third-line anticonvulsant medication is recommended. Notably, third- and fourth-line antiepileptics will be less efficacious. Dilantin is a less favorable option during status epilepticus due to its cardiovascular effects, especially with a rapid infusion.

Paralytic medications are contraindicated in status epilepticus. Motor activity will stop, masking ongoing seizure. If a paralytic is needed for successful intubation, use a short-acting paralytic such as succinylcholine. Succinylcholine is contraindicated in status epilepticus due to the risk of hyperkalemia. If anticonvulsants fail to stop seizure activity, general anesthetic doses of propofol, midazolam, phenobarbital, or inhaled anesthetic gases are the final option. Refractory status epilepticus can be fatal.

Guillain–Barré Syndrome

Guillain–Barré syndrome (GBS) is an immune-mediated neuropathy that carries a very high morbidity and mortality if not identified and treated promptly. GBS is a post-infection disease process with up to 70% of patients reporting an illness within 6 weeks preceding symptom onset. Respiratory and gastrointestinal illnesses are the most frequently reported. There was an increase in GBS cases following the A/H1N1 flu vaccine in 1976, however since then there are reports of one case of GBS for every 1 million doses of flu vaccine administered.

The risk is higher to contract GBS after having flu than from a vaccine. The incidence is slightly higher in males than in females.[3,16]

The disease follows a linear course, usually reaching its peak at approximately 4 weeks. If the symptoms wax and wane or continue to progress longer than 4 weeks an alternative diagnosis should be sought. The most common form of GBS presents as an ascending weakness starting in the lower body and progressing cephalically. Hyporeflexia or areflexia is usually present. Allowed to progress unchecked, GBS will lead to near total paralysis. Cranial nerve involvement leads to dysphagia. Additionally, dysautonomia can cause cardiac arrhythmias and unstable blood pressure. Mechanical ventilation is required in up to 30% of patients.[3,16]

GBS is essentially a diagnosis of exclusion. Nerve conduction studies may help distinguish GBS from other myopathies. Examination of the cerebral spinal fluid will show a normal white blood cell count with an elevated protein level in 80% of patients, but this does not appear until approximately 2 weeks into the disease progression.[3,16]

Intravenous immunoglobulin (IVIg) or plasmapheresis are currently the only two treatments available for GBS. Early treatment initiation can abort the progression of the disease. Early treatment can be completed on an outpatient basis. Roughly 80% of patients treated early will recover full function within 6 months. However, if the disease progresses to the need for mechanical ventilation, the course of the disease can require months of hospitalization and a prolonged recovery.

In the transport environment, the patient will require close monitoring for airway clearance and ineffective ventilation requiring intubation. Cardiac and blood pressure monitoring is required for rapid identification and intervention of dysautonomia.

Amyotrophic Lateral Sclerosis (ALS)

ALS is a fatal neuromuscular disease. Most patients die within 2–5 years from diagnosis. Although the exact pathology is not fully understood, ALS is caused by degeneration of the motor pathways leading to paralysis. It is a diagnosis of exclusion which unfortunately can lead to a prolonged delay in diagnosis. Risk factors include advancing age, family history, and the presence of over 120 identified genetic mutations.[3,17,18]

The most common form involves both upper and lower motor neurons. The initial presentation is complaints of gradual weakness. As the weakness progresses the patient will lose the muscle strength to speak, cough, gag, sneeze, swallow, urinate and defecate. Frontotemporal dementia is present in 20%–50% of patients. Other symptoms that may accompany ALS are hypersalivation, pseudobulbar affect, cognitive impairment, and depression.

There are multiple ongoing studies but there is no cure for ALS. Three medications, riluzole, edaravone, and sodium phenylbutyrate/taurursodiol, have been approved by the FDA. These medications provide a modest benefit in functional decline.

Care is focused on symptom management and palliative care. Depending upon the patient's wishes, a percutaneous feeding tube, noninvasive positive-pressure ventilation, and intubation with mechanical ventilation will eventually be required. Most patients will ultimately succumb to respiratory failure.

Transport clinicians may be called to transport a patient with ALS to a higher level of care or a skilled nursing facility, hospice, or home for comfort care. Airway and ventilation management is the focus of care during transport. For longer-range fixed-wing transports, oral care, positioning, and nutrition may be needed. It is important to understand the patient's care decisions prior to initiating transport. A pre-mission plan is made with the patient of actions to be taken if there is a change in the patient's condition during transport.

Cauda Equina Syndrome

The spinal cord ends at L1 or L2. The cauda equina is a cluster of nerve roots continuing down from the spinal cord. Compression of the cauda equina causes back pain, bilateral leg and foot weakness, urinary retention or incontinence, bowel incontinence, and saddle numbness. Traumatic injury, herniated discs, spinal infections, and malignant tumors are a few of the causes of cauda equina syndrome. Emergently, dexamethasone is administered to reduce inflammation and pain while being transferred for definitive treatment. Surgical decompression within 48 hours of onset improves neurologic recovery from herniation and traumatic injury. Antibiotics are urgently administered for infections. Tumors are rarely primary spinal cord tumors. Rather they are malignant extensions of a primary cancer elsewhere in the body. It is not uncommon for the cauda equina symptoms to prompt the patient to seek care only to discover they have cancer.[1,3]

Decision-Making in Neurologic Emergencies

Neurologic disorders often cause a rapidly progressing deterioration in the patient's condition. If the patient survives the acute insult, the cost to quality of life may be high. The long-term outcome may include persistent coma, ventilator dependence, paralysis and a protracted course ending in death. The transport team helps to determine the patient's/family's wishes for life-prolonging interventions prior to embarking on the patient transport. Is the patient's condition stable enough to handle the stress and stimuli of transport? Does a patient with advancing ALS wish to be intubated or would they prefer palliative care without intubation? Is it ethically and medically sound to transport a patient who is brain dead (Box 7.5) Set the mission up for success by having the difficult conversation and know the expected outcome.[3,13,19,20]

• **BOX 7.5** **Brain Death Testing**

- Irreversible coma with known cause
- Absence of CNS-depressant drugs
- Absence of paralytic drugs
- Normothermia
- No endocrine, electrolyte or metabolic abnormalities
- Systolic BP ≥100 mmHg
- No spontaneous respirations with apnea testing
- Pupils non-reactive
- Absent corneal, gag, cough reflexes
- Oculocephalic reflex absent
- Oculovestibular reflex absent
- Absence of motor response to deep central noxious stimuli (spinal reflexes are permissible)

Summary

Transport teams are dispatched to provide rapid transport of patients with neurologic emergencies. These conditions place a significant burden on quality of life. Morbidity and mortality are high. Prompt recognition of a neurologic emergency and swift intervention by the transport crew throughout the patient mission are necessary for optimal patient outcomes.

References

1. Hartjes TM, ed. *AACN Core Curriculum for Progressive and Critical Care Nursing.* 8th ed. Elsevier; 2023.
2. Hall JE, Hall ME. *Guyton and Hall Textbook of Medical Physiology.* 14th ed. Elsevier; 2021.
3. Hickey JV, Strayer AL, eds. *The Clinical Practice of Neurological and Neurosurgical Nursing.* 8th ed. Wolter Kluwer; 2020.
4. Anestis DM, Tsitsopoulos PP, Tsonidis CA, Foroglou N. The current significance of the FOUR score: a systematic review and critical analysis of the literature. *J Neurol Sci.* 2020;409:116600. doi: 10.1016/j.jns.2019.116600
5. Foo CC, Loan JJM, Brennan PM. The relationship of the FOUR score to patient outcome: a systematic review. *J Neurotrauma.* 2019;36(17):2469–2483. doi: 10.1089/neu.2018.6243
6. Cook AM, Jones GM, Hawryluk GW, et al. Guidelines for the acute treatment of cerebral edema in neurocritical care patients. *Neurocrit Care.* 2020;32(3):647–666.
7. Torbey MT, Bosel J, Rhoney DH, et al. Evidence-based guidelines for the management of large hemispheric infarction. *Neuorcrit Care.* 2015;22:146–164.
8. ASTNA; Holleran RS, Wolfe AC, Frakes MA, eds. *Patient Transport: Principles and Practice.* 5th ed. St. Louis, MO: Elsevier; 2017.
9. Oh S, Delic JJ. Hyperosmolar therapy in the management of intracranial hypertension. *AACN Adv Crit Care.* 2022;33(1):5–10.
10. Centers for Disease Control and Prevention. Stroke Facts. CDC; April 5, 2022. Available at: https://www.cdc/gpve/stroke/facts.htm.
11. Ashcraft S, Wilson S, Nystrom K, Dusenbury W, Wira C. Care of the patient with acute ischemic stroke (prehospital and acute phase of care): update to the 2009 comprehensive nursing care scientific statement. *Stroke.* 2021;52(5):e164-e178. doi: 10.1161/STR.0000000000000356
12. American Stroke Association. *Guidelines for the Early Management of Patients with Acute Ischemic Stroke: 2019 Update to the 2018 Guidelines for the Early Management of Acute Ischemic Stroke.* American Heart Association; 2020.
13. Greenberg SM, Ziai WC, Cordonnier C, et al. 2022 Guideline for the management of patients with spontaneous intracerebral hemorrhage: a guideline from the American Heart Association/American Stoke Association. *Stroke.* 2022;53:e282-e361. doi: 10.1161/STR.0000000000000407
14. Glauser T, Shinnar S, Gloss D, et al. Evidence-based guideline: Treatment of convulsive status epilepticus in children and adults: report of the guideline committee of the American Epilepsy Society. *Epilepsy Curr.* 2016;16(1):48–61.
15. University of Virginia. Established Status Epilepticus Treatment Trial (ESETT) (ClinicalTrials.gov Identifier: NCT01960075). Clinacaltrials.gov. 2021. Available at: https://clinicaltrials.gov/ct2/show/results/NCT01960075?view=results.
16. Nguyen TP, Taylor RS. Guillain Barré Syndrome. In: StatPearls [Internet]. Treasure Island, FL: Stat Pearls Publishing; July 4, 2022. Available at: https://www.ncbi.nlm.nih.gov/books/NBK532254/.
17. Chen JJ. Overview of current and emerging therapies for amyotrophic lateral sclerosis. *Am J Manag Care.* 2020;26(9):S139–S145.
18. Lexicomp. Riverwoods, IL: Wolters Kluwer Health, Inc. Available at: http://online.lexi.com.
19. American Academy of Neurology (AAN). Update: determining brain death in adults. *Neurology.* 2010;74:1911–1918.
20. Omelianchuk A, Bernat J, Caplan A, et al. Revise the Uniform Determination of Death Act to align the law with practice through neurorespiratory criteria. *Neurology.* 2020;98(13):532–536. doi: 10.1212/WNL.0000000000200024

8

Cardiovascular Emergencies

ROGER L. LAYELL

COMPETENCIES

1. Perform a detailed cardiovascular assessment before, during, and after transport.
2. Identify patients with acute cardiac events and provide appropriate treatment.
3. Recognize the potential for lethal events and initiate appropriate interventions.
4. Recognize the pitfalls of invasive hemodynamic monitoring during transport.
5. State specific treatment for patients with acute cardiac events and hemodynamic abnormalities.

Introduction

Cardiovascular emergencies will challenge even the most experienced transport team. Critical care transport of patients with acute cardiovascular events requires rapid assessment and critical thinking skills to provide life-saving treatment. The demand for medical transport of patients who are dependent on invasive devices and new sophisticated technology has continued to increase over time.[1] This chapter describes advances in clinical care for patients with acute coronary syndromes (ACS) including acute myocardial infarction (AMI), cardiogenic shock, heart failure (HF), aortic dissection, and other manifestations of cardiovascular disease, with a focus on assessment and management relative to the medical transport environment.

Individuals experiencing acute cardiac events, decompensated HF, or an aortic dissection in a small, isolated, resource-limited, community-based hospital often require rapid critical care transfer to a tertiary care facility for further evaluation and emergent intervention. Transport of these critically ill patients involves several issues unique to the transport environment, which include the potential effects of altitude and the difficulty associated with the initiation of resuscitative interventions in a limited space and uncontrolled environment, such as in an aircraft or in the back of a transport vehicle.

Alterations of Cardiovascular Physiology at High Altitudes

One of the greatest threats to patients with cardiovascular disease is hypoxia. Decompensation of patients with acute cardiovascular disease during transport at high altitudes is generally caused by hypoxic hypoxia, which is defined as an oxygen deficiency in the body tissues, sufficient enough to cause impaired function.[1,2] Individual patient tolerances vary, but patients with cardiac disease are usually at risk for compromise when the cabin pressure exceeds 6000 feet. Physiologic changes occur as barometric pressure decreases, resulting in a lower partial pressure of oxygen. This reduction in the amount of oxygen in the blood decreases oxygen availability to the tissues. As altitude increases, the availability of oxygen for gas exchange decreases, causing a reduction in oxygen saturation. Compensatory mechanisms are activated in an effort to maintain adequate oxygen delivery to the tissues. These include increases in heart rate (HR), respiratory rate, and cardiac output (CO). This increased workload on the heart increases myocardial oxygen consumption and necessitates the need for increased blood flow to the heart muscle.

In healthy individuals, cardiac reserve allows the body to compensate for reduced blood flow to the tissues by altering HR and stroke volume (SV). Blood flow to the heart muscle is also increased by dilating the coronary artery microvasculature. Cardiovascular disease may limit a patient's ability to maximize CO in response to an increase in oxygen demand. Patients with coronary artery disease (CAD) who are unable to compensate for the increased workload imposed on the heart because of decreased oxygen tension at high altitudes may experience chest pain, cardiac dysrhythmias, HF, pulmonary edema, or even cardiac arrest.[2–4]

Supplemental oxygen should be given to patients during transport when indicated. The current 2020 American Heart Association (AHA) Guidelines Update for Cardiopulmonary Resuscitation and Emergency Cardiovascular Care continues to recommend arterial oxygen saturation (SaO_2) of greater than 93%.[5] The potential detrimental effects of altitude can be minimized by administering supplemental oxygen and aircraft pressurization at higher altitudes. In fixed-wing transport, limiting cabin altitude to a maximum of 6000 feet has been shown to eliminate problems for patients with cardiovascular disease.[3] Cabin pressure is not a fixed variable and may need to be adjusted to accommodate the patient's condition. Cabin pressure can be adjusted to as low as sea level; however, a decrease in cabin pressure may come at the expense of travel time at a lower altitude. Flights at lower altitudes may result in decreased speeds and therefore longer flights with an increased need for refueling stops during the trip. This will lengthen the time a patient is out of a controlled environment.

Decisions regarding altitude restrictions or limitations must be based on patient history, current clinical condition, and pilot-in-command expertise and judgment. These decisions need to be evaluated throughout the mission and may need to be adjusted as a result of continued in-flight patient surveillance.[3,6,7]

Special Considerations for Cardiopulmonary Resuscitation in the Transport Environment

Cardiac arrest is of special concern to those involved in the transport of critically ill patients. Cardiopulmonary resuscitation (CPR) in the confined space of an aircraft cabin or ground transport vehicle is both difficult and challenging. Advanced cardiac life support (ACLS) guidelines are used as the standard of practice for resuscitation of the patient in cardiac arrest by most transport programs.[5] Team members are expected to have current verification of ACLS skills through the AHA to participate in patient care within the transport environment.[5–7] Detailed pre-transport assessment, planning, and intervention along with prompt correction of dysrhythmias, repletion of electrolytes, and continuous maintenance of adequate oxygenation and ventilation may help to prevent the need for resuscitation during transport.

Transport teams must maintain a state of perpetual readiness for emergencies such as cardiac arrest. Preparation includes ensuring the proper functioning of resuscitation equipment and that an adequate oxygen supply is readily available. ACLS drugs should be well labeled, not expired, and ready for quick administration. Generally, the number of crew members available to perform basic and advanced life support resuscitation is limited to only two medically trained personnel. Resuscitation roles and responsibilities must be well defined for effective and rapid response during an emergency.[8]

Cardiopulmonary Resuscitation and Defibrillation During Transport

High-quality CPR and defibrillation are the two interventions that have been shown to increase neurologically intact survival.[9]

High-quality, uninterrupted CPR is essential for improved survival from cardiac arrest. Manual chest compressions remain the standard of care for the treatment of cardiac arrest.[9] The performance of manual CPR during out-of-hospital cardiac arrest is often suboptimal and affects survival.[10,11] Providing high-quality, effective CPR in a moving ambulance or in an aircraft during a flight can be challenging and often dangerous for the providers. Transport personnel should aim to provide the best-quality CPR possible within the constraints and limitations of their operating environment. The 2020 AHA Guidelines Update for Cardiopulmonary Resuscitation and Emergency Cardiovascular Care identifies specific settings in which the use of mechanical CPR devices may be considered as a strategy for delivering high-quality compressions during CPR.[5] Specific settings identified include prolonged CPR, situations in which the number of rescuers is limited, during hypothermic cardiac arrest, in the angiography suite, during preparation for extracorporeal CPR, and in moving ambulances.[5,12] In these guidelines, the AHA stresses the importance of limiting interruptions in CPR during deployment and removal of these devices.

There are many benefits to using mechanical CPR devices in the resource-challenged, transport environment. Mechanical CPR can improve the consistency of chest compressions (rate and depth), minimize interruptions in chest compressions, reduce rescuer fatigue during prolonged resuscitation, and allow for CPR to continue during patient transfer.[12] The use of these devices will allow providers to complete other necessary tasks and eliminate the safety concerns related to the performance of CPR by an unrestrained crew in a moving vehicle or aircraft. The use of these devices requires a commitment to training and quality review.[8]

Special consideration should be given to transport vehicle configuration in anticipation of the potential need for CPR and resuscitation during transport. The position and height of the stretcher in relation to the transport crew is important. It must allow the crew the ability to change positions, facilitating proper hand and arm positioning during chest compressions. A well-designed configuration minimizes the need for crew members to extend or release restraint devices during the administration of therapeutic interventions.[6,7]

Defibrillation During Transport

The most critical factor in the determination of the success of a resuscitative effort is time to restoration of effective spontaneous circulation.[9–11] Immediate defibrillation is the priority in the treatment of confirmed ventricular fibrillation (VF) and pulseless ventricular tachycardia (VT).[5,9–11] The close-quarters, metallic composition of transport vehicles, and proximity of vital electronic equipment, particularly in the rotor-wing environment, previously generated concern among transport personnel about the safety of defibrillation in this environment. Holleran addressed the potential electrical risks of airborne defibrillation and showed that defibrillation with modern equipment in a medically equipped twin-engine helicopter is safe.[6] Despite cramped quarters and sensitive electrical equipment, defibrillation can be performed without hesitation, whether the aircraft is on the ground or in the air, provided that standard defibrillation precautions are observed. The transport crew should use self-adhesive defibrillation pads and follow the ACLS defibrillation standards for the selection of energy levels.[5] The crew should inform the pilot before defibrillation and maintain clearance from the patient and stretcher when discharging the current.

Temporary Pacing During Transport

Temporary pacing is used when the heart's normal conduction system fails to produce myocardial contraction, resulting in hemodynamic instability.[13] It is indicated when a patient's HR is too slow or too high to maintain adequate CO, or in those at risk for developing significant bradycardias. The purpose of pacing is to reestablish normal hemodynamics in a compromised heart that is beating either too fast or too slow. During transport, transcutaneous pacing may be used until a transvenous pacemaker can be inserted. Ventricular pacing is used more often in emergent situations, but atrial or atrioventricular (AV) sequential may be indicated in some settings.[13]

Transcutaneous Pacing

Transcutaneous pacing (TCP) is indicated for many types of dysrhythmias in the transport setting. Atrioventricular blocks are a common cause of symptomatic bradycardia and can result from the following etiologies: infections, inflammation, ischemia, degenerative, metabolic, and vagotonic responses resulting in increased vagal tone.[14,15]

TCP provides immediate, temporary pacing during critical situations, without the risks associated with placing an invasive pacemaker. It is an external, rapid, noninvasive, and time-saving method to pace the heart.[13] This temporary method stimulates ventricular myocardial depolarization through the chest wall via two large electrodes that are placed on the anterior and posterior chest wall or on the anterior and left lateral positions. These are placed in addition to the standard electrodes placed for cardiac monitoring. These patches are attached by a cable to an external pulse generator. Energy (milliamps [mA]) is delivered to the myocardium via the external pulse generator based on the set rate, sensitivity, and output. TCP is a quick method for pacing, but it also requires a significant amount of energy to achieve capture and successful pacing of the heart. Patient discomfort is common and will require the use of medications for pain and sedation. The reliability of TCP is dependent on the skin-to-pad contact and the thoracic impedance that must be overcome during pacing. Because of these limitations, TCP should only be considered as a temporary method of pacing until a more definitive treatment with a transvenous or permanent pacemaker can be achieved. TCP should be performed according to current ACLS protocols.[5]

TCP requires electromechanical capture which occurs when the pacer stimulus produces a myocardial contraction. This is evidenced by the presence of a pulse associated with a QRS seen on the electrocardiogram (ECG). The patient will receive no benefit if electrical and mechanical capture is not occurring. Typically, it has been taught that mechanical capture is verified by the presence of a carotid or radial pulse, but the clinician needs to be sure that they are palpating a pulse and not a pseudo pulse produced by muscle twitching resulting from the pacer stimulus. One of the most definitive ways of verifying mechanical capture from TCP would be the presence of an arterial line waveform.[14] However, the next best verification of mechanical capture is by the presence of heart tones. Heart tones can be assessed with auscultation of a stethoscope or by Doppler in the transport setting. Heart tones are produced by the opening and closing of valves due to pressure differential changes. Additionally, utilizing the waveform plethysmograph from the oxygen saturation monitor can allow for monitoring of mechanical capture during transport when evaluating for heart tones is not possible.[13] A plethysmograph can measure variations in volume inside an organ or the entire body. The pulse oximeter is able to measure the amount of hemoglobin that is presumably saturated with oxygen. The photoplethysmograph is a plethysmograph utilizing optical techniques and is also a pulse oximeter that quantifies oxygen saturation levels. This device is capable of quantifying the arterial blood volume with each beat.

External pacemakers are typically programmed to default to the synchronous mode, allowing the transcutaneous pacemaker to effectively support the patient's underlying rhythm. The synchronous mode is a demand mode that fires only when a QRS complex is not sensed within a specific time range. Alternatively, the asynchronous mode is a fixed mode that will fire regardless of the patient's native intrinsic rhythm.[13]

Transvenous Pacing

Transvenous pacing is indicated when more prolonged pacing is required.[15] It is commonly used for short-term management of symptomatic bradycardias, either as a bridge to permanent pacing or for self-limited bradycardias. Transvenous pacing is more reliable than TCP because a pacer lead is directly in contact with the myocardium. This method of pacing is more reliable than TCP but requires the placement of pacing wires by an experienced physician. A pacing lead wire is inserted through a vein into the right atrium or right ventricle.[15] Once inserted, the lead wires are attached to a battery-operated, external pulse generator. The transport crew should become familiar with the types of transvenous pacemakers that are used by local hospitals.

Before leaving the referring facility, the pacemaker setting should be verified. These settings include the rate, sensitivity (mV), and output (mA). Mechanical capture should be confirmed by the presence of a pulse. Problems encountered during transvenous pacing include lead disconnection from the generator and battery failure. Additional batteries should be taken on all transports. The transport crew must know how to reattach loosened lead wires and how to change the battery of the pacemaker if warranted during transport.[6,7]

Complications that may be encountered during transport include sensing problems, failure to capture, myocardial penetration, and cardiac tamponade. Pacemaker malfunctions include failure to sense or failure to capture. Under-sensing or failure to sense occurs when the pacemaker does not see the native cardiac activity and pacing occurs randomly in the middle of, or after, a P wave or QRS complex. It may be caused by malposition of the catheter, poor intracardiac signal quality, or generator malfunction. Under-sensing is managed by turning the sensitivity setting of the pulse generator to the full-demand position.[13] Oversensing, which results in pauses in the paced rhythm, can result from sensing of atrial electrical activity if the pacing lead is positioned near the tricuspid valve, from sensing of T waves; or from sensing voltage transients that are the result of lead wire fracture, environmental influences, or signals from the generator. The problem of oversensing can be resolved by turning the sensitivity setting toward the asynchronous position until the unwanted signals are no longer sensed.[13] Failure to sense will cause the pacer to fire regardless of the patient's underlying rhythm which can possibly result in an R-on-T phenomenon. Simply put, this means the synchronous pacer is now delivering pacer spikes in an asynchronous type of fashion.

Failure to capture during transvenous pacing can be related to the patient's clinical condition or to the mechanics of the pacing unit. Clinical conditions resulting in loss of capture include acidosis, hypoxia, antiarrhythmic drugs, and electrolyte imbalances. Mechanical causes of loss of capture include poor endocardial contact, lead fracture or dislodgment, or myocardial perforation. The pacer output (mA) should be increased while the underlying cause is identified and treated. Most authors suggest setting the output to three times the initial threshold to prevent later loss of capture. Failure to capture can be related to a malposition of the lead, resulting in poor endocardial contact, catheter dislodgment, fracture, or to an increase in the myocardial stimulation threshold. It is identified by a pacing spike on the ECG without a P wave or QRS complex. To resolve this problem, the current output should be increased until consistent capture occurs. If electrolyte imbalance is the underlying problem, then it should be corrected. The position of the lead should be checked and repositioned if necessary.

Myocardial penetration or perforation can occur when the pacing wire is inadvertently placed into the pericardial sac. This can be identified by a pericardial friction rub and often a squeaking systolic sound or murmur.[15] If the pacing wire has migrated, it should be repositioned. If cardiac tamponade occurs in association with perforation, immediate pericardiocentesis should be performed. If a pericardiocentesis is not in your scope of practice, continue aggressive fluid resuscitation.

Targeted Temperature Management

The new AHA guidelines recommend that targeted temperature management should be used in comatose, adult patients who achieve the return of spontaneous circulation after cardiac arrest.[5] Comatose patients are defined as those without any meaningful response to verbal commands. A constantly maintained temperature between 32°C and 36°C is recommended for at least 24 hours.[9–11] The induction of this mild-to-moderate hypothermia in comatose patients after cardiac arrest has been shown to be beneficial with improved neurologic outcomes and reduced mortality.[9,11] Currently, the routine prehospital administration of cold intravenous (IV) fluids is not recommended because available evidence suggests there is no direct benefit and that there may be some potentially harmful effects.[5,9,10,16]

Acute Coronary Syndrome

ACS comprises a spectrum of clinical conditions caused by varying degrees of coronary artery occlusion. The three presentations of ACS include unstable angina, acute non–ST-elevation MI (NSTEMI), and acute ST-elevation MI (STEMI).[17] ACS may result from a variety of conditions in which coronary arteries are narrowed or occluded by clots, plaque (fat), or spasm. Any of these syndromes may cause sudden cardiac death.[17,18]

Pathophysiologic Factors

An abrupt change in the caliber of a coronary artery can occur as a result of a coronary blood vessel spasm or the abrupt worsening of an atherosclerotic plaque. Atherosclerotic plaques can suddenly become more narrowed because of the formation of an atheroma in the wall of the vessel or the formation of a thrombus on the surface of a damaged plaque.[19]

ACS begins with a disruption of the endothelium overlying an atherosclerotic lesion. Lesions more likely to be involved in ACS are the mild-to-moderate lesions with thin fibrous tissue caps. The continuum of unstable angina, acute NSTEMI, and acute STEMI is, in truth, a varying degree of the same underlying problem: a mild-to-moderate lipid-laden atherosclerotic plaque that suddenly ruptures exposing the underlying cholesterol gruel to the circulating blood and setting in place multiple mechanisms that attempt to repair the damaged vessel wall.[20] Platelets, once activated, bind to exposed areas of the vessel wall. More platelets are drawn to the area, and the activated platelets begin to bind to each other via receptors on their surface, known as glycoprotein IIb/IIIa receptors. The activation of platelets during this process causes a release of regulatory substances, which cause further aggregation of platelets and vasoconstriction. Platelet activation also leads to the secretion of vasoconstriction substances, which limit blood flow in the affected coronary artery.[21] At the same time, the clotting cascade is activated, leading to the formation of thrombin. Thrombin is a potent stimulant of platelet activation and is responsible for the conversion of fibrinogen in the bloodstream to fibrin. As platelets accumulate in the area, a platelet plug forms, which itself can intermittently occlude flow in the coronary. As this mass of platelets becomes organized, fibrin interconnects, resulting in the formation of a stable blood clot, or thrombus.[20]

Once platelets have aggregated on the surface of the ruptured plaque, the competition between antithrombotic and thrombotic processes in the body becomes intense. The vessel may reocclude at any time or heal without further symptoms, or the ruptured plaque/platelet plug may be incorporated into the atherosclerotic plaque, contributing to the progressive growth of atherosclerotic CAD.[21]

The degree to which a coronary artery is occluded and whether or not it remains occluded by this process subsequently determines in which part of the continuum of ACS an event is classified. For example:

1. One event is unstable angina caused by an acute change in the caliber of a coronary artery resulting from plaque rupture and thrombus formation.[21] If transient occlusion of a coronary artery by activated platelets at the site of a ruptured plaque occurs with subsequent recanalization of the vessel, the patient may be symptomatic at rest (while the coronary is occluded) and have symptoms that resolve spontaneously with re-cannulation of the vessel. Transient ECG changes may occur while the patient is symptomatic, but the episode is often too short to show either ECG changes or evidence of myocardial injury.

2. An event classified as an NSTEMI infarction begins in the same manner, but either occlusion of the coronary is prolonged (with myocardial necrosis) or distal embolization of small platelet clumps occurs, leading to occlusion of smaller distal coronary branches and therefore myocardial necrosis. Spontaneous recanalization may occur, but biochemical evidence of myocardial necrosis is found (troponin, CPK-MB). In both of these instances, a significantly narrowed coronary artery (although recanalized) remains, and therapy is aimed at keeping the activated platelets present on the artery surface from progressing into a stable thrombus.

3. Acute STEMI represents the syndrome of acute plaque rupture, which continues to its ultimate endpoint, an organized thrombus made up of activated platelets with cross-linked fibrin, resulting in a stable thrombus. These patients have continued chest pain and associated ST segment elevation because of injury caused by total occlusion of coronary blood flow. At this point, therapy must be aimed at immediate reperfusion.

Diagnosis, Assessment, and Treatment

The diagnosis of ACS is based on patient presentation, serum markers of cardiac injury, and findings on a 12-lead ECG. It is important to exclude other nonischemic causes of chest pain including aortic dissection, esophageal rupture, and pulmonary embolism.[18]

The initial assessment should include an evaluation of chest pain and other associated signs and symptoms. Chest pain can be evaluated by using the OPQRST mnemonic. This involves assessing onset, provocation and palliation, quality, radiation, site, and time course. A quick, focused examination should be done by transport crews to determine the presence of other conditions that may complicate the management of these patients. These include evaluation for HF, cardiogenic shock, or other causes of hemodynamic compromise. A 12-lead ECG should quickly be obtained to determine whether ECG changes consistent with ACS are present.

ECG changes indicative of unstable angina or NSTEMI include ST depression and inverted T waves, without the presence of Q waves. ECG changes seen with STEMI include ST elevation ≥1 mm in two contiguous leads or ≥2 mm in V1 and V2.[5] The Smith–Modified Sgarbossa criteria is utilized in identifying STEMI in patients with preexisting left bundle branch block (LBBB). The Smith–Modified Sgarbossa criteria provide a sensitivity of 80% and specificity of 99% when analyzed against the original Sgarbossa criteria which only produced a sensitivity of 20% and specificity of 98%.[22] The Smith–Modified Sgarbossa criteria for diagnosis of an AMI in the setting of a preexisting LBBB requires the following three criteria to make the diagnosis: (1) One lead or more with concordant ST segment elevation of at least 1 mm; (2) one lead or more in leads V1–V3 with concordant ST segment depression; (3) one lead or more with at least 1 mm of ST segment elevation and corresponding excessive discordant ST elevation as delineated by ST segment elevation of greater than 25% of the depth of the antecedent S-wave.[22] If any of these criteria are met the sensitivity is 80% and the specificity is 99% in satisfying the diagnostic values for the identification of an acute MI in a preexisting LBBB.[22] Laboratory values including electrolytes, coagulation studies, hemoglobin and hematocrit, and cardiac biomarkers including troponin and CPK-MB should be reviewed for abnormalities.

Treatment goals in ACS include quick identification of the cause of the chest discomfort and aggressive management using evidence-based interventions.[18] Initial management involves rapid assessment and treatment of airway, breathing, and circulation (ABCs). Continuous cardiac monitoring, oxygen saturation, supplemental oxygen, as indicated, and IV access should always be continued during transport. The current 2020 AHA Guidelines Update for Cardiopulmonary Resuscitation and Emergency Cardiovascular Care continues to recommend an arterial oxygen saturation of greater than 93%.[5] Cardiac dysrhythmias should be treated according to ACLS protocols. Combi-pads should be placed and available for defibrillation and pacing if needed. Resuscitation equipment and emergency medications should also be readily available.

Immediate treatment of ACS includes the administration of oxygen, aspirin, nitroglycerin (NTG), and morphine as outlined in the ACS ACLS protocol.[5,18] A major goal in the treatment of ACS is to augment the anticoagulant properties that the body possesses and to interfere with the clot formation process. ACSs begin primarily as a process mediated by activated platelets; therefore, therapeutic strategies are aimed at inhibition of platelets and interference with platelet-to-platelet interactions. Initial pharmacologic treatment begins with the administration of 325 mg of non–enteric-coated aspirin (ASA). Aspirin is a potent inhibitor of thromboxane, a stimulated platelet aggregation. Aspirin has clearly been shown to decrease MI and death in patients who present to the hospital with ACS.[18]

NTG works by relaxing vascular smooth muscle, leading to both arterial and venous vasodilatation. Venodilatation results in decreased preload and a decrease in ventricular wall tension. Arterial vasodilatation leads to a decrease in systemic blood pressure (BP). These actions work to decrease myocardial oxygen consumption and demand. Coronary vasodilatation also occurs, leading to increased myocardial oxygen supply. Initially, three sublingual NTG tablets (0.4 mg) or one to two sprays are given under the tongue every 3–5 minutes for ongoing symptoms as tolerated by the patient or until the pain is relieved. A nitroglycerin infusion is usually initiated if the pain is not relieved by initial sublingual

doses (unless contraindicated). The infusion dose of nitroglycerin is based on your program's protocols. NTG is contraindication if a phosphodiesterase inhibitor has been taken within the last 24–36 hours depending on the specific medication.[23] It should be used with extreme caution in patients with an inferior wall MI with right ventricular (RV) infarction, hypotension (systolic BP [SBP] <90 mmHg), tachycardia, and bradycardia.

Morphine or fentanyl, which are narcotic analgesic agents, may also be used to treat the pain associated with ACS. Usually, 2–4 mg IV is given with repeated doses as indicated for ongoing chest pain per individual program protocols. Morphine helps to decrease the workload on the heart by reducing sympathetic stimulation caused by pain and anxiety.

Other medications that may be used for the treatment of ACS include beta-blockers, heparin, and glycoprotein IIb/IIIa inhibitors. Beta-blockers work by decreasing myocardial oxygen demand. These agents interrupt sympathetic impulses by competing with the neurotransmitter norepinephrine at the beta-sympathetic nerve endings. Beta-receptor inhibition results in decreased HR, decreased myocardial contractility, and slowed impulse transmission through the cardiac conduction system. These effects lead to decreased myocardial oxygen consumption. In addition, beta-blockers decrease MI size and improve survival rates because of a decreased incidence of myocardial rupture and VF.[22]

Heparin is a potent anticoagulant that augments the body's ability to reduce thrombin generation and fibrin formation. Heparin does not dissolve a clot that has already formed; however, it does halt the propagation of existing clots or any new clots. Clinical evidence supports the use of heparin in ACSs.[18] The transport team should follow individual program protocols.

The glycoprotein IIb/IIIa receptors on the surface of platelets are responsible for the attachment of platelets to one another. Drugs that inhibit this process block the common final pathway of platelet aggregation; therefore, they are inhibitors of the formation of thrombus. The agents currently in use, such as abciximab, eptifibatide, and tirofiban, all have different mechanisms of action, dosing strategies, and half-lives. A review of these drugs is not included because it is beyond the intended scope of this chapter. These medications, which have become an important part of the treatment of patients with ACSs, should be familiar to transport personnel. Current AHA 2020 guidelines recommend the use of glycoprotein IIb/IIIa inhibitors in addition to aspirin and heparin for patients with an NSTEMI or refractory ischemia.[5]

Acute Myocardial Infarction

Assessment and Diagnosis

According to the AHA/ACC/ESC/WHF acute myocardial infarctions can be categorized as either type 1 or type 2. Atherosclerotic plaque rupture is responsible for type 1 myocardial infarctions.[24] The criteria for detecting type 1 myocardial infarctions include observation in the oscillations of cTn ranges with at least one reading above the 99th percentile and at least one of the following additional findings: manifestations of new-onset myocardial ischemia, recently developed ischemic electrocardiographic changes, the evolution of pathologic Q waves. Additionally, imaging affirmation of new forfeiture of workable myocardium or regional wall movement malformation in a fashion harmonious with ischemic physiology.[24]

The criteria for the detection of type 2 myocardial infarctions include the following: oscillations of the cTn values with a minimum of one value greater than the 99th percentile URL with evidence of myocardial oxygen demand superseding the supply not pertaining to coronary thrombosis requiring a minimum of one of the following: manifestations of new-onset myocardial ischemia; recently developed ischemic electrocardiographic changes; the evolution of pathologic Q waves.[24] Just as seen with type 1, type 2 must have additional imaging affirmation of new forfeiture of workable myocardium or regional wall movement malformation in a fashion harmonious with ischemic physiology.[24]

An acute myocardial infarction occurs because of coronary artery occlusion from a thrombus forming on the surface of a ruptured atherosclerotic plaque. When flow no longer exists in the coronary artery, the entire distribution of that coronary artery is at risk for injury or myocardial cell death. Initially, that wall of the heart becomes stiff and then stops moving, which results in a loss of left ventricular ejection fraction, potentially leading to significant valvular dysfunction and ventricular arrhythmias. The length of interruption in coronary blood flow will determine the resultant extent of myocardial injury and damage.

The cardiac blood supply is made up of three principal coronary arteries supplying nutrients during diastole. These vessels, the first branches off of the aorta, originate from the coronary ostia at the level of the aortic valve cusps. The left main coronary artery divides into the left anterior descending (LAD) and the left circumflex arteries. The LAD supplies the anterior surface of the heart, the anterior two-thirds of the septum, and part of the lateral wall. The LAD distribution is represented on the surface ECG in the V or chest leads. The circumflex coronary artery supplies branches to the lateral and posterior surfaces of the heart. The circumflex is not well represented on the standard ECG. Changes caused by ischemia or infarction in the circumflex coronary artery may be seen in the lateral (I, aVL, and V5, V6) leads or in the posterior wall by inference from changes in the V1, V2, and V3 leads, which appear as ST segment depression that is actually elevation on the posterior surface of the heart.

In 85% of patients, the right coronary artery (RCA) supplies blood to the inferior surface of the heart and to the posterior third of the interventricular septum by way of one of its branches, the posterior descending coronary artery. These areas of the heart are represented on the ECG as the inferior leads which are II, III, and aVF. On the way to the inferior surface of the heart, the RCA is also responsible for supplying blood flow to the right ventricle. When an inferior wall MI is seen it is important to do a right-sided 12-lead ECG to search for the concurrent presence of an RV infarct because the RV is also supplied by the RCA. If an RV infarct is present, ST elevation will be seen in V4R. The maintenance of RV preload, with the administration of fluids, is the initial therapy for support of RV infarction. Positive inotropic agents, such as dobutamine or milrinone, may be indicated to augment the contractility of the damaged RV.[25] Nitrates and other drugs that decrease preload should be used with caution because they may cause decreased CO and BP.

ECG changes seen with STEMI include ST elevation greater than or equal to 1 mm in two contiguous leads (leads that represent an area of the heart that is supplied by a single coronary), or greater than or equal to 2 mm in V2 and V3. A full discussion of 12-lead interpretation is beyond the scope of this chapter. Ongoing chest pain associated with 12-lead ECG changes that show ST segment elevation in contiguous leads known as an acute injury pattern together makes the diagnosis of an AMI. ST segment elevation on the ECG represents ischemia, injury, and subsequent myocardial cell necrosis in the area of the occluded coronary artery.[26]

Initial assessment of patients with suspected AMI should include a detailed history, evaluation of chest pain and other associated signs and symptoms, and assessment for other concurrent conditions that could complicate management such as HF or cardiogenic shock. Chest pain can be quickly evaluated by using the OPQRST mnemonic. Patients who present with an AMI describe chest heaviness, discomfort, or pressure, often associated with shortness of breath (SOB), diaphoresis, nausea, and vomiting. The discomfort may radiate to the neck, jaw, or arms. Excessive sympathetic stimulation may result in an elevated BP and an increased HR. The patient should be evaluated for the presence of an S3, rales, or distended neck veins, which indicate the presence of HF caused by either severe left ventricular failure from the AMI or flash pulmonary edema resulting from the acute onset of severe mitral regurgitation.[27] The patient should also be evaluated for contraindications for specific types of therapy such as fibrinolytic administration.

Cardiac troponin is a molecular marker released when myocardial cells become damaged, therefore identifying myocardial tissue decay. Troponin is a predictable molecular marker for distinguishing those patients who are highly probable to have negative consequences when acute myocardial infarction is suspected.[28] The evolution of the high-sensitivity troponin assay permits the recognition of minor myocardial insults, therefore increasing the probability of identifying discreet myocardial infarctions.[29] Evidence has shown that high-sensitive cardiac troponin levels are higher in men than in women.[30] A patient with non–ST-elevation myocardial infarction will display inconsistent molecular marker concentrations and fluctuations, even when using the same high-sensitive troponin testing. This occurs due to high-sensitive troponin levels being dependent upon the patient's age, sex, and any pre-existing comorbidities.[31] The American College of Cardiology (ACC) and American Heart Association (AHA) provides a Class I recommendation to measure cardiac troponin in subjects with chest pain and further endorses the use of high-sensitive cardiac troponin assays.[32]

Atypical Symptoms

Atypical symptoms can include but are not limited to abdominal, back, or urinary complaints, dyspnea, central nervous system concerns, and even nonspecific problems.[33,34] The typical symptoms of an acute myocardial infarction include sudden onset of substernal chest discomfort, accompanied by diaphoresis, and radiating pain to the neck, back, jaw, and left arm. However, subtle atypical symptoms can be present in women, diabetic and/or elderly patients, and others that can sometimes go unnoticed.[35–39] Atypical symptoms of acute myocardial infarction occur more often in women than in men, leading to a delay in the diagnosis and treatment of these women compared to men.[33,35] These atypical symptoms include complaints of acid reflux or back pain.[33–35] Women and diabetics may present with unexplained belching which is indicative of an inferior wall myocardial infarction.[37–39] Patients at risk for presenting with atypical chest pain include those with a history of high blood pressure, chronic kidney disease, and a history of myocardial infarction. Patients with risk factors for atypical chest pain should be evaluated when presenting with unexplained nonexertional dyspnea. Female patients, especially elderly, are more prone to presenting with atypical chest pain when having an acute myocardial event.[33,35] Hiccups, which are usually considered harmless and self-resolving, may become persistent or intractable and are often overlooked as an underlying cardiovascular-related symptom.[36–39] The 12-lead electrocardiogram continues as the first-line diagnostic tool for predicting myocardial infarction, due to its ease of access and application.[34]

STEMI Equivalents

STEMI equivalents are electrocardiographic findings that can identify patients that are in the pre-infarction phase of a serious myocardial infarction.[40] Earlier identification of STEMI equivalents often allows for early intervention which can prevent myocardial damage. One major difference between a STEMI equivalent and an acute STEMI is that these findings can be identified in a patient who is asymptomatic.[40] Wellen's syndrome is considered a warning sign for a consequential proximal left anterior descending coronary artery stenosis, potentially resulting in a substantial anterior wall infarct if undetected.[41] Wellen's syndrome is identified on the 12-lead ECG by deep, wide, inverted downsloping of the T-waves in lead V1–V4, signaling myocardial ischemia.[41]

DeWinter T-waves are another pre-infarction indicator involving the proximal left anterior descending artery; however, the morphology of the T-wave is slightly different from those observed in Wellen's syndrome. When DeWinter T-waves are present there will be concave upward sloping of at least 1 mm within the depressed ST segment. Again, these findings will be identified in leads V1–V4 with the upward sloping beginning at the J-point with uniform tall and remarkable T-waves.[41]

According to the Fourth Universal Definition of Myocardial Infarction, lead aVR is allocated as a STEMI equivalent when there is ST segment elevation, along with certain additional repolarization patterns.[24] When there is ST segment elevation in lead aVR, this suggests ischemia of the entire myocardium, often correlated to obstructive coronary artery disease.[42] The presence of ST segment elevation in either lead aVR and/or V1, along with six other surface leads, having greater than 1 mm of ST segment depression, is classified as a STEMI equivalent.[42]

Management of AMI

Management of acute myocardial infarction has dramatically changed over the last decade because of improvements in pharmacologic support, hemodynamic monitoring, mechanical and surgical support, and the development of ventricular assist devices (VADs). Once the diagnosis of an AMI is clear, it should immediately prompt the decision of reperfusion therapy with primary angioplasty and associated pharmacologic therapy.

In AMI patients, the preferred reperfusion strategy is the restoration of the normal blood flow in the infarct-related artery using primary percutaneous coronary intervention (PCI). It is recommended that fibrinolytic agents be used if PCI is unavailable in patients within 120 minutes without contraindications to the use of these drugs.[18]

Critical care transport is essential for the rapid transport of these patients to tertiary institutions with angioplasty facilities. Acknowledgment of the presence of an AMI in the pre-hospital setting or at a referring institution should prompt the receiving institution to activate its cardiac catheterization laboratory staff. This process can be facilitated by transport personnel who can take AMI patients directly to the cardiac catheterization laboratory to reduce the "door to catheter" time. Direct physician-to-physician contact and the timely fax of electrocardiographic results can avoid unnecessary delays in reperfusion therapy.

As with the other types of acute coronary syndrome, an AMI begins as a platelet problem but evolves into a process that ends in the formation of a thrombus through the formation and infiltration of the platelet plug by fibrin cross-links. The initial treatment goals are therefore similar to those for other ACS conditions. The use of aspirin, heparin, and glycoprotein IIb/IIIa inhibitors in addition to a definitive reperfusion strategy, such as emergent angioplasty, are the basic concepts of AMI therapy. Fibrinolytic therapy destroys fibrin in the intracoronary thrombus. In doing so, activated platelets are released from the thrombus. These activated platelets can reassemble and reocclude the vessel if adjunctive anticoagulation and antiplatelet strategies are not used. Oral antiplatelets will also be given in addition to ASA, including clopidogrel, ticagrelor, and prasugrel.

Agents such as beta-blockers, NTG, and morphine sulfate for pain control are important to decrease myocardial oxygen demand. In patients with adequate BP, IV morphine sulfate and IV NTG therapy can be used for pain control. Beta-blockers (metoprolol) can help decrease myocardial oxygen demand in the patient with no contraindication (i.e., severe congestive HF, bradycardia, or diffuse wheezing).

Emergency *coronary artery bypass grafting (CABG) surgery* is performed in the setting of an AMI for patients with severe left main disease, failed angioplasty, and multivessel CAD not amenable to percutaneous revascularization. The time needed to activate a pump team and to place patients on bypass limits CABG as an initial strategy for reperfusion. Critical care transfer of these patients via air or ground is essential, and the transport crew should be knowledgeable and skilled in the care of these challenging patients.

Dysrhythmias

Serious electrical abnormalities of the HR and rhythm are classified as dysrhythmias.[43] The function of the heart's electrical system is to transmit electrical impulses from the sinoatrial node (SA) to the atria and ventricles, causing contraction and delivery of blood to the lungs and body.

Altered blood flow to the myocardium during AMI or other cardiac conditions can affect the heart's conduction system leading to dysrhythmias. Dysrhythmias are usually classified as being too fast (*tachycardia*) or too slow (*bradycardia*); in regularity, one or more beats occurring earlier or later than expected; or in a different pattern of activation of the cardiac muscle.[43] Dysrhythmias can originate in any area of the heart. They are usually divided into those that start in the atrium, the AV node, or the ventricle.

Identification of the origin of the dysrhythmias is based on the following[26]:

1. Rate: Normal is 60 to 100 beats/min, slow is less than 60 beats/min, and fast is greater than 100 beats/min (in adults).
2. Rhythm: Regular or irregular.
3. P waves: Present, morphology, one P wave before every QRS complex.
4. PR interval duration: Normal, shortened, or prolonged; normal is 0.12 to 0.20 seconds.
5. QRS morphology and duration: Normal duration is 0.06 to 0.12 seconds. Does QRS follow every P wave?

Pathophysiologic Factors

Cells that conduct the electrical current through the heart are known as pacemaker or automatic cells. The normal pacemaker of the heart, the SA node, is located at the junction of the superior vena cava and the right atrium. An electric impulse is initiated at this node and travels through the internodal pathways to the AV node. The AV node is located in the right atrium, directly above the tricuspid valve and anterior to the coronary sinus. The electrical impulse travels through the AV node and then moves through a common bundle of His, which divides almost immediately into the right and left bundles. The left bundle divides further to form two direct pathways to the anterior and posterior papillary muscles. The electrical impulse then permeates the many small fibers of the Purkinje network, beginning at the endocardium and ending in the ventricular myocardium.[15]

The primary pacemaker of the heart is the SA node, which normally paces the heart at a rate of 60 to 100 beats/min. Secondary pacemakers include the AV junction with an inherent rate of 40 to 60 beats/min and the ventricles with an inherent rate of 20 to 40 beats/min. Dysrhythmias are the result of an irritable focus or foci in the electrical conduction system. Several mechanisms contribute to the development of dysrhythmias. The ischemic process and post-necrotic entities and underlying cardiac disease may enhance myocardial electrical instability leading to dysrhythmias. In addition, the development and treatment of myocardial failure result in mechanical dysfunction, metabolic changes, and electrolyte shifts as well as contribute to rhythm disturbances. Invasive cardiac instrumentation or pharmacologic therapies also have the potential to provoke serious dysrhythmias.

Dysrhythmias Originating in the Sinoatrial Node

Sinus Tachycardia

Sinus tachycardia originates in the SA and is characterized by an HR greater than 100 beats/min. It is a physiologic response to the body's demand for increased oxygen caused by conditions such as anxiety, exercise, smoking, infection, anemia, hypotension, and hyperthyroidism. Treatment is directed toward correcting the underlying cause of the tachycardia, as opposed to correcting the rapid HR. CO may be reduced as a result of decreased ventricular filling with rates greater than 180 beats/min, leading to further ischemia and tissue damage during AMI. IV or oral beta-blockers may be used when the tachycardia produces symptoms, as long as the underlying cause is corrected first.[26,44]

Sinus Bradycardia

Sinus bradycardia originating in the SA is defined as an HR less than 60 beats/min. Relative bradycardia involves an HR that is not sufficient enough to maintain adequate CO and may be greater than 60 beats/min.[45] Sinus bradycardia may be caused by disease of the SA node, hypoxia, normal athletic heart, vagal stimulation, AMI, or various medications. Patients with asymptomatic bradycardia require no treatment and should be observed for decompensation. Those that become symptomatic as HR falls, usually below 50 beats/min, will require treatment because of decreased CO and coronary perfusion. They may become hypotensive, have altered mental status, complain of chest pain and SOB, or have signs and symptoms of HF.[45] It is important to distinguish between asymptomatic and symptomatic bradycardia to determine when treatment is required.

The current AHA 2020 guidelines should be used for the treatment of symptomatic bradycardia, beginning with the administration of IV atropine.[5] The first dose is usually 0.5 mg IV, and it may be repeated every 3–5 minutes to a maximum dose of 3 mg. Atropine enhances sinus node automaticity and AV conduction. If atropine is ineffective, prepare for TCP or the initiation of a vasopressor infusion using either dopamine or epinephrine. TCP should be started immediately if IV access is not available.

Ultimately these patients may require transvenous pacing. The use of lidocaine can be lethal to a patient with bradycardia when the bradycardia is a ventricular escape rhythm.[46]

Dysrhythmias Originating in Atria

Supraventricular Arrhythmias

Supraventricular arrhythmias originate above the ventricle and reflect atrial irritability. An ectopic pacemaker outside the SA node, in the atria or AV junction, takes over at a rate of 150–250 beats/min. It is referred to as paroxysmal supraventricular tachycardia (SVT) when it starts and ends abruptly. Atrial tachycardia, atrial flutter, and atrial fibrillation (AF) are examples of these dysrhythmias.[26]

Atrial Tachycardia

Atrial tachycardia is a regular rhythm, greater than 150 beats/min, and is usually associated with a narrow QRS complex. The QRS may be prolonged if a bundle branch block or aberrant conduction is present. An impulse originating outside the SA node in the atria takes over as the pacemaker of the heart. The HR is usually between 160 and 240 beats/min. P waves precede the QRS but are often obscured because of the rapid HR.[26]

Atrial Flutter

Atrial flutter presents as a series of rapid, regular flutter waves, often described as sawtooth in appearance. An ectopic pacemaker outside the SA node in the atria takes over as the pacemaker with an atrial rate of 220–350 beats/min. The ventricular rhythm is usually regular if the AV conduction ratio is constant, but it may be irregular if there is variable conduction through the AV node.[47]

Atrial Fibrillation

Atrial fibrillation (AF) occurs when multiple atrial ectopic atrial pacemakers fire chaotically in rapid succession with a usual atrial rate of 350–600 beats/min.[44,47] Impulses are randomly conducted through the AV node to the ventricles, resulting in a typically irregular ventricular response. Atrial fibrillation is often described as being irregularly irregular. AF results in loss of effective atrial contraction (atrial kick), which may reduce CO by as much as 25%, and also promotes mural thrombus formation.[47]

Treatment of Supraventricular Tachycardia

Treatment of supraventricular dysrhythmias begins with determining whether the patient is stable or unstable, and then providing treatment based on clinical condition and identified rhythm. The objectives of treatment are to control the rate, convert the rhythm, and use anticoagulation therapy when appropriate. Unstable patients have signs and symptoms such as altered mental status, hypotension, or chest pain attributed to the existing tachycardia. Patients who are symptomatic must be treated immediately to reverse the consequences of increased workload on the heart and reduced CO. These patients require immediate cardioversion as outlined in ACLS guidelines. The rhythm should be evaluated if the patient is stable, and pharmacologic treatment is indicated according to ACLS guidelines.[5] Initial treatment of stable SVT includes vagal maneuvers and administration of IV adenosine. Adenosine will not terminate atrial flutter or AF, but will help to slow AV conduction. Slowing AV conduction will assist in the identification of flutter or fibrillation waves. Beta-blockers and calcium channel blockers may also be used if indicated.

Dysrhythmias Originating in the Atrioventricular Node

First-Degree Atrioventricular Block

First-degree AV block is characterized by a constant prolongation of the PR interval greater than 0.20 seconds. There is a constant delay in the conduction of an impulse through the AV node. P waves are identical and precede every QRS complex. First-degree AV block has been associated with congenital structural heart disease such as endocardial cushion defects. Other causes include ischemia, anoxia, digitalis toxicity, and AV node malfunction. It is rarely treated, but the cause should be determined and corrected.

Second-Degree Atrioventricular Block

Mobitz type I (Wenckebach AV block) is characterized by the progressive lengthening of the PR intervals until a QRS complex is completely dropped, and the cycle is repeated. Each atrial impulse takes progressively longer to travel through the AV node until conduction is completely blocked. This is a less serious form of second-degree AV block and usually does not require treatment unless the patient becomes symptomatic.

Mobitz type II is recognized when the P waves are periodically blocked from conduction to the ventricles without a progressive prolongation of the PR interval. In this type of block, the PR interval of all conducted beats is constant. The P waves are identical and precede each QRS complex when they are present. Mobitz type II is more serious than Mobitz type I and often progresses to third-degree AV block. If the patient is symptomatic, immediate treatment with pacing or beta-adrenergic support (dopamine or epinephrine infusions) may be required as outlined in the current ACLS guidelines.[5] Atropine is usually ineffective in reversing type II AV blocks with widened QRS complexes.[43]

Third-Degree Atrioventricular Block or Complete Heart Block

Third-degree AV block is a potentially lethal conduction abnormality characterized by separate and independent atrial and ventricular activity. Either sinus or ectopic atrial pacemakers control the atria, and a pacemaker that is distal to the AV block controls the ventricles. The ECG shows completely dissociated P waves and QRS complexes. Immediate treatment in symptomatic third-degree AV block involves the use of TCP or a transvenous pacemaker, if available. Pharmacologic therapy can include atropine at 0.5–1.0 mg (although normally ineffective unless the QRS is narrow) or the initiation of a vasopressor infusion using either dopamine or epinephrine.[43,47] Dopamine infusions are started at a rate of 2–20 mcg/kg/min and epinephrine infusion at a rate of 2–10 mcg/min and titrated to patient response. Ultimately these patients will require transvenous pacing.

Dysrhythmias Originating in Ventricles

Ventricular Arrhythmias

Ventricular ectopic activity is a common phenomenon in AMI, and *ventricular arrhythmias* are the major cause of sudden cardiac death in the United States.[48] The most common cause of ventricular arrhythmia is ischemic CAD. Ventricular arrhythmias arise in the ventricles beyond the bifurcation of the bundle of His.

Death from a ventricular arrhythmia occurs through its interference with the cardiac pumping function. Several conditions that occur during ventricular arrhythmias contribute to the decrease in CO, which in turn can cause syncope and lead to cardiac arrest. The loss of the normal AV sequence is associated with a significant decrease in CO. The rate of the ventricular arrhythmia also determines hemodynamic instability. A rate below 150 beats/min does not usually cause hemodynamic compromise if the duration is short. If the VT exceeds 200 beats/min, significant symptoms are usually present and can include dyspnea, lightheadedness, loss of vision, syncope, and cardiac arrest. Patients with ventricular tachyarrhythmias should be closely monitored because they have an increased risk of progression to VF, especially with a history of compromised ejection fraction.

Ventricular Tachycardia

VT originates from an ectopic pacemaker in the ventricles, usually with a rate of 150–250 beats/min.[49] The QRS complexes appear wide and bizarre. Any tachycardia with a QRS complex exceeding 120 milliseconds in duration is labeled as a wide complex tachycardia.[47] Ventricular fibrillation is labelled as a wide-complex tachycardia and is the result of chaotic disturbance easily recognized by a ventricular rate exceeding 300 with no regularity. Ventricular fibrillation is a lethal rhythm if not identified and treated immediately. The rhythm may be well tolerated or associated with hemodynamic compromise. Current emphasis related to treatment methods is still placed on whether the patient's condition is deemed stable or unstable, and with or without a pulse.[5] In the assessment of the patient in VT, instability is determined by symptoms displayed such as chest pain, hypotension, decreased level of consciousness, shock, SOB, or pulmonary congestion that can be attributed to the rapid HR, usually greater than 150 beats/min. If the patient's condition is determined to be unstable, the rhythm is wide and regular (monomorphic), and pulses are detected, then immediate synchronized cardioversion is indicated. If the rhythm is wide but irregular (polymorphic) with pulses present, defibrillation instead of cardioversion should be instituted. VT without pulses should be immediately defibrillated according to current ACLS guidelines.[5] In stable patients, VT is first treated with pharmacologic agents. The current ACLS guidelines recommend the use of amiodarone, procainamide, and sotalol as the antiarrhythmics of choice at this time. Lidocaine can also be used as an alternative agent in these stable patients. Magnesium should be considered in the patient with torsades de pointes. Current ACLS guidelines for specific algorithms should be used for the treatment of all dysrhythmias.

Ventricular Fibrillation

VF is chaotic depolarization from multiple ectopic pacemakers in the ventricles. No effective contraction occurs, which results in severe hemodynamic compromise caused by a lack of CO. It is characterized by rapid, abnormal, fine, or coarse fibrillatory waves, and the absence of QRS complexes. VF is the most common mechanism of cardiac arrest from myocardial ischemia or infarction. The best treatment for VF is early, high-energy unsynchronized defibrillation. High-quality CPR should be performed until defibrillation is available. If defibrillation fails, start pharmacologic treatment with epinephrine 1 mg IV pushes every 3–5 minutes. Vasopressin was removed from the most current ACLS guidelines because it was found to offer no advantage over epinephrine in cardiac arrest.[5] Antiarrhythmic drugs including amiodarone and lidocaine may also be given during cardiac arrest from VF between each countershock. Again, adherence to current ACLS guidelines regarding CPR, defibrillation, and pharmacotherapy is important.

Pulseless Electrical Activity and Asystole

Pulseless electrical activity (PEA) is defined as any organized rhythm without a pulse, where there is electrical activity but no mechanical contraction of the heart. The QRS complex may be wide or narrow, fast, or slow, and regular or irregular. This excludes asystole, VF, and VT without a pulse. Asystole is characterized by an absence of ventricular contraction and CO without a pulse. The ECG will show a flat line with no discernible electrical activity, and no pulse will be present. Both PEA and asystole are life-threatening conditions, resulting in death unless they are quickly treated. Treatment for both PEA and asystole begins with high-quality CPR followed by the administration of 1 mg of epinephrine IV or interosseous every 3–5 minutes. CPR should not be interrupted during resuscitation. If during resuscitation a shockable rhythm arises, immediate defibrillation should be instituted. The current ACLS guidelines do not recommend the use of TCP for patients in asystole. Efforts should be focused on the quick identification of reversible causes using the Hs (hypovolemia, hypoxia, hypo/hyperkalemia, hydrogen ion [acidosis], and hypothermia) and Ts (tension pneumothorax, tamponade [cardiac], toxins, and thrombosis [coronary and pulmonary]), as outlined in the current ACLS guidelines. Reversible causes must be rapidly searched for and treated immediately to have a successful resuscitation.

Implantable Cardioverter-Defibrillators

Implantable cardioverter-defibrillators (ICDs) are an accepted treatment regimen for repressing sudden cardiac death.[34] According to the AHA/ACC/HRS, placement of an ICD is intended for primary prevention of those who have not yet suffered sudden cardiac arrest or had prolonged ventricular tachycardia, however, they are at high risk for developing sudden cardiac arrest.[35,36] The AHA/ACC/HRS recognizes placement of an ICD for secondary prevention of those who have previously suffered cardiac arrest, had prolonged ventricular tachycardia, or ventricular arrhythmias invoking syncope.[35,36] Ventricular arrhythmias are classified as those that arise either from the ventricular myocardium or the His–Purkinje system. Rhythms included in this category are ventricular tachycardia, ventricular fibrillation, ventricular flutter, and premature ventricular contractions. Approximately 70% of patients suffering from cardiac arrest were noted to have been in ventricular fibrillation.[36] ICD implementation in patients with long QT syndrome or who are at high risk for developing long QT syndrome will have a reduction in mortality from this therapy.[37] Patients who have pathologic Q-waves, identifying dead infarcted cardiac tissue, on their ECG have benefited from ICD placement. Increased mortality has been noted in patients who have pathologic Q-waves as the result of arrhythmias, which are preventable with ICD placement.[38] ICD insertion in patients with Brugada syndrome (see later in this chapter) can decrease the risk of sudden cardiac death, by cardioverting occurrences of ventricular fibrillation.[39] Placement of an ICD is the primary treatment in individuals diagnosed with arrhythmogenic right ventricular cardiomyopathy.[40]

When transporting a patient with an ICD in place who goes into cardiac arrest, manual defibrillation is indicated. There are no contraindications to defibrillation, even with an ICD in place. Patients that have a pacemaker or ICD in place do not affect the indication or efficaciousness of the course of action when a shockable rhythm is identified.[50]

Complications from ICD Placement

There are, however, difficulties with ICD therapy, mostly correlated with the implementation of and prolonged habitation of transvenous leads in the cardiovascular structural system.[34] Typically, ICD implementation is performed in the location known as the safety triangle, which is bordered by the pectoralis major, latissimus dorsi, and nipple line at the base of the axilla. Complications can occur when placement is outside these parameters, potentially causing damage to underlying vascular structures.[41] When ICDs are placed there is the risk for complications, which occur in about 20% of cases. Complications occurring from ICD placement can range from mild to severe. A minor complication could be inaccurate, shallow placement, whereas a severe complication could include vascular damage.[42] Cardiac perforation is a serious complication and is noted to occur in approximately 5% of cases.[43]

Patients with ICDs can potentially suffer an electrical storm, which is intractable episodes of ventricular tachycardia or ventricular fibrillation over a short period, subsequently resulting in the continuous firing of the ICD. The occurrence of an electrical storm generally comes from individuals with underlying cardiomyopathies.[44] These patients may or may not require hemodynamic management for stabilization, however, this must be addressed in the initial treatment phase. Once stabilized, the patient's ICD may be interrogated, where it will be reprogrammed, to lessen the ongoing shocks. After the initial stabilization occurs, uncovering the potential triggers should then take precedence. Triggers may include electrolyte disturbances, antiarrhythmic medication therapy, myocardial ischemia, or heart failure.[44] Suppression of sympathetic nervous system stimulation is key to the initial management of those suffering from an electrical storm and can be managed with beta-blocker therapy or the denervation of sympathetic cardiac fibers.[44,45] Electrical shocks result in cellular destruction in the ventricular myocardium, significant irregularities in calcium balancing, and free radical damage.[45]

Cardiogenic Shock

Cardiogenic shock is a clinical condition of extreme pump failure leading to an inability of the heart to perfuse the vital organs. It is pump failure that results in inadequate tissue perfusion. Classic signs of cardiogenic shock include significant systemic hypotension and evidence of end-organ hypoperfusion, such as altered mentation and low urine output.[50–54] Hemodynamic parameters are often used to define this condition. These include persistent SBP of less than 80–90 mmHg or a mean arterial pressure (MAP) of 30 mmHg lower than baseline, a reduced cardiac index (CI) of less than 1.8 L/min per square meter without support or less than 2–2.2 L/min per square meter with support, and elevated ventricular filling pressures (pulmonary artery wedge pressure [PAWP] of >18 mmHg).[55] Often this diagnosis is made using a pulmonary artery catheter (PAC), which allows for measurement of both CI and filling pressures (PAWP). An alternative method involves using echocardiography. The most common cause of cardiogenic shock is MI in which there is extensive ischemic damage involving greater than 40% of the left ventricle.[51,52,56,57]

During the past two decades, the primary goal of therapy for patients with AMI has been to manage or prevent pump failure. Because the amount of ventricular failure is directly related to the extent of infarction, therapies aimed at limiting MI size and early revascularization are imperative in reducing the incidence and extent of pump failure.

There are many other causes of cardiogenic shock, including severe RV infarction, acute exacerbation of severe HF, stunned myocardium as a result of cardiac arrest or hypotension, advanced septic shock, significant dysrhythmias, valvular disorders, ruptured ventricular wall aneurysm, cardiac tamponade, and tension pneumothorax.[51,52,56]

Pathophysiologic Factors

Cardiogenic shock results when the heart is unable to pump blood forward, resulting in a decreased SV, CO, and tissue perfusion. Oxygen delivery falls causing a reduction in the delivery of oxygen and nutrients to the tissues. Ultimately, end-organ damage and multisystem organ failure occur if this process is not reversed.

Assessment and Diagnosis

Cardiogenic shock is usually diagnosed based on clinical presentation and physical findings. The classic presentation includes severe systemic hypotension, signs of tissue hypoperfusion (altered mental status, cold, clammy skin, decreased urine output, and metabolic acidosis), and respiratory distress caused by pulmonary congestion. Patients in cardiogenic shock appear acutely ill and are in acute distress. They may complain of difficulty breathing and chest pain. Physical examination often reveals profound hypotension, signs of peripheral hypoperfusion, jugular venous distension (JVD), hypoxemia, acidosis, rales, and oliguria.[51,53] They often have an ashen or cyanotic appearance, and the skin is cool and clammy with mottled extremities. Some patients have a depressed sensorium, resulting from hypoxemia. Pulses may be irregular if dysrhythmias are present, and peripheral pulses are faint and rapid. JVD is usually present. A repeat 12-lead ECG should be done to look for the presence of ischemia, injury, and infarct. A PAC may be placed in patients who do not respond to initial resuscitative efforts to allow for monitoring and guidance therapy related to CO and cardiac filling pressures.

Hemodynamically, patients in cardiogenic shock manifest marked hypotension, with an SBP of 80–90 mmHg, or MAP of 30 mmHg lower than baseline, a reduced CI of less than 1.8 L/min per square meter without support or less than 2.0–2.2 L/min per square meter with support, abnormal mental status; cold, clammy skin; decreased urinary output (UO), elevated HRs, and a PAWP of greater than 18 mmHg.[55] They may also exhibit pulmonary congestion, arterial hypoxemia, and evidence of metabolic acidosis (low serum bicarb and elevated serum lactate). Dysrhythmias often occur as a result of hypoxemia, and the chest x-ray (CXR) may reveal pulmonary vascular congestion.

Patients in cardiogenic shock require frequent assessment of hemodynamic parameters, including BP, HR, and pulmonary artery pressures (if a PAC is present). They should be frequently assessed for peripheral perfusion, presence of edema, color and warmth of skin, blood gases, hemoglobin, and hematocrit to assess oxygen-carrying capacity and function.

Management

Initial management of cardiogenic shock includes early identification and rapid, aggressive stabilization before the onset of hypotension. Severe hypotension and hypoperfusion are treated with both pharmacologic and nonpharmacologic methods of circulatory support. Specific issues to be addressed include correction of hypoxemia, correction of electrolyte levels and acid–base balance, maximization of volume status, treatment of sustained dysrhythmias, inotropic and vasopressor support, early revascularization, and consideration of intra-aortic balloon pump (IABP) support and the use of VADs. Oxygenation and airway support are imperative, and correction of hypoxemia may include intubation and mechanical ventilation. Patients with severe pulmonary congestion will require intubation and the use of positive end-expiratory pressure (PEEP). Electrolyte imbalances, such as hypokalemia and hypomagnesemia, create vulnerability to ventricular dysrhythmias, whereas acidosis may depress myocardial contractility.[51]

Maximization of volume status necessitates fluid resuscitation unless pulmonary edema is present. PAWP should be maintained at the lowest value that results in adequate CO. Intake and output should be monitored carefully. Patients with inferior wall myocardial infarction often have an associated RV infarction. The maintenance of RV preload, with the administration of fluids, is the initial therapy for support of RV infarction. Discreet fluid boluses such as 250 mL of isotonic saline can be used with careful evaluation after each bolus to determine whether CO and perfusion have improved. Frequent assessment of PAWP and CO is essential. Pulmonary edema may result in the setting of overzealous, unmonitored fluid administration. Antiarrhythmic drugs, cardioversion, and pacing should be used promptly as necessary to correct any dysrhythmias or heart blocks that affect CO. Inotropic agents and vasopressors should be initiated for cardiovascular support in the presence of inadequate tissue perfusion with adequate intravascular volume. Nitrates, beta-blockers, and angiotensin-converting enzyme (ACE) inhibitors, normally used to improve outcomes after AMI, can worsen hypotension and should be avoided in true cardiogenic shock. Mechanical circulatory support, IABP, and VADs may be needed to stabilize patient conditions until coronary angioplasty and can be used as a bridge to surgical revascularization or heart transplantation.

Pharmacologic Therapy

It is essential to aggressively treat severe hypotension and tissue hypoperfusion in cardiogenic shock to maintain vital organ perfusion. Pharmacologic management includes the use of both inotropic and vasopressor agents. Severe hypotension leads to hypoxemia and lactic acidosis, which may decrease responsiveness to vasopressors as well as cause further myocardial depression. Vasopressors used for the initial treatment of hypotension include norepinephrine and dopamine. The effect of dopamine is dose-dependent. In higher doses, usually greater than 10 mcg/kg/min, it acts as an alpha-agonist causing vasoconstriction. Norepinephrine has both alpha-agonist and some beta-agonist activity resulting in potent vasoconstriction as well as some positive inotropic effects. Some evidence suggests that outcomes may be better with norepinephrine versus dopamine.[54]

Dobutamine is a positive inotropic agent that can be used in patients that have an SBP greater than 80 mmHg when CI is low and PAWP is high. This drug improves CO by increasing myocardial contractility. An alternative to this inotropic agent is milrinone. It is both a positive inotrope agent as well as a vasodilator. It is important to remember that dobutamine and milrinone do not reverse the hypotension that is seen in post-MI shock. Generally, vasopressors are used in patients who have severe hypotension, and a positive inotropic agent is used when severe hypotension is not present. Both of these agents are often used in patients with cardiogenic shock.

Patients who are not hypotensive but in a low CO state may also require afterload reduction with vasodilators to decrease the workload on the heart. Vasodilators should be used with extreme caution because they can cause further hypotension and a decrease in coronary blood flow. Vasodilators are used to increase forward flow by reducing afterload; these drugs include sodium nitroprusside and NTG. Sodium nitroprusside reduces afterload by decreasing filling pressures and can also increase SV. NTG reduces PAWP and left ventricular filling pressure and redistributes coronary blood flow to the ischemic area. Diuretic therapy is limited to treating pulmonary congestion and decreasing intravascular volume, improving oxygenation.[57]

Intra-Aortic Balloon Pump Counterpulsation

When pharmacologic support and adjunctive therapies fail to improve low CO and poor perfusion associated with cardiogenic shock, an IABP may be used as a temporary stabilizing therapy.

In the setting of cardiogenic shock complicated by AMI, the optimal strategy involves revascularization and adjunctive IABP support. Coronary reperfusion can be achieved by PCI, emergent CABG, or by fibrinolysis. Primary PCI is the preferred method of revascularization if it can be implemented within 90–120 minutes of initial hospital presentation.[18] Ideally, it should be performed within 90 minutes of first medical contact.[5,18] IABP can be used effectively to stabilize patients before angiography and revascularization. Stabilization with IABP and appropriate hemodynamic management, followed by transfer to a tertiary care facility, is the treatment option for those facilities without direct angioplasty capability.[18] There is further discussion of IABP counterpulsation in Chapter 9.

Heart Failure

Definition and Pathophysiologic Factors

Heart failure (HF) is common and potentially fatal in the critically ill. It occurs when the heart is unable to pump sufficient blood to meet the metabolic needs of the body, resulting in inadequate tissue perfusion.[46,55] Any condition that decreases the heart's ability to pump can cause HF. Blood begins to back up into the pulmonary and/or systemic circulations. Signs and symptoms seen in HF are the result of the accumulation of fluid behind the left or right ventricle or both. This results in congestion of the vascular system draining into the heart. The most common causes of HF are left ventricular systolic (inability to pump blood forward) and diastolic dysfunction (impaired ventricular filling). Damage to the myocardium for any reason will result in the failure of the heart as an effective pump. There are many causes of HF, including prolonged myocardial ischemia or infarct, heart valve disorders, conduction defects, wall damage from cardiomyopathies, and hypertension.[46] HF is a progressive, debilitating condition that ultimately results in death unless the patient is a candidate for a cardiac transplant.

Assessment and Diagnosis

A careful history usually reveals the cause of HF, such as MI, hypertension, or valvular disorders. Left ventricular dysfunction from CAD and advanced age are the primary risk factors that contribute to the development of HF. Other risk factors include diabetes, angina, hypertension, a history of cigarette smoking, obesity, elevated high-density lipoprotein, abnormally high or low hematocrit levels, proteinuria, and a history of CAD or previous MI. The patient presents with SOB, which begins initially with exertion and progresses to SOB at rest. In severe HF, the patient has orthopnea and must sit upright or lean over a table to breathe.

Physical examination reveals signs and symptoms resulting from excess fluid accumulation behind the left or right ventricles. In RV failure, JVD, elevated central venous pressure (CVP), hepatomegaly, and peripheral pitting edema without venous insufficiency may be present. In left ventricular failure, dyspnea at rest, orthopnea, cough, fatigue, and weakness, elevated PAWP, laterally placed point of maximal intensity, and an S3 gallop may be present.[46]

Electrocardiographic monitoring may show the development of dysrhythmias such as AF, complete heart block, and rapid tachycardia, which could exacerbate pump failure. Laboratory data are nonspecific, although arterial hypoxemia and metabolic acidosis are common, and respiratory alkalosis may be present with significant tachypnea. Chest x-rays can reveal cardiomegaly and may show pulmonary vascular congestion and interstitial edema. Invasive monitoring reveals an elevated right atrial (RA) and PAWP, elevated systemic vascular resistance (SVR), and low CO.[46] Transport crews must remain alert to factors that can aggravate the underlying cardiac dysfunction. These factors include the extension of active ischemia or infarction, uncontrolled hypertension, or heavy alcohol consumption. Viral infections and cases of pneumonia frequently trigger the onset of symptoms and may necessitate weeks of close supervision for recovery, if recovery is even possible. AF, which can cause or result from worsening failure, warrants the restoration of normal sinus rhythm to improve cardiac function. Obesity is both a primary cause and an aggravating factor for HF. Orthopnea is a sensitive symptom of elevated filling pressures, and the degree of orthopnea parallels the amount of increased pressure. JVD indicates the presence of elevated resting filling pressures. Peripheral edema may be seen in those with chronic HF. Weight gain may indicate an impending episode of HF. Abdominal symptoms can result from hepatic congestion. Once the patient is determined to be in failure, they must be evaluated for manifestations of hypoperfusion. Evidence of hypoperfusion includes low BP, narrow pulse pressure, cool extremities, and altered mentation.

Management

Knowledge of precipitating factors, physical findings, and past management of HF will assist in the treatment of these complex and challenging patients. Management of HF focuses on the reduction of preload for relief of pulmonary edema, reduction of afterload with vasodilators to enhance SV, and use of positive inotropic agents to enhance contractile function. IV diuretics and nitrates are used for preload reduction. Afterload reducing agents and ACE inhibitors are used in the chronic, as opposed to the acute, setting. Inotropic agents are rarely used to enhance contractility because of the increase in myocardial oxygen demand unless shock is present.[46] Currently, beta-blockers are used to improve LV performance and improve survival.[58]

Oxygenation and ventilation are the first priorities in the management of HF patients. The airway should be rapidly assessed and stabilized in patients presenting with acute dyspnea. Supplemental oxygen and assisted ventilation should be provided when indicated. Routine use of oxygen is not recommended unless hypoxemia (an SaO_2 of <94%) is present.[58–61]

Noninvasive ventilation (NIV) is indicated as the optimal choice of initial treatment in those patients with sudden onset cardiogenic pulmonary edema.[59,60] Patients with respiratory failure who fail NIV or have contraindications to its use should be intubated. PEEP is used to improve oxygenation when patients are mechanically ventilated. Pulse oximetry and waveform capnography measuring end-tidal CO_2 should be used to monitor ventilation and oxygenation during transport. Continuous ECG monitoring is needed to monitor for dysrhythmias that may occur as a result of electrolyte imbalances. Strict intake and output measurements must be maintained and recorded. Responses to medications should be closely evaluated and documented. All medication infusions should be maintained on IV pumps and titrated as indicated based on patient condition.

Structural Heart Disease

The normal heart valve can be defined as a slender, pliable, structural tissue that permits the passage of blood in one pathway and inhibits the retrograde flow of blood. In the acute setting of regurgitant structural heart disease lesions, the provider must consider several key factors in the care of these patients. Regurgitant valves are floppy and do not want to close and stay shut. The predominant cause of mitral regurgitation is due to a defective valve or chordae and secondary causes result from disorders of the left atrium or left ventricle. The leading cause of moderate-to-severe mechanical heart disease in adults over the age of 55 is mitral valve regurgitation.[47] Secondary mitral valve regurgitation occurs in between 10% to 60% of cases in post-myocardial infarction patients and greater than 50% of the time in those with dilated cardiomyopathy.[48] Acute myocardial infarctions can cause ischemic mitral valve regurgitation, especially with inferior and lateral wall infarcts. During an inferior or lateral wall infarct, the mitral valve can become ischemic because one of the coronary arteries responsible for supplying blood in these areas of the heart provides the blood supply to the posterior-medial papillary muscle, which is the most prone to rupture since it only has a single blood supply.

Treatment is primarily based upon optimizing treatment of heart failure. In mitral valve regurgitation, an elevated dynamic course is affected by loading conditions like elevated blood pressure, and fluid overload, which can exacerbate regurgitation and shunting of blood.[48]

Tricuspid regurgitation occurs frequently in those patients with extreme progressive mitral valve regurgitation.[49] The tricuspid and mitral valves are atrioventricular valves located between the atria and the ventricles. Tricuspid valve regurgitation allows the backflow of blood back into the right atrium. Aortic regurgitation is another type of mechanical heart disease that is identified by retrograde blood flow from the aorta into the left ventricle, occurring during the diastolic phase of the cardiac cycle. The aortic valve root or the aortic valve itself is primarily affected by the various etiologies that cause aortic regurgitation. The etiology and gravity of the aortic regurgitation are best identified by echocardiography.[51]

In mitral and aortic valve regurgitation, an elevated dynamic course is affected by loading conditions like elevated blood pressure and fluid overload, which can exacerbate regurgitation and shunting of blood. These regurgitant lesions are sensitive to elevated afterloads; therefore, maintaining the minimal MAP required for organ perfusion will reduce valvular backflow.

The semilunar valves of the heart include the pulmonic and aortic valves. A stenotic valve is a valve that is stiff and does not want to open, and when opened, it tries to stay open and does not want to close.

The typical aortic valve is composed of three cusps, right, left, and posterior. These three cusps are respectively all the same size. Many cases of aortic stenosis can be correlated to a pathology involving the cusp. There are three commonly identified reasons for aortic stenosis: calcified degrading due to age, hereditary bicuspid aortic valve, and those occurring after an inflammatory valve disease. The structural causes of stenosis in the three situations are calcification, fibrosis, and connection binding.[56] A simplified explanation of aortic stenosis would be to think of a drink bottle that is full, which, when turned upside down with the lid removed and squeezed with excessive force, can be emptied very quickly. However, if the lid is placed on the drink bottle, with one small slit placed in it, that same drink bottled when turned upside down will be much harder to empty when squeezed with excessive force. This is what happens with the left ventricle when it tries ejecting blood through a stenotic aortic valve.

Acute Pericarditis

Pericarditis refers to inflammation of the pericardial sac. It is one of the most common disorders involving the pericardium, and it has many different causes. The pericardium is a closed fibrous sac that surrounds the heart. It consists of an inner serous membrane, called the visceral pericardium, which closely adheres to the superficial myocardium and coronary vessels. The fibrous outer layer that surrounds the heart is the parietal pericardium. The space between the visceral and parietal layers normally contains 10–20 mL of pericardial fluid that acts as a lubricant between the contracting surfaces. The exact role of the pericardium is unclear; however, it is believed to serve as a lubrication system, ensuring that cardiac motion is unimpaired by surrounding mediastinal structures. Because the pericardium resists stretching, it functions as a protective mechanism to prevent sudden dilation of the heart. The pericardium may also protect the heart from infection.

Pericarditis is often associated with AMI. It results from an extension of the infarction to the epicardial area and is associated with an inflammatory response localized to the pericardium bordering the infarction. It may also be a delayed response to a more generalized inflammatory process, such as in Dressler's syndrome. Other common conditions associated with the development of pericarditis include infection, collagen vascular diseases, uremia, malignancy, drug therapy, and trauma.[62,63]

Assessment and Diagnosis

Pericarditis may present as an isolated process or be a manifestation of another underlying condition.[62,63] The presentation of pericardial heart disease depends on the pericardium's response to injury and the subsequent effect on cardiac function. The presentation will vary depending on the underlying cause. Diagnosis and recognition of acute pericarditis in the emergent situation are largely dependent on a patient history of pleuritic chest pain and the presence of a pericardial friction rub.[62,63] Typical chest pain is described as severe, sharp, and substernal and increases with inspiration or in the reclining position. This pain may be further aggravated by coughing or movement and is reduced when the patient sits up and leans forward. Sitting up and leaning forward reduces pressure on the parietal pericardium, allowing for splinting of the diaphragm.[64] Substernal pain may radiate to the neck, shoulder, and back. It is important to distinguish chest pain caused by pericarditis from that of other life-threatening conditions such as MI, aortic dissection, and pulmonary embolism.

Physical examination reveals a pericardial friction rub that may be heard at various times and in various locations during the patient's course. This is highly specific to pericarditis. The friction rub resembles a high-pitched grating or scratching sound. It is best heard with the diaphragm of the stethoscope placed at the lower left sternal border or apex with the patient sitting up and leaning forward during expiration. Pericardial friction rubs may be distinguished from pleural rubs by having patients hold their breath during auscultation. Pleural rubs will disappear during this period because they are caused by friction between the inflamed visceral and parietal pleura. A pericardial friction rub will continue to be heard because it is caused by friction between the two inflamed layers of the pericardium. The presence of a friction rub does not exclude the presence of a large pericardial effusion or tamponade. Associated signs and symptoms of pericarditis include fever and leukocytosis, dyspnea related to increased pain with inspiration, dysphagia related to irritation of the esophagus by the posterior pericardium, and sinus tachycardia. A normal BP should be present, without a paradoxical pulse or venous distension.

ECG changes that may be seen include ST elevation and atypical T wave abnormalities caused by inflammation of the epicardium. Diffuse ST segment elevation across most leads of the 12-lead ECG in conjunction with PR segment depression is the typical ECG presentation.

The typical 12-lead ECG presentation of a patient with acute pericarditis is a new onset of global ST segment elevation or a depressed PR segment. The 12-lead ECG is considered the primary diagnostic tool for identifying acute pericarditis.[65] In approximately 40% of patients with pericarditis, ECG changes may be atypical. The patient can have ST segment elevation that does not geographically correlate to making a diagnosis of a STEMI. Simply put, the elevation may be sporadic and not be seen in contiguous leads as they would with the typical AMI.[66] These changes can appear and then disappear depending on the position of the patient. Considering that the pericardium is electrically silent, ECG changes can occur as the result of an inflamed epicardium, subsequently affecting the myocardium and therefore suggesting coinciding involvement of the myocardium versus uncomplicated pericarditis.[66] The most ominous symptom of acute pericarditis is the rapid onset of sharp chest pain. In some cases, the pain can present differently, however having the patient lean forward will improve the pain. This pain has a linear relationship with deep inspiration, tussis, and even presents with hiccups. Occasionally, the patient can experience pain that radiates into the trapezius ridge.[66]

Management

Careful evaluation should be done to distinguish pericarditis from other life-threatening conditions such as MI, aortic dissection, and pulmonary embolism. Most patients with pericarditis can be managed with medical therapy. Treatment is focused on relief of pain and resolution of the underlying inflammation. This is accomplished by treating with nonsteroidal anti-inflammatory drugs (NSAIDs) unless they are contraindications. These include ibuprofen, indomethacin, and aspirin. Ketorolac, a parenteral NSAID, has also been found to be effective in the treatment of pericarditis.[67] It is also recommended that patients receiving aspirin or NSAIDs also receive a proton pump inhibitor for

gastrointestinal protection.[63] During transport, a major priority of care is appropriate pain control and continued reduction of inflammation using the prescribed NSAID agents. Narcotic analgesia agents such as morphine or fentanyl should be considered for additional control of pain. Patients should be monitored for complications of pericarditis, such as pericardial effusion, which can rapidly accumulate resulting in cardiac tamponade.

Infective Endocarditis

The endocardium is the narrow, smooth tissue that inlays the inner chambers of the myocardium, forming the plane of the valves. When these structures become infected, the result is termed endocarditis. In several studies there are multiple causes of the illness, however the most prevailing cause of infective endocarditis is *Staphylococcus aureus*.[66] When bacteria are introduced into the bloodstream from things like periodontal disease, intravenous drug abuse, and implanted cardiovascular devices, infective endocarditis can manifest. The bacteria can become attached, as vegetations, to the valves and result in the endocardium becoming infected.[66] Presently, blood chemistry analysis and obtaining cultures from the heart valves are the primary identifiers for uncovering the contributing pathogen. The importance of this information allows clinicians to utilize the most optimal antimicrobial therapy for treating patients with infective endocarditis.[68] Nonbacterial thrombotic endocarditis is considered an infrequent illness, resulting from sterile formed vegetations.[69]

Patients at Risk for Infective Endocarditis

Patients with predisposing cardiovascular conditions, specifically those with structural heart disease, like surgically implanted prosthetic valves, aortic stenosis, and a prior history of endocarditis, are at high risk for infective endocarditis. Additionally, endovascular hardware insertion like a pacemaker or PICC line, intravenous drug use, and hemodialysis patients are at risk for infective endocarditis.[69]

Assessment Finding Indicative of Infective Endocarditis

Infective endocarditis patients will generally present with a temperature above 38°C. Additionally, the patient may present with a new regurgitant murmur. Localized erythema at the site of a pacemaker or indwelling catheter indicates the potential for infection. Some classic signs like splinter hemorrhages, conjunctival petechiae, Janeway lesions, or Osler's nodes may be seen with infective endocarditis. Even nonspecific signs indicating flu-like symptoms such as malaise, nocturnal hyperhidrosis, rigors, cephalgia, and myalgia can be symptoms of infective endocarditis.[70]

Treatment for Infective Endocarditis

Antibiotic therapy is indicated in the treatment of infective endocarditis with a variety of different medications like vancomycin, cefazolin, nafcillin, ceftriaxone, daptomycin, ampicillin-sulbactam or gentamicin. Any of these therapies may be used in conjunction with each other depending on the specifics of the underlying cause of the infection. Ultimately, the patient will require surgical intervention to remove the vegetation from the heart valve.[70]

Cardiac Effusion and Tamponade

The pericardium is a closed, fibrous sac surrounding the heart, consisting of a visceral and parietal layer. The space between the two layers normally contains between 10 and 20 mL of pericardial fluid that acts as a lubricant between the contracting surfaces. Pericardial *effusion* is present when there is an accumulation of more than the normal amount of fluid in this sac. Pericardial effusions may occur rapidly or over time. Effusions can be caused by any pericardial condition, such as acute pericarditis, post-MI or cardiac surgery, infection, aortic dissection extending proximally into the pericardium, collagen vascular disease, and chest trauma.[64,67]

Cardiac tamponade occurs when the accumulation of fluid results in increased pressure and subsequent compression of all chambers of the heart to such an extent that early diastolic filling diminishes, and CO is significantly compromised.[71]

Pathophysiologic Factors

The hemodynamic effects of effusion are related to the speed of accumulation of the fluid. Rapid accumulation of 150–200 mL may produce acute cardiac tamponade; in contrast, large pericardial effusions, which develop slowly, can be totally asymptomatic. Under normal conditions, between 10 and 20 mL of fluid may be present in the pericardial space. The development of a larger volume of fluid may result from pericardial inflammation of any cause, HF, traumatic injury to the heart, aortic dissection, or neoplasm. Accumulation of additional fluid in the pericardial sac begins to impede cardiac filling as intrapericardial pressure begins to rise. This leads to impaired CO, which ultimately results in cardiac tamponade.[71]

Assessment and Diagnosis

Mild-to-moderate pericardial effusions may not produce symptoms. If the fluid accumulates slowly, the fairly noncompliant pericardium stretches to accommodate the increasing volume with little or no rise in intrapericardial pressure until it reaches a size where it can no longer stretch. However, if the fluid accumulates rapidly, a small volume can be life-threatening. The clinical diagnosis of tamponade is usually made based on history and physical findings. Clinical symptoms of cardiac tamponade are related to systemic venous congestion, a reduction in cardiac SV, and respiratory effects of impaired ventricular filling. Early tamponade manifests as tachycardia, tachypnea, edema, and elevated venous pressure. The classic signs, described as Beck's triad, include distended neck veins resulting from elevated CVP, decreased BP, and muffled heart sounds. Pulsus paradoxus (abnormal fall in systolic pressure during inspiration caused by differential filling of the ventricles) may be present. The ECG will typically show sinus tachycardia and low voltage. Electrical alternans, a beat-to-beat alteration in the QRS complex, may also be present, reflecting the movement of the heart in the pericardial fluid.[71] Chest x-rays may show a widening cardiac silhouette with a clear lung field. Echocardiography is the recommended method for rapid and accurate diagnosis of tamponade, if available.

Cardiac tamponade from trauma is usually the result of penetrating injuries, but blunt injury may also cause the pericardium to fill with blood from either injury to the heart itself or from the surrounding great vessels. Cardiac tamponade should be suspected in any trauma patient with PEA or lack of response to volume resuscitation.[66] If early signs of cardiac tamponade are not treated, severe hypotension and RA and RV collapse occur, resulting in profound circulatory failure and shock.

Management

Emergent evacuation of the pericardial fluid is definitive therapy in the presence of acute cardiac tamponade. Hemodynamic support during the preparation of the patient for pericardiocentesis includes administration of blood, plasma, normal saline solution, or lactated Ringer's solution. Pericardiocentesis is accomplished with needle aspiration of pericardial fluid via the subxiphoid method. Removal of even small amounts of fluid will result in temporary relief of symptoms. A positive pericardiocentesis caused by trauma necessitates an open thoracotomy for definitive treatment.

Hypertensive Crisis

Hypertensive crisis is a potentially life-threatening complication of hypertension. It may occur in patients with or without chronic hypertension. Patients without prior hypertension may not tolerate BP levels as high as those patients with chronic hypertension.

The presence of end-organ damage determines whether the crisis is defined as urgent or emergent. Critical elevation of the BP without end-organ damage is considered a hypertensive urgency and can be treated with oral medication over the course of 24–48 hours.[72] Those with severe hypertension and manifestations of acute, ongoing end-organ injury are said to have a hypertensive emergency. A hypertensive emergency requires an immediate reduction in BP to prevent end-organ damage.[72] The SBP often exceeds 200 mmHg, with a diastolic BP greater than 120 mmHg. No predetermined criteria exist for the level of BP necessary to produce a hypertensive emergency because an acute rise in BP from a normal baseline may produce symptoms of end-organ damage. This may occur in pregnant patients who develop eclampsia. The rate of increase of the BP and the difference between the patient's usual level and the level present during the crisis are the more important factors. A hypertensive crisis is a rapid progressive rise in BP sufficient to cause potentially irreversible damage to vital organs. The major organs at risk are the brain, heart, and kidneys. A variety of serious end-organ effects are associated with hypertension. These include CAD, ischemic and hemorrhagic stroke, aortic dissection, renal failure, and HF. A hypertensive crisis may cause aortic dissection, cerebral hemorrhage, renal failure, and left-sided HF.[72]

Assessment and Diagnosis

There are many risk factors for hypertension including advanced age, family history of hypertension, race, high sodium intake, excess alcohol use, excess weight, diabetes, dyslipidemia, renal disease, sleep apnea, endocrine disorders, various medications, and physical inactivity. Hypertensive emergencies are diagnosed based on the presence of severe hypertension with manifestations of end-organ damage.

The purpose of the physical examination is to identify signs of end-organ damage. Retinopathy, congestive HF, arrhythmias, or focal neurologic deficits may be present on clinical examination. Funduscopic examination findings consistent with retinopathy include retinal hemorrhages, papilledema, and exudates. Palpitations, angina, or congestive HF can present with cardiovascular decompensation. Signs and symptoms of left ventricular failure include chest pain, dyspnea, pink frothy sputum, rales, and bronchospasm. Neurologic symptoms may include altered mental status, headache, nausea, and seizures.[73]

Hypertensive encephalopathy is one of the most severe complications seen in hypertensive emergencies. It is characterized by the presence of progressive central nervous system signs and symptoms, including severe headache, nausea, vomiting, and visual difficulties. Focal neurologic findings can include blindness, seizures, aphasia, and hemiparesis. If left untreated, symptoms may progress to convulsions, stupor, coma, and death. Hypertensive emergencies are often caused by mismanagement or patient nonadherence to treatment regimens.

Management

Therapy should be based on the clinical situation, critical organ involvement, and the desired time frame for lowering the BP. Identification of the specific antihypertensive agent and BP goals for optimal management varies depending on the specifics of the hypertensive emergency. Immediate, but careful reduction in BP is indicated. Rapid, uncontrolled BP reduction may result in ischemic damage to vascular beds that are accustomed to a higher BP. The majority of hypertensive emergencies can be managed by lowering mean arterial BP gradually by 10%–20% in the first hour and by a further 5%–15% over the next 23 hours.[72] The major exceptions to this include patients with ischemic strokes, acute aortic dissections, and non-traumatic hemorrhagic strokes.[72,74] Target BP goals should be known before departing the referring facility.

Frequent, accurate BP measurement is often difficult during transport. Arterial pressure monitoring will provide the easiest and most accurate method for monitoring BP. Monitoring cardiac rhythm, level of consciousness, and assessment for signs of impending pulmonary edema or cardiac failure will help the transport team evaluate whether the antihypertensive agents are effective. Several parenteral and oral agents are available to use in a hypertensive crisis. The choice of drug is dependent on the type of hypertensive crisis and the specific medications that are available. Examples of antihypertensive drugs that can be given IV include sodium nitroprusside, NTG, nicardipine, labetalol, esmolol, clevidipine, fenoldopam, hydralazine, and phentolamine. These are generally used in hypertensive emergencies. Oral agents are generally reserved for use in hypertensive urgencies in which there is hypertension but no signs of end-organ damage.

Sodium nitroprusside is one of the more common agents used to treat hypertensive emergencies. It acts by direct peripheral vasodilation with balanced effects on arterial and venous blood vessels. The antihypertensive effect of IV sodium nitroprusside is apparent in seconds and is dose-dependent. Once the drug is discontinued, the pressure will rapidly rise to the previous level in 1–10 minutes. Infusion rates must be closely monitored to avoid sudden fluctuations in BP.

Hemodynamic Monitoring in Cardiovascular Assessment

Critical care transport requires specialized knowledge and skills related to hemodynamic monitoring. The use of these technologies allows for the assessment of cardiopulmonary status and responses to therapy. Clinicians must be familiar with hemodynamic monitoring technologies and have the knowledge and skill to provide safe and effective care during transport. Space limitations, noise levels, and vibration in the transport environment may complicate the use of sophisticated hemodynamic monitoring equipment. Transport team members must refine their use of visual and tactile assessment skills for clinical patient evaluation. These skills should be used in conjunction with hemodynamic monitoring.

Cardiac Output

The circulatory system is responsible for maintaining adequate perfusion so that oxygen and nutrients are delivered to the tissues, meeting the metabolic needs of the body. Hemodynamic monitoring assists in the identification and timely initiation of interventions aimed at maintaining or restoring adequate tissue perfusion.

Cardiac output (CO), defined as the amount of blood ejected from the heart into the systemic circulation per minute, is a major contributor to maintaining adequate oxygen delivery to the tissues. The normal range for CO is 4–8 L/min.[75] Cardiac index (CI) is determined by dividing CO by body surface area (BSA). BSA is based on height and weight. CI is a more precise measurement of cardiac performance because it allows for differences in body size. Normal CI ranges from 2.5 to 4 L/min per square meter.[75]

CO is determined by heart rate (HR) and stroke volume (SV). The SV, which is the amount of blood ejected from the heart per heartbeat, is dependent on preload, afterload, and contractility. Preload can be defined as the amount of blood in the ventricles at end-diastole. Increased preload causes the cardiac muscle to stretch, resulting in an increase in the force of the following cardiac contraction. Starling's law states that an increase in preload or stretch will result in an increase in the subsequent force of contraction, improving CO.[76] Afterload is the amount of resistance the ventricles must overcome to eject their contents into the systemic or pulmonary circulations. Contractility is the force of ventricular contraction. It is determined by the amount of muscle fiber shortening that is needed to cause the force of contraction in the absence of changes in preload and afterload.

Invasive Hemodynamic Monitoring

Invasive hemodynamic monitoring is used to monitor a patient's hemodynamic state and allows for the assessment of volume status and administration of fluids and medications. Invasive measurements are obtained using a fluid-filled, pressure monitoring system. The insertion of invasive lines should be done by qualified physicians or designated personnel who have validated skills and practice with these lines. Appropriate setup and maintenance of the pressure monitoring system are critical for obtaining accurate and reliable measurements. Transport crews must be familiar with hemodynamic monitoring technologies and have the knowledge and skill to provide safe and effective care during transport. These include the use of arterial lines, central venous catheters (CVCs), and PACs. Transports of these patients require careful monitoring and maintenance of the invasive lines to prevent accidental movement or dislodgement.

Basics of Pressure Monitoring

Invasive measurements are obtained using a fluid-filled, pressure monitoring system. Waveforms that are generated by the heart (mechanical signal) are detected by the pressure transducer and converted to an electrical signal that is displayed on the bedside or transport monitor.

Ensuring Accurate Measurements Setup

Appropriate setup and maintenance of the pressure monitoring system are critical for obtaining accurate and reliable measurements. This system consists of pressure tubing with a transducer and flush device, a flush solution, a pressure bag, and a reusable pressure cable. Noncompliant pressure tubing should be used between the transducer and the invasive catheter so that the physiologic signal is transmitted without distortion. Soft, compliant IV tubing should not be used because it may absorb a portion of the generated signal before it reaches the transducer leading to inaccurate pressure readings. A continuous flush system must be used to maintain the patency of the system and minimize clot formation.[77] Most often this is accomplished by placing the flush bag into a pressure bag that is inflated to 300 mmHg. This allows the system to be flushed at a constant rate of 3 mL/h. An alternative method involves placing the system on an infusion pump to maintain the patency of the system. This is often done in small children and neonates. The system should be flushed to gravity including all ports before attaching to the invasive line. Gravity flushing prevents microbubble formation in the system. All stopcock ports should be flushed, and any air removed from the system. Air bubbles present anywhere in the system will cause distortion of the signal, resulting in inaccurate measurements.[77] Once the system has been flushed to gravity, and all air eliminated from the system, it should be placed into the pressure bag and inflated to 300 mmHg. Now the pressure monitoring system is ready to be attached to the invasive line once it has been placed into the patient.

Leveling and Zeroing

The system must be leveled and zeroed to obtain accurate pressure measurement. The patient should be placed supine with the head of the bed flat or elevated 45 degrees.[76–79] Leveling eliminates the effects of the weight of the fluid-filled catheter tubing and fluid column.[67] This involves placing the air–fluid interface of the stopcock closest to the transducer at the phlebostatic axis (Figs. 8.1 and 8.2). The phlebostatic axis is used as the zero-reference point and is considered to be at the level of the atria.[76–78] It is defined as the intersection of the fourth intercostal space and the mid-chest (midway between the anterior and posterior chest walls; see Fig. 8.1). Marking the phlebostatic axis with an X on the chest will allow for future identification of this reference point. A carpenter level or laser level should be used to align the air–fluid interface with the phlebostatic axis. The system must be releveled with every position change to obtain accurate values. A 2-mmHg error can result from every inch of discrepancy between the phlebostatic axis and the air–fluid interface.[75] If the air–fluid interface is above the phlebostatic axis, then erroneously low values result; if it is below the phlebostatic axis, then erroneously high values will result because of the effects of hydrostatic pressure.[80]

In the transport environment, an effective strategy involves taping the transducer at the phlebostatic axis until the patient arrives at the receiving facility. This will eliminate the need to relevel with every position change. Zeroing and leveling of the system to the phlebostatic axis eliminates the effects of hydrostatic and atmospheric pressure. It assures that only heart or vessel pressures are measured. It is important to reconfirm that the appropriate pressure waveform is seen on the monitor screen after zeroing the system. Zeroing should be done once the pressure system is

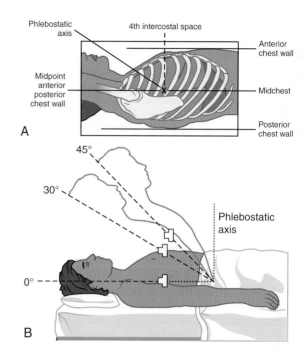

• **Fig. 8.1 A, B,** Location of the phlebostatic axis. (From Lough ME. *Hemodynamic Monitoring: Evolving Technologies and Clinical Practice.* St. Louis, MO: Elsevier; 2016.)

attached to the transport monitor and any time questionable values are displayed. Once the invasive catheter is placed, the pre-primed fluid-filled pressure monitoring system should be attached, making sure the pressure bag is inflated to 300 mmHg.

Reading Pressure Waveforms

All pressure measurements should be obtained at end-expiration. End-expiration is the point in the respiratory cycle in which there is the least effect of intrathoracic (pleural) pressure on intracardiac pressures.[76–79]

Dynamic Response Testing (Square Wave Test)

Dynamic response testing determines the system's ability to accurately reproduce a physiologic signal. The dynamic response should be assessed for all pressure monitoring systems using the square wave test. During a square wave test, the fluctuations that result from a fast flush are analyzed. If an optimal square wave results, the system is assumed to be able to accurately record the patient's pressure waveform during monitoring.[76–79]

Selected Invasive Pressure Monitoring Technologies

Transport crews must have the knowledge and skills to safely care for patients with invasive pressure monitoring technologies including arterial lines, CVC lines, and PACs. This includes setup, zeroing and leveling of the hemodynamic monitoring system.

Arterial Pressure Monitoring

Arterial lines are inserted when continuous BP monitoring is required or when frequent arterial blood gas analysis is indicated. Continuous monitoring of BP allows for timely titration of vasoactive and antihypertensive infusions. Common sites for insertion include the radial, femoral, brachial, and dorsalis pedis arteries.

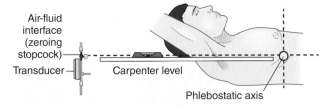

• **Fig. 8.2** Air–fluid interface. (From Rabbani Hagler D, Hagler D. Assessment: cardiovascular system. In: Harding MM, ed. *Lewis's Medical-Surgical Nursing: Assessment and Management of Clinical Problems*, 12th ed. Elsevier; 2023.)

The radial artery is the most frequently used site because the hand has a secondary source of blood supply from the ulnar artery. It also runs over a bone, allowing for compression of the site in case of bleeding.[77] Complications of arterial lines include limb ischemia, infection, and bleeding.[77]

Transport crews are usually not trained and credentialed to place arterial lines but must be familiar with the setup, maintenance, and interpretation of values. The pressure monitoring system is set up and maintained as previously described. The use of this pressure monitoring system allows for direct, real-time, and continuous monitoring of systolic and diastolic pressures as well as MAP. In adults, the previously described pressure bag setup with a continuous flush device should be used to maintain catheter patency to prevent clot formation.

Central Venous Pressure Monitoring

CVP monitoring allows for the assessment of right heart hemodynamics and may aid in evaluating responses to therapy. CVP is monitored using a fluid-filled pressure monitoring system that is attached to the distal port of the CVC. This allows for continuous monitoring of the CVP. Normal CVP ranges from 2 to 8 mmHg in adults.[76] Serial measurements and trending of this value are recommended over interpreting a single static value. CVP measurements should be obtained at end-expiration. The system must be set up correctly, leveled, and zeroed to obtain accurate measurements. The use of CVCs provides access to the central circulation for providing fluids, medications, venous blood sampling, and monitoring the CVP, if indicated. Common sites include the right internal jugular, subclavian, and femoral veins. Complications include pneumothorax, hemothorax, infection, and bleeding.

Pulmonary Artery Monitoring

This invasive technology allows for direct measurement of RA pressure, pulmonary artery pressure, PAWP, and CO as well as the calculation of systemic and pulmonary vascular resistance. Some specialized catheters also allow for intracardiac pacing, continuous measurement of CO, and fiberoptic measurement of continuous mixed venous oxygen saturation (SvO_2).

Transport crews must be competent in the use and clinical application of hemodynamic values and waveforms obtained from PACs. It is critical to understand the principles of the proper placement and the potential for migration of the catheter that can lead to life-threatening pulmonary artery infarct or rupture.[74] This includes an understanding of its various lumens or ports and the use of pressure monitoring systems. Values obtained with a PAC provide information that may be trended to improve the care of patients with hemodynamic stability.

A PAC is a flow-directed, multi-lumen, balloon-tipped catheter inserted into the right side of the heart (pulmonary artery). It is used to assess volume status, administer fluids and medications, and assess CO in the critically ill.[76–79] The balloon at the tip of the catheter allows blood flow to float the catheter through the vena cava into the heart, terminating in the pulmonary artery (Fig. 8.3). The standard 7.5 Fr PAC has four lumens, is 110 cm in length, and has black markings every 10 cm starting at the distal tip of the catheter (Fig. 8.4). These markings are helpful for positioning during insertion as well as establishing the insertion depth once the catheter has been placed. Catheters that are placed from the subclavian vein should have an insertion depth of 35–50 cm, those placed from the internal jugular vein should have an insertion depth of 40–55 cm, and those placed via the femoral vein should be at 60 cm, 70 cm from the right antecubital fossa and 80 cm from the left antecubital fossa.[79] The catheter has multiple lumens or ports, including the proximal injectate port, pulmonary artery distal port, balloon inflation port, and thermistor connector. Some PACs have additional infusion ports that can be used for the administration of fluids and medications. The proximal port opens up in the right atrium and is used to monitor RA pressure and for injection of a fluid bolus during intermittent CO measurement. The distal port opens up in the pulmonary artery and is used to monitor systolic, mean, and diastolic pressures in the pulmonary artery. This port also allows for sampling of mixed venous blood. Both of these ports should be transduced using a pressure monitoring system so that there is a continuous display of the values and waveforms on the monitor. The balloon inflation port is used to obtain a PAWP, which is obtained by slowly inflating the balloon with air, using a preset 1.5-mL syringe until the pulmonary artery pressure converts to a PAWP waveform (Fig. 8.5). Normally it should take between 1.25 and 1.5 mL of air to convert from a pulmonary artery to a PAWP waveform.[79] The balloon should not be inflated for more than 2–4 respiratory cycles (8–15 seconds), and once a PAWP reading is obtained, it should be passively deflated by removing the syringe from the balloon port. Active deflation by pulling back on the syringe may result in tearing of the balloon. Pulmonary rupture resulting in life-threatening hemorrhage may result from prolonged balloon inflation.[81] The thermistor port allows for monitoring of a temperature change during bolus CO measurement and for the monitoring of core body temperature.

Complications include dysrhythmias, pulmonary artery rupture, pulmonary infarct, embolic events, and infection. Routine use of these catheters has decreased over the years, but the transport crew may still encounter their use in select populations including patients with cardiogenic shock, complicated MI and HF, trauma, acute respiratory distress syndrome, and pulmonary hypertension.[82] Because of this, transport crews should be familiar

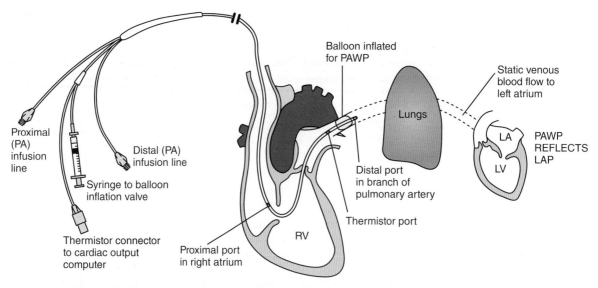

• **Fig. 8.3** Position of pulmonary artery in the heart. (From Preuss T, Wiegard DL. Single-pressure and multiple pressure transducer systems. In: Wiegard DL, ed. *AACN Procedure Manual for Critical Care*. 4th ed. St. Louis, MO: Elsevier/Saunders; 2011.)

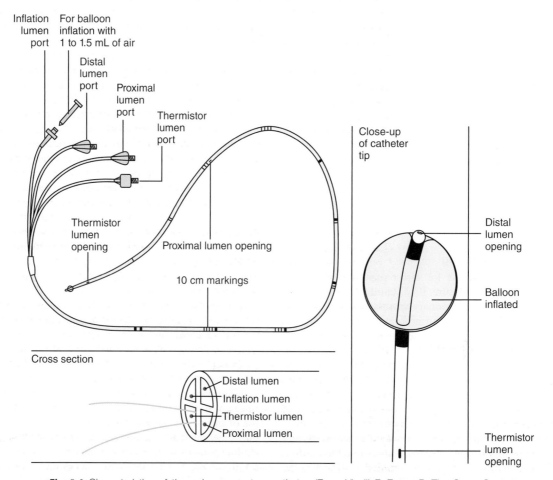

• **Fig. 8.4** Characteristics of the pulmonary artery catheter. (From Visalli F, Evans P. The Swan-Ganz catheter: a program for teaching safe effective use. *Nursing*. 1981;81(11):42-47.)

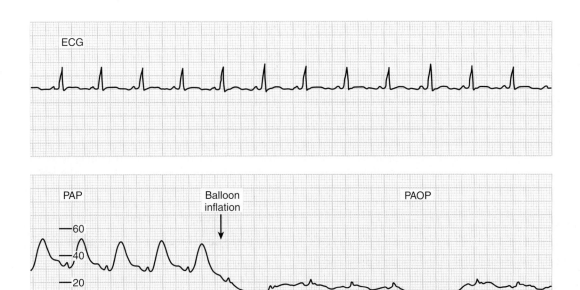

• **Fig. 8.5** Change of pulmonary artery waveform to pulmonary artery wedge pressure waveform. (From Wiegand DL. *AACN Procedure Manual for Progressive and Critical Care.* 8th ed. St. Louis, MO: Elsevier.)

with normal values and waveform morphology for each of the measurements obtained with a PAC.

Verification of correct PAC position is made using CXR and waveform analysis. Dysrhythmias may result if the catheter is pulled back into the right ventricle. A catheter that is positioned too distal into the pulmonary artery may become spontaneously wedged, resulting in a pulmonary infarct or rupture.[82] Steps must be taken to ensure accurate measurement of hemodynamic values including appropriate setup, leveling, zeroing, validating correct catheter position, and assessing the dynamic response of the pressure monitoring system.

Transport considerations specific to PACs include the following: (1) documentation of insertion depth to allow for identification of catheter migration; (2) always transducing the distal port using a pressure monitoring system, confirming the presence of a pulmonary artery waveform; and (3) watching for catheter migration. Catheters that migrate proximally into the RV or that become permanently wedged must be repositioned to prevent life-threatening complications including dysrhythmias and pulmonary artery rupture. In the event the catheter migrates, have the patient reposition if possible and reassess or withdraw the catheter slightly and observe waveform. Advancing the catheter can potentially result in harm. Repositioning the catheter should be done following specific programs, procedures, and protocols, such as (4) verifying that the balloon is deflated by removing the syringe and allowing for passive deflation, (5) taking the original 1.5-mL syringe with the catheter, (6) never flushing the catheter in a wedged position, and (7) never using the distal port to administer fluids or medications other than the saline flush at 1–3 mL/h.

General Transport Safety and Consideration (Invasive Hemodynamic Lines)

On arrival at the bedside, the transport crew should evaluate the pressure monitoring setup, hemodynamic waveforms, and values being obtained with invasive hemodynamic technologies. The catheter site and insertion depth (CVC and PACs) should be documented and the CXR reviewed for placement if available. The

catheter site should be assessed and covered with an occlusive dressing. Catheters must be secured, and the patency of all ports confirmed before changing over to the transport monitor. Vented caps on stopcock ports should be replaced with sterile, nonvented caps to prevent accidental blood loss or infection. Excess tubing and stopcocks should be removed from the pressure monitoring system to reduce distortion in the system. Once the invasive line is connected to the transport monitor, it should be zeroed and leveled to the phlebostatic axis. The pressure bag should be inflated to 300 mmHg and monitored periodically during transport to maintain the patency of the system. Waveforms and hemodynamic data should be evaluated during transport. The distal port of all PACs must be transduced with a pressure monitoring system to monitor for catheter migration. Monitor alarms should be set to alert the transport crew that a change in the patient's condition has occurred or that the catheter has migrated or become dislodged. Potential complications that can occur during transport include catheter migration or dislodgement, clot formation at the catheter tip, and hemorrhage from line disconnection. Loss of distal circulation can occur with arterial lines. Direct pressure should be held to the site of any dislodged catheter until bleeding stops.

Less Invasive Hemodynamic Monitoring

Less invasive hemodynamic monitoring technologies now allow for the evaluation of flow-determined hemodynamic parameters in the critically ill. Some of these include CO, SV, pulse pressure variation, and SV variation. Most of these systems are based on arterial waveform analysis in which SV is estimated based on variation in the pulse waveform.[81] These less invasive hemodynamic technologies differ in several ways including the algorithm used to determine the values, the way the information from the arterial waveform is transformed, the requirement for calibration, the required site for arterial catheter placement, and the accuracy with which the parameters such as CO are achieved.[81] Several of the currently available technologies that analyze the arterial pulse wave morphology include the FloTrac (Edwards Lifesciences Corporation, Irvine, California), PiCCO (Pulsion, Feldkirchen,

Germany), and LiDCO (LiDCO Ltd, London, United Kingdom) systems.[83] An accurate arterial waveform is required to obtain valid data from these technologies. These systems use the previously described fluid-filled arterial line setup. The system should be leveled and zeroed to the phlebostatic axis. Distortion of the arterial waveform caused by technical issues, such as inaccurate leveling to the phlebostatic axis, over or under damping, or from dysrhythmias, may result in erroneous values.[84] Because these systems are based on the arterial waveform, it is imperative that an accurate arterial waveform be achieved for accurate measurement of SV and therefore CO. Currently, an additional monitor is required for these technologies.

Noninvasive Hemodynamic Monitoring

Noninvasive methods used to assess the hemodynamic status of the patient include the monitoring of the capillary refill, pulse rate and quality, BP, mentation, UO, and skin temperature. Mental status changes are important when determining the patient's overall condition. Significant changes in mentation occur in shock when the flow is compromised to the vital organs. Skin temperature and color, capillary refill, and UO in the absence of renal disease reflect tissue perfusion as it relates to CO and intravascular volume. A combination of noninvasive methods such as capillary refill time, quality of the heart rate, and quality of the pulse or pulse contour should be used in conjunction with hemodynamic monitoring to assess the adequacy of CO during the transport of critically ill patients.

BP measurements are frequently used to make a clinical decision during transport. The gold standard for monitoring BP is direct measurement using an arterial pressure monitoring system.[77] Direct BP monitoring via an arterial line is more accurate than indirect pressures specifically in the presence of hypertension, hypothermia, and shock.[76–79] Unfortunately, invasive arterial pressure monitoring is not always feasible in the transport environment. Because of this, noninvasive or indirect BP monitoring is frequently relied on for measurements of BP. BP can be obtained noninvasively using mechanical Doppler augmentation, automated BP devices (NIBP), or palpation of the radial pulse with a sphygmomanometer and cuff. These noninvasive, indirect measures assess flow, whereas direct arterial pressure monitoring measures pressure. It is important to keep in mind that direct and indirect measures will not always correlate because of the differences between measuring flow versus pressure. Inaccuracies in noninvasive BP monitoring frequently occur because of inappropriate cuff size or positioning of the extremity during BP measurement. The BP cuff width should be 40% of the arm circumference or one that covers two-thirds of the extremity being used.[75,85] Using a cuff that is too large will result in erroneously low readings. A cuff that is too small will result in erroneously high readings. Because of this, the transport crew should carry several sizes of cuffs to accommodate for patient size and age. Accuracy is also affected by the position of the extremity in which the BP is being taken. The extremity should be positioned at the phlebostatic axis (mid-chest level) for accurate BP reading. Elevation of the extremity above the phlebostatic axis will result in erroneously low values and if placed below this level will result in erroneously high values. Although BP measuring devices can be useful for monitoring trends in the patient's hemodynamic status, the patient's hemodynamic status should be evaluated with multiple methods rather than one specific parameter such as BP.

The stresses of flight, such as the effect of vibration on biomedical equipment and electromagnetic interference, have not been defined totally.[86] Thus transport crews must use a combination of invasive and noninvasive assessment methods to evaluate patient status throughout the transport process.

ETCO₂ for Monitoring Cardiac Output

As clinicians, we have been using the measurement of end-tidal CO_2 (ETCO$_2$) on the capnograph during CPR to evaluate the effectiveness of the chest compressions, which gives us an estimate of cardiac output and organ perfusion during that time. We know that an ETCO$_2$ of less than 10 mmHg is correlated with poor quality chest compression and that a major spike in the ETCO$_2$ is an indicator of return of spontaneous circulation (ROSC).[83] Respectively, an ETCO$_2$ of 20 mmHg can be achieved if quality chest compressions are provided, which provides an estimate of the cardiac index in the range of 1.6–1.9 L/min/m^2.[84] According to the current ACLS guidelines, optional chest compressions are being provided if the ETCO$_2$ is 10–20 mmHg.[84] However, the ETCO$_2$ is an underutilized, noninvasive measuring tool for estimating cardiac output in the critical care transport setting of patients with a perfusing pulse. The continuous waveform provided by the capnograph can provide trending values that correlate with the cardiac output. If adequate ventilation is maintained, the ETCO$_2$ delivers a persistent inclination of pulmonary blood flow, thereby an approximation of cardiac output. It has been demonstrated that ETCO$_2$ can be beneficial in approximating a modification in cardiac output.[86] Utilizing the Fick principles to the exhaled respiratory gases permits calculating cardiac output by evaluating oxygen consumption, and the variation of arterial and venous blood oxygen elements.[87]

Plethysmograph Utilization for Monitoring Cardiac Output

The plethysmograph, which comes standard on many critical care ECG monitoring devices, is a graphical display of the perfusion index. The perfusion index is the correlation of pulsating blood flow to the nonpulsating static flow to the peripheral tissues of the body, like the ear lobe, fingertips, or toes.[88] The perfusion index is an indicator used to evaluate the pulse strength at the site of sensor placement. The value range of the perfusion index is from 0.02%, indicating a very weak thready pulse, to 20%, which identifies a very strong and bounding pulse. The dependability of the perfusion index can fluctuate according to the physiologic conditions of the patient as well as the site placement for the monitoring device.[88]

Brugada Syndrome

Brugada syndrome is a genetic mutation consistent with sodium channel neuropathy, subsequently involving the specific gene *SCN5A*.[89,90] There are two essential elements required for Brugada syndrome to exist: an abatement in retaining depolarization and anatomic irregularities due to interstitial fibrosis.[91] Brugada syndrome can occur in those who inherit the disorder, however it can occur with no family history but have exacerbating factors such as fever, illness, or pharmacologically induced.[92] The Brugada syndrome ECG presentation can present from certain electrolyte irregularities, cocaine toxicity, cannabis use, and specific sodium channel blockers utilized in antiarrhythmic therapy.[93] Roughly 13% of Brugada syndrome incidents have been correlated with functional loss of modifications in the myocardial calcium channels, thereby reducing depolarization.[93] The genetic mutation phenotype Brugada syndrome occurs about 10 times more often in men than it does in women.[94] Electrolyte deficiencies are responsible for producing the right bundle branch block ECG pattern associated with Brugada syndrome. These deficiencies allow the left ventricle to depolarize first, instead of simultaneously, the way they should under normal physiologic circumstances.

Brugada syndrome may produce syncope, palpitation, or sudden cardiac death in the clinical setting.[92,93] Brugada syndrome can manifest from being asymptomatic to the ancillary ECG findings produced.[93] The long-lasting effects that Brugada syndrome can leave on patients include left ventricular hypertrophy and cardiomyopathies, like arrhythmogenic cardiomyopathy.[93] Brugada syndrome is a deviant pattern of ST segment elevation noted in the right precordial leads on a 12-lead ECG, that causes a high occurrence of sudden cardiac death.[94] Brugada syndrome has a distinct pattern of acclivous ST segment elevation and can be noted in leads V1–V4. Brugada syndrome type 1, known as coved-type,[95] is identified by the convexity in the shape of the ascending S wave within the rSr pattern in the right precordial leads.[96] The second type of Brugada syndrome is known as saddle-back-type, which is characterized again by a convexly shaped ST segment in the right precordial leads V1, V2, or V3, however, with this type, there are noted perpendicular T-waves.[97] The morphology of the T wave is another distinct difference between Brugada type 1 and type 2. In type 1 the T wave will have a declivous deflection; in type 2 the T wave will have an acclivous deflection.[97] These arrhythmias emerge from a disproportion amidst the depolarization and repolarization currents, inflected by the cardiac action potential.[93]

The website www.brugadadrugs.org contains a directory of medications that should be circumvented in patients with Brugada syndrome.[94,98,99] Medications like procainamide, propranolol, phenytoin, metoclopramide, propofol and tramadol are specific regimens that critical care providers should avoid administering in patients with Brugada syndrome.[98,99] Quinidine, an antiarrhythmic medication, has been shown as a treatment regimen for Brugada, due to its ability to lower the probability of ventricular fibrillation.[92,98,99] Lidocaine or amiodarone are available options for the treatment of Brugada syndrome-related ventricular fibrillation.[100] However, it is recommended to utilize one or the other of these medications in treating arrhythmias resulting from Brugada, since they produce different effects on the cardiac action potential.

Preexcitation Syndromes

The normal excitation of the myocardium begins in the sinoatrial node, then transmits through both atria via the internodal tracts. Atrial depolarization is then extended to the atrioventricular node, advancing through the bundle of His onto Purkinje fibers which are made up of the bundle branches. Preexcitation syndromes occur due to an early incitement of the ventricles by an impulse traveling through an aberrant tract, resulting in the averment of physiologic impeding in the atrioventricular junction. Preexcitation syndromes occur because these electrical tracts are either partially or entirely separate from the typical transmission pathways.[101] Furthermore, specific labelling of preexcitation syndromes has been developed based on whether the rhythm is generated via a forward-flowing ventricular tract or reverse-flowing atrial stimulation through an aberrant tract.[101]

There are two main preexcitation syndromes that critical care providers may encounter: those are Wolff–Parkinson–White (WPW) and Lown–Ganong–Levine (LGL). Preexcitation syndromes produce tachyarrhythmias. Wolff–Parkinson–White syndrome is seen more often with atrial fibrillation and LGL is seen more with supraventricular tachycardia. WPW is a preexcitation syndrome, producing life-threatening arrhythmias due to divergent cardiac electrical transmissions via aberrant pathways within the myocardium. The signature electrocardiographic feature of WPW is a shortened PR interval coupled with a rapidly acclivous widened QRS complex, better known as a "delta wave" in the presence of a sinus rhythm.[102]

Lown–Ganong–Levine syndrome involves an aberrant conduction tract that marginally or altogether diverts the atrioventricular node producing a straight triggering of the bundle of His by the sinoatrial node.[101] LGL and WPW syndromes can have the same mirroring clinical manifestations, sometimes making them hard to differentiate. One distinction between the two is that LGL will not possess the rapidly acclivous widened QRS complex that WPW possesses but will have a short PR interval. The distinction in the respective transmission speed of the atrioventricular node as opposed to the aberrant pathway influences the magnitude of preexcitation and variable revelation on the electrocardiogram.[103] The terminal vectors of the QRS are a representation of preexcitation of the ventricles, therefore, signifying potential clues for diagnosing abnormal or undiscovered preexcitation.[103] Preexcitation disorders may pose concerns, simply because symptoms may go unrecognized and in certain cases cease to exist.[104] Symptoms observed with these preexcitation syndromes include, but are not limited to, palpitations, dyspnea, tinnitus, dizziness, syncope, diplopia, and cardiac arrest.[102] Additionally, diagnosis via electrocardiographic interpretation often goes unrecognized.[103]

In cases with suspected ST-elevation myocardial infarction that have preexisting preexcitation syndromes, diagnoses may be ambiguous. STEMIs produce predominant repolarization irregularities that could be concealed due to ancillary ST segment and T wave variations, which are ancillary repolarization anomalies, generated by preexcitation syndromes.[105] The proportion of preexcitation is determined by the respective participation of the AV node and aberrant tract depolarization, cumulating in ventricular incitement.[105] Definitive delta waves can conceal pathologic Q waves and declivous delta waves can mimic the Q wave. Repeated electrocardiograms can assist in diagnosing STEMI in preexcitation syndromes.[106]

The most efficacious and definitive therapy for treating preexcitation syndromes is an ablation of the aberrant tract.[107] This intervention will be performed by an interventional cardiologist at a tertiary hospital. However, the critical care provider may be requested to transport these patients to those facilities and manage the patient in receiving definitive care. If the patient is not symptomatic, they do not require immediate therapy and should only be monitored during transport.[102] If the patient is symptomatic, and requires intervention, a few of the treatments for the patient with preexcitation syndromes and atrioventricular reentrant tachycardias that critical care providers may utilize include beta-blocker therapies like propranolol and metoprolol, which has an effective rate of between 50% to 90%.[107] Additionally, procainamide is another recommended medication in treating retrograde AV nodal reentry tachycardias.[102]

AV nodal blocking agents are however contraindicated in the presence of preexcitation and atrial fibrillation.[108] When the aberrant conducting pathway has the potential for accelerated forward transmission, accelerated atrial arrhythmias may be transmitted to the ventricle inciting accelerated ventricular rates that can degenerate, resulting in ventricular fibrillation.[102] This rationale is why

AV nodal blocking agents are contraindicated in these situations, because of aberrant accessory pathways and accelerated atrial rhythms, such as atrial fibrillation, atrial flutter, or atrial tachycardia. Depending on the underlying arrhythmia, this variation of arrhythmias will present as a wide complex tachycardia and can be either regular or irregular.[102]

When the impulse of the nerve fibers is transmitted in the typical direction with AV nodal reentry tachycardia and Wolff–Parkinson–White syndrome, as seen by evidence on the electrocardiogram, only then can AV nodal inhibiting agents such as beta-blockers, diltiazem, verapamil, or digoxin be considered.[103]

Critical Care Transport of the Cardiovascular Patient

Specialized skills and knowledge are required for the transport of patients with cardiovascular emergencies. Proper patient preparation, stabilization, and resuscitation should be performed during the transport of these challenging and critically ill patients. This should include assessment, planning, intervention, and evaluation.

Assessment

Assessment of the cardiovascular patient begins with the initial information elicited from the referring agency by dispatch personnel. This information can be invaluable for evaluating the best vehicle for patient transport and is helpful for air transport (especially when flying in an aircraft with limited space and weight restrictions), for anticipating in-flight emergencies, and for preparing the receiving agency for the patient. Time en route to the referring agency can be spent developing a preliminary plan of care based on initial information obtained from dispatch and the referring agency when available.

For the cardiovascular patient, assessment and preparation for transport are directed toward recognition, prevention, and correction of hypoxia and maintenance of adequate tissue perfusion and CO. The amount of time spent on assessment of the cardiovascular patient depends on the severity of the illness and the need for rapid intervention. The transport crew should obtain as much information as possible to provide safe and efficient transport to a definitive care institution and to ensure continuity of care.

A brief history of the event may be elicited from the patient, family members, or referring agency personnel. A general appraisal of the patient can be made while approaching the bedside and observing at that time the skin color, diaphoresis, activity or position of comfort, and respiratory distress. This should include observing for the presence of IV drug infusions, the amount of oxygen that is being delivered, the presence of invasive hemodynamic monitoring lines, and the cardiac rhythm displayed on the monitor. Initial perception of the situation helps to organize and direct the management of the patient for efficient and safe transport.

The physical examination is often abbreviated because of time constraints and is based on the transport crew's judgment in determining what information is vital for transport. Hands-on assessment of the patient includes confirmation of vital signs and hemodynamic readings and the identification of implications for continued emergency care. Initial evaluation of airway, breathing, and circulation (ABC) is of paramount importance. If the patient is not in immediate need of CPR, the overall cardiovascular status should be evaluated. Any necessary procedures should be performed at this time, such as intubation, IV or central line insertion, chest thoracostomy tube insertion, or additional therapeutic interventions as indicated.

Planning and Intervention

Adequate management and preparation of the patient for transport can greatly reduce the need for resuscitative measures en route to receiving facilities. Planning care for the transport of the critical cardiovascular patient includes anticipating complications that may occur as a result of the disease process. This requires a strong critical care knowledge base and ongoing competency in the transport of the critically ill.

Evaluation

Throughout the transport process, the transport team must systematically evaluate the patient's progress, analyze data, and modify the plan of care based on the patient's response to therapy. In the transport environment, continual assessment and monitoring of the patient provide data regarding the success or failure of each intervention.

Summary

Technological advancement is driving the medical industry, which in turn affects air and ground medical transportation programs. The critical care transportation industry must adapt to and be proficient with the ever-changing technology that patients and their families are using in their communities. Chapter 9 contains a thorough explanation of the current methods used for the mechanical management of the patient with cardiovascular disease. One day these patients will inevitably need emergent transportation, and critical care transport programs must be delivered and personnel prepared to provide optimal patient care.

References

1. Geller BJ, Sinha SS, Kapur NK, et al. Escalating and de-escalating temporary mechanical circulatory support in cardiogenic shock: a scientific statement from the American Heart Association. *Circulation*. 2022;146(6):e50–e68.
2. Storz JF, Scott GR. Life ascending: mechanism and process in physiological adaptation to high-altitude hypoxia. *Ann Rev Ecol Evol System*. 2019;50:503. doi: 10.1146/annurev-ecolsys-110218-025014
3. Damergis JA. Physiological parameter changes of high altitude and their correlation with acute mountain sickness. *Ann Emerg Med*. 2008;51(4):536.
4. Erdmann JS. Effects of exposure to altitude on men with coronary artery disease and impaired left ventricular function. *Am J Cardiol*. 1998;81(3):266–270.
5. AHA. *Advanced Cardiovascular Life Support Provider Manual*. Dallas, TX: American Heart Association; 2020.
6. Holleran RS, Wolfe AC, Frakes MA. *ASTNA Patient Transport: Principles and Practices*. 5th ed. St Louis, MO: Mosby Elsevier; 2017.

7. Treadwell T, Santiago JP. *Standards for Critical Care and Specialty Transport.* Aurora, CO: Air & Surface Transport Nurses Association; 2019.

8. Dismukes RK, Kochan JA, Goldsmith TE. Flight crew errors in challenging and stressful situations. *Aviat Psychol Appl Human Factors.* 2018;8(1):35–46. doi: 10.1027/2192-0923/a000129

9. Rasmussen TP, Bullis TC, Girotra S. Targeted temperature management for treatment of cardiac arrest. *Curr Treat Opt Cardiovasc Med.* 2019;22(11). doi: 10.1007/s11936-020-00846-6

10. Lüsebrink E, Binzenhöfer L, Kellnar A, et al. Targeted temperature management in postresuscitation care after incorporating results of the TTM2 Trial. *J Am Heart Assoc.* 2022;11:e026539.

11. Olasveengen TM, Mancini ME, Perkins GD, et al. Adult Basic Life Support: 2020 international consensus on cardiopulmonary resuscitation and emergency cardiovascular care science with treatment recommendations. *Circulation.* 2020;142(16 suppl 1):S41–S91.

12. Seewald S, Obermaier M, Leferimg R, et al. Application of mechanical cardiopulmonary resuscitation devices and their value in out-of-hospital cardiac arrest: a retrospective analysis of the German Resuscitation Registry. *PLoS ONE.* 2019;14(1):e0208113.

13. Adams A, Adams C. Transcutaneous pacing: an emergency nurse's guide. *J Emerg Nurs.* 2021;47(2):326–330. doi: 10.1016/j.jen.2020.11.003

14. Hulleman M, Mes H, Blom MT, Koster RW. Conduction disorders in bradysystolic out-of-hospital cardiac arrest. *Resuscitation.* 2016; 106:113–119.

15. Kusumoto F, Schoenfeld M, Barrett C, et al. 2018 ACC/AHA/HRS Guideline on the Evaluation and Management of Patients With Bradycardia and Cardiac Conduction Delay: Executive Summary. *J Am Coll Cardiol.* 2019;74(7):932–978.

16. Szarpak L, Filipiak KJ, Mosteller L, et al. Survival, neurological and safety outcomes after out of hospital cardiac arrest treated by using prehospital therapeutic hypothermia: a systematic review and meta-analysis. *Am J Emerg Med.* 2021;42:168–177. doi: 10.1016/j.ajem.2020.02.019

17. Makki N, Brennan TM, Girotra S. Acute coronary syndrome. *J Intens Care Med.* 2015;30(4):186–200. doi: 10.1177/08850666 13503294

18. Gulati M, Levy PD, Mukherjee D, et al. AHA/ACC/ASE/CHEST/ SAEM/SCCT/SCMR Guideline for the Evaluation and Diagnosis of Chest Pain: a report of the American College of Cardiology/ American Heart Association Joint Committee on Clinical Practice Guidelines. *Circulation.* 2021;144(22):e368–e454. doi: 10.1161/ CIR.0000000000001029

19. Oikonomou E, Leopoulou M, Theofilis P. A link between inflammation and thrombosis in atherosclerotic cardiovascular diseases: clinical and therapeutic implications. *Atherosclerosis.* 2020;309:16-26.

20. Libby P, Pasterkamp G, Crea F, Jang I. Reassessing the mechanisms of acute coronary syndromes: the vulnerable plaque and superficial erosion. *Circ Res.* 2019;124(1):150–160.

21. Papapanagiotou A, Daskalakis G, Siasos G, Gargalionis A, Papavassiliou AG. The role of platelets in cardiovascular disease: molecular mechanisms. *Curr Pharm Design.* 2016;22(29):4493-4505.

22. Borovac JA, Orsolic A, Miric D, Glavas D. The use of Smith-modified Sgarbossa criteria to diagnose an extensive anterior acute myocardial infarction in a patient presenting with a left bundle branch block. *J Electrocardiol.* 2021;64:80–84. doi: 10.1016/j.jelectrocard.2020.12.002

23. Kim KH, Kerndt CC, Adnan G, Schaller DJ. Nitroglycerin. In: StatPearls [Internet]. Treasure Island, FL,: StatPearls Publishing; 2022 Jan-. [updated 2022, Sep 27]. Available at: https://www.ncbi.nlm.nih.gov/books/NBK482382/.

24. Thygesen K, Alpert JS, Jaffe AS, et al; Executive Group on behalf of the Joint European Society of Cardiology (ESC)/American College of Cardiology (ACC)/American Heart Association (AHA)/World Heart Federation (WHF) Task Force for the Universal Definition of Myocardial Infarction. Fourth Universal Definition of Myocardial Infarction. *J Am Coll Cardiol.* 2018;72(18):2231–2264. doi: 10.1016/j.jacc.2018.08.1038

25. Ayers JK. Maani CV. Milrinone. In: StatPearls [Internet]. Treasure Island, FL: StatPearls Publishing; 2022 Jan [updated 2022, Sep 6]. Available at: https://www.ncbi.nlm.nih.gov/books/NBK532943/.

26. Dubin D. *Rapid Interpretation of EKGs.* 6th ed. Tampa, FL: Cover Publishing Company; 2000.

27. Kasper DL. *Harrison's Principles of Internal Medicine.* 19th ed. New York: McGraw–Hill Medical; 2015.

28. Sörensen NA, Ludwig S, Makarova N, et al. Prognostic value of a novel and established high-sensitivity troponin I assay in patients presenting with suspected myocardial infarction. *Biomolecules.* 2019;9(9):469.

29. Neumann JT, Twerenbold R, Ojeda F, et al. Application of high-sensitivity troponin in suspected myocardial infarction. *N Engl J Med.* 2019;380(26):2529–2540.

30. Zhao Y, Izadnegahdar M, Lee MK, et al. High-sensitivity cardiac troponin—optimizing the diagnosis of acute myocardial infarction/ injury in women (CODE-MI): rationale and design for a multi-center, stepped-wedge, cluster-randomized trial. *Am Heart J.* 2020;229:18–28.

31. Clerico A, Zaninotto M, Aimo A, et al. Use of high-sensitivity cardiac troponins in the emergency department for the early rule-in and rule-out of acute myocardial infarction without persistent ST-segment elevation in Italy. *Clin Chem Lab Med.* 2022;60(2):169–182.

32. Sandoval Y, Apple FS, Mahler SA, Body R, Collinson PO, Jaffe AS, International Federation of Clinical Chemistry and Laboratory Medicine Committee on the Clinical Application of Cardiac Biomarkers. High-sensitivity cardiac troponin and the 2021 AHA/ACC/ASE/CHEST/SAEM/SCCT/SCMR guidelines for the evaluation and diagnosis of acute chest pain. *Circulation.* 2022;10:1161.

33. Møller AL, Mills EHA, Gnesin F, et al. Impact of myocardial infarction symptom presentation on emergency response and survival. *Eur Heart J Acute Cardiovasc Care.* 2021;10(10):1150–1159. doi: 10.1093/ehjacc/zuab023

34. Miranda DF, Lobo AS, Walsh B, Sandoval Y, Smith SW. New insights into the use of the 12-lead electrocardiogram for diagnosing acute myocardial infarction in the emergency department. *Can J Cardiol.* 2018;34(2):132-145. doi: 10.1016/j.cjca.2017.11.011

35. DeVon HA, Mirzaei S, Zègre-Hemsey J. Typical and atypical symptoms of acute coronary syndrome: time to retire the terms? *J Am Heart Assoc.* 2020;9(7):e015539.

36. Lee J-W, Moon JS, Kang DR, et al. Clinical impact of atypical chest pain and diabetes mellitus in patients with acute myocardial infarction from prospective KAMIR-NIH Registry. *J Clin Med.* 2020; 9(2):505. doi: 10.3390/jcm9020505

37. Zhang F, Tongo ND, Hastings V, et al. ST-Segment elevation myocardial infarction with acute stent thrombosis presenting as intractable hiccups: aAn unusual case. *Am J Case Rep.* 2017;18:467–471. doi: 10.12659/ajcr.903345

38. Gao H, Zhang B, Song L, Yao S, Zhang Z, Bai M. Acute proximal left anterior descending thrombosis manifested by persistent hiccups: a case report. *Medicine.* 2019;98(48):e18096. doi: 10.1097/ MD.0000000000018096

39. Hovey J, Perwez T, Regula P, Chaucer B, Nagalapuram V. Acute coronary syndrome presenting with hiccups. *Cureus.* 2021;13(7): e16244. doi: 10.7759/cureus.16244

40. Layell R. Recognizing STEMI equivalents, identifying myocardial infarction vs other coronary syndromes. *EMS World Magazine.* 2020;49(2):26–29.

41. Kyaw K, Latt H, Aung SSM, Tun NM, Phoo WY, Yin HH. Atypical presentation of acute coronary syndrome and importance of Wellen's syndrome. *Am J Case Rep.* 2018;19:199–202. doi: 10.12659/ ajcr.907992

42. Ko W, Hurng G, Zhou R, Dai X. A systematic approach to evaluate patients presenting with ST-segment elevation in lead aVR: a case series. *Cureus.* 2020;12(11):e11800. doi: 10.7759/cureus.11800

43. Hoff J. Evaluation and interventional management of cardiac dysrhythmias. *Surg Clin.* 2022;102(3):365-391.

44. Hammond BB, Zimmermann PG, eds. *Sheehy's Manual of Emergency Care*. 7th ed. St. Louis, MO: Emergency Nurses Association. Elsevier/Mosby; 2013.

45. Ye F, Winchester D, Stalvey C, et al. Proposed mechanisms of relative bradycardia. *Medical Hypothesis*. 2018;119:63–67. doi: 10.1016/j.mehy.2018.07.014

46. Papadakis MA. *Current Medical Diagnosis and Treatment 2016*. 55th ed. New York: McGraw-Hill; 2016.

47. Wesley K. In *Huszar's Basic Dysrhythmias and Acute Coronary Syndromes: Interpretation and Management*. 4th ed. St. Louis, MO: Elsevier/Mosby; 2011.

48. Al-Khatib SM, Stevenson WG, Ackerman MJ, et al. AHA/ACC/HRS Guideline for management of patients with ventricular arrhythmias and the prevention of sudden cardiac death: a report of the American College of Cardiology/American Heart Association Task Force on clinical practice guidelines. *J Am Coll Cardiol*. 2018;72(14):e91–e220.

49. Foglesong A, Mathew D. Pulseless ventricular tachycardia. In: StatPearls [Internet]. Treasure Island, FL: StatPearls Publishing; 2022 Jan [updated 2022, Aug 1]. Available at: https://www.ncbi.nlm.nih.gov/books/NBK554467/.

50. Goyal A, Chhabra L, Joseph C, Sciammarella JC, Cooper JS. Defibrillation. In: StatPearls [Internet]. Treasure Island, FL: StatPearls Publishing; 2022 Jan [updated 2022 Aug 10]. Available at: https://www.ncbi.nlm.nih.gov/books/NBK499899/.

51. Tehrani BN, Truesdell AG, Psotka MA, et al. A standard and comprehensive approach to the management of cardiogenic shock. *JACC Heart Fail*. 2020;8(11):879-891. doi: 10.1016/j.jchf.2020.09.005

52. Hashmi KA, Abbas K, Hashmi AA, et al. In-hospital mortality of patients with cardiogenic shock after acute myocardial infarction; impact of early revascularization. *BMC Res Notes*. 2018;11:721. doi: 10.1186/s13104-018-3830-7

53. Jentzer JC, Burstein B, Diepen SV, et al. Defining shock and pre-shock for mortality risk stratification in cardiac intensive care unit patients. *Circ Heart Fail*. 2021;14(1):e007678. doi: 10.1161/CIRCHEARTFAILURE.120.007678

54. Lim JY, Park SJ, Kim HJ, et al. Comparison of dopamine versus norepinephrine in circulatory shock after cardiac surgery: a randomized controlled trial. *J Cardiac Surg*. 2021;36(10):3711–3718.

55. Aimo A, Castiglione V, Borrelli C, et al. Oxidative stress and inflammation in the evolution of heart failure: from pathophysiology to therapeutic strategies. *Eur J Prevent Cardiol*. 2020;27(5):494–510.

56. Brener MI, Rosenblum HR, Burkhoff D. Pathophysiology and advanced hemodynamic assessment of cardiogenic shock. *Methodist Debakey Cardiovasc J*. 2020;16(1):7–15.

57. Kapur NK, Thayer KL, Zweck E. Cardiogenic shock in the setting of acute myocardial infarction. *Methodist Debakey Cardiovasc J*. 2020;16(1):16–21. doi: 10.14797/mdcj-16-1-16

58. Ajam T, Ajam S, Devaraj S, Fudim M, Kamalesh M. Effect on mortality of higher versus lower beta blocker (metoprolol succinate or carvedilol) dose in patients with heart failure. *Am J Cardiol*. 2018;122(6):994–998.

59. Masip, J. Noninvasive ventilation in acute heart failure. *Curr Heart Fail Rep*. 2019;16:89–97. doi: 10.1007/s11897-019-00429-y

60. Heart Failure Society of America, Lindenfeld J, Albert NM, et al. Heart Failure Society of America 2010 Comprehensive Heart Failure Practice Guideline. *J Card Fail*. 2010;16(6):e1–e194.

61. Berbenetz N, Wang Y, Brown J, et al. Non-invasive positive pressure ventilation (CPAP or bilevel NPPV) for cardiogenic pulmonary edema. *Cochrane Database Syst Rev*. 2019;4:CD005351.

62. Ismail TF. Acute pericarditis: update on diagnosis and management. *Clin Med (Lond)*. 2020;20(1):PMC6964178.

63. Mcnamara N, Ibrahim A, Satti Z, Ibrahim M, Kiernan TJ. Acute pericarditis: a review of current diagnostic and management guidelines. *Future Cardiol*. 2019;15(2):119–126. doi: 10.2217/fca-2017-0102

64. Spodick DH. Acute, clinically noneffusive ("dry") pericarditis. In: Spodick DH, ed. *The Pericardium: A Comprehensive Textbook*. New York: Marcel Dekker; 1997.

65. Rajani R, Klein JL. Infective endocarditis: a contemporary update. *Clin Med (Lond)*. 2020;20(1):31–35. doi: 10.7861/clinmed.cme.20.1.1

66. Satriano UM, Nenna A, Spadaccio C, et al. Guidelines on prosthetic heart valve management in infective endocarditis: a narrative review comparing American Heart Association/American College of Cardiology and European Society of Cardiology guidelines. Ann Transl Med. 2020;8(23):1625. doi: 10.21037/atm-20-5134

67. Hurrell H, Roberts-Thomson R, Prendergast BD. Non-infective endocarditis. *Heart*. 2020;106(13):1023–1029.

68. Rodríguez-García R, Rodríguez-Esteban MÁ, Fernández-Suárez J, et al. Evaluation of 16S rDNA heart tissue PCR as a complement to blood cultures for the routine etiological diagnosis of infective endocarditis. *Diagnostics*. 2021;11(8):1372. doi: 10.3390/diagnostics11081372

69. Iung B, Duval X. Infective endocarditis: innovations in the management of an old disease. *Nat Rev Cardiol*. 2019;16(10):623–635. doi: 10.1038/s41569-019-0215-0

70. Long B, Koyfman A. Infectious endocarditis: an update for emergency clinicians. *Am J Emerg Med*. 2018;36(9):1686–1692. doi: 10.1016/j.ajem.2018.06.074

71. Alerhand S, Adrian RJ, Long B, Avila J. Pericardial tamponade: a comprehensive emergency medicine and echocardiography review. *Am J Emerg Med*. 2022;58:159–174.

72. Van den Born VKH, Lip GYH, Brguljan-Hitij J, et al. ESC Council on Hypertension position document on the management of hypertensive emergencies. *Eur Heart J Cardiovasc Pharmacother*. 2019;5(1):37–46.

73. Fukui T. Management of acute aortic dissection and thoracic aortic rupture. *J Intens Care*. 2018;6:15.

74. Jen JP, Malik A, Lewis G, Holloway B. Non-traumatic thoracic aortic emergencies: imaging diagnosis and management. *Br J Hosp Med (Lond)*. 2020;81(10):1–12.

75. Nguyen LS, Squara P. Non-invasive monitoring of cardiac output in critical care medicine. *Front Med*. 2017;4:200.

76. Lough ME. *Hemodynamic Monitoring: Evolving Technologies and Clinical Practice*. St. Louis, MO: Elsevier; 2016.

77. Pierre L, Pasrija D, Keenaghan M. Arterial lines. In: StatPearls [Internet]. Treasure Island, FL: StatPearls Publishing; 2022 Jan [updated 2022, May 8]. Available at: https://www.ncbi.nlm.nih.gov/books/NBK499989/.

78. Thanachartwet V, Wattanathum A, Sahassananda D, et al. Dynamic measurement of hemodynamic parameters and cardiac preload in adults with dengue: a prospective observational study. *PLoS One*. 2016;11(5):e0156135. doi: 10.1371/journal.pone.0156135

79. Edward Lifesciences. Normal hemodynamic parameters and laboratory values. 2022. Available at: https://education.edwards.com/normal-hemodynamic-parameters-pocket-card/1167897#.

80. Layell R. Recognition and care of aortic dissection. If it looks like a STEMI plus a CVA, be vigilant for this life threat. *EMS World Magazine*. 2021;50 (5):40–43.

81. Rodriguez Ziccardi M, Khalid N. Pulmonary artery catheterization. In: StatPearls [Internet]. Treasure Island, FL: StatPearls Publishing; 2022 Jan [updated 2022,Jul 18]. Available at: https://www.ncbi.nlm.nih.gov/books/NBK482170/.

82. Nair R, Lamaa N. Pulmonary capillary wedge pressure. In: StatPearls [Internet]. Treasure Island, FL: StatPearls Publishing; 2022 Jan [updated 2022, Apr 21]. Available at: https://www.ncbi.nlm.nih.gov/books/NBK557748/.

83. Sandroni C, De Santis P, D'Arrigo S. Capnography during cardiac arrest. *Resuscitation*. 2018;132:73–77.

84. Herndon A, Moore A. End tidal CO_2 in cardiac arrest. [NUEM Blog. Expert Commentary by Trueger NS]. 2018. Available at: http://www.nuemblog.com/blog/ETCO2.

85. Ringrose JS, Padwel R. Automated blood pressure measuring devices: how are they clinically validated for accuracy? *J Human Hypertens*. 2023:37(2):101–107.

86. Kerslake I, Kelly F. Uses of capnography in the critical care unit. *BJA Education.* 2017;17(5):178–183.

87. Nguyen LS, Squara P. Non-invasive monitoring of cardiac output in critical care medicine. *Front Med.* 2017;4:200.

88. Amperor Direct USA. What is perfusion index (PI). 2022. Available at: https://www.amperordirect.com/pc/help-pulse-oximeter/z-what-is-pi.html.

89. El Sayed M, Goyal A, Callahan AL. Brugada syndrome. In: StatPearls [Internet]. Treasure Island, FL: StatPearls Publishing; 2022 Jan [updated 2023, Aug 8]. Available at: https://www.ncbi.nlm.nih.gov/books/NBK519568/.

90. Hosseini SM, Kim R, Udupa S, Costain G, Jobling R, Liston E. National Institutes of Health Clinical Genome Resource Consortium. Reappraisal of reported genes for sudden arrhythmic death: evidence-based evaluation of gene validity for Brugada syndrome. *Circulation.* 2018;138(12):1195–1205.

91. Blok M, Boukens BJ. Mechanisms of arrhythmias in the Brugada syndrome. *Int J Mol Sci.* 2020;21(19):7051. doi: 10.3390/ijms21197051

92. Mankbadi M, Hassan S, McGee M, et al. Brugada syndrome: the role of risk stratification in selecting patients for implantable cardioverter-defibrillator placement. *Cureus.* 2018;10(6):e2799.

93. Cerrone M, Costa S, Delmar M. The genetics of Brugada syndrome. *Ann Rev Genomics Human Genet.* 2022;23:255–274.

94. Attard A, Stanniland C, Attard S, Iles A, Rajappan K. Brugada syndrome: should we be screening patients before prescribing psychotropic medication? *Ther Adv Psychopharmacol.* 2022;12:20451253211067017. doi: 10.1177/20451253211067017

95. Boncoraglio MT, Esteves J, Pereira F, et al. Brugada pattern: unraveling possible cardiac manifestation of SARS-CoV-2 infection. *J Med Cases.* 2021;12(5):173–176. doi: 10.14740/jmc3644

96. Baranchuk A, Enriquez A, Villuendas R, de Luna AB. Differential diagnosis of rSr' pattern in leads V1–V2. Comprehensive review and proposed algorithm. *Ann Noninvas Electrocardiol.* 2015;20(1):7–17. doi: 10.1111/anec.12241

97. Korlipara H, Korlipara G, Pentyala S. Brugada syndrome. *Acta Cardiol.* 2021;76(8):805–824. doi: 10.1080/00015385.2020.1790823

98. Postema PG, Wolpert C, Amin AS, et al. Drugs and Brugada syndrome patients: review of the literature, recommendations, and an up-to-date website (www.brugadadrugs.org). *Heart Rhythm.* 2009;6(9):1335–41. doi: 10.1016/j.hrthm.2009.07.002

99. Smith Jr LD, Gast S, Guy, DF. Brugada syndrome: fatal consequences of a must-not-miss diagnosis. *Crit Care Nurse.* 2021;41(5):15–22.

100. Aleksandrowicz D. Amiodarone or lidocaine, that is the question – pharmacological therapy of refractory ventricular fibrillation associated with Brugada syndrome. *Resuscitation.* 2021;169:76–77.

101. Soos MP, McComb D. Lown Ganong Levine syndrome. In: StatPearls [Internet]. Treasure Island, FL: StatPearls Publishing; 2022 Jan [updated 2022, Oct 2]. Available at: https://www.ncbi.nlm.nih.gov/books/NBK546711/.

102. Chhabra L, Goyal A, Benham MD. Wolff–Parkinson–White syndrome. In: StatPearls [Internet]. Treasure Island, FL: StatPearls Publishing; 2022 Jan [updated 2022, May 22]. Available at: https://www.ncbi.nlm.nih.gov/books/NBK554437/.

103. Xu Z, Liu R, Chang Q, Li C. Preexcitation syndrome: experimental study on the electrocardiogram of antegradely conducting accessory pathway. *BMC Cardiovasc Disord.* 2018;18(1):100.

104. Rubio Campal JM, Blanco AM, Calero LB, et al. Comparison of outcomes of catheter ablation in asymptomatic versus symptomatic preexcitation to guidelines and beyond. *Am J Cardiol.* 2021;161:51–55. doi: 10.1016/j.amjcard.2021.08.051

105. Rajendran K, Thankachan A, Sreedharan MK, Salam A. Preexcitation syndrome presenting with acute myocardial infarction. *BMJ Case Rep.* 2022;15(7):e250667.

106. Page RL, Joglar JA, Caldwell MA, et al. Evidence Review Committee Chair: 2015 ACC/AHA/HRS guideline for the management of adult patients with supraventricular tachycardia: a report of the American College of Cardiology/American Heart Association Task Force on Clinical Practice Guidelines and the Heart Rhythm Society. *Circulation.* 2016;133(14):e506–74.

107. Stasiak A, Niewiadomska-Jarosik K, Kędziora P. Clinical course and treatment of children and adolescents with the preexcitation syndrome – own studies. *Dev Period Med.* 2018; 22(2):113–122.

108. Coppola G, Corrado E, Curnis A, et al. Update on Brugada syndrome 2019. *Curr Prob Cardiol.* 2021;46(3):100454.

9

Mechanical Circulatory Support Devices in Transport

ASHLEY M. CHITTY, TONYA I. ELLIOTT, LESLIE C. SWEET, AND ALLEN C. WOLFE JR.

COMPETENCIES

1. Identify the indications for use of mechanical circulatory support devices.
2. Verbalize an assessment of the patient with a mechanical circulatory support device.
3. Manage specific mechanical circulatory support devices before, during, and after the transport process.

Mechanical circulatory support (MCS) is indicated in patients who, despite optimal medical management, remain in cardiogenic shock or refractory advanced heart failure. This chapter will review the current MCS devices (MCSDs) for both acute and chronic support, patient assessment and management while on these devices, and the related transport considerations and recommendations.

Background

Over the past decades, several medical breakthroughs led to improved patient outcomes while on MCSDs allowing for thousands of patients to be treated with MCSDs annually. Improved diagnostics and treatments for heart disease have facilitated earlier recognition of patients with advanced heart failure and identification of those eligible for MCS, both acute and chronic devices, which has subsequently improved overall clinical outcomes. Additionally, the evolution of MCS designs, including smaller pumps and improved hemocompatibility, has broadened patient eligibility for MCS and improved long-term survival on device. Currently there are thousands of patients living in the community on durable MCS devices, some hundreds of miles from the implanting hospital. With the increased use of temporary MCS devices in the setting of acute heart failure as well, the need for trained transport clinicians is growing.

Safe transport of this critically ill patient population involves training, planning, communication, and vigilant assessment. Transport clinicians at a large referral hospital were able to demonstrate successful outcomes after transporting patients supported on acute MCS over long distances.[1] At this single-center study, patient survival was equivalent to registry results from the Extracorporeal Life Support Organization (ELSO) demonstrating the feasibility of safe MCS transport.

Cardiac congenital anomalies alter blood flow through the cardiopulmonary system rendering pediatric patients unable to oxygenate and/or circulate blood in a manner compatible with life. These children require extracorporeal membrane oxygenation (ECMO) until a more permanent therapy for heart failure can be provided, such as long-term ventricular assist devices (VAD) and heart transplantation. Transporting pediatric patients on ECMO to VAD and heart transplant centers is paramount to survival. Coppola et al. provided a review of decades of cases in which pediatric patients in cardiogenic shock were transported on ECMO with comparable outcomes to patients supported on ECMO within their institution.[2] These studies demonstrated the need to have knowledgeable transport services readily available to safely transport critically ill patients on MCSD.

Indications for Ventricular Assist Device Therapy

MCS is indicated when patients suffer decompensated acute or chronic heart failure refractory to conventional pharmacologic and mechanical therapies such that hospital discharge is not feasible, or frequent rehospitalizations are needed to stabilize patient symptoms. Cardiac transplant is the current gold standard for treating patients with end-stage heart failure who are deemed eligible, and it offers a 50% survival rate at 13 years post transplant.[3,4] Durable VADs can provide improved quality of life when compared to advanced heart failure and are readily available (unlike waiting for a suitable donor organ) and without the side effects of immunosuppressive therapy. The indications for VAD implantation include the following: (1) bridge to recovery (BTR); (2) bridge to more definitive therapy; (3) short-term support, formerly bridge to transplant (BTT); and (4) long-term support, formerly destination therapy (DT).

Bridge to recovery (BTR) refers to MCS that allows the heart to "rest". Given time to rest, the native heart function may then recover and adequately support circulation, allowing for explantation of the device. Initially, this indication was thought to be limited to acute cardiogenic shock and temporary support, but clinical experience has shown in a small cohort of patients that myocardial recovery may be achieved with a longer duration of support provided by long-term "durable" devices.[5,6]

Bridge to definitive therapy describes the use of a short-term device to temporarily support the failing heart through an acute event. After patients are stabilized, cardiac function may be more thoroughly evaluated to determine whether the insult is reversible, or whether a more definitive, long-term therapy is indicated. Definitive therapy strategies may include more conventional percutaneous coronary interventions, coronary artery bypass graft surgery, cardiac transplantation, or long-term VAD support.

Short-term support (BTT) refers to the implantation of a durable VAD in transplant candidates whose heart becomes refractory to conventional pharmacologic support and for whom a suitable donor heart has not yet become available. The VAD is intended to provide adequate circulatory support and improved end-organ perfusion until a donor heart becomes available. It is then removed along with the native heart during the transplant surgery. Current data from the United Network of Organ Sharing (UNOS) Registry shows that there are almost three times as many heart transplant candidates as there are recipients, reaffirming the ongoing shortage of available donor organs.[3,7] The reduction in pre-transplant mortality is attributable to multiple factors, including the use of VADs to bridge these patients. In 2018, UNOS redefined donor allocation for hearts to favor transplanting the sickest patients first. This new allocation system favors support on temporary devices.[3,7] Table 9.1 shows the breakdown of MCS use for BTT up to 2018, as the outcomes data takes years to manifest.[8] Donor-to-candidate volume mismatch and the allocation system policies have produced an increasing number of BTT patients on short-term MCSDs.

Long-term support (DT) describes the use of a VAD to sustain circulatory support in patients with medically refractory advanced heart failure who are deemed ineligible for cardiac transplant because of other comorbidities or who have declined listing for transplant. Historically, these patients would be sent home, if possible, with palliative or hospice care for the duration of their lives. With the advent of dischargeable, durable devices, these patients may be adequately sustained on VADs and still be active members of their families and communities. Observational data from the MOMENTUM trial demonstrated that 58.4% of HeartMate 3 patients were alive 5 years post implant.[9] These data also reveal that 54% of patients (composite outcome includes patients who went on to transplant and explant for recovery) were free from stroke and pump exchange surgery.[9] Data from a large multicenter national registry (Interagency Registry for Mechanically Assisted Circulatory Support; INTERMACS) revealed sustained improvement in quality of life in patients who remained free from complications, such as strokes.[10] Ultimately, these reductions in complications across both studies translate to improved patient experience and a better quality of life.

The Basics

MCSDs are designed to support the pumping function of a failing heart, whether the etiology is acute cardiogenic shock or severe chronic cardiomyopathy. These devices may be separated into two major categories: short-term or acute devices and long-term, durable devices.[11] Temporary, short-term support can be provided by an intra-aortic balloon pump (IABP), ECMO, and acute continuous flow VADs (e.g., Impella Heart Pump [Abiomed, Inc.; Danvers, MA], CentriMag Acute Circulatory Support System [Thoratec Corporation | Abbott, Inc.; Pleasanton, CA]). Support on these devices confines patients to the hospital until a more definitive, dischargeable device can be implanted or the support can be weaned.

Patients may be discharged into the community on durable devices such as a *total artificial heart (TAH)* and *ventricular assist devices (VADs)*. The TAH (SynCardia Systems, Inc.; Tucson, AZ) is a device that completely *replaces* the native heart physically and functionally. Implantation of a TAH involves removal of the native heart, specifically the right and left ventricles, similar to cardiac transplantation. The TAH is attached to the atria and great vessels of the native heart (pulmonary artery [PA] and aorta), with complete excision of the remaining heart muscle. Because of the size of a TAH, patients must have adequate thoracic space to accommodate the pump. TAHs are indicated for patients with medically refractory biventricular heart failure. Because the TAH replaces both ventricles, should the driver/console fail, there is no native heart or native function to provide circulatory support, so the device must be manually pumped (only available for the Companion Driver [SynCardia] used when patients are inpatients) or the driver is exchanged to the portable backup driver (Freedom Portable Driver [SynCardia] used in the community).

VADs, such as the HeartMate II and HeartMate 3 left ventricular assist devices (Thoratech Corporation | Abbott Inc.; Pleasanton, CA) and the HeartWare HVAD system (Medtronic; Minneapolis, MN), are designed to *assist* the native heart in pumping adequate blood to vital body organs. The native heart remains intact, and the VAD is attached to the appropriate heart chambers and great vessels. The degree of circulatory support

TABLE 9.1	Adult Heart Transplants: Recipient Characteristics (Transplants January 1992 to June 2018)			
	Jan 1992 to Dec 2000 (N = 37,616)	Jan 2001 to Dec 2009 (N = 33,588)	Jan 2010 to Jun 2018 (N = 36,830)	P-Value
Inotrope use	46.7%[a]	43.4%	35.7%	<0.0001
IABP use	6.0%	6.2%	6.6%	0.0672
ECMO use	0.2%[b]	0.7%	1.1%	<0.0001
VAD	—	18.9%	40.4%	<0.0001
TAH	—	0.7%	1.3%	
BiVAD	—	3.3%	2.7%	
No MCS use	—	77.2%	55.6%	

[a]Based on Apr 1994 to Dec 2000 transplants.
[b]Based on Apr 1996 to Dec 2000 transplants.
BiVAD, Biventricular assist device; *ECMO*, extracorporeal membrane oxygenation; *IABP*, intra-aortic balloon pump; *MCS*, mechanical circulatory support; *TAH*, total artificial heart; *VAD*, ventricular assist device.
From ISHLT International Registry for Heart and Lung Transplantation 2021. *J Heart Lung Transplant.* 2021;40(10):1023–1072.

provided by the VAD varies depending on the design of the VAD and the pumping capabilities of the native heart. VADs are referenced based on the side of the heart receiving support. When VADs support the right side of the heart, the pumps are referred to as *right ventricular assist devices* (RVADs), and VADs that support the left side of the heart are LVADs. When the technology is used to support both sides of the heart, it is referred to as a *biventricular assist device* (BVAD or BiVAD) and can be two of the same VAD devices or two different VAD devices (a hybrid configuration).[12] With full BiVAD support, patients in sustained ventricular fibrillation are usually coherent as the arrhythmia is clinically insignificant because of adequate circulation from the BiVAD system.

Device Characteristics and Designs

VAD technology has evolved significantly over recent years. The earliest designs of MCS included roller pumps for cardiopulmonary bypass (CPB) and the IABP for cardiogenic shock. Although the use of IABPs for acute cardiogenic shock may increase cardiac output (CO) by 10%–15%, a significant mortality rate remains in shock patients. Both CPB and IABPs are limited in the duration of support that they can provide.

Pulsatile flow pumps or VADs (PF-VADs) are devices that are considered *fill-to-empty* or *volume-displacement pumps*. The most widely used pulsatile VAD was the extended vented electric (XVE) LVAD, now obsolete. Pulsatile pumps have a blood sac or chamber in which blood collects before being ejected into the circulation, similar to the native heart's diastole and systole. The rate at which these devices pump depends on filling of the blood chambers and does not necessarily correlate with the patient's native heartbeat. Unlike an IABP with electrocardiogram (ECG) tracing capabilities, any apparent synchrony of pumping rates between PF-VADs and the native heart is coincidental. These devices have inflow and outflow valves to ensure unidirectional blood flow through the pump. The mechanics that create pulsatility are prone to wear and tear over time, leading to pump failure. The size of the XVE LVAD was also prohibitive for implant in patients with small body habitus. Hence, durable volume displacement VADs were abandoned and replaced with impellers that spin continuously.

Continuous flow pumps or VADs (CF-VADs) pull blood from the left ventricle (LV) then push it into the aorta continuously, creating pulseless flow. CF-VADs do not have a blood-collecting chamber or unidirectional valves, and they do not pause for optimal filling. They do have inflow and outflow cannulas but instead of a blood chamber they contain a high-speed impeller. The impeller is similar to a turbine engine or propeller. Because CF-VADs draw blood continuously from the supported ventricle, pulsatility of the sustained circulation may be dampened significantly. For example, if the VAD is supporting the left side of the heart, then a peripheral pulse may be difficult to palpate, requiring reliance on more basic assessment skills of adequate circulation (e.g., capillary bed refill, adequate mentation, urine output).

CF-VADs may be further differentiated into axial and centrifugal flow pumps. The CF-VAD impeller uses rotational energy to propel blood through the pump. It may be cylindrical or disk shaped, and uses blades or vanes to direct the blood flow forward. CF-VADs are also valveless, so a pump stop or inadequate speed may be associated with retrograde flow.

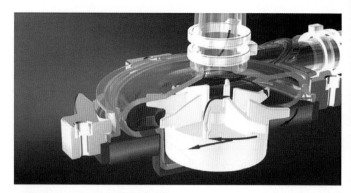

• **Fig. 9.1** Blood flow through an axial flow impeller. (Reproduced with permission of Abbott, © 2024. All rights reserved.)

The blood flow path of the axial flow devices is linear across the cylindrical impeller, relying on circumferential energy (Fig. 9.1). The rotational speed of an axial flow device is typically 8000 to 15,000 rotations per minute (rpm). The blood flow path of the centrifugal flow devices involves a 90-degree turn through the disk impeller via the perpendicular inflow and outflow ports, combining both centrifugal and circumferential energy to propel the blood forward (Fig. 9.2). The rotational speed of the centrifugal pump is typically 2000–6000 rpm. In addition, the centrifugal blood pump impeller is magnetically and/or hydrodynamically suspended (elevated by the blood flow through the pump), which eliminates the amount of contacting mechanical surfaces that otherwise could wear with time.[13] Hence, centrifugal pumps are often referred to as "wearless" pumps. As the technology advances, these devices, inherent to their design, have become smaller, more energy-efficient, and have fewer contacting parts. The benefits of these advances are that the pumps will likely last longer and can be implanted in a wider range of body sizes, which makes the technology more accessible to more patients.

Temporary Devices for Acute Cardiogenic Shock

Temporary devices used for acute cardiogenic shock are indicated for immediate stabilization of the patient's condition, with an average projected support time of 7–10 days. Common indications for these devices include acute cardiogenic shock associated with myocardial infarction (MI), postcardiotomy shock, viral myocarditis, and temporary right ventricular failure (RVF) associated with implantation of a permanent LVAD. The advantage of these short-term devices is that they allow the clinical team the opportunity to stabilize patients, allowing time to fully assess the clinical pathology and etiology of the cardiogenic shock, and the most appropriate course for further therapy. Strategies at this time include the addition of maximal pharmacologic therapies and possibly interventional procedures to improve circulation and optimize the potential for recovery and removal of the VAD versus confirming that the VAD cannot be weaned. In the latter case, the next strategies are to consider eligibility for cardiac transplant versus long-term VAD therapy. In extreme cases, withdrawal of

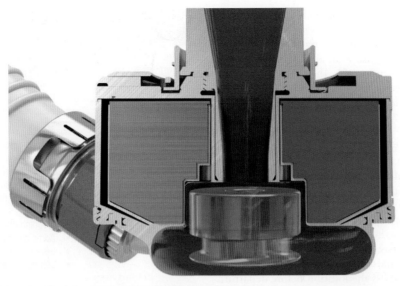

• **Fig. 9.2** Blood flow through a centrifugal flow impeller. (Reproduced with permission of Abbott, © 2024. All rights reserved.)

pharmacologic and mechanical support may be warranted and requested by next of kin.

Typical acute cardiogenic shock devices that may necessitate medical transport are the IABP, ECMO, Impella Heart Pumps (Abiomed, Inc.; Danvers, MA), and the CentriMag Acute Circulatory Support System (Thoratec Corporation | Abbott, Inc.; Pleasanton, CA). The major components of these blood pumps typically include cannulas and blood tubing that are attached to the native circulation (i.e., major blood vessels versus the heart) and then to the blood pump; and the console that runs the pump and provides electrical power to the system, with backup batteries for patient transportation while on support. All of these devices currently require systemic anticoagulation to minimize the potential for thrombus formation and occlusion in balance with avoiding excessive bleeding. In that acute temporary devices are inherently prone to increase the risk of bleeding due to damage of clotting factors, judicious use of blood transfusions is important to avoid related complications such as subsequent right heart failure, and increased allosensitization. Heparin is used most often, although an alternative agent such as argatroban or bivalirudin may be needed if the patient has tested positive for heparin-induced thrombocytopenia (HIT).

Intra-aortic Balloon Pump (IABP)

The Pathophysiology

The myocardium is supplied by the coronary arteries which carry oxygen-rich blood from the root of the aorta. During ventricular contraction, known as systole, the subendocardial coronary vessels are compressed due to high ventricular pressures causing coronary blood flow to pause. As a result, coronary perfusion occurs during ventricular relaxation, known as diastole. The principle of intra-aortic balloon pump counterpulsation is to improve the ventricular performance of a failing heart by increasing myocardial oxygen supply through coronary perfusion and reducing myocardial oxygen demand (Table 9.2).[14]

Secondary Effects of Intra-aortic Balloon Pump Support

The catheter's balloon is timed to inflate and deflate in synchrony with the cardiac cycle. This counterpulsation increases myocardial oxygen supply while decreasing the myocardial demand and afterload of the heart. When the balloon inflates during diastole, the left ventricle is relaxed and the aortic valve is closed, which increases oxygenated blood flow into the coronary arteries. This blood displacement not only improves the myocardial oxygen supply, but also increases aortic diastolic pressure.

| TABLE 9.2 | Secondary Effects of Intra-aortic Balloon Pump Support |||||||||

	CLINICAL PARAMETER								
	CO	SV	LVEF	CPP	Systemic Perfusion	HR	PCWP	SVR
Secondary effect	↑	↑	↑	↑	↑	↓	↓	↓

CO, Cardiac output; *CPP*, coronary perfusion pressure; *HR*, heart rate; *LVEF*, left ventricular ejection fraction; *PCWP*, pulmonary capillary wedge pressure; *SV*, stroke volume; *SVR*, systemic vascular resistance.

This effect is called diastolic augmentation. Helium gas is used to inflate the balloon because of its low viscosity which allows it to travel quickly through the long connecting tubes with minimal turbulence and has a lower risk than air of causing an embolism should the balloon rupture.[15] The IABP console is modified and designed specifically for transport outside the hospital setting. The indications and contraindications are listed in Table 9.3.

Catheter and Console Operations

The IABP catheter is usually inserted in the femoral artery at the bedside with placement confirmed by chest x-ray or under fluoroscopy. The catheter's balloon consists of a polyurethane membrane (balloon) positioned in the descending thoracic aorta (Fig. 9.3). If positioned properly, the radiopaque markers at the tip should be about 2 cm distally to the origin of the subclavian artery (typically between the second and third intercostal space) and the catheter base should lie above the renal arteries. The transport team should assess the location before departure. This can be easily done by verbally asking the referring MD for affirmation of placement or by evaluating the chest x-ray. The catheter size is determined by the inserting physician and is based on the patient's body size. It is labeled at the base of the catheter which is sutured externally near the femoral artery or entrance point if the femoral is not an option (axillary artery, subclavian artery). The size and volume in milliliters are on this label.

The catheter is connected to a pump console that monitors heart rate and arterial blood pressure. There are two different types of catheters. The one most commonly encountered is the fiberoptic catheter. A fiberoptic manometer is located at the tip of the catheter's balloon. It provides accurate, fast, high-quality hemodynamic measurements. Therefore, this is the most accurate measure of blood pressure. This allows for

TABLE 9.3	Indications and Contraindications for Intra-aortic Balloon Pump
Indications for temporary use	• Intractable angina • Cardiogenic shock • Complications of acute myocardial infarction • Complicated angioplasty • Refractory myocardial ischemia
Contraindications	Absolute: • > mild aortic regurgitation • Aortic dissection • Aortic aneurysm (significant) • Severe sepsis • Irreversible brain damage Relative: • Bleeding disorder • Aortic atheroma • Severe peripheral artery disease • Left ventricular outflow

Data from Intra-aortic Balloon Pump. https://www.aats.org/tsra-primer-intra-aortic-balloon-pump.

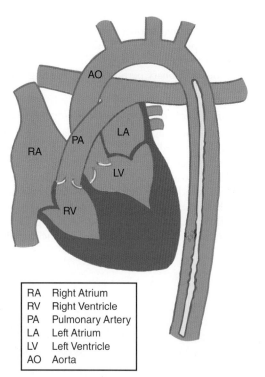

RA Right Atrium
RV Right Ventricle
PA Pulmonary Artery
LA Left Atrium
LV Left Ventricle
AO Aorta

The IABP is deflated during systole, as the heart contracts.

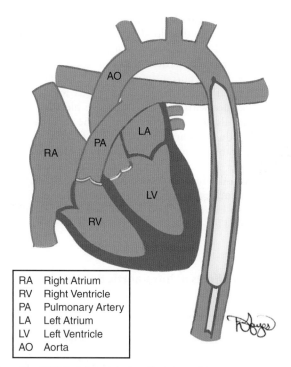

RA Right Atrium
RV Right Ventricle
PA Pulmonary Artery
LA Left Atrium
LV Left Ventricle
AO Aorta

The IABP is inflated during diastole as it improves coronary circulation.

• **Fig. 9.3** Placement of intra-aortic balloon pump (IABP) balloon-tipped catheter. The goal of inflation is to produce a rapid rise in aortic pressure, which optimizes diastolic augmentation and increases oxygen supply to the coronaries. During deflation, the reduction in end aortic diastolic pressure (afterload) causes improved cardiac performance. (Courtesy David Hayes.)

the software algorithm to measure key markers in the waveform analysis and optimize left ventricular support. The timing algorithms are updated continually, allowing for optimal inflation and deflation. The timing adapts to changes in both heart rate and ECG rhythm on a beat-to-beat basis.[16,17] The console has colorful display panels combined with pneumatic and electronic innovations. They have cardiosynchronization capabilities with auto-select trigger selection and timing. The IABP adapts its deflation automatically while supporting ventricular ectopy or other arrhythmias.[16] If the timing is not correct, several physiologic changes can occur, as outlined in Table 9.4.

TABLE 9.4   Intra-aortic Balloon Pump Timing Errors

Timing Error	Effect
Early inflation	Premature closure of the aortic valve causing aortic regurgitation Increase in MVO$_2$ demand Aortic regurgitation Potential increase of PCWP Increased afterload
Late inflation	Suboptimal coronary perfusion
Early deflation	Retrograde coronary blood flow Suboptimal coronary perfusion and cause angina Suboptimal afterload reduction Increase in MVO$_2$

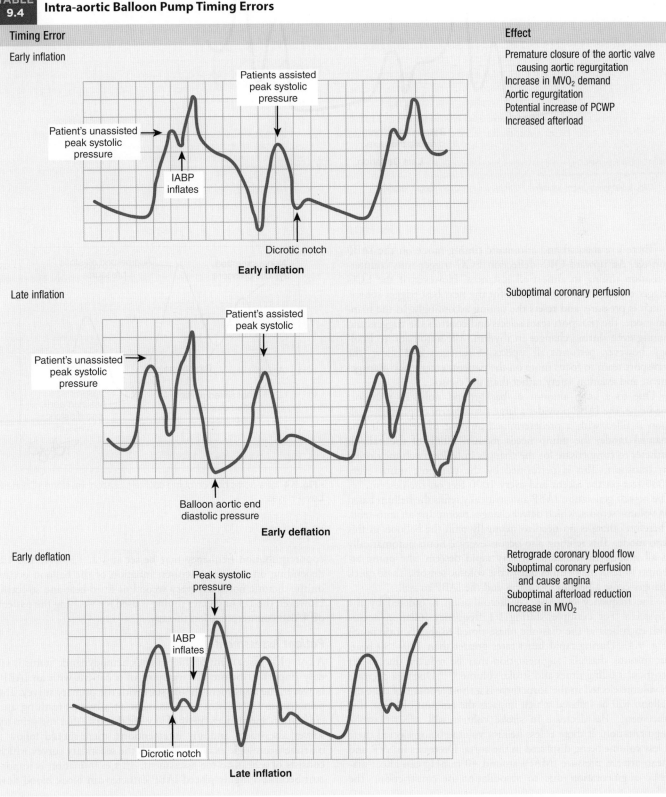

Early inflation

Late inflation

Early deflation

Continued

TABLE 9.4	Intra-aortic Balloon Pump Timing Errors—cont'd	
Timing Error		**Effect**
Late deflation 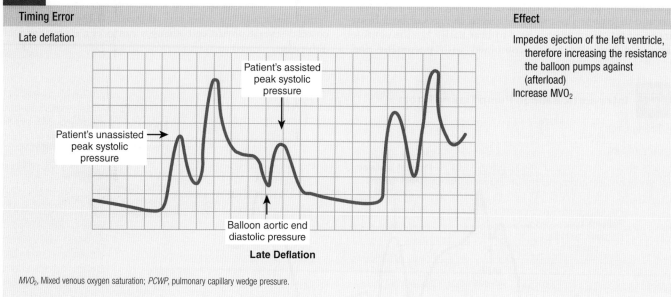 **Late Deflation**		Impedes ejection of the left ventricle, therefore increasing the resistance the balloon pumps against (afterload) Increase MVO$_2$

MVO_2, Mixed venous oxygen saturation; *PCWP*, pulmonary capillary wedge pressure.

There is a manual and automatic timing mode on the IABP console. An upward QRS deflection ECG trigger runs counterpulsation timing in almost all instances. However, if the ECG trigger is lost, the pump searches for the next best trigger source, which is pressure, and resets the timing accordingly. In the manual mode, the transport team selects and controls the triggers and timing even during changes in rhythm. The automatic technology, however, performs all aspects of function and allows the transport team to focus more on the patient, emergency management, and aviation safety rather than the console.

Due to a large amount of background noise in transport medicine, the IABP provides a large visual alarm display. The balloon is filled with a predetermined amount of helium. In the manual mode, the pump needs manual filling of the balloon catheter to compensate for the changes in balloon volume during air transport. This is performed by the transport teams every 2000 feet on the ascent and every 1000 feet on the descent.[16,17] The newest generation IABP automatically refills the helium based on volume sensors, which detect changes prompting an auto-refill. Therefore, there is no need to manually refill the balloon in this auto mode. This refilling also occurs every 2 hours automatically in all modes. In situations of very rapid descent, the pump attempts to refill many times due to the volume sensors. These quick changes cause a helium loss alarm and the IABP to stall.

The frequency of IABP counterpulsation is ordered by the physician. For example, during 1:1 frequency inflation occurs with each beat at the diastolic phase timed to the dicrotic notch (Fig. 9.4). During rapid heart rates greater than 120–130 beats per minute, diastolic augmentation may be reduced due to left ventricular filling times and stroke volume.[16,18] Due to a decrease in volume ejected in the aorta there is a short amount of time the balloon will be inflated which impacts the amount of blood displacement. The decrease in stroke volume will affect diastolic augmentation. If there is less helium volume being ejected there is less volume being displaced in the aorta. Decreases in SVR and mean arterial pressure (MAP) around 40 mmHg can affect diastolic augmentation due to vasodilation or constriction. The

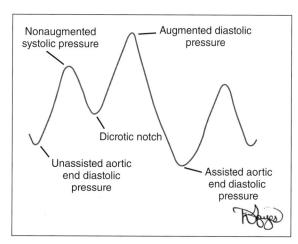

• **Fig. 9.4** Intra-aortic balloon pump counterpulsation waveform. (Courtesy David Hayes.)

counterpulsation frequency may be set at 1:2, 1:3, 1:4, and 1:8 depending on the manufacturer. Inflation of the balloon occurs on the dicrotic notch on every second or third beat and so forth. However, the 1:3 or greater timing is used for weaning the patient off IABP counterpulsation therapy.

Patient Assessment

A complete assessment of the patient's hemodynamic status is vitally important before the transport of a patient with an IABP; however, the assessment should start with the primary survey. The primary survey consists of assessment of airway, breathing and circulation and management of any life threats. After the primary survey assessment and any interventions, there should follow a baseline neurologic examination with the secondary survey which consists of a head-to-toe assessment. This examination is important because a highly placed IABP catheter can block blood flow to the left subclavian artery, left common carotid artery, and vessels of the left arm.

The hemodynamic assessment should consist of an evaluation of the patient's cardiac output (CO), cardiac index (CI), systemic vascular resistance (SVR), pulmonary vascular resistance (PVR), and other pulmonary artery catheter (PAC) data, if available. The assessment of the IABP includes diastolic augmentation, pump timing, and any alarms. Auscultation of heart sounds should occur on standby of the console for a brief period so that the sounds are heard. In air and ground transport, hearing capabilities are impaired; therefore, all the important sound-assessed information should be obtained before leaving the referring facility. Blood samples drawn through the IABP catheter should be avoided. Assessment of left brachial pulse helps with assessment of the position of the catheter. Anuria or oliguria may be indicators of the catheter being too low unless hypoperfusion is the culprit.

Laboratory values are an important part of the patient assessment of a patient receiving IABP therapy. The review may include the most recent complete blood count (CBC), prothrombin time (PT), partial thromboplastin time (PTT), platelet counts, and a basic metabolic panel. If oozing at the insertion site is present or occurs, the patient may receive an infusion of clotting factors and the transport team may consider careful placement of a bag of intravenous (IV) fluids over the exit site. This provides light pressure without interfering with the counterpulsation of the IABP. The oozing is most likely the result of the decrease in platelets caused by IABP counterpulsation or anticoagulation effects from other medications. The head of the bed or stretcher should be less than 30 degrees to prevent occlusion of the catheter at the femoral artery site. Light restraints or sedation may help keep the leg with the catheter secured to prevent accidental dislodgement or interference with console functioning. The diameter of the catheter varies from patient to patient; therefore, assessment of distal pulses is important to ensure perfusion of extremities. An occlusion can cause ischemia and result in clot formation, decreased circulation, and total arterial occlusion causing possible limb amputation if the IABP is not repositioned or removed. The transport team should perform a thorough assessment and relay

any complications from IABP therapy to the accepting physician with documentation in the chart.

Transport Considerations

Transport considerations for IABP patients are detailed in Table 9.5.

Management of IABP Emergencies in Transport

The common emergencies most frequently seen in IABP patients in transport are detailed in Table 9.6.

Extracorporeal Membrane Oxygenation (ECMO)

Heart transplant remains the gold standard for treating end-stage, advanced heart failure in eligible candidates. Organ Procurement and Transplantation Network (OPTN) and UNOS establish national policies to ensure fair organ allocation, which were updated in 2022, as previously mentioned. Under these new OPTN guidelines patients supported on ECMO will be given priority listing status (status 1).[19] Hence, more transplant-listed patients who decompensate quickly from cardiogenic shock will be considered for ECMO and may then require transport to the transplanting center to be registered as a candidate on the transplant waiting list with urgent upgrade to status 1.

Indications for ECMO

ECMO is used in patients in emergently decompensating cardiac, cardiopulmonary, or pulmonary failure. Candidates for ECMO support include patients who experience cardiac and/or pulmonary collapse. Each ECMO center has their own policies/guidelines regarding indications and contraindications of placing a patient on ECMO. The commonly found indications and contraindications can be found in Table 9.7.

ECMO System

The inflow cannula for ECMO drains blood from the venous circulation into the circuit. A centrifugal pump head then pumps the blood through the system and the oxygenator, ultimately

TABLE 9.5	Transport Considerations for Intra-aortic Balloon Pump Patients
Transport Vehicle	Assure sufficient batteries and the inverter is operable and charges the console. Assure the console is properly secured per the program aviation standards.
Equipment	Adapters are necessary backup equipment along with a 60-mL syringe, cables, extra helium, and batteries. The Arrow (Teleflex) and Maquet Cardiosave (Getinge) insertion kits are supplied with adapters that allow for transport teams to connect the male–female connection tubing to allow transfer from one machine to another. Blood pressure readings should be taken from the IABP console and not the NIBP cuff or manually. The highest pressure sensed or heard is diastolic augmentation, not systolic. Therefore, documentation of the NIBP or manual pressures provides inaccurate information. Inability to calibrate the fiberoptic balloon – use an alternative source such as radial arterial line.
Helium	Note the helium icon on the console to assess the amount of helium available. Please note the valve on the tank must be turned off for refilling and the number of auto-fills should be tracked on some IABP consoles. It will affect the overall supply. At altitudes greater than 10,000 feet in an unpressurized cabin, the fiberoptic catheters may be altered and inoperable. They are more accurate below 10,000 feet.[2,5] Temperature extremes (affects IABP functioning and tubing elasticity). Environmental care should be provided to prevent detrimental effects.
Assessment	Consider positioning the patient in a slight lateral position to prevent pressure area relief. Reassessment of mental status due to potential stroke, and migration of IABP.

IABP, Intra-aortic balloon pump; *NIBP*, noninvasive blood pressure.

TABLE 9.6 Intra-aortic Balloon Pump Emergencies

Problem	Intervention
Ventricular fibrillation or pulseless ventricular tachycardia arrest	Follow ACLS or program guidelines. Stopping the pump is not necessary. Pump is grounded and can accommodate electrical shocks.
Cardiopulmonary arrest: asystole or pulseless electrical activity	Begin ACLS or program guidelines and place the pump on pressure mode during compressions. IABP pump will continue to pump with compressions as pressure is sensed.
Power failure	Attach a 60-mL syringe to the proximal stopcock. Inflate the IABP catheter with 40 mL of air or helium and immediately aspirate once every 5 minutes to prevent clot formation on the catheter while IABP is inactive.
Diastolic hypertension	Provide afterload reduction medication or decrease augmentation volume in IABP if possible.
Rapid heart rate greater than 130 bpm	Treat the origin of the tachycardia.
Balloon rupture (evidenced by blood in the sheath but the helium can dehydrate the blood causing it to present as rust-colored flakes, loss gas alarm)	Stop the pump immediately; clamp the catheter. Position patient in the flat position. IABP needs to be removed as soon as possible to decrease the chance of entrapment of the balloon.
Balloon migration. Upward: occlusion of the left subclavian and carotid artery. Downward: occlusion of renal or mesenteric arteries (decrease in urinary output or abdominal pain)	Notify physician to plan for re-siting of the balloon.

ACLS, Advanced cardiac life support; *IABP*, intra-aortic balloon pump.

TABLE 9.7 Indications and Contraindications for ECMO

Indications	
	• Cardiogenic shock/severe cardiac failure
	• Postcardiotomy with inability to wean off cardiopulmonary bypass
	• Post heart transplant with graft failure
	• Bridge to transplant
	• Periprocedural support for high-risk cardiac interventions
	• Massive pulmonary embolism
	• Massive hemoptysis/pulmonary hemorrhage
	• Acute anaphylaxis
	• Peripartum cardiomyopathy
	• Sepsis with severe cardiac depression
	• Cardiac index <2 L/min/m^2
	• Persistent cardiopulmonary arrest despite traditional resuscitative efforts
Contraindications	**Absolute:** • Unrecoverable heart and not a candidate for transplant or ventricular assist device • Chronic organ dysfunction (emphysema, cirrhosis, renal failure) • Prolonged cardiopulmonary resuscitation without adequate tissue perfusion • Aortic dissection • Severe aortic valve regurgitation • Current intracranial hemorrhage **Contraindications to ECLS – ECPR:** • Initial rhythm asystole • Age >80 years • Chest compressions not initialed within 10 min of arrest • Cardiopulmonary resuscitation >60 min before implanting ECMO • Preexisting severe neurological disease • Any absolute contraindications as listed previously

Examples of indications and contraindications for venovenous (VV) ECMO and venoarterial (VA) ECMO. This does not represent an exhaustive list of indications/contraindications for either modality.
As per ELSO guidelines: the primary indication for ECLS is acute severe heart and/or lung failure with high mortality risk despite optimal conventional therapy.
ECLS is considered at 50% mortality risk. ECLS is indicated in most circumstances at 80% mortality risk.
ECLS, Extracorporeal life support; *ECMO*, extracorporeal membrane oxygenation; *ECPR*, extracorporeal cardiopulmonary resuscitation; *ELSO*, Extracorporeal Life Support Organization.
Modified from Zeidman AD. Extracorporeal membrane oxygenation and continuous kidney replacement therapy: technology and outcomes – a narrative review. *Adv Chron Kidney Dis*. 2021;28(1): 29–36.

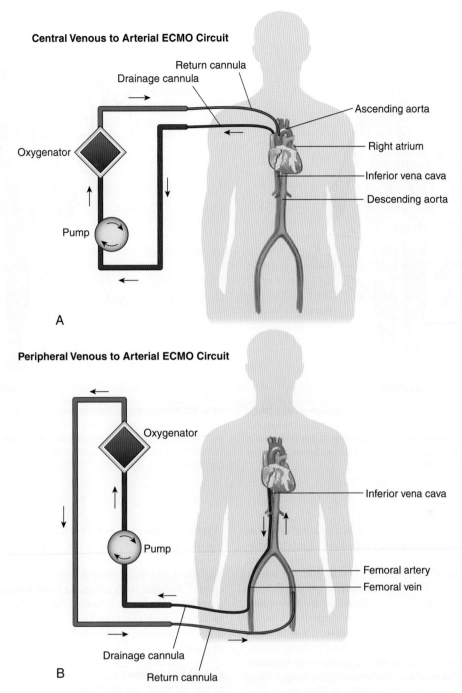

Central Venous to Arterial ECMO Circuit

Return cannula

Drainage cannula

Oxygenator

Pump

Ascending aorta

Right atrium

Inferior vena cava

Descending aorta

A

Peripheral Venous to Arterial ECMO Circuit

Oxygenator

Pump

Inferior vena cava

Femoral artery

Femoral vein

Drainage cannula

Return cannula

B

• **Fig. 9.5** Overview of an extracorporeal membrane oxygenation (ECMO) circuit. Central (**A**) and peripheral (**B**) placement of an ECMO circuit.   (Modified from Hung M, Vuylsteke A, Valchanov K. Extracorporeal membrane oxygenation coming to an ICU near you. J *Intensive Care Soc.* 2012;13(1):31–38.)

returning the oxygenated blood to the patient (Fig. 9.5). Cannula placement is based on the patient's need for pulmonary vs. cardiopulmonary support. Cannulation can be either a single site or dual site. For cardiac and cardiopulmonary failure, the cannulas drain from the venous system (e.g., inferior vena cava [IVC] or right atrium via the femoral or jugular veins) into the circuit then return through the arterial system (e.g., ascending aorta for central ECMO, femoral artery or subclavian artery for peripheral ECMO). This approach is known as venous–arterial or venoarterial (VA)

ECMO (Fig. 9.6). Usually, in adult patients the inflow cannula (venous) is 19–25 Fr cannula and the return (arterial) is 15–23 Fr cannula.[20] Cannula sizes are determined by the patient size, and desired ECMO flow requirements.

In patients with pulmonary or ventilatory failure, the cannulas drain from the venous system (e.g., femoral and/or jugular vein) into the circuit and return oxygenated blood back into the venous system. This approach is known as venous–venous or venovenous (VV) ECMO (Fig. 9.7). A distal perfusion catheter is often placed

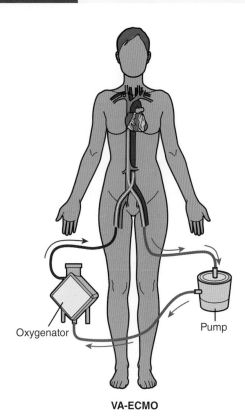

VA-ECMO

• **Fig. 9.6** Venoarterial extracorporeal membrane oxygenation (VA ECMO) circuit cannulation scheme. (Modified from Squiers JJ, Lima B, DiMaio JM. Contemporary extracorporeal membrane oxygenation therapy in adults: Fundamental principles and systematic review of the evidence. *J Thorac Cardiovasc Surg.* 2016;152(1):20–32.)

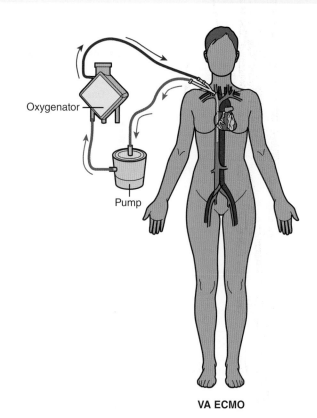

VA ECMO

• **Fig. 9.7** Venovenous extracorporeal membrane oxygenation (VV ECMO) circuit cannulation scheme. (Modified from Squiers JJ, Lima B, DiMaio JM. Contemporary extracorporeal membrane oxygenation therapy in adults: Fundamental principles and systematic review of the evidence. *J Thorac Cardiovasc Surg.* 2016;152(1):20–32.)

during the ECMO cannulation procedure in the same artery as the arterial cannula to ensure adequate blood flow in this extremity, preventing limb ischemia (Fig. 9.8). Usually, in adult patients the inflow cannula (venous) is 23–31 Fr cannula and the return (venous, internal jugular) is 15–19 Fr cannula.[20]

ECMO patients are at risk for thromboembolism formation, thus an anticoagulant is administered to prevent thrombus. Unfractionated heparin is the most commonly administered anticoagulant.[21] It is important to monitor for the effects of anticoagulation during transport. The transport team should monitor the cannulation sites for bleeding and swelling, abdominal girth, output from any drainage systems such as urinary catheters or chest tubes, sanguineous secretions from the endotracheal tube, and perform serial neurological assessments.

ECMO Components

The ECMO system consists of one bifurcated/dual lumen or two separate cannulas, the pump, a membrane oxygenator, the circuit tubing, a control panel, an oxygen source ideally with a blender, and a power cable. Transport teams should carry an emergency kit, including but not limited to a hand crank (if applicable), sterile shears, clamps, connectors, fluid, backup primed circuit and console.[22] Organizations should have a checklist to ensure equipment is present and not expired.

The ECMO system removes carbon dioxide and oxygenates the blood through the membrane oxygenator (Fig. 9.9). ECMO support allows for ventilatory setting changes that reduce inhaled oxygen requirements and positive end-expiratory pressure, reducing the risk of barotrauma. The effects of hyperoxia are still being researched, but the limited research has indicated that hyperoxia may decrease cardiac output and increase systemic vascular resistance.[23] Patients with advanced heart failure tend to be the most sensitive to the hemodynamic effects of hyperoxia, in comparison to patients with other etiologies.[23] Hyperoxia can cause worsening lung function due to impaired gas exchange and decreased ciliary efficacy.

ECMO Parameters

In VV ECMO, the flow supports oxygenation while VA ECMO supports cardiac output. Rotations per minute are adjusted to obtain the desired flow. Adult ECMO flows are usually 4–6 L/min. The listed measures and pressures are for the portable centrifugal pump, Cardiohelp System (Maquet | Getinge; Wayne, NJ). Venous pressure (pVen) measures the blood inlet pressure, normally −50 to −80 mmHg. A pVen greater than −100 mmHg may indicate hypovolemia or vasodilatation. When pVen exceeds −100 mmHg a chugging or a chatter may occur. Arterial pressure (pArt) is measured on the post-oxygenator side and measures the pressure in the return/outlet cannula. The pArt usually measures less than 250 mmHg. A rapid increase in the pArt may indicate an occluded or kinked return cannula. Delta Pressure (Δp) measures the pressure across the membrane, the difference between the initial pressure (pInt) and the pArt. A Δp greater than 50 mmHg may indicate a blood clot.

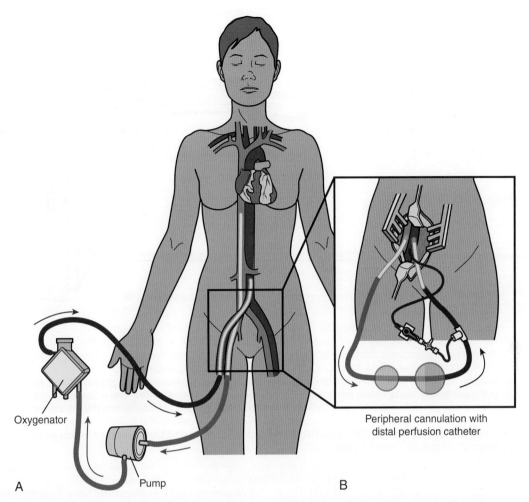

• **Fig. 9.8** Basic cannulation for VA ECMO support. **A,** Peripheral cannulation. **B,** Peripheral cannulation with distal perfusion catheter. (Modified from Keebler ME, Haddad EV, Choi CW, et al. Venoarterial extracorporeal membrane oxygenation in cardiogenic shock. *JACC Heart Fail.* 2018;6(6):503–516.)

Oxygenator

Pump

A

Peripheral cannulation with distal perfusion catheter

B

ECMO Transport Considerations

The Extracorporeal Life Support Organization (ELSO) has developed guidelines for transporting patients on ECMO. The guidelines and transport are available online in the ASAIO Journal.[22] Patients may need to be emergently transported to a center that has the capacity to implant ECMO, or if already supported on ECMO, may need to go to a center with access to transplant or durable VADs.

Transport of ECMO patients requires conscientious coordination and careful considerations in comparison to transportation of routine critical care patients. It is recommended that, prior to transport, the transport team, sending facility, and receiving facility should have a discussion regarding the potential risks and benefits of transport by air vs. ground, and specific patient needs during transport. The distance between centers and weather conditions impacts which mode of transport is appropriate, so careful planning is required. During colder months the transport team needs to consider temperature and wind chill, for without an ECMO heater, the patient's core temperature decreases rapidly causing arrhythmias or coagulation issues. An ECMO cooler should be considered for transports performed in extreme heat climates. The weight of the additional equipment added to the

aircraft and crew member weights need to be relayed and discussed with the pilot for aircraft weight and balance calculations as soon as possible.

Equipment considerations must include the ability to provide power to the circuit and to have a redundant system in the event of device malfunction. For long-distance transfers, consider attaching not only the ECMO system, but the monitor and pumps to a power source. Redundant systems include but are not limited to a primed backup ECMO circuit, adequate oxygen supply for both the ventilator and ECMO circuit, and an increased amount of medication to allow for maximum titration of drips if needed. If transporting a patient by air, ensure you allow for unexpected, prolonged ground transfer time due to unforeseen circumstances such as traffic, EMS delays, or unanticipated weather. If the transport team does have point-of-care lab capabilities, the team should consider having a discussion with the accompanying perfusionist/ECMO specialist about the estimated transport time and potential need for labs during transport and their ability to bring a point-of-care lab device. Many ECMO patients have coagulopathies, so the transport team should discuss the need for additional blood products to ensure adequate blood volume. ECMO lines should be evaluated

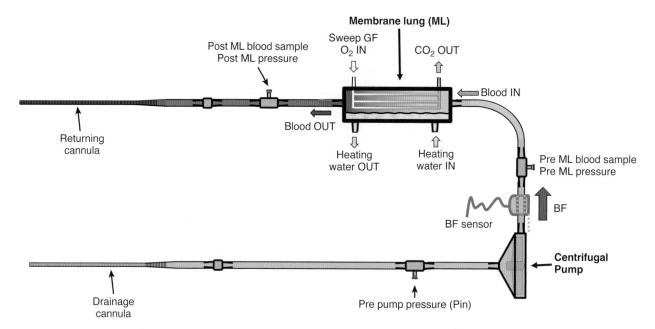

• **Fig. 9.9** Schematic of a basic circuit for venovenous extracorporeal membrane oxygenation (VV ECMO). From the drainage to the returning cannula, a basic circuit for VV ECMO includes a connector with stopcock for drainage pressure monitoring (pre-pump pressure or Pin); the centrifugal pump; a flow sensor for monitoring blood flow (*BF*); a connector with stopcock for monitoring pressure and sampling for gas analysis of the input blood (pre-membrane lung [*ML*] pressure); the membrane lung oxygenator (*ML*) (inlet and outlet port for blood, sweep gas flow (*GF*), and heating water are represented); and a connector with stopcock for monitoring pressure and obtaining samples for gas analysis of blood leaving the oxygenator (post-membrane lung [*ML*] pressure). (From Pesenti A, Grasselli G, Zanella A, et al. Extracorporeal support of gas exchange. In Schnapp LM, Stapleton RD, Broaddus VC, et al., eds, *Murray & Nadel's Textbook of Respiratory Medicine*. 7th ed. Elsevier; 2022.)

after all patient movements to ensure the absence of kinks and compression on the tubing.

Management of ECMO Emergencies in Transport

Emergencies in ECMO patients during transport are uncommon and can be stressful since time is of the essence during these emergencies. Many emergencies can be avoided; these procedures should be discussed and practiced routinely.

When emergencies occur, clinicians should follow policies or guidelines from the device manufacturer or their institution. If the ECMO pump fails, immediately clamp tubing both pre and post oxygenator, place the circuit on the hand crank (if applicable), check the tubing for air bubbles and clots, remove the clamps and start cranking at the same RPMs prior to the failure while troubleshooting the failed pump or obtaining a backup pump. The pump can fail due to battery failure or decoupling of the centrifugal pump.

ECMO Transport Team Model

There are many different models and team configurations utilized for ECMO transports based on the patient's needs and space constraints. The most common rotor wing transport team makeup for a patient already on ECMO consists of two transport team members, and a perfusionist or ECMO specialist who will manage the ECMO circuit during the transport. When space allows in alternate transplant vehicles, e.g., critical care vehicles or fixed wing aircraft, consider allowing for more personnel; the team may select to have a respiratory therapist or physician to accompany the team and patient.

Extracorporeal Cardiopulmonary Resuscitation (ECPR)

ECPR is the placement of VA ECMO during cardiopulmonary resuscitation or intermittent return of spontaneous circulation (ROSC).[24] ECPR's purpose is to support end-organ perfusion while evaluating and treating reversible conditions.[24] ECPR should be considered in select patients who have failed conventional cardiopulmonary resuscitation (CCPR).[25] In October 2022, the Extracorporeal Life Support Organization data reported out of 12,125 adult patients 42% survived ECLS (Extracorporeal Life Support), and 30% survived hospital discharge or transfer.[26] Many institutions with ECPR programs have their own variation of ECPR inclusion criteria. Inclusion criteria defined by the Extracorporeal Life Support Organization for ECPR are age less than 70 years, bystander CPR within 5 minutes of arrest, initial cardiac rhythm of ventricular fibrillation/pulseless ventricular tachycardia/pulseless electrical activity, less than 60 minutes from arrest to ECMO blood flow, end-tidal CO_2 ($ETCO_2$) >10 mmHg during CCPR, or intermittent ROSC/recurrent ventricular fibrillation.[27] Quickly evaluating and identifying a cardiac arrest patient as a potential ECMO candidate with minimal scene time is paramount for improved patient outcomes. The use of supraglottic airway versus endotracheal intubation remains controversial, and the data remain mixed.[28]

Prehospital or scene ECMO is the future of ECMO. The Minnesota Mobile Resuscitation Consortium was the first "community-wide ECMO-facilitated resuscitation program" in the United States.[29] Many out-of-hospital cardiac arrest (OHCA) patients are excluded solely based on their inability to be transported and arrive at an ECPR center within the desired time for favorable outcomes. To increase accessibility to ECPR centers Helicopter-Borne ECPR teams have been developed to reach these remote OHCA patients. Helicopter-Borne ECPR teams are currently being utilized in the Netherlands, Switzerland, and France.

ECMO – Special Considerations

Improvement in ECMO technology led to an expanded use as a treatment option in the acute setting of medically refractory cardiogenic shock and heart failure patients. Impella Heart Pumps provide another option for prophylactic device support for high-risk percutaneous angioplasty procedures, as well as support of severe left or right heart failure as a bridge to more definitive therapy. The continuous flow physiology on ECMO support does not offload the left ventricle thereby hampering ventricular recovery and allows blood to congest in the lungs. A novel strategy being evaluated is to offload the ventricle with an Impella device in combination with VA ECMO, colloquially referred to as ECMELLA.[11] Transport of these patients involves careful attention to both device platforms.

Impella Heart Pumps

Impella System Components

The Impella Heart Pumps are catheter-based devices that are indicated for temporary support in the setting of refractory cardiogenic shock following cardiac surgery and acute MI. The device is intended to support circulation for hours to days, allowing the ventricle to rest and recover. The Impella devices are microaxial catheters that are placed percutaneously in the femoral or axillary artery and guided to the heart. The devices provide LV support by directly unloading blood from the left side of the heart, resulting in a decrease in LV end-diastolic volume and end-diastolic pressure, and increasing aortic pressure and flow.

There are five Impella left-sided support catheters: Impella 2.5, 5.0, LD; CP with SmartAssist optical sensor; and 5.5 with Smart-Assist optical sensor. Support depends on the device and can provide flow rates between 2.5 L/min and 6 L/min. Impella CP may be used to support circulation during high-risk cardiac catheterization procedures. Impella 5.5 and LD devices are placed by cardiac surgeons through a graft anastomosed into the axillary artery or ascending aorta. The Impella RP is a right ventricular support system and is inserted percutaneously into the femoral vein and guided up to the PA. The Impella RP is indicated for patients who develop right heart failure following LVAD implant, cardiac transplant, cardiac surgery, or an MI, and delivers blood flow up to 4 L/min.

The Impella system has three components: the motorized catheter/pump, the purge system, and the automated Impella controller (AIC). The catheter has an inlet port through which blood flows into the catheter to the impeller. The impeller spins thousands of times a minute to accelerate blood flow through the catheter, ejecting it out the outlet port into the great vessel. For LV support, the inlet port is located within the LV, whereas the Impella RP has the inlet port within the IVC. The outlet ports are in the aorta and PA, respectively (Fig. 9.10). These catheters are inserted under fluoroscopy to ensure proper positioning of the catheter and the inlet and outlet ports, and are anchored to the groin with sutures. The Impella 5.5 and LD catheter will exit on the chest.

The motor housing sits just above the outlet area on the cannula. Proximal to the motor housing is a fiberoptic pressure sensor that monitors pressure seen in the aorta and ventricle relative to

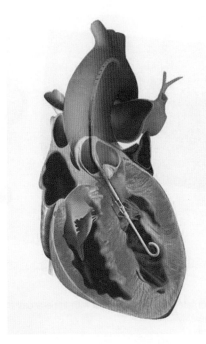

• **Fig. 9.10** Impella catheter placement. (Courtesy Abiomed, Inc.)

the placement of the catheter across the valve. The sensor readings create a waveform that is displayed on the AIC and indicates proper placement of the catheter. There is a repositioning sheath on the catheter to limit the incidence of limb ischemia and catheter migration. The red plug on the back end of the Impella houses a memory chip and pressure transducer, which remembers the setting when transferring consoles.

The Impella catheter is connected to the purge system. The purge system has a bag of IV fluid (typically heparinized dextrose solution) attached to the purge cassette, which is then loaded into the AIC, and attached to the catheter on the other side. The purge cassette flushes the catheter with the viscous IV fluid to reduce the risk of clot formation and prevent blood from entering the motor housing.

The catheter is attached externally to the AIC (Fig. 9.11), which performs three functions: it facilitates user interface to monitor and control the device, it delivers the purge fluid to the catheter, and it has a backup power supply. The AIC allows for the speed of the impeller rotation to be adjusted to control the intensity of ventricular emptying. The system displays the speed with Performance Levels or "P levels": zero (P-0 = no rotation) is the lowest, ranging from P-1 at 10,000 rpm to P-9 over 30,000 rpm.

Information obtained from the AIC or monitor includes the placement signal derived from the pressure gradient detected by the optical sensor in the catheter. The placement signal is used to determine the location of the sensor in relation to the aortic valve. Aortic pressure waveforms confirm the inlet and outlet positions on opposite sides of the aortic valve for left support. The motor current waveform is also displayed, along with the flow rate in liters per minute, purge system flow (mL/h), power status (AC or battery), and any active alarms.

Patient Management

The implanting center will set the P level, which should not be adjusted during transport except in two situations. Suction events are the most common clinical issues causing alarms. A suction event indicates that the impeller is offloading more blood than the

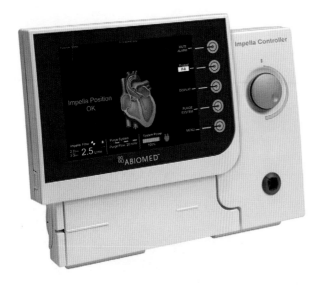

• **Fig. 9.11** Automated controller for use with Impella catheter. (Courtesy Abiomed, Danvers, MA.)

amount filling the ventricle. This can result in collapse of the ventricle/vessel or the catheter tip sucking up against the inside of the heart. Reducing the P by one or two levels allows for better filling. If a patient's condition deteriorates during transport requiring cardiopulmonary resuscitation, then the P level should be reduced to P-2.

Patients on these systems are anticoagulated to prevent thromboembolic events. The manufacturer recommends an activated clotting time (ACT) of 160–180 seconds.

Transport Considerations

The manufacturer of the Impella devices recommends that transport personnel receive training from the company.[30] This includes an overview of the device key features in patient management, training, and emergencies:

1. Description of the device
2. Evaluation of the parameters and waveforms
3. Stabilization of the catheter insertion site
4. Loading and unloading of the AIC
5. Use of flight mode with enhanced software on the AIC
6. Monitoring of patient and parameters during transport
7. Emergency interventions

Monitoring the AIC involves evaluation of the waveforms. The motor current is monitored to determine whether the pump is placed correctly across the valve. Any alarms indicative of loss of motor current or malpositioning of the catheter should be considered a high priority or critical alarm and be addressed promptly per the device manual.[31] If this occurs, then the patient should be treated medically because he or she is not being supported by the device.

Patients may be transported via ground or air, including fixed-wing aircraft and helicopters. Do not raise the head of the bed above 30 degrees and consider a knee immobilizer to stabilize the catheter placement. Do not reposition the catheter in the aircraft; this should occur in the accepting facility under fluoroscopy or echocardiogram. Monitor the exit site for bleeding and hematoma formation and assess the distal pulses.

The AIC can operate the system on a battery for 60 minutes and will beep intermittently as a reminder. The internal battery

must be charged for 5 hours for the system to run for 1 hour. The device should be attached to AC power when in the vehicle or at the referring facility. When loading the device into the transport vehicle, make sure the engine is running and the inverter is operational before attaching to AC power. This will prevent a significant drain on the transport vehicle battery and affect its ability to start. The AIC is on a cart that has to be secured in the transport vehicle to prevent rolling and possible catheter dislodgement. The method will vary by transport provider.

Manufacturer guidelines for transport recommend ensuring the following before leaving with the patient:

1. Communication of transfer to manufacturer's Clinical Support Center.
2. Peel-Away sheath has been removed, repositioning sheath in place; Tuohy–Borst valve securely locked.
3. Slack removed during implant or after any repositioning events.
4. Ensure repositioning sheath angle of entry is maintained by adding folded 4×4s as necessary; blue suture pad secured to patient's leg using forward suture.
5. Knee immobilizer in place; Impella catheter secured within it.
6. Insertion site intact? Any oozing?
7. Centimeter marker on catheter showing CM at exit site. (Assure catheter stabilized.)
8. Purge solution hanging is D5W with 25 U/mL heparin (note if another purge solution is hanging; D5W with 50 U/mL heparin is acceptable).
9. **Emergency Considerations:** If chest compressions are medically indicated, know how to reduce support to P-2.

Refer to Box 9.1 for key points and considerations for transport of an Impella-supported patient.

• BOX 9.1 Key Points for Impella Transport

1. Ensure the transport team has been trained in the care of patients with Impella support. Resources include:
   a. Abiomed Regional Clinical Support team
   b. Abiomed website
   c. Literature review: Impella in Transport: physiology, mechanics, complications, and transport considerations (see Gottula, 2022).
2. Know the type of catheter and expected flows.
3. Ensure flow sheets for documentation of device parameters are available on craft.
4. Ensure emergency contact information is on the craft: Abiomed On-Call Support, implanting and receiving facilities.
5. Check anticoagulation status and ACT goal with implanting center.
6. Assess the patient by checking the insertion site for hematoma or bleeding.
7. Maintain the angle of the catheter at the insertion site with a gauze roll.
8. Check for peripheral pulses.
9. Immobilize the knee on the inserted side and ensure head of bed is not greater than 30°.
10. Mark the Impella catheter at the skin site to allow for quick visual assessment of any displacement of the catheter.
11. On the craft, hang purge solution to decrease risk of air in line.
12. Secure AIC with bed mount bracket to stretcher.
13. If Impella is used in a hybrid configuration, ensure the transport team knows the essentials of that system, usually ECMO.

ACT, Activated coagulation time; *AIC*, automated Impella controller; *ECMO*, extracorporeal membrane oxygenation.
From Gottula A, Shah C, Milligan J, et al. Impella in transport: physiology, mechanics, complications, and transport considerations. *Air Med J.* 2022;41(1):114–127.

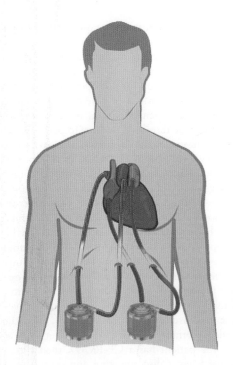

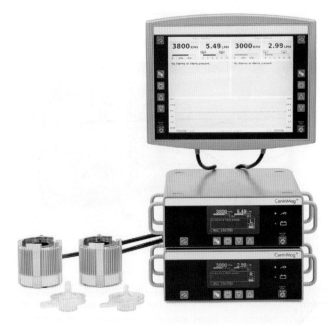

CentriMag Acute Circulatory Support System

The CentriMag Acute Circulatory Support System is a short-term, extracorporeal, magnetically levitated centrifugal blood pump capable of providing RVAD, LVAD, or BiVAD support. The blood pump typically provides 4 to 5 L/min blood flow, with normal pump speeds of 3000–4000 rpm. The CentriMag System is approved for 30 days of circulatory support.

Implantation of the CentriMag Blood Pump is most often performed intraoperatively via a sternotomy, with venous and arterial cannulation of the RA and PA, respectively, for RVAD support and, similarly, the left atrium (LA) and aorta for LVAD support (Fig. 9.12). Percutaneous placement may be performed with femoral venous and arterial access for inflow and outflow cannulation, respectively.

The components of the CentriMag System include: the blood pump, which contains the magnetically suspended impeller; the motor, which houses and drives the pump; the blood cannula, which connects the pump to the patient; an ultrasonic flow probe, which provides a direct measurement of the pump flows; and the console and backup console, capable of supporting one blood pump per console.

The blood pump is locked into the pump motor, which in turn is mounted on a bracket attached to a bedside pole. Locking of the blood pump into the motor is critical to ensure proper function of the system. A motor cable attaches the motor and blood pump to the console, which is secured on a bedside stand. If a BiVAD is implanted, then two consoles and two pump motors are needed for the two blood pumps, with backup consoles available for emergency support (Fig. 9.13).

The ultrasonic flow probe is placed directly onto the outflow blood tubing providing the unique ability to directly measure flow, whereas other MCS systems calculate blood flow based on pump/clinical parameters. The flow probe can also detect retrograde flow and alarm accordingly. The location of the flow probe should be changed regularly by approximately 1 cm to avoid creating a cinched area in the tubing, in which blood flow could slow and become susceptible to thrombus formation. The console display screen provides the pump speed, pump flow, power source and status, and alarm messages. Console adjustments include the ability to adjust the speed ranges from 500 to 5000 rpm, along with low- and high-flow alarm triggers.

Assessment of the CentriMag Blood Pump includes monitoring patient hemodynamics; recognizing that the continuous flow pump may dampen arterial waveforms and minimize palpable pulses in the patient with LVAD support; and monitoring for suction events as demonstrated by blood tubing chattering, presence of air in the tubing, and drops in pump flows. The blood tubing must be free of kinking and obstruction at all times, specifically on the inflow side, to help prevent air from entraining in the cannula. Prevention of suction is achieved with improving blood volume and decreasing pump speed. Full anticoagulation is required for the CentriMag System, with systemic IV agents (e.g., heparin or argatroban if the patient is HIT positive). Monitoring for thrombus formation or fibrin layering includes a focus on the tubing connections, which are frequently secured with tie-bands, and the blood pump. If the pump must be stopped at any time, then a tubing clamp must be applied to the outflow graft before turning off the pump. An extra motor, console, and flow probe should be available at all times for the patient with CentriMag Blood Pump support (Fig. 9.14).

Table 9.8 provides a brief overview of all the acute cardiogenic shock devices discussed in this section.

Interfacility Transport Considerations and Assessment of Acute VADs

The transport of acute VADs requires competent clinicians. The transport crew should have critical care experience and be trained on the management of VADs or plan to transport a third rider

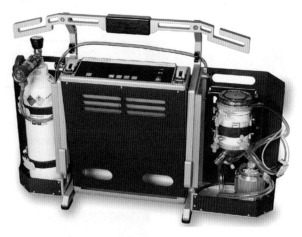

• **Fig. 9.14** CentriMag 2nd Generation System on CMS Transporter. (Reproduced with permission of Abbott, © 2024. All rights reserved.)

who is considered the expert during the transport. As more community hospitals implant VADs, the need for transport to more definitive centers for heart transplantation or more permanent devices is warranted. Before any transport on any device, an assessment for ensuring a properly functioning inverter is crucial. Consult the operational manual for specific information, which may vary with each device, and have clamps and heparin available for the transport. Of note, the weight and space issues are also important for rotor-wing and fixed-wing transports.

The physical assessment of the patient includes the primary and secondary survey with a review and analysis of laboratory values, advanced hemodynamics, adequate perfusion indicators, and adequate ventilation. In addition, auscultation of native heart sounds is recommended because peripheral pulses may be difficult to palpate if a centrifugal device is used. An assessment of device alarms and battery status should also be included, with review of the device display screen to obtain more specific information

about device performance, including pump flow, rate, and speed. These data should be reviewed with a physician to ensure that specific device parameters are maintained.

As patients may have recently had surgical placement of the MCS system, consideration for postoperative assessment and care must be provided. Regardless of whether a patient has a stable (closed) or unstable (open) sternum, the sternum is weakened, and a plan should be discussed on how to perform external compressions in the event of an emergency. The patients are typically sedated with IV medications. Therefore, it is important to ascertain the pre-implant Glasgow Coma Score to compare it with newer findings should the patient awake during transport.

Vasoactive medications, PA catheter, ventilator, and systemic anticoagulation are common in all patients with temporary MCS devices. The higher-than-normal clotting time may be related to the earlier operating room procedure (MCS implantation). The ACT goal needs to be stated by the implanting team. It is common for patients to have chest tubes which should be monitored carefully for increased bleeding. Epicardial pacing wires may be in place and used if temporary pacing is needed. If a patient has an implantable cardioverter defibrillator (ICD), then the transport crews should ascertain from records whether it is activated or disabled. If the patient has a CF-RVAD, then extreme caution should be used when disconnecting any central vascular access device and exchanging IV bags to prevent air from entering the circulatory system if the lines are left uncapped. The most common postoperative issues facing acute patients with VADs are bleeding, arrhythmias, cardiac tamponade, hemodynamic instability, and sepsis. Other potential complications include acute respiratory distress syndrome, pulmonary embolism, and hypothermia related to heat loss from the external pump tubing.

When transporting patients on devices with externally exposed cannulas and/or blood tubing, additional precautions must be considered. The external cannulas should be visible at all times, due to possibility of kinking and subsequent air entrainment. Ensure that the straps that secure the patient to the transport

TABLE 9.8	Acute Cardiogenic Shock Devices: Characteristics and Features		
	ECMO	**Impella**	**CentriMag**
Type	Centrifugal	Microaxial	Centrifugal
Ventricle support	BiVAD	LVAD, RVAD, BiVAD	LVAD, RVAD, BiVAD
Rate/speed	1000–4000 rpm	10,000–33,000 rpm	1000–5500 rpm
Flow (L/min)	3–4	2.5–6	4–5, maximum 9.9
Flow probe	Yes	No	Yes
Internal backup console	No	No	No
Console backup battery (minutes)	90	60	Primary 60; backup 120
Manual pump	Yes	No	No
Defibrillation/cardioversion	—	Yes	Yes, without disconnect
CPR	Per physician only	Per physician	Per physician
Anticoagulation	Heparin	Heparin	Heparin

BiVAD, Biventricular assist device; *CPR*, cardiopulmonary resuscitation; *ECMO*, extracorporeal membrane oxygenation; *LVAD*, left ventricular assist device; *rpm*, rotations per minute; *RVAD*, right ventricular assist device.

stretcher do not kink or compress the cannulas. In emergency situations in which pump function is considered compromised, only the outflow cannula should be clamped. Clamping the inflow cannula can result in air entrainment within the system. Additionally, inherent in the acute indication design, these devices are typically intended to be temporary and may therefore be susceptible to movement and/or dislodgement. It is imperative that stable positioning of the cannulas and catheters are a high priority throughout transport. Consideration of immobilization of the blood tubing as well as the affected patient limb, if appropriate, should be included in the planning phases of transport, along with methods for securing the console near the patient.

Durable Devices for Refractory Advanced Heart Failure

Total Artificial Hearts

The *SynCardia temporary Total Artificial Heart (TAH-t)*, an artificial heart (Fig. 9.15) currently available in the United States, received approval from the Food and Drug Administration (FDA) in October 2004 as a bridge to transplant. It is the only durable, dischargeable device that is pulsatile. The device consists of blood pumps with one percutaneous pneumatic cable per pump and the external hospital-based (Companion 2 Hospital Driver) and portable (Freedom Portable Driver) consoles. The 70-mL blood pump is sized for adults and a 50-mL blood pump for a smaller patient cohort.

The TAH-t is capable of improving CO and end-organ perfusion, with pump flows up to 9.5 L/min. The pump rate is fixed, but the blood sacs can accommodate an increased blood volume return, as with exercise, allowing for an increased CO. Patients supported by the TAH-t no longer need inotrope, pacemaker, and/or defibrillator support. To optimize pump performance, the

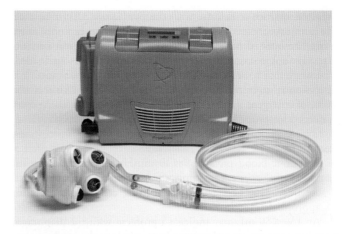

• **Fig. 9.16** Freedom Portable Driver with the SynCardia temporary Total Artificial Heart. (Courtesy of syncardia.com.)

Companion 2 Hospital Driver allows the clinicians to adjust the pump parameters while in the hospital, including pump rate, left and right pump and vacuum pressures, and a percentage of time in systole.

The Freedom Portable Driver (Fig. 9.16) is the portable pneumatic driver for the SynCardia TAH-t, which allows patients to be discharged home on support. It can be carried in a backpack or shoulder bag, and runs on electricity, batteries, or a car battery. The system needs two batteries to function, each with a 2-hour capacity. The driver's display screen provides the pump rate in beats per minute, fill volume (FV), and CO when the display button is pushed. The pump rate is a fixed setting adjusted by the implanting center with special equipment and cannot be altered in the field. The default beats per minute is 125 and is the common setting to help fill and empty the TAH-t. The FV maximum is 70 mL, but it is usually maintained at approximately 60 mL.[32] CO should be sufficient to restore stable outputs and is usually more than 4 L/min. The driver also contains an internal backup system, which is activated automatically if the primary system fails, triggering an alarm until the console is replaced by the backup console; otherwise, no lights or sounds are active on the driver unless there is an alarm.

Patient Assessment

The TAH-t creates pulsatile blood flow so that patients have a systolic and diastolic pressure. The chest should be auscultated to ensure pump function, even though the TAH-t can be heard just standing at the bedside. Because the TAH-t replaces the native ventricles, patients do not have an ECG tracing; hence, there is no need to monitor the ECG or place electrodes. Clinical assessment, then, is focused on the blood pressure and the TAH-t parameters on the Freedom Portable Driver console, with the target parameters outlined in Table 9.9.

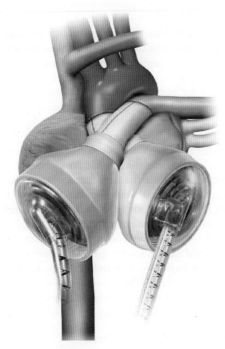

• **Fig. 9.15** SynCardia temporary Total Artificial Heart (TAH-t). (Courtesy of syncardia.com.)

TABLE 9.9	Clinical Targets for the SynCardia Temporary Total Artificial Heart (TAH-t)		
Blood Pressure	TAH-t bpm	TAH-t FV	TAH-t CO
<140 mmHg	~120 bpm	>50 mL	>3.5 L/min

bpm, Beats per minute; *CO*, cardiac output; *FV*, fill volume.

Fluid balance is delicate with the SynCardia TAH-t because the pump ventricles are stiff; therefore, the system can only move a fixed amount of blood. Judicious use of fluids to treat patients is paramount to ensuring that patients are not volume-overloaded.

Ensure that backup batteries are present during transport. It is also essential to bring the backup Freedom Portable Driver in the event of emergent need to switch drivers, and 12V vehicle power is needed for proper operation.

Parameters

1. A systolic blood pressure >140 mmHg will result in an inability of the system to empty efficiently and requires immediate treatment. Contact the implanting center for orders for appropriate medications.
2. An FV <50 mL may indicate a problem with the diaphragm within the pump and necessitate a switch to the implant console. The patient should be transported to the implant center as soon as possible.
3. CO <3.5 L/min is an emergency:
   Vasopressor agents are to be avoided.
   Chest compressions are contraindicated. Emergency action for a malfunction of the Freedom Drive is to exchange it.
   Defibrillation is not effective because there are no native ventricles.
   Contact the implanting center for instructions while the patient is emergently transported to that center.

Emergency Transport Considerations

For an emergent transport, transport teams unfamiliar with the device should transport the patient's significant other to assist in management of the device. Assess if the significant other has been trained on the device at the implantation center and if they are able to assist with management of the device. Another option is to ask the conscious patient questions about the operation and emergency management of the device, such as how to change the batteries or exchange the Freedom Portable Driver if necessary. This will provide a quick review of the basics to transport the patient "emergently" from point A to point B.

There are three *alarms* on the Freedom Portable Driver: battery status, temperature, and fault. The only way to silence these alarms is to resolve the issue. Transport teams should reference the Freedom Driver System Operator Manual or emergency medical services (EMS) VAD field guides to troubleshoot these alarms.[33]

Continuous Flow Devices

The first generation VADs were pulsatile, and due to wear-and-tear and pump size issues, the volume displacement pumps have become obsolete. The currently available long-term VADs are CF-VADs intended for LVAD support. The components of these systems are: the blood pump, with an inflow cannula and an outflow graft; the controller, which runs the pump and provides device status and alarm indicators; and the power sources. The power sources include wall units or AC adaptors for use at night, and batteries for untethered operation. As the pumps are designed for long-term operation and the risk of failure is minimal, there are no external hand pumps as the impeller speeds are in excess of 2000 rpms.

Blood flow dynamics through the pumps are impacted by the differential pressures at the inflow (LV) and outflow (aorta) cannulas and are therefore preload-dependent and afterload-sensitive. The higher differential pressure (higher aortic pressure relative to ventricular pressure) results in a lower pump outflow. Conversely, the lower differential pressure (increased ventricular pressure relative

to aortic pressure) results in a higher pump outflow. Hence, systemic hypertension, for example, will diminish the pump output. Anticoagulation of these devices currently includes at least one antiplatelet (usually aspirin) and antithrombin therapy (warfarin).

The physiologic and subsequent geometric changes that occur with LV support may perpetuate RVF, prompting the need for additional inotropic support or even temporary mechanical support for the RV. If necessary, it is possible to support the RV with a temporary device and the LV with a durable device. The temporary RVAD may then be weaned and explanted after several days of RV myocardial rest.

Another feature of the CF-VADs is that they are valveless. Because these devices draw blood continuously through the pump, valvular assurance of unidirectional blood flow is not needed. However, without valves and with no mechanism for manually running the pump, pump failure and subsequent stoppage may potentially result in significant retrograde blood flow (approximately 1–2 L/min) from the aorta back through the pump into the LV. Hence, efforts to prevent device failure have a heightened importance.

Axial Flow Ventricular Assist Devices

The *axial flow VADs* are continuous flow blood pumps with a linear blood path across the impeller. Two axial flow long-term blood pumps currently available in the United States are the HeartMate II Left Ventricular Assist System (LVAS) and the Jarvik 2000 Ventricular Assist Device.

HeartMate II LVAD

The *HeartMate II LVAD* (Thoratech Corporation | Abbott Inc.; Pleasanton, CA) is an axial flow ventricular assist device with its inflow cannula and outflow graft attached to the left ventricular apex and ascending aorta, respectively, with placement of the blood pump in a subdiaphragmatic, preperitoneal pocket (Fig. 9.17). The inflow cannula has a textured surface intended to stimulate the development of a biological (pseudo-intimal) layer to help reduce the risk for thrombus formation on the cannula. The driveline is tunneled across the abdomen and exits through the skin, connecting the implanted pump to the external components of the system.

The HeartMate II system controller monitors the system, provides alarm and power statuses, and transmits power from the power source to the pump. The display button on the controller screen will allow the user to toggle through pump parameters, including speed, flow, and pulsatility index (PI), and power usage in watts. This allows the provider to assess the VAD performance. Alarms and lights along with messages in the display alert providers to pump issues and instruct the providers on actions to be taken.

The controller has two power cables that connect to either the electrical power module, mobile power unit (MPU) or to portable batteries with battery clips. The green light on the controller confirms that both power connections are good. The batteries can provide up to 10–12 hours of power, depending on power usage. The controller and power source are kept close to the patient, along with the backup controller and batteries. In the event of a primary controller malfunction, the controllers must be exchanged. Although the controller icons include the pump running symbol, confirmation should also be made by auscultating the chest.

Jarvik 2000 Ventricular Assist Device

The *Jarvik 2000* (Jarvik Heart, Inc., New York, NY) axial flow pump has several nuances that differentiate it from the other axial

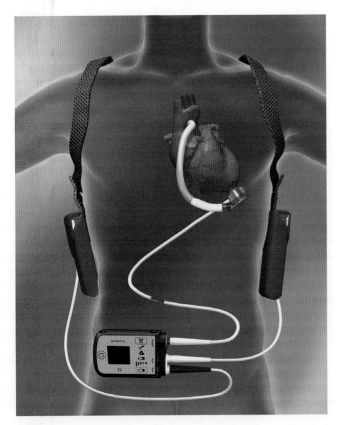

• **Fig. 9.17** Implantation approach of the HeartMate II Left Ventricular Assist System. (Reproduced with permission of Abbott, © 2024. All rights reserved.)

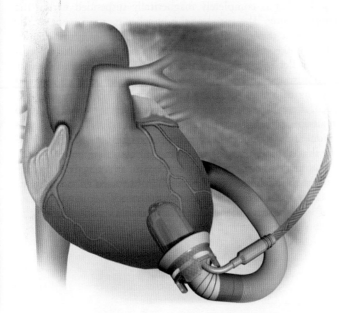

• **Fig. 9.18** Implantation approach for the Jarvik 2000 Ventricular Assist Device. (Courtesy Robert Jarvik, MD.)

flow pumps. The inflow cannula contains the impeller, which is placed directly into the LV apex (Fig. 9.18). The potential advantage of this intraventricular placement is that the pump pocket used by the other devices is obviated, as is the potential for pump pocket infections. Furthermore, the absence of a separate inflow cannula eliminates that component and its associated risk for

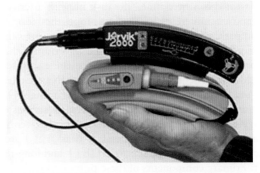

• **Fig. 9.19** Jarvik 2000 VAD controller and battery. (Courtesy of Robert Jarvik, MD.)

pump thrombosis. The outflow graft is anastomosed to the aorta. Another nuance of the Jarvik 2000 is tunneling of the driveline. As a part of the current US clinical trial, the driveline may be tunneled through the abdomen, as with other CF-VADs, or it may be tunneled under the skin to a pedestal located behind the ear, an approach thought to potentially decrease the risk of driveline infection, now being evaluated in the clinical trial.[34]

Similar to other LVAD controllers, the Jarvik 2000 controller provides power to the pump, and monitors and triggers alarm statuses (Fig. 9.19). In addition to these standard features, the Jarvik 2000 controller uniquely allows the patient the ability to manually adjust the speed of the pump to accommodate the body's physiological demands (e.g., lower speeds for rest, intermediate speeds for everyday activity, higher speeds for strenuous activity). The speed-adjustment knob is located on the side of the controller next to the speed settings indicator. The speed settings are numbered 1 to 5, with 1000-rpm incremental speed rates per speed setting, ranging from 8000 to 12,000 rpm. The speed rates correlate with a volume of augmented blood flow, which is not necessarily actual blood flow.

Adequate filling of the blood pump affects the pump flow, as with any of the other devices. A setting of 1 provides an estimated augmented blood volume of 1–2 L/min, whereas a setting of 5 provides an estimated augmented blood volume of 5–7 L/min. The watts used to drive the pump are indicated on the controller and range from 3 to 13. The intermittent low-speed (ILS) function allows the controller to lower the pump speed intermittently to facilitate washing of the aortic valve and root with native heart ejection to help prevent pump thrombosis.[35] The cables that connect the pump to the external components include an extension cable with a retractable coil that allows up to an additional 6 feet from the patient to the controller.

The Jarvik 2000 is designed to be powered by battery sources only and not electricity. The pump may be attached to the battery recharger for battery support, but it does not draw electricity even though the battery charger is plugged into a wall socket. The two types of battery sources for the Jarvik pump are the portable batteries that provide up to 7–12 hours of support per battery and the reserve batteries that provide up to 24 hours of support. All of the batteries recharge by being plugged into electricity.

Centrifugal Flow Rotary Pumps

The centrifugal blood pumps are continuous flow pumps with disk impellers that are magnetically and/or hydrodynamically suspended. These pump designs suggest a "wearless" system with maximal durability because there are no contacting mechanical parts to wear down over time. The disk impeller uses both centrifugal and circumferential energy to propel the blood through the blood path, which includes a perpendicular turn as the blood enters and exits the impeller. Centrifugal flow pumps that transport providers may encounter in the field include the HeartWare HVAD System (Medtronic; Minneapolis, MN; see HeartWare HVAD section for updated information regarding FDA recall notices), and the HeartMate 3 Left Ventricular Assist System (Abbott Inc.; Pleasanton, CA). Both pumps received commercial approval (Conformité Européenne: CE Mark) in Europe and FDA approval in the US for short-term/BTT and long-term/DT support. Primary components of these pumps, as with their axial flow pump predecessors, include the blood pump, the external controller, and the power source. Similarly, the pump flow dynamics of the centrifugal LVAD are sensitive to the differential pressure relationships of the inflow and outflow cannulas, and to preload and afterload. Additionally, these devices currently require both antithrombin and antiplatelet therapy.

HeartWare HVAD System

The HeartWare HVAD centrifugal pump has an impeller suspended within the pump using both magnetic and hydrodynamic (blood flow) forces and is implanted within the pericardial space (Fig. 9.20), with outflow graft anastomosis to the ascending aorta and subcutaneous driveline tunneling to either the right or left upper quadrant of the abdomen. The driveline is significantly smaller than its predecessors and is connected to the external controller (Fig. 9.21), which is then connected to the appropriate power source.

The controller provides important pump information including the pump speed, flow, and watts parameters; waveform peaks and troughs; alarm settings, and messages and interventions to correct them; and power source and status. A unique characteristic of this pump is that the patient's hematocrit (Hct) value is entered into the controller at the implanting center using the

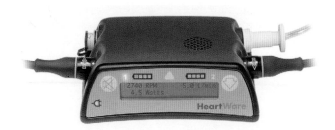

• **Fig. 9.21** HeartWare HVAD System controller. (Courtesy Medtronic, Minneapolis, MN.)

System Monitor. The Hct value (a measure of blood viscosity) is combined with pump speed and watts to provide a highly accurate calculated pump flow.[36] As such, an incorrect entry of the patient's Hct or an outdated value may affect the flow estimate and trigger an inappropriate low- or high-flow alarm. HVAD pump speeds typically range between 2500 and 3200 rpms. The Lavare Cycle, when activated by the clinician, provides automatic periodic speed variation intended to reduce the potential for blood stasis within the ventricle.

Power sources include external batteries, AC adaptor to an electrical outlet, and a direct current (DC) adaptor to a car outlet. One battery provides 4–6 hours of support and will automatically switch over to the fully charged battery when necessary. External batteries are recharged by a portable battery charger.

HeartMate 3 Left Ventricular Assist Device

The HeartMate 3 LVAD (Fig. 9.22) is a centrifugal VAD with an impeller that is completely magnetically suspended within the pump housing. The speed of the impeller rotation is set by the clinicians at the implanting center and is usually approximately 4800–5600 rpm. An additional design feature is that the speed of the impeller pulses up and down 30 times a minute or every 2 seconds, disrupting the blood movement inside the pump and reducing thrombus formation. Because of this small variation in speed, there is a different characteristic to the sound of the pump on auscultation. This pulsation, however, cannot be felt with palpation, and happens so quickly that it is not captured by the setting that displays the speed on the controller.

Another design modification is the modular driveline. A known device complication is damage to the external driveline,

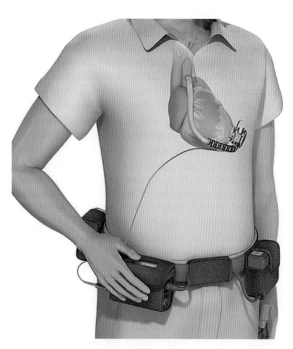

• **Fig. 9.20** HeartWare HVAD System. (Courtesy Medtronic, Minneapolis, MN.)

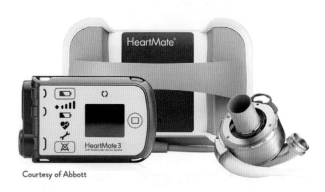

Courtesy of Abbott

• **Fig. 9.22** HeartMate 3 LVAD System and controller. (Reproduced with permission of Abbott, © 2024. All rights reserved.)

resulting in pump stoppage. The modular driveline allows clinicians to replace the external portion of the driveline by unlocking the connection and attaching a new driveline. This connection point needs to be protected from accidental stress and disconnection. The connection is a heavy, metal two-piece section on the driveline. It should be inspected to ensure that a yellow ring between the two metal pieces cannot be seen. If the yellow ring is visualized, then stabilize the connection and contact the implanting center for instructions on ensuring that the two metal halves are screwed together.

The interface on the controller for the HeartMate 3 LVAD is very similar to that of the HeartMate II LVAD. The controllers for the two systems can be distinguished by the color scheme of the body of the controller. The back of the HeartMate 3 pocket controller is black, which allows the care team to quickly identify that the patient has a HeartMate 3 simply by looking at the controller. The back of the HeartMate II controller is white. All external components are similar in appearance and operation as with the HeartMate II.

Table 9.10 provides a brief overview of all the chronic heart failure devices discussed in this section.

Interfacility or Scene Transport Considerations and Assessment of Long-Term VADs

The number of patients discharged in the community with VADs has increased in recent years. Because heart failure can be treated with VADs and the improved durability of the devices means longer support times, transport crews are likely to encounter this patient population. Most of these patients have long-term devices with more stable conditions, unlike their acute VAD counterparts who are more likely being transported in the immediate postoperative period. Some of the more stable patients have had their devices for weeks or months, and others for years. With the increased number of VAD options, transport crews are challenged to remain competent on all of them. Therefore, the educational leadership of these programs must ascertain which devices are in their area and develop training programs accordingly.

Patient Assessment

As many patients attempt to normalize their appearance when managing the equipment, identifying that a supported patient actually has a CF-VAD may be the first assessment challenge. If any of the external components are seen, quickly confirm if the patient has a VAD because this will dramatically change your assessment.

Once it is determined that the patient has a CF-VAD, the patient assessment will need to be modified due to continuous flow physiology. Auscultate the chest to listen for native heart sounds and the pump. Because a pulse oximeter uses the surge in blood flow during systole to calculate an accurate saturation, it may not be accurate in these patients, so clinical decisions should not be based on this number. Peripheral blood pressures must be measured using a sphygmomanometer, a Doppler flow probe, and gel. Automated blood pressure machines rely on pulsatility, which is dependent on the native heart function and filling. Assessing the patient's level of consciousness, skin color and temperature, cardiac rhythm, and signs of dehydration versus volume overload are important first steps.

It is important to know the model of the device, whether it is axial or centrifugal flow, and whether backup equipment is readily available. Having the contact information from the implanting center will be especially helpful. If the site can be contacted, then the clinicians may be able to provide patient-specific information to help with the clinical assessment and

TABLE 9.10	Refractory Advanced Heart Failure Devices: Characteristics and Features				
	SynCardia TAH-t	HeartMate II LVAD	Jarvik 2000 VAD	HeartWare HVAD System	HeartMate 3 LVAD
Type	Volume displacement	Axial	Axial	Centrifugal	Centrifugal
Ventricle support	TAH	LVAD	LVAD	LVAD	LVAD
Typical rate/speed	120–135 bpm	8000–12,000 rpm	8000–12,000 rpm	2400–3000 rpm	4000–9000 rpm
Flow (L/min)	4.9–9.5	4–10	Up to 8	2–10	4–10
Motor current (watts)	Not displayed	6–8	3–10	2.5–8.5	4–8
Built-in backup controller	Backup motor	Yes	No	No	Yes
Battery support (hours/battery set)	2	10–12	7–12	8–12	8–12
Manual pump	No	No	No	No	No
Defibrillation/ cardioversion	No	Yes	Yes	Yes	Yes
CPR	No	Per physician	Per physician	Per physician	Per physician
Antithrombin	Yes	Yes	Yes	Yes	Yes
Antiplatelet	Yes	Yes	Yes	Yes	Yes

bpm, Beats per minute; *CPR*, cardiopulmonary resuscitation; *LVAD*, left ventricular assist device; *rpm*, rotations per minute; *TAH*, total artificial heart.

management. The controller will provide VAD parameters, which are important to monitor and trend throughout the transport. The controller can also be helpful during alarm conditions, because it may provide information about troubleshooting the alarm and specific actions to take. Controller alarms need to be reported immediately to the implanting center.

Low-flow alarms occur with poor filling of the pump or obstruction to emptying. The Mechanical Circulatory Assist Guidelines from the International Society of Heart Lung Transplant state several etiologies that result in poor pump filling. These patient–pump interface issues can be summarized in an acronym SHAB DORC:

S: Sepsis or sedation: Assess the patient for signs and symptoms of infection, and/or use of sedatives that can cause vasodilatation.

H: Hypertension: Mean arterial pressure (MAP) >90 mmHg may create too much resistance, limiting forward blood flow through the pump; typical MAP target is 65–85 mmHg.

A: Arrhythmias: Obtain rhythm strip to assess for arrhythmias as ineffective RV function will decrease LVAD filling.

B: Bleeding: Approximately 25%–30% of all patients with VADs experience gastrointestinal (GI) bleeding.[37]

D: Dehydration: This may be the result of aggressive diuretic regimen or poor oral intake.

O: Overdrive: The speed is too fast for the patient's current volume status, or there is an obstruction, especially seen in the immediate postoperative period caused by tamponade.

R: Right heart failure.

C: Clot: Clot formation inside the pump is a possible complication and can change the blood flow dynamics through the pump.

Patient monitoring and management should include establishing IV access, monitoring heart rhythm, and obtaining results of the most recent blood tests to include CBC, blood chemistries, and international normalized ratio (INR).

VAD Assessment

Assessment of the device function includes review of the VAD parameters (speed, flow, PI, power) displayed on the controller. The VAD parameters should be monitored frequently and routinely for the duration of the transport. The pump flow is the amount of blood flow through the pump, which is calculated by the system in liters per minute (L/min). The Jarvik 2000 LVAD, as previously described, does not provide a calculated measure of flow; rather, it provides a dial setting associated with an estimate of augmented flow volume.

The pump speed is how fast the impeller inside the pump is spinning and is measured in rotations per minute (rpm). The pump speed is set at the implanting center and is a fixed speed. Only the Jarvik 2000 LVAD has the ability to adjust the speed outside of the hospital setting.

The power is how much energy in watts the pump uses to rotate the impeller to move the blood flow at the set speed. The HeartMate devices have an additional parameter, the PI, which is a unitless measure that reflects the native heart pulsatility seen by the pump, commonly ranging from 3 to 6. If it is outside of this range, then consider the pump is not filling or emptying adequately. Reference the above referenced SHAB DORC for troubleshooting clinical implications.

In addition to the pump parameters, the controllers or consoles for each VAD are designed to provide information to clinicians on their display screens regarding urgent or emergent conditions that require interventions. Alarms are announced

through audible alerts and/or illuminated lights on the controllers/consoles. Each system has a way to differentiate noncritical versus hazard alarms based on the warning signals. The battery status is typically monitored by the controller or console and should be checked frequently to avoid power interruption. If the battery power reaches a critical low level and needs to be replaced, be sure to replace the low battery with a new one from the patient's back-up supply.

Disconnect and reconnect one battery at a time. It is important to avoid disconnecting both power sources at one time as that will stop the pump. Ensure that all connections are properly aligned prior to securing the connection. Issues with connections or component functionality will trigger alarms. Contact the implanting center to obtain instructions on how to intervene.

The alarm guides for each device may be accessed by referring to the device-specific manufacturer website, which is the most reliable source of current information. Additionally, the International Society of Heart and Lung Transplantation MCS guidelines published in 2013[38] reference the use of the EMS VAD field guides as a resource for providers interfacing with VAD equipment. The VAD coordinator professional organization, the International Consortium of Circulatory Assist Clinicians, has endorsed the use of the field guides as best practice. The most current versions of the field guides are available electronically on http://www.mylvad.com or https://iccac.global/public/documents.

The patients are instructed to always carry a travel bag with the necessary back-up equipment needed to manage the device in an emergency. This bag should contain extra batteries, backup controllers, and other specific equipment for the device. Also inside the travel kit is a reference card for the alarms and contact information for the patient's VAD program team to contact for patient management. This travel bag and equipment should always be transported with the patient. The patient is also instructed to be in the company of another person who is trained in emergency management of the device. If an emergency arises that renders the patient unconscious, then the secondary caregiver should take over management of the pump. The secondary caregiver must also be transported if weight and space allow.

Emergency Considerations

Emergent assessment and proper intervention when VAD patients are unconscious is challenging because the pulseless state is expected. A rapid assessment is made to determine whether the unconscious VAD patient suffers from cardiogenic shock (RV collapse, VAD equipment malfunction), metabolic dysregulation (abnormal blood sugar, drug overdose), or a neurologic event (e.g., stroke or cerebrovascular accident [CVA]). Assessment of the $ETCO_2$ can provide valuable information regarding perfusion. The decision to initiate chest compressions must be made by assessing the patient's level of consciousness and MAP, and VAD auscultation and alarms. Chest compressions are indicated when VAD patients are unconscious and have evidence of poor perfusion such as a MAP <50 mmHg and a lack of pump function.[39] In these instances follow ACLS or program guidelines.

Additional Patient Considerations

The patients who require readmission to the local hospital do so for multiple reasons. *VAD malfunctions* must quickly be assessed to determine if external peripheral component replacement will reestablish safe function. Patients should have a travel bag or back-pack with extra batteries and controllers readily available for component replacement. Should the backup components need to be used, patients must return to the implanting center for equipment replacement as soon as possible.

VAD related complications can be associated with hemocompatibility issues leading to clotting or bleeding such as pump thrombosis, strokes, or GI bleeding.[40] The first step is to contact the implanting VAD center for all management of bleeding, clotting or volume issues. There is a delicate balance between clotting and bleeding that is achieved by maintaining VAD patients on a therapeutic dose of warfarin, monitored by INR levels, usually targeting 2.0–3.0.[41] Supra- or subtherapeutic INR levels put patients at an increased risk for these hemocompatibility complications. VAD patients are also at an increased risk for GI bleeds compared to other patients on warfarin because pump support is often associated with arteriovenous malformations in the vessels of mucosal membranes (ENT, GI, and genitourinary systems). The pumps also damage the von Willebrand factor (vWF) in the blood. This blood clotting factor helps platelets stick to damaged blood vessels preventing blood loss. VAD patients may then ooze blood from small blood vessels along the GI tract, resulting in significant blood loss sometimes over a short period of time.

In addition to stringent anticoagulation management, blood pressure management is also important as both of those may impact the incidence of stroke in VAD patients. Hence, it is important to monitor the MAP closely to maintain a target of 65–85 mmHg.[38] Another pump-related complication is infection, especially around the pump and/or driveline. Meticulous care of the driveline exit site is required to decrease the risk of infection. Stabilization of the driveline prior to transport will reduce the risk of trauma to the exit site, a leading cause of infection.

Historical Context and Future Direction

Historical Perspective

The history of mechanical circulatory support devices (MCSDs) originated around the mid-1960s, when Dr. Michael DeBakey implanted the first successful cardiac assist device in a young woman who could not be weaned from cardiopulmonary bypass (CPB). Having been supported for 10 days[42] as a bridge to recovery, she was ultimately discharged home. This landmark success fueled further interest in the development and use of MSCDs for end-stage heart failure. Researchers and physicians directed their focus to total replacement of the failing heart with the use of a TAH, with the first successful implant by Dr. Denton Cooley in 1969 (the Liotta heart). The Jarvik-7 TAH, designed in collaboration with Dr. Robert Jarvik and colleagues, was implanted in 1982 by Dr. William DeVries and provided an unprecedented 112 days of full support in an elderly dentist, Dr. Barney Clark, before he succumbed to multiple complications.[42,43] Since then, through enhancements and modifications, the Jarvik-7 has evolved into the SynCardia temporary TAH being used for BTT today.

Concurrently, advancements in immunosuppression therapy placed heart transplantation as the gold standard for end-stage heart failure for the lucky few, as a disproportionate number of transplant candidates compared to available donor organs resulted in patient deaths on the waiting list.[44] This disparity heightened the need for developing readily available VAD technology capable of sustaining patients awaiting a donor organ, as well as providing lifetime support for those deemed ineligible for transplant, DT. Inherent limitations of a TAH prompted the field to focus on developing smaller, durable technology to *assist* the failing heart versus completely replacing it.[42]

The early VAD designs were fill-to-empty, volume displacement pumps, and were used as BTT originally in clinical trials.[45] With further enhancements, they allowed VAD-supported patients to be discharged home into the community,[42] which not only significantly improved the patient's quality of life, but also required community support, education, and training.

The success of BTT trials prompted investigation into the DT indication for patients deemed ineligible for transplant. The Randomized Evaluation of Mechanical Assistance for the Treatment of Congestive Heart Failure (REMATCH) clinical trial demonstrated that the HeartMate Extended Vented Electric Left Ventricular Assist System (HeartMate XVE LVAS; Thoratec Corporation, Pleasanton, CA) significantly improved survival and quality of life compared with optimal medical management in this very ill patient cohort. The survival benefit was limited (52% and 23% at 1 and 2 years post implant), and device comorbidities were significant enough that the clinical community continued to develop improvements and alternative technologies.[42,46] The goal became to develop smaller pumps, with increased durability and hemocompatibility, decreased power demands, ideally without drivelines, and associated with minimal comorbidities and improved clinical outcomes, including quality of life. These efforts have led to the continuous flow VADs that are now used as outlined previously in this chapter.

In tandem with the durable VAD evolution, development of the IABP began in the late 1950s with Dr. Dwight Harken, who described the method of counterpulsation, with removal of a portion of blood volume during systole to be rapidly replaced during diastole.[47] Complications arose in the early experience, but by the early 1960s, Dr. Spyridon Moulopolous developed a simple, effective, and affordable circulatory assist device to treat LVF, known today as the IABP.[10,48,49] His groundbreaking work supporting cardiogenic shock patients with the IABP[5] paved the way for additional research, including Dr. Adrian Kantrowitz's work in the late 1960s, demonstrating that counterpulsation was able to reverse cardiogenic shock with both hemodynamic and clinical improvement.[48]

In summary, the evolution of MCSDs has created a more sophisticated set of treatment strategies to offer complicated advanced heart failure and cardiogenic shock patients who are supported with both air and surface transport.

Future Innovations

The future of MCS support is to provide totally implantable circulatory support with smaller, more durable systems free of transcutaneous drivelines, and with improved hemocompatibility resulting in fewer device-related complications. As an alternative or adjunctive option for refractory heart failure, the quest for MCS is to design mechanical support devices that are durable, applicable to multiple body sizes, easy to implant, easy to manage technically and clinically, with minimal concurrent medication requirements including anticoagulation therapy, and suitable for all refractory heart failure indications.

• BOX 9.2   Checklist Review for Mechanical Circulatory Support Device Transport

1. Can I do external cardiopulmonary resuscitation?
2. If not, is a hand pump or external device available for use?
3. If the device slows down (low flow state), what alarms are triggered?
4. How can I speed up the rate of the device?
5. Do I need to use heparinization for the patient if the device slows down?
6. Can the patient undergo defibrillation while connected to the device?
7. If the patient can undergo defibrillation, does anything need to be disconnected before defibrillation?
8. Does the patient have a pulse with this device?
9. What are acceptable vital sign parameters?
10. Can this patient be externally paced?

Summary

The use of VADs will only increase as the technology continues to evolve and improve. The next frontier of MCSD projects to be smaller, more energy-efficient, and possibly less invasively implanted, with the hope of wireless energy transfer technology to eradicate the transcutaneous driveline. The potential for easier technology with easier implantation approaches allows smaller hospitals the opportunity to implant these devices and potentially transport these patients to larger facilities. This progress will have a significant impact on the volume of critical care air and surface transports. As this occurs, transport teams must remain competent in MCSD transport and develop specific policies and guidelines related to the management and transport of this special patient population. Because the number of devices in this country is expanding, most prehospital and transport personnel cannot remain comfortably competent with the nuances of them all.

Box 9.2 outlines a series of questions each transport team member can ask the patient, secondary caregiver, or knowledgeable provider to ensure safe and swift transport by the teams. Answers to these questions provide the information needed to safely transport patients with MCSDs during an interfacility or scene flight if a situation occurs in which a patient presents with an unfamiliar device.

REFERENCES

1. Oesterling A, Bott S, Davis E. Outcomes from long-distance interfacility transport of adult patients on acute mechanical circulatory support. *Air Medical J.* 2022;41(2):233–236.
2. Coppola AP, Tyree M, Larry K, DiGeronimo R. A 22-year experience in global transport extracorporeal membrane oxygenation. *J Ped Surg.* 2008;43(1):46–52.
3. Colvin M, Smith JM, Skeans MA, et al. OPTN/SRTR Annual Data Report 2020: Heart. *Am J of Transplant.* 2022;22(S2):350–437.
4. Moayedi Y, Fan CPS, Cherikh WS, et al. Transplant outcomes. *Circ Heart Fail.* 2019;12:e006218. doi: 10.1161/CIRCHEARTFAILURE.119.00621
5. Farrar DJ, Holman WR, McBride LR, et al. Long-term follow-up of Thoratec ventricular assist device bridge-to-recovery patients successfully removed from support after recovery of ventricular function. *J Heart Lung Transplant.* 2002;21(5):516–521.
6. Wood C, Maiorana A, Larbalestier R, et al. First successful bridge to myocardial recovery with a HeartWare HVAD. *J Heart Lung Transplant.* 2008;27(6):695–700.
7. Organ Procurement and Transplantation Network and the Scientific Registry of Transplant Recipients. OPTN/SRTR 2020 Annual Data Report Heart. *Am J Transplant.* 2022;22(suppl 2):350–437. doi: 10.1111/ajt.16977
8. Khush KK, Hsich E, Potena L. The International Thoracic Organ Transplant Registry of the International Society for Heart and Lung Transplantation: Thirty-eighth adult heart transplantation report – 2021; Focus on recipient characteristics. *J Heart Lung Transplant.* 2021;40(10):1023–1034.
9. Mehra M, Goldstein D, Cleveland J, et al. Five-year outcomes with patients with fully magnetically levitated vs axial flow LVAD devices in the MOMENTUM 3 randomized trial. *JAMA.* 2022;328(12):1233–1242.
10. Grady K, Fazeli P, Kirklin J, Pamboukian S, White-Williams C. Factors associated with health-related quality of life 2 years after LVAD implantation: insights from INTERMACS. *J Am Heart Assoc.* 2021;10(14):e021196. doi: 10.1611/JAHA.121.021196
11. Baran D, Jaiswal A, Henning F, Patapov E. Temporary mechanical circulatory support: devices, outcomes and future directions. *J Heart Lung Transplant.* 2022;41(6):678–691.
12. Samuels LE, Shemanski KA, Casanova-Ghosh E, et al. Hybrid ventricular assist device: HeartMate XVE LVAD and Abiomed AB5000 RVAD. *ASAIO J.* 2008;54(3):332–334.
13. Moazmi N, Fukamachi K, Kobayashi M, et. al. Axial and centrifugal continuous-flow rotary pumps: a translation from pump mechanics to clinical practice. *J Heart Lung Transplant.* 2013;32(1):1–11.
14. Gravelee GP, Davis RF, Stammers AH, et al. *Cardiopulmonary Bypass: Principles and Practice.* 3rd ed. New York: Lippincott, Williams & Wilkins; 2008.
15. Hardy N, Starr N, Cosgrave J, Madhavan P. Intra-aortic balloon pump entrapment and surgical removal: a case report. *Eur Heart J.* 2017;1(1):ytx002. doi: 10.1093/ehjcr/ytx002
16. Cardiosave IABP Operation – Transport: Quick Reference Guide. Wayne, NJ: Maquet | Getinge Group; 2021. Available at: https://getinge.training/wp-content/uploads/2021/02/Cardiosave-IAB-Operation-Transport-Quick-Reference-Guide-MCV00020163_REVC.pdf.
17. Arrow AutoCat 2 Wave IABP Abbreviated: Operation and Troubleshooting Guide. Research Triangle Park, NC: Teleflex. 2013. Available at: https://nanopdf.com/download/arrow-autocat-2-wave-iabp-abbreviated_pdf.
18. González LS, Grady M. Intra-aortic balloon pump counterpulsation: technical function, management, and clinical indications. *Int Anesthesiol Clin.* 2022;60(4):16–23. doi: 10.1097/aia.0000000000000379
19. OPTN Heart Transplantation Committee. Guidance and Policy Clarifications Addressing Adult Heart Allocation Policy. OPTN Heart Transplantation Committee; 2020. p 94.
20. Pavlushkov E, Berman M, Valchanov K. Cannulation techniques for extracorporeal life support. *Ann Transl Med.* 2017;5(4):70. doi: 10.21037/atm.2016.11.47
21. Al-Jazairi A, Raslan S, Al-Mehizia R, et al. Performance assessment of a multifaceted unfractionated heparin dosing protocol in adult patients on extracorporeal membrane oxygenator. *Ann Pharmacother.* 2021;55(5):592–604. doi: 10.1177/1060028020960409
22. Labib A, August E, Agerstrand C, et al. Extracorporeal life support organization guideline for transport and retrieval of adult and pediatric patients with ECMO support. *ASAIO J.* 2022;68(4):447–455. doi: 10.1097/mat.0000000000001653
23. Smit B, Smulders YM, van der Wouden JC, Oudemans-van Straaten HM, Spoelstra-de Man AME. Hemodynamic effects of

acute hyperoxia: systematic review and meta-analysis. *Crit Care.* 2018;22(1):45. doi: 10.1186/s13054-018-1968-2

24. Ozturk Z, Kesici S, Ertugrul L, et al. Resuscitating the resuscitation: a single-centre experience on extracorporeal cardiopulmonary resuscitation. *J Paediatr Child Health.* 2023;59(2):335–340. doi: 10.1111/jpc.16295

25. Kim H, Cho YH. Role of extracorporeal cardiopulmonary resuscitation in adults. *Acute Crit Care.* 2020;35:1–9. doi: 10.4266/acc.2020.00080

26. ELSO. ECMO | Extracorporeal Membrane Oxygenation. ECLS International Summary of Statistics. 2022. Available at: https://www.elso.org/registry/internationalsummaryandreports/internationalsummary.aspx.

27. Richardson ASC, Tonna JE, Nanjayya V, et al. Extracorporeal cardiopulmonary resuscitation in adults. Interim Guideline Consensus Statement From the Extracorporeal Life Support Organization. *ASAIO J.* 2021;67:221–228. doi: 10.1097/mat.0000000000001344

28. Lyng JW, Baldino KT, Braude D, et al. Prehospital supraglottic airways: an NAEMSP position statement and resource document. *Prehosp Emerg Care.* 2022;26:32–41. doi: 10.1080/10903127.2021.1983680

29. Bartos JA, Frascone RJ, Conterato M, et al. The Minnesota mobile extracorporeal cardiopulmonary resuscitation consortium for treatment of out-of-hospital refractory ventricular fibrillation: Program description, performance, and outcomes. *eClinicalMedicine.* 2020;29–30:100632.

30. Abiomed. Impella Education, Patient Management: Transporting a Patient on Impella Heart Pump Support. 2021. Available at: https://www.heartrecovery.com/education/education-library/qsv-transport-training.

31. Abiomed. Impella Ventricular Support Systems for Use during Cardiogenic Shock and High-Risk PCI: Instructions for Use and Clinical Reference Manual. Danvers, MA: Abiomed; 2022. Available at: Abiomed Heart Recovery: Education and Training. Available at: https://www.heartrecovery.com/education.

32. Slepian MJ, Smith RG, and Copeland JG. The SynCardia CardioWest Total Artificial Heart. In: Baughman KL, Baumgartner WA, eds. *Treatment of Advanced Heart Disease.* Boca Raton, FL: Taylor & Francis; 2006.

33. SynCardia. TAH Manual. Tucson, AZ: SynCardia Systems; 2014.

34. ClinicalTrials.gov. Evaluation of the Jarvik 2000 Left Ventricular Assist System with Post-Auricular Connector-Destination Therapy Study. [Last update posted 2024-03-20] Available at: https://clinicaltrials.gov/ct2/show/study/NCT01627821.

35. Selzman CH, Feller ED, Walker JC, et al. The Jarvik 2000 left ventricular assist device: results of the United States bridge to transplant trial. *ASAIO J.* 2023;69(2):174–182. doi:10.1097/MAT.0000000000001750

36. Hayward C, Adachi I, Baudart, S, et al. Global best practices consensus: long-term management of patients with hybrid centrifugal flow left ventricular assist device support. *J Thorac Cardiovasc Surg.* 2022;164:1120–1137.

37. Mehra MR, Uriel N, Naka Y, et al. A fully magnetically levitated left ventricular assist device-final report. *N Engl J Med.* 2019;380:1618–1627.

38. Feldmen D, Pamboukian SV, Teuteberg JJ, et al. The 2013 International Society of Heart and Lung Transplantation guidelines for mechanical circulatory support. *J Heart Lung Transplant.* 2013;32(2):121–146.

39. Givertz M, DeFilippis E, Colvin M, Darling C, Elliott T. HFSA/SAEM/ISHLT Clinical expert consensus document on the emergency management of patients with VADs. *J Card Fail.* 2019:25(7):494–515.

40. Trinquero P, Pirotte A, Gallagher L, Iwaki K, Beach C, Wilcox J. Left ventricular assist device management in the emergency department. *West J Emerg Med.* 2018;19(5):834–841.

41. Macaluso GP, Pagani FD, Slaughter MS, et al. Time in therapeutic range significantly impacts survival and adverse events in destination therapy patients. *ASAIO J.* 2022;68:14–20.

42. Kirklin JK, Frazier OH. Developmental history of mechanical circulatory support. In: Frazier OH, Kirklin JK, eds. *ISHLT Monograph Series Mechanical Circulatory Support.* Vol 1. Philadelphia, PA: Elsevier; 2006.

43. Devries W. The permanent artificial heart: four case reports. *JAMA.* 1988;259(6):849–859.

44. American Heart Association. *Heart Disease and Stroke Statistics: 2005 Update.* Dallas, TX: American Heart Association; 2005.

45. Portner P, Oyer P, McGregor C. First human use of an electrically powered implantable ventricular assist system. *Artif Organs.* 1985; 9(a):36.

46. Rose EC, Gelijns AC, Maskowitz AJ, et al. For the REMATCH Study Group: Long-term use of a left ventricular assist device for end-stage heart failure. *N Engl J Med.* 2001;345(20):1435–1443.

47. Overwalder PJ. Intra-aortic balloon pump (IABP) counterpulsation. *Intern J Thoracic Cardiovasc Surg.* 1999;2(2):2–2.

48. Bolooki H. *Clinical Application of the Intraaortic Balloon Pump.* Armonk, NY: Futura Publishing; 1998.

49. Moulopoulos SD, Topaz S, Kolff WJ. Diastolic balloon pumping (with carbon dioxide) in the aorta – a mechanical assistance to the failing circulation. *Am Heart J.* 1962;63:669–675. doi: 10.1016/0002-8703(62)90012-1

Reference Manuals

Abbott. CentriMag Blood Pump: Instructions for use. Pleasanton, CA: Abbott, Inc.; 2019.

Abbott. 2nd Generation CentriMag System Operating Manual. Pleasanton, CA: Abbott, Inc.; 2019.

Abbott. HeartMate II Left Ventricular Assist System: Instructions for use. Pleasanton, CA: Abbott, Inc.; 2020.

Abbott. HeartMate 3TM Left Ventricular Assist System: Instructions for Use. Pleasanton, CA: Abbott; 2022.

Abiomed. Clinical Education and Training: Hub–Spoke Transfer. Version 5. https://www.abiomed.com.

Abiomed. Impella RP with SmartAssist System with the Automated Impella Controller. Danvers, MA: Abiomed, Inc; 2022.

Abiomed. Impella Ventricular Support Systems for Use during Cardiogenic Shock and High-Risk PCI: Instructions for Use and Clinical Reference Manual. Danvers, MA: Abiomed, Inc; 2022. Heart Recovery: Education and Training. Available at: https://www.heartrecovery.com/education.

Jarvik. Jarvik 2000 Operator Manual. New York: Jarvik Heart, Inc; 2009.

Jarvik. Jarvik 2000 Patient Handbook. New York: Jarvik Heart, Inc; 2009.

Maquet. Cardiosave IABP Operation – Transport. Quick Reference Guide. Wayne, NJ: Maquet | Getinge; n.d.

Medtronic. HeartWare HVAD System Instructions for Use. M017474c001. Rev 1. Miami Lakes, FL: HeartWare, Inc. | Medtronic; 2021.

OPTN Heart Transplantation Committee. Guidance and Policy Clarifications Addressing Adult Heart Allocation Policy. OPTN Heart Transplantation Committee; 2020.

SynCardia. SynCardia Temporary Total Artificial Heart (TAH-t) with the Freedom Driver System Operator Manual. Tucson, AZ: SynCardia Systems, Inc; 2005.

Teleflex. Arrow IABP Class Room. flexLearning. Available at: https://flexlearning.jimdo.com/arrow-iabp-class-room/.

COMPETENCIES

1. Discuss the anatomy and physiology of the pulmonary system.
2. Understand the oxyhemoglobin dissociation curve.
3. Identify strategies for assessment and monitoring pulmonary function.

4. Describe common respiratory emergencies and their associated pathophysiologies, as well as strategies for management or intervention.

This chapter provides an overview of pulmonary emergencies in the transport setting. It begins with a brief review of anatomy and physiology, which serves as the foundation for actions taken by the transport clinician. From there the concept of acute respiratory failure is outlined, focusing both on monitoring and intervention. Lastly, the etiology, pathophysiology, assessment, and treatment of common pulmonary emergencies is presented.

Anatomy and Physiology

Thoracic Cage and Musculature

The lungs reside in and are connected to the thoracic cavity, which protects the cardiopulmonary structures and other organs. The skeletal framework includes the ribs, sternum, costal cartilages, and the posterior thoracic vertebrae. Two layers line the surface of the lung: the visceral pleura, which covers the outermost lining of the lung, and the parietal pleura, which lines the thoracic wall. Between the two pleural linings is a space that contains approximately 20 mL of serous fluid that acts as a lubricant. This fluid allows the two linings to smoothly glide over each other during inspiration and exhalation. In addition, these thoracic structures allow for a pressure gradient to manifest with muscle contraction facilitating the process of ventilation. Other organs found in the thorax include the esophagus, thymus gland, lymphatic vessels, and nerves.[1-4]

The diaphragm is a dome-shaped muscle that separates the abdominal and thoracic cavities. Working alongside the diaphragm are the external intercostal muscles, which lie between the ribs. At rest, contraction of the diaphragm and external intercostal muscles represents the active phase of inhalation. As the diaphragm contracts and descends inferiorly and as the intercostal muscles contract to lift the ribs and expand the diameter of the chest wall, a negative pressure gradient is created, and air is inspired. As the diaphragm and intercostals relax, the diaphragm naturally ascends, and the chest wall collapses in with relaxation

of the external intercostals. This causes an increase in the intrapleural and intra-alveolar pressure and an outflow of air from the lungs.[1-5]

Normally, the diaphragm and intercostal muscles can provide adequate ventilation without recruiting other muscles to aid in the process. Breathing can be facilitated by or augmented with the use of accessory muscles, either via a conscious decision or due to distress from acute or chronic pathophysiologic processes. Accessory muscles can be further classified by the part of the breathing cycle in which they are utilized: inspiration versus expiration. The inspiratory accessory muscles include the scalene, sternocleidomastoid, trapezius, pectoralis, and external intercostal muscle. The contraction of these muscles helps to increase the diameter of the chest which assists in creating a larger pressure gradient between the intrapleural pressure and outside environment. On the expiratory side are the abdominal muscles and internal intercostal muscles. These muscles are enlisted when airway resistance is heightened; the muscles are used to push up on the diaphragm or decrease the lateral and anteroposterior diameter of the chest.[1,2,4]

Failure of the diaphragm and accessory muscles to maintain adequate movement of air will eventually result in a state of respiratory failure and both an inadequate delivery of oxygen and build-up of carbon dioxide. For this reason, it is important for the clinician to monitor the effort of breathing, observing the use of accessory muscles, and intervening before these systems reach fatigue.[5]

Airways, Lungs, and Vasculature

At the macroscopic level, breathing occurs in the lungs. The lungs are a pair of pyramid-shaped organs that contain a large epithelial surface across which gas exchange occurs. Air makes its way into the lungs from the upper airway and the incrementally smaller passageways of the lower airway: trachea, right and left mainstem bronchi, bronchioles, and alveolar ducts. The lungs also house supportive structures that maintain the integrity of the airway, vasculature that permits both perfusion and gas exchange, and adaptive mechanisms that attempt to maintain normal function at baseline and during injury or illness. Each of these components represents an area in which pathophysiologic processes can occur.[6]

Air passes to each lung from the trachea via the right and left mainstem bronchi. The trachea splits into the mainstem bronchi at the carina, which is the bifurcation within the lower airway, at the level of the Angle of Louis or approximately at the second rib. The right mainstem bronchus extends from the trachea at an angle of around 20–30 degrees in comparison to the left, which is about 45–55 degrees. This explains the important assessment for endobronchial placement of any artificial airway to assure that the patient's lungs are inflating equally bilaterally and that adequate gas exchange is occurring with the provision of effective ventilation.[1–4]

The right and left mainstem bronchi branch further into distal bronchi and bronchioles. The lobar bronchi divide into segmental bronchi, which are excellent anatomic identification markers for sites of infections or lung masses. The next two divisions after the subsegmental bronchi include the bronchioles and terminal bronchioles. Distal to the terminal bronchioles are the respiratory zones where alveolar budding begins and gas exchange occurs. The next three regions, the respiratory bronchioles, alveolar ducts, and alveolar sacs, are also referred to as the acini, and they are the primary structures within the lungs.

Moving distally through the lower airway and past the bronchioles are the acini, which are the primary structures within the lungs. As noted above, they include the respiratory bronchioles, alveolar ducts, and alveolar sacs. At this point in the tracheobronchial tree, the size of the respiratory bronchioles decreases in diameter and continues to bifurcate further into three to four generations. The alveolar ducts and alveolar sacs interface with the pulmonary capillary membrane where the major transaction of oxygen and carbon dioxide takes place. The alveolar sacs are made up of type I and type II cells. Type I cells are squamous epithelial cells and type II cells are granular pneumocytes. Type II cells exhibit several functions, including the production of surfactant and surfactant-associated proteins, division and differentiation into type I cells that may have been damaged, and transport of sodium and water toward the endothelial cells and blood to help minimize fluid accumulation in the alveolar space. Surfactant produced by these type II cells decreases surface tension and helps prevent alveolar collapse. There are approximately 270–300 million alveoli in an average-sized adult, with the total surface area equivalent to the size of a tennis court.[1–4]

The pulmonary capillary membrane, as described above, interfaces with the alveoli via a network of vascular beds. This allows for gases to diffuse across the alveolar–capillary membrane to facilitate both ventilation and oxygenation, both of which are described in the following sections. The efficacy of gas diffusion across the alveolar–capillary membrane is dependent on several factors and often dictates interventions in the clinical setting. Some of these factors include partial pressure of gases, alveolar surface area, driving pressure, and the thickness of the alveolar–capillary membrane.[2]

Lung Volumes and Capacities

Tidal volume is the amount of air that moves in and out of the lungs with each breath. This term, however, describes only one aspect of the overall picture. As shown in Fig. 10.1, the body is able to inhale and exhale a quantity of air in excess of normal tidal volume. The additional capacity can be used based on physiologic need (i.e., metabolic acidosis) or due to conscious effort (i.e., forced expiration).[7]

One limiting value is total lung capacity (TLC), which is the maximum amount of air that the lungs can hold. Physiologic and pathophysiologic factors vary from one individual to the next because of differences in age, height, gender, and ethnicity. Furthermore, there are certain chronic disease processes (such as emphysema) and acute pathologies (such as pulmonary edema) that impact these values.

In relation to patient presentation and treatment, the important thing to note is that the body possesses a capacity for ventilation that exceeds normal use. This means that a patient who needs more volume may be able to compensate unassisted. This ability is limited by physiology and constrained by fatigue that may eventually impede compensation. For this reason, it is important for the transport clinician to monitor ventilatory effort to identify when compensation is occurring and when it may begin to fail.

Ventilation

Ventilation is the gross movement of air into and out of the airways with breathing. Adequate ventilation contributes to the

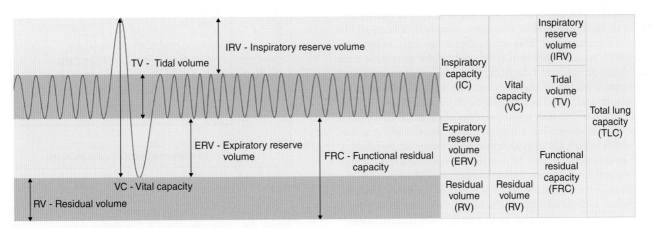

• **Fig.10.1** Lung volumes and lung capacities. (From https://commons.wikimedia.org/wiki/File:Lung Volume.jpg.)

movement of oxygen throughout the body, and it rids the body of carbon dioxide. The movement of carbon dioxide out of the body is an important concept in ventilation. Carbon dioxide is created during the process of cellular respiration, and it diffuses into the bloodstream where it binds to hemoglobin and is then transported to the lungs. When carbaminohemoglobin, hemoglobin bound with carbon dioxide, passes through the pulmonary capillaries, the carbon dioxide is released into the bloodstream, diffuses across the alveolar–capillary membrane, and is exhaled into the environment. Because this process occurs in a predictable fashion, measuring the amount of carbon dioxide in exhaled air allows clinicians to evaluate the efficacy of ventilation. Ventilatory failure is often defined as PCO_2 of greater than 50 mmHg.[1,5]

Ventilation is the product of both respiratory rate and tidal volume and carbon dioxide elimination does require movement. If ventilation is inadequate, the patient can compensate by either increasing the rate of breathing or by increasing the depth of breaths. Observing for these changes will clue the clinician to suspect an underlying pathophysiologic process.[5] Effective ventilation depends on several factors, including a patent airway, intact thoracic cage, the integrity of the alveolar–capillary membrane, normal lung compliance, appropriate airway resistance, and adequate nutrition. Ventilation is regulated by the brain and requires a healthy central nervous system to ensure adequate and automatic ventilation to support the needs of the body.

Oxygenation

The delivery of oxygen to the tissues is vital for normal physiologic processes to occur. Tissue cells utilize oxygen as an energy source in order to perform basic functions and to maintain homeostasis. Onboarding oxygen into the blood requires three general steps: the movement of oxygen into the lungs by ventilation or diffusion, the movement of oxygen from the air into the lungs, across the alveolar capillary membrane, and into the blood, and finally the loading and unloading of oxygen onto hemoglobin molecules in the blood.

For gas exchange to occur once oxygen is into the alveoli, several steps are involved. In the lungs, a gas molecule must diffuse through the alveolar–capillary membrane, which is composed of (1) the liquid lining of the intra-alveolar membrane, (2) the alveolar epithelial cell, (3) the basement membrane of the alveolar epithelial cell, (4) loose connective tissue (the interstitial space), (5) the basement membrane of the capillary endothelium, (6) the capillary endothelium. Once oxygen has diffused into the plasma in the capillary blood, it must cross the erythrocyte membrane, and the intracellular fluid in the erythrocyte until a hemoglobin molecule is encountered. This occurs almost instantly, in approximately 0.25 second. Diffusion is affected by the alveolar surface area, driving pressure, and the thickness of the alveolar capillary.[2,4]

Oxygen is carried in the blood in two ways: dissolved in the blood plasma and bound to hemoglobin. At physiologic partial pressure of oxygen (PO_2), only a small amount of oxygen is dissolved in plasma because oxygen has a low solubility. Interestingly, it is that value which is used for clinical definition of oxygenation failure, a PO_2 variously defined as <50 mmHg or <60 mmHg.[1] Oxygen must first make its way into the bloodstream via diffusion across the alveolar–capillary membrane where it is picked up by, or binds to, hemoglobin. Diffusion is the process of gas molecules moving from an area of higher concentration to an area of lower concentration.[8]

Oxygen delivery is the product of cardiac output (CO) and total arterial oxygen content ($DO_2 = CO \times CaO_2$). Cardiac output is based on stroke volume and heart rate, whereas CaO_2 is derived from the amount of dissolved oxygen plus the total hemoglobin content, oxygen binding capacity of hemoglobin, and the hemoglobin's oxygen saturation. Specifically, the oxygen carrying capacity equation is: $CaO_2 = (1.39 \times Hb \times SpO_2/100) + (0.003 \times PO_2)$. Under normal physiologic conditions, the tissues use 250–300 mL O_2 per minute; this leaves the remaining three-fourths in available reserve to be employed during periods of increased metabolic demand.[9]

In the event this reserve of oxygen is unable to meet the demands of the body, the system compensates by increasing cardiac output to augment delivery. This is manifested by an increase in cardiac output and can be observed clinically by an increase in heart rate or tachycardia. It is often accompanied by a comparable mechanism to increase ventilation and can be observed as an increase in respiratory rate. The clinician can further this process by administering supplemental oxygen and implementing interventions to facilitate the movement of oxygen.

The Oxyhemoglobin Dissociation Curve

The oxygen–hemoglobin (oxyhemoglobin) dissociation curve illustrates the relationship between the hemoglobin saturation of oxygen and PaO_2. This curve depicts the ability of hemoglobin to bind and release oxygen into the tissues and changes under certain physiologic conditions. The relationship between oxygen content and the pressure of oxygen in the blood is not linear. The upper portion of the curve is relatively flat and shows that small changes in PaO_2 have little effect on the percentage saturation in hemoglobin. However, when looking at the PaO_2 as it drops below 60 mmHg, there is a drastic drop in the saturation of hemoglobin. This emphasizes the importance of maintaining a PaO_2 greater than 60 mmHg in clinical practice. There are many factors that influence the oxyhemoglobin dissociation curve and affect the loading and unloading of oxygen. These include the pH, temperature, 2,3-diphosphoglycerate (2,3-DPG), abnormal hemoglobin, and carbon dioxide (Fig. 10.2).[1,2,4,10]

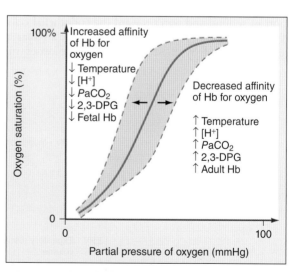

• **Fig. 10.2** Oxyhemoglobin dissociation curve relates oxygen saturation and partial pressure of oxygen in the blood. The curve is affected by many variables. *2,3 DPG*, 2,3-Diphosphoglycerate; *Hb*, haemoglobin. (Modified from Davies JD, Dexter AM. Bedside monitoring of pulmonary function. In: Moore FA, Bellomo R, Marini JJ, et al., eds. *Textbook of Critical Care*. 8th ed. Elsevier; 2024. Figure 33.3.)

The oxyhemoglobin dissociation curve is important to consider when evaluating the accuracy of pulse oximetry. A shift in the curve can change the SpO_2 despite no change in PaO_2. For example, in respiratory acidosis, a right shift will occur which results in a decreased SpO_2 but no change in PaO_2. It is important to have an understanding of the oxyhemoglobin dissociation curve to create a broader clinical perspective when assessing patients and creating treatment plans. Relying too heavily on devices and monitoring systems does not create a thorough representation of the patient's condition. Knowledge of the dissociation curve can help the transport clinician anticipate change and make adjustments to combat a worsening condition.[1,2,4,7]

There are several factors that impact the ability of hemoglobin to bind oxygen in the blood. In general terms, management of and consideration for the oxyhemoglobin dissociation is a balancing act. Increased binding, commonly described as a left shift in the context of the graphic shown above, results in more oxygen being carried to the tissues where it can be utilized. Tightly-held oxygen is not released as readily, therefore a shift too far to the left can be counterproductive. Conversely, a right shift allows oxygen to be released more readily, but a shift too far results in oxygen being released before it reaches the tissues where it is needed. The state of oxygen binding and hemoglobin affinity varies within the bloodstream—it is not uniform. The state of the oxyhemoglobin dissociation curve varies from the lungs to the tissues with an ideal state being that in which oxygen is effectively bound centrally and then readily released at sites where it is needed by tissues. While it may be tempting to consider the curve as a general concept, recognize that it is a dynamic process constantly in transition.[5]

Let's return to specific factors that affect this process: pH, temperature, presence of 2,3-DPG, the state of hemoglobin itself, and carbon dioxide all influence the oxyhemoglobin dissociation curve. The pH of blood is a measurement of the hydrogen ion concentration in the blood. It is used to express a state of acidity or alkalinity. As the hydrogen ion concentration increases, there is a decrease in the pH, a state of acidity, and a subsequent decrease in the affinity for oxygen, which leads to the hemoglobin giving up oxygen to the tissues. This is represented by a right-sided shift in the oxyhemoglobin dissociation curve. Conversely, because there is a decrease in hydrogen ions, the pH increases, and physiologically there is an increased affinity of hemoglobin for oxygen, augmenting its uptake from the alveoli.[1,2,4]

As body temperature rises, such as during exercise or during an increased metabolic state, there is a shift to the right in the curve and oxygen is released to the tissues. A shift to the left due to a drop in temperature, as in a state of hypothermia, would not allow oxygen to be released to the tissues as readily.[1,2,4]

2,3-DPG is a phosphate found in large quantities in the red blood cells, and it impacts the affinity of hemoglobin for extracting and utilizing oxygen. An increase in 2,3-DPG will shift the curve to the right, and low levels will result in a left-sided shift. Its presence is oftentimes referred to as a chisel aiding in the drop-off of oxygen to the tissues. Factors such as hypoxia and the presence of anemia lead to increased 2,3-DPG levels. Another consideration is that packed red blood cells (PRBCs) are preserved with citrate, which can decrease levels of 2,3-DPG in transfused blood; this can lead to an increased affinity or left shift which impairs oxygen unloading or delivery.[11]

Abnormalities in the hemoglobin molecule can also affect oxygen loading and unloading. Structural abnormalities occur when the amino acid sequence changes the shape of the molecule's polypeptide chains, altering it from its normal parameters and functioning.[5] By altering the shape of the molecule, there is a tendency for changes in oxygen affinity. Carboxyhemoglobin, methemoglobin, and fetal hemoglobin all cause a left-sided shift and an increased oxygen affinity.[1] Increasing the affinity for oxygen improves the ability to pick up oxygen at the level of the lungs, but the opposite occurs with the ability to drop that oxygen off to the tissues, which becomes impaired. A left-shift could be the result of processes like hypothermia, hypocapnia, and low levels of 2,3-DPG, as was mentioned above.

As carbon dioxide levels increase, the blood becomes more acidotic, which causes a right-sided shift of the dissociation curve. This acidotic state is created by the reaction between carbon dioxide and water forming carbonic acid, with the end result being a drop in pH. This inverse ratio of pH and PCO_2 is termed the Bohr effect. To simplify, a right-sided shift means it becomes more difficult to collect oxygen but easier to drop it off to the tissues. A decreasing PCO_2 leads to an alkalotic state, increased O_2 affinity, and a left-sided shift.[1]

Ventilation–Perfusion Matching

Alveolar ventilation is the volume per minute that reaches the alveoli and physiologically takes part in the process of gas exchange. The variables that make up the total in this equation are tidal volume, respiratory rate, and dead space. This is approximately 4 L/min.[1]

Perfusion is the amount of blood flow to the respiratory capillaries. Normally, the amount of blood that perfuses the alveoli is 5 L/min (i.e., cardiac output). In a perfect physiologic state, the ventilation of every alveolus is matched by an equivalent of perfusion, resulting in an average ventilation–perfusion (V̇/Q) ratio of 4:5 or 0.8.[1,2,4]

This relationship can be altered by a multitude of disease states and physiologic conditions. When inadequate ventilation occurs relative to a normal state of perfusion, as occurs in pneumonia, the V̇/Q ratio is said to be low and is referred to as a shunt. Pulmonary shunting can be subdivided into relative and absolute shunts, and the latter can be further divided into anatomic and capillary shunting. A shunting effect can essentially impact oxygen uptake causing an impairment in gas exchange resulting in hypoxia. The severity of the shunt depends on whether oxygen therapy is initiated and effective. As the V̇/Q ratio lowers, the less responsive it will be to oxygen therapy. In an absolute shunt, it will be completely unresponsive to oxygen. An anatomic shunt exists when blood travels from the right side of the heart to the left side without undergoing gas exchange, such as is seen with a congenital heart defect.[1,2,4,6]

When there is normal ventilation or an increase in ventilation causing abnormal or compromised perfusion, a mismatch occurs. The classic example would be a pulmonary embolus, which causes an increase in the V̇/Q ratio; this has also been referred to as dead space ventilation. As the name implies, dead space is the volume of air that does not come in contact with the pulmonary capillary blood and is essentially wasted. Anatomic dead space consists of the volume of air that does not participate in gas exchange and is approximated by 2 mL/kg or 1 mL/lb.[2,6]

In the setting of poorly ventilated arterioles, constriction occurs, diverting the blood to better-ventilated areas. Similarly, inadequately perfused alveoli weaken and collapse, causing atelectasis or alveolar consolidation. This causes a diversion of airflow to more effectively perfused areas. This is a natural process known as hypoxic pulmonary vasoconstriction and helps to compensate for imbalanced ratios.

Distribution of the ventilation and perfusion is heavily weighted by gravity. It can, however, be used to maximize the V̇/Q̇ ratio in the compromised lung. By placing the patient in a position where the functional alveoli are in the dependent position and the affected units are elevated, ventilation and blood flow can be maximized, improving gas exchange. This is something to take into consideration when positioning patients in the critical care transport environment. Suboptimal positioning could contribute to poor ventilation and perfusion which can be detrimental to the patient and cause deterioration.[1,2,4]

Monitoring

In the transport environment, ongoing assessment and measurement of respiratory functioning is essential to detecting acute changes in the patient's condition and pulmonary functioning. Anticipating and identifying potential deterioration and respiratory compromise can be done using both noninvasive and invasive means. Pressure monitoring of the airway and vascular system are more invasive ways to track these changes and often require invasive vascular access. Other examples of monitoring include pulse oximetry, end-tidal capnography, electrocardiograms (ECGs), blood draws, blood gases, and pulmonary function testing.

Pulse Oximetry

The primary tool used to monitor oxygenation in the prehospital setting is pulse oximetry. The pulse oximeter uses light to determine to what extent hemoglobin is saturated with oxygen. A probe is placed on a specific region of the body, such as the finger or earlobe, and specific wavelengths of light are emitted between the surfaces of the probe. As light is absorbed by oxygenated and deoxygenated hemoglobin, the device measures how much light passes through from one side of the sensor to the other and is able to extrapolate a value to describe what percentage of hemoglobin is carrying oxygen. A normal value for this saturation of peripheral oxygen (SpO_2) is 94%–99%.[13]

In clinical practice, pulse oximetry is often utilized as the objective measure of oxygenation, therefore oxygen administration might be warranted with values below 94%. Similarly, with a value of 100% oxygen may be withheld to avoid potential adverse effects associated with a high SpO_2. It is important to note that pulse oximetry should not be used in isolation to assess the patient's oxygenation. Physical signs of hypoxia, which can occur independent of a low SpO_2, include cyanosis, tachycardia, restlessness, confusion, and respiratory distress. Treatment for hypoxia, regardless of how it is inferred, depends on underlying pathology and is described in the subsequent sections.[14]

Correct measurement of SpO_2 depends on several factors: adequate perfusion with pulsatile flow, correct placement on the body (i.e. different probes are designed for different areas), normal body temperature, variables that might physically obstruct the measurement (i.e., nail polish or dirt). Dyshemoglobinopathies, such as methemoglobinemia or carbon monoxide poisoning, will render oximetry values inaccurate. Quantitative values reported by pulse oximeters may underestimate the degree of hypoxia in patients with darker skin. For all of these reasons, it is important to consider the quantitative value afforded by the pulse oximeter in the overall context of patient presentation.[15]

End-Tidal Carbon Dioxide

End-tidal carbon dioxide ($ETCO_2$) is a technology that allows the clinician to measure the amount and pattern of carbon dioxide (CO_2) in exhaled air. The value of assessing CO_2 in exhaled air is based on the idea that CO_2 is produced in the body and delivered to the lungs in a predictable manner. Monitoring exhaled CO_2 allows the clinician to assess efficacy of ventilation and the processes that contribute to effective ventilation (i.e., perfusion and metabolism). This is particularly relevant to the management of pulmonary emergencies in transport.[16]

$ETCO_2$ is measured by placing a sensor that measures the partial pressure of CO_2 at a location where exhaled air passes through. In the intubated patient, the sensor is placed in the ventilator circuit just distal to the endotracheal tube. In the spontaneously breathing patient, however, the sensor can be placed at the nares or oropharynx. The former is often referred to as mainstream, the latter as sidestream. It is important to note, however, that a sidestream sensor placed at the nares may underestimate $ETCO_2$ in the patient that is exhaling primarily at the mouth.[16]

$ETCO_2$ includes both quantitative and qualitative components. The quantitative value is the peak partial pressure of CO_2 during exhalation. A normal value is 35–45 mmHg, however that value does not accurately reflect plasma $PCO2$. Delivery of CO_2 to the lungs for exhalation is dependent on adequate perfusion, so in a low cardiac output state, $ETCO_2$ will fall below the expected range. Other physiological changes affect the difference between arterial and end-tidal carbon dioxide measurements as well, both increasing and decreasing the difference. It is important to recognize that these other, unpredictable, factors can lead to inappropriate, possibly detrimental, changes when $PETCO_2$ is used to guide mechanical ventilation.[17]

The qualitative component is a waveform that shows the change in partial pressure over time throughout the expiratory phase. This is helpful for evaluating airway appliance placement, integrity of a ventilation circuit, and resistance to exhalation.

Blood Gases

Another tool used to evaluate both oxygenation and ventilation is blood gas analysis. This technology measures pH and concentrations of gases in a blood sample; these values can then be compared to normal ranges to identify specific processes, both pathophysiologic and compensatory.[5] The interpretation of arterial blood gases is discussed in Chapter 8 and Chapter 9 in the context of mechanical ventilation, but recognize that blood gases can also be measured in both mixed venous and venous blood samples as well—this potentially facilitates use in the transport setting when access to arterial samples may not be possible.[18]

Blood gas measurements represent pH and ventilation more effectively than they do oxygenation, because tissue oxygen delivery is more a function of hemoglobin saturation, as discussed earlier. They also reflect physiology only at the single snapshot in time when the gas was drawn, which may not be the steady state for a patient.

Electrocardiogram

Electrocardiogram (ECG or EKG) or cardiac monitoring is another tool commonly used in the transport setting to monitor trends in patient status over time and identify specific pathophysiologic processes. Details of ECG interpretation in the context of cardiac emergencies is discussed in Chapter 8, but there are some concepts specific to pulmonary emergencies that warrant discussion here.

In general terms, cardiac monitoring allows the clinician to observe trends in patient presentation. As it relates to pulmonary emergencies, it is important to monitor for progression toward acute respiratory failure. While the most common metrics for evaluating this progression are the degree of oxygenation (via SpO_2 and/or PaO_2) and ventilation (via $ETCO_2$ and/or ventilatory parameters), tachycardia may accompany respiratory distress, and bradycardia may correlate with respiratory failure. There are also specific patterns associated with certain pulmonary emergencies. These are discussed further in the following sections but include examples such as patterns associated with pulmonary embolism,[19] pulmonary hypertension,[20] and chronic obstructive pulmonary disease,[21] among others.

Oxygen and Ventilation Support

It is common for critically ill or injured patients to require oxygen therapy to support adequate tissue oxygenation. Oxygen delivery systems are classified into two categories: high-flow systems and low-flow systems.

Low-flow systems are devices that deliver oxygen at or below the patient's physiologic need. This type of system allows the patient to draw supplemental oxygen from the apparatus in addition to room or ambient air external to the device. In this type of system, the patient's minute ventilation directly impacts the concentration of oxygen that is inspired because the patient with a high minute ventilation entrains a greater amount of room air per minute.[22–24] For example, with 15 L/min of low-flow oxygen therapy, a patient with a high minute ventilation of 20 L/min inspires less oxygen, as percentage of overall air taken in, than a patient with a lower minute ventilation of 10 L/min.[24,25] Examples of low-flow oxygen delivery systems include nasal cannulas, simple face masks, and nonrebreather or partial nonrebreather masks.

High-flow oxygen systems deliver oxygen above the patient's physiologic minute ventilation. The result of this is that FiO_2 is less dependent on the patient's ventilatory pattern. Flow exceeding the patient's intrinsic minute ventilation reduces physiologic dead space, delivers oxygen via a partial pressure gradient, and can generate a small amount of end-expiratory pressure.

While oxygen therapy is indicated for hypoxic respiratory failure and to prevent deterioration toward acute respiratory failure, there are times when supporting the movement of air, rather than the composition of that air, is the treatment of choice. While oxygen therapy and ventilatory support are frequently used simultaneously, each focuses on a different component of the overall breathing process.

At its most basic level, ventilatory support involves interventions to allow or facilitate the gross movement of air into the lungs. A simple head-tilt-chin-lift or modified jaw-thrust could be considered ventilatory support. These concepts and other techniques, ranging from nasal or oropharyngeal airways to endotracheal intubation, are commonly discussed in the context of airway management. Positive-pressure ventilation, whether provided by noninvasive means or a tracheal tube, allows for the manipulation of mean airway pressure to support oxygenation and of minute ventilation to support carbon dioxide removal.

On occasion, support for oxygenation and ventilation requires restoration of the basic anatomy of the thorax. For example, a flail segment in the thoracic cage can impair effective negative-pressure ventilation and requires some kind of stabilization. When the potential space between the visceral and parietal pleura is replaced with actual space by fluid, blood, air, or infectious exudate, lung volumes are lost and, in extreme cases, airway and vascular anatomy is distorted. In these cases, thoracotomy or thoracostomy to remove the space-occupying material can be indicated.

In addition to airway management techniques, there are other ways a patient's pulmonary health can be supported. A combination of techniques may be the best and most effective approach to clearing secretions. All of these tools can be utilized to enhance pulmonary hygiene by mobilizing secretions, decreasing viscosity, and fragmenting mucus plugs.

Pulmonary hygiene utilizes the body's own mechanisms, as well as supplementary devices, to assist in the clearance of mucus and secretions. Moisture and mucolytics can help to decrease secretion viscosity. Other therapies and equipment that can help facilitate mobility and clearance of secretions include chest physiotherapy, vibratory devices, and breath-stacking or lung recruitment with cough assistance, glossopharyngeal breathing, positional drainage, and pressure resistance.[26]

Humidity is an effective tool that can prevent constriction and narrowing of the airway. Dry, cool gases delivered to the patient, especially at high flow rates, can prevent mucous mobility, create more viscous secretions, and potentiate mucous plugging and respiratory compromise. Providing humidity to the lungs is important for lung compliance, especially for individuals who have chronic conditions such as asthma. Asthmatics may have an increased potential for bronchospasm when the airway is too dry.

Acute Respiratory Distress Syndrome

Pathophysiology

Acute respiratory distress syndrome (ARDS) is a lung injury that has several causes, and it is a condition that can be difficult to treat and can be fatal. ARDS may arise due to complications related to another disease process or injury, but the most common cause is severe sepsis with a pulmonary source of infection.[27] While sepsis is the most common risk factor worldwide, there are a number of other associated risk factors including certain chronic and acute disease states, age, sex, ethnicity/race, and lifestyle factors.[28] The syndrome is a condition characterized by diffuse inflammation of the lung that causes severe and often fatal hypoxemia and respiratory failure.[29] Poor diffusion of gas across the alveolar capillary membrane further damages the lung tissue, increasing edema, and decreasing oxygen levels in the blood. Poor oxygenation is usually due to mismatched and intrapulmonary shunting.

The alterations in pulmonary vascular permeability change lung structure and function in two phases. The first phase includes the initiation of an exudative state with an overwhelming expression of proinflammatory responses. Damage to the pulmonary endothelium and epithelium ensues, and fluid begins to accumulate in the alveoli. Phase two causes extensive pulmonary fibrosis and loss of normal alveolar structure, weakening the muscles of the respiratory system.[23,30] The outstanding characteristic of ARDS is hypoxemia refractory to oxygen therapy. Because ARDS can accompany other disease states or injuries, the transport clinician must consider both the patient's current condition along with the pathophysiology of the underlying problem. Acute respiratory distress syndrome has a mortality rate of approximately 46%, and survivors of the condition commonly reduces intrapulmonary shunting. Additionally, this positioning improves secretion mobilization.[29] The prone position is not tolerable or appropriate for all patients, and it may be contraindicated in some patients. such as those with increased intracranial pressure, spinal cord injuries, major abdominal surgeries, or severe hemodynamic instability (Fig. 10.3). The movement of patients into and out of prone position, and the transport of patients in prone position both engender risk when not performed in a planned manner by experienced teams.[32,33]

Fluid balance is an important factor to consider, with general recommendations of remaining fluid-neutral or net-negative in hemodynamically stable patients.[28] In ARDS, the pulmonary capillary membrane is impaired, allowing fluid to leak into the alveoli. A patient may require intravenous (IV) crystalloids, vasopressors, inotropes, and diuretics to aid in the maintenance of effective tissue perfusion, fluid balance, and fluid distribution.

Inhaled pulmonary vasodilators such as nitric oxide and, increasingly, prostacyclin agents such as epoprostenol, may be

experience residual lung damage and long-term, ongoing health complications.[28]

The consensus definition for ARDS, often called the Berlin definition, describes several criteria: timing, chest imaging, origin of edema, and oxygenation (Box 10.1). These features necessarily describe essential examination elements.

Interventions

ARDS is a complex condition which makes it challenging to manage. A primary goal of therapy should include avoiding ventilator-induced lung injury by using a lung-protective ventilation strategy whenever possible. The genesis of lung-protective ventilation is with studies on mortality in ARDS, and lung-protective ventilation is discussed in detail in Chapter 9.

Positive end-expiratory pressure (PEEP) is added to mechanical ventilation in an attempt to improve arterial oxygenation. PEEP increases the functional residual capacity of the lung, reduces closing volume, and improves overall lung compliance. Additionally, PEEP reduces mismatching, mitigates end-expiratory alveolar collapse, maintains alveolar recruitment, and can reduce ventilator-induced lung injury (VILI). Reducing atelectasis with PEEP may also more evenly distribute inflation stress produced by repetitive opening and closing of alveolar structures during ventilation. As the disease process worsens and lung compliance decreases, higher levels of PEEP may be needed to maintain oxygenation levels. The management of the ventilated patient with ARDS is oxygenation support with high PEEP and low lung protective volumes to prevent higher-than-desired peak inspiratory pressures. Higher peak pressures can cause complications such as spontaneous pneumothorax.[1,23,30,31]

Hypoxemia at this state is severe, and supplemental oxygen is necessary. The oxygen delivery system and amount of FiO$_2$ used depends on the patient's condition. Advanced ventilation strategies may need to be employed to improve oxygenation of the ARDS patient. These patients can be difficult to oxygenate and ventilate, and because of this, priority to oxygenate takes precedence over ventilation, and permissive hypercapnia may be accepted.

There are physiological and outcome benefits to placing ARDS patients in a prone position. Proning a patient improves perfusion to the less damaged areas of the lungs, decreases mismatching, and

Supine Position

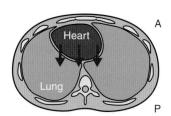

Gravitational pressure of heart and mediastinum on the lungs.

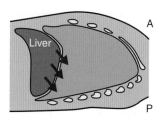

Compressive effects of the abdominal organs on the lungs.

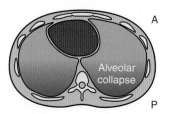

Expansion of the chest wall and overall less homogeneous chest wall compliance.

Prone Position

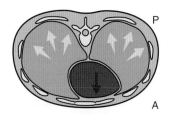

Decreased gravitational pressure of heart and mediastinum on the lungs.

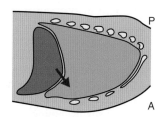

Decreased compressive effects of the abdominal organs on the lungs.

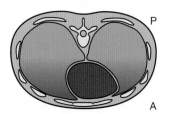

More homogeneous chest wall compliance due to restriction of anterior chest wall movement.

• **Fig. 10.3** Physiologic effects of prone positioning. (Modified from Venus K, Munshi L, Fralick M. Prone positioning for patients with hypoxic respiratory failure related to COVID-19. *CMAJ.* 2020;192(47):E1532–E1537.)

beneficial for some patients with ARDS.[34,35] ARDS patients sometimes require cannulation for extracorporeal membrane oxygenation.[36]

Chronic Obstructive Pulmonary Diseases

Pathophysiology

Chronic obstructive pulmonary disease (COPD) represents the spectrum of asthma, chronic bronchitis, and emphysema.[31] Emphysema and chronic bronchitis coexisting to some extent is not unusual, and while each entity is discussed separately in this textbook, it is important to remember that both can be present in the same patient simultaneously.

In the transport environment, a clinician may need to consider altitude when ventilating patients and managing cardiac output. A patient with COPD may have limited ability to increase ventilation and cardiac output in response to stress, which is why knowledge of altitude and flight physiology may be an important factor to consider.[1]

Asthma is the restriction of airflow secondary to airway inflammation, and it is a recurrent and to some extent, reversible obstructive pulmonary disorder. The characteristics of asthma include airway inflammation, increased airway responsiveness to various stimuli, airway bronchoconstriction, and increased mucous production.[37] Asthma predisposes individuals to other diseases in the COPD spectrum.[26] The prevalence and severity of the condition has increased in recent years, and there are a number of contributing factors for this, including genetics, lifestyle factors, diet, tobacco use and exposure, air pollutants, allergen exposure, malnutrition, obesity, perinatal risks, and prematurity, among others.[38]

Airway responsiveness can be triggered by various stimuli, and the result is an inflammatory response. With this response comes cellular infiltration and mucosal edema causing hyperreactivity and contraction of smooth muscle and an overproduction of mucus. Clearance of these secretions is diminished due to the edema, and this causes abnormalities, increased airway resistance and bronchospasm, and hyperinflation of the lungs with an increase in residual volume. Status asthmaticus is a severe attack that is refractory to bronchodilator therapy.[23]

Chronic bronchitis is defined as having a productive cough for at least three consecutive months and for two successive years, in which the cough cannot be attributed to any other cause. Several contributing factors are known to be instrumental in the etiology of chronic bronchitis. Smoking and inhaled pollutants contain irritants that aid in the pathologic changes that contribute to exacerbations, recurrent infections, and hospitalizations. Secondhand smoking and work-related environments can also be influential and directly related to the origin of the disease process.[3]

In chronic bronchitis, pathologic changes are common to the large- and medium-size airways, which have direct implications to the distal airways. External irritants cause chronic inflammation and bronchospasm, reducing the cross-sectional diameter in the airways. This chronic inflammatory state leads to a hypersecretion of copious amounts of sputum in which the body's normal protective mechanisms become easily overwhelmed and ineffective from impairment of the mucociliary blanket. This can progress to partial or complete airway blockage. These manifestations can occur with or without measurable airflow obstruction. The progressive result of these combinations of factors can lead to hypercapnia and hypoxia. Assessments and interventions for the chronic bronchitis patient are discussed below in conjunction with the discussion of

emphysema, as they closely align and may be assessed and treated in a similar capacity.

Emphysema is an alveolar disease state that is defined as the presence of a permanent enlargement of the airspaces distal to the terminal bronchioles, accompanied by destruction of their walls and without obvious fibrosis.[1] In other words, the alveoli erode, the airspaces become enlarged, break down, and become thin-walled. This destabilizes the bronchioles, and the lungs begin losing the elastic recoil they naturally exhibit, which leaves the airways weak and easily collapsible, causing the trapping of gas.[26] Factors that contribute to the development of emphysema include smoking, inhaled pollutants, occupational hazards, gender, socio-economic factors, and alpha-1 antitrypsin deficiency.[1,3]

Years before symptom onset, pathological changes can be occurring. The alveoli are damaged or destroyed and the airspaces beyond the terminal bronchioles are enlarged. This leads to an increase in the ratio of air to lung tissue in the alveoli, and once the alveolar–capillary interface becomes anatomically altered, the gas exchange is impaired. As the proximal structures to the alveolus fail to keep the airways open, the expiratory phase becomes essential to CO_2 elimination, as the resistance to airflow increases. This allows air to be trapped in the alveoli increasing residual volumes. Typically, the patient's vital capacity is close to normal until the disease has advanced to a severe stage.[1,3]

Assessment

The history is important to understanding the primary etiology of the disease. Minor pulmonary infections, stress, changes in weather, or continued exposure to environmental pollutants (including smoking) can easily exacerbate the condition. The patient's subjective assessment of the condition is important for determining the usual status of the disease, and the historical hospitalization course will aid in the severity of the current pulmonary state. The clinician should assess similar questions as addressed above in the asthmatic patient regarding hospitalization and intubation. The patient may report increased dyspnea, change in sputum production, or an increase in the malaise that may accompany the disease.[37]

The transport clinician's assessment should include a careful history to identify precipitating factors. For instance, a viral illness or other environmental exposure may precede the acute exacerbation of asthma—the patient may report an initial cough or dyspnea, and someone with a long history of asthma can usually "rank" the relative severity of the exacerbation as compared to prior episodes. The assessment should also include a thorough medication history that includes timing and dosage of inhalers, bronchodilators, steroids, and the like. Other useful history questions that relate specifically to individuals with COPD-categorized illnesses include any previous intensive care unit admissions and previous intubations. This can help the transport clinician gauge how severe this patient's condition may become and the process in which it may develop. The information obtained in the history will improve the clinician's ability to anticipate and adapt to the ever-changing circumstances that can occur in asthmatic patients.

On physical examination, clinicians may recognize different degrees of distress based on the severity of the current episode. Tachypnea, tachycardia, elevated respiratory rate, wheezing, and a prolonged expiratory phase are not uncommon, and some individuals will not be able to complete full sentences without becoming breathless. If no wheezing is heard and the patient has difficulty talking, the transport clinician should consider the situation emergent and anticipate rapid deterioration. The absence of wheezing may indicate that the patient is not able to ventilate sufficiently to produce breath sounds; this is sometimes referred to as "silent chest," an ominous sign due to hyperinflation of the chest causing an inability to transmit sound.[26] Inspiratory retractions may be seen, as may the use of accessory muscles. The blood pressure may be variable, and pulsus paradoxus may be present. Cyanosis and lethargy are late signs and necessitate immediate attention and intervention.[23]

To determine the severity of the asthmatic episode, diagnostic studies are performed. Resistance to airflow is measured with spirometry or a peak flow meter. Spirometric measurement of forced expiratory volume in 1 second (FEV_1) is done before and after asthma treatments to ascertain treatment success. Peak expiratory flow rate can be accomplished with a handheld meter and has been used to determine whether arterial blood gas (ABG) measurement is necessary.[37,40] Pulmonary function testing is helpful with management and monitoring; however, clinical presentation is key for identification in an acute case.

In addition to measurement of resistance to airflow, chest radiography is a common diagnostic tool that may be used if other parameters are abnormal. ABG measurements may be helpful in severe asthma patients.

In chronic bronchitis, pathologic changes are common to the large- and medium-size airways, which have direct implications to the distal airways. External irritants cause chronic inflammation and bronchospasm, reducing the cross-sectional diameter in the airways. This chronic inflammatory state leads to a hypersecretion of copious amounts of sputum in which the body's normal protective mechanisms become easily overwhelmed and ineffective from impairment of the mucociliary blanket. This can progress to partial or complete airway blockage. These manifestations can occur with or without measurable airflow obstruction. The progressive result of these combinations of factors can lead to hypercapnia and hypoxia. Assessments and interventions for the chronic bronchitis patient are discussed below in conjunction with the discussion of emphysema, as they closely align and may be assessed and treated in a similar capacity.

The clinical presentation of chronic bronchitis and emphysema each have individual characteristics that may overlap, with many patients having a combination of the two diseases. Physical examination may reveal rhonchi, expiratory wheezes, or diminished breath sounds. Rales may be present during a state of pulmonary infections. Accessory muscles for inspiration and expiration are actively used due to the increased work of breathing. Tachycardia and the presence of dysrhythmias are not uncommon in either condition. In the emphysema patient, the thorax is hyperresonant to percussion because of hyperinflation of the alveoli, and the anterior posterior diameter of the chest is increased, which can also lead to muffled heart sounds. Observation of the patient's respiratory pattern may reveal pursed-lips with a prolonged expiratory phase.

The patient frequently wants to sit upright and lean forward, with their hands on the knees in a tripod position. This positioning aids in the stability of the accessory muscles and should be allowed for patient comfort whenever possible. Emphysema patients are often referred to as "pink puffers" because they are markedly dyspneic and can maintain a relatively normal arterial oxygenation level in less severe stages. Conversely, patients with chronic bronchitis are frequently referred to as "blue bloaters" because they appear edematous and cyanotic. These patients tend to have a larger physical build and tend to be overweight. A chronic, loose productive cough is a classic presentation.[1,3,4]

In any COPD patient, mental status is an important component of the transport team's objective assessment of the patient. Retention of CO_2 occurs in the later stages of the disease processes, and once the CO_2 level in the arterial circulation increases beyond the baseline level, one of the first signs is behavioral and emotional changes. These may vary from confusion, irritability, and a decrease in intellectual performance caused by obtundation. Any alterations should be aggressively investigated and treated. When available, ABG results contain valuable information revealing the extent of distress or failure, but it is important that clinicians use this as supplementary information and "match" this with the patient's clinical condition. Other worthy common laboratory findings may include polycythemia, hypochloremia (as HCO_3- rises), and hypernatremia.[18]

Radiologic findings for patients with chronic bronchitis may include translucent lung fields, fibrotic-appearing lung markings caused by bronchial thickening, depressed or flattened diaphragms, and right atrial enlargement (cor pulmonale). The patient with emphysema may also show similar manifestations, such as translucency, flattened diaphragms, and occasional atrial and ventricular enlargement, along with a narrowed heart silhouette.[3]

ECG findings in advanced stages of these disease states may show low-voltage complexes, right axis deviation, and flattened or inverted P waves in I and aVL. These common diagnostic tools may be available during interfacility transfers and benefit in the continuity of care when combined with a thorough patient assessment. The transport clinician should verify which procedures or labs have been performed and discuss any significant data or imaging results prior to transport to understand the extent to which the process has progressed.

Interventions

Acute interventions for asthma are directed toward management of inflammation and reversal of bronchoconstriction. Initial actions should include ensuring airway patency and providing supplemental oxygen, as well as determining possible causes and eliminating those stimulants as able.

Medications used to treat asthma are divided into two categories: controller and rescue medications. Controller medications include orally inhaled corticosteroids, leukotriene modifiers, mast cell stabilizers, and systemic corticosteroids. Rescue medications include inhaled beta-2 agonists, inhaled anticholinergics, systemic corticosteroids, and magnesium sulfate. Antibiotics are not indicated for routine asthma exacerbation, and should be reserved for patients with evidence of pneumonia. Asthma patients who require intubation have increased mortality rates.[37]

Patients with obstructive lung diseases may live at varying baseline levels of hypoxia, and this should be considered when determining how much supplemental oxygen should be administered. Supplemental oxygen is given to correct the patient's hypoxia to return the patient to their baseline level. It should be noted that the peripheral chemoreceptors are located at the bifurcations of the aortic arteries and the aortic arch. These chemoreceptors are responsive to low levels of oxygen in the arterial blood and become active only when the PaO_2 is less than approximately 60 mmHg. However, the major influence of stimulation, received by the medulla, is excessive levels of hydrogen ions from the cerebrospinal fluid by the central chemoreceptors.

This hypoxic response is far slower than signals sent by the central chemoreceptors.[8]

Other approaches to the care of the COPD patient should be based on clinical presentation and assessment. Once again, patient positioning and nonpharmacological interventions should be explored in combination with medication management. In acute management, short-acting beta-2 agonists are commonly used for bronchial smooth muscle relaxation in addition to anticholinergics such as ipratropium bromide. Systemic glucocorticosteroids can also be implemented because of the inflammatory process; however, the onset of action is usually within 1–2 hours. This population of patients oftentimes is already on combination long-acting beta-2 agonist/glucocorticosteroids, long-acting anticholinergics, and uncommonly methylxanthines. The patient may need assistance with removal of secretions via nasotracheal suctioning or endotracheal suctioning when intubated. IV fluids for rehydration may be necessary, and these should be administered cautiously in the presence of heart failure. Antibiotic therapy and expectorants are frequently utilized because of recurrent infections.

During exacerbations, attention to support for both oxygenation and ventilation is important. Noninvasive ventilation has been used with extreme success in curbing the progression of distress for patients with all forms of COPD, including asthma.

Hemoptysis

Pathophysiology

Hemoptysis is the coughing or spitting up of blood arising from the respiratory tract. The amount of blood expelled can vary widely from scant amounts of sputum streaked with blood to massive pulmonary hemorrhage. Any volume of hemoptysis is considered abnormal. The most common etiologies of hemoptysis are tuberculosis, cancer, bronchiectasis, lung abscess, and acute bronchitis. For patients with massive hemorrhage, the bronchial vasculature is the most common source, followed by the pulmonary vasculature. Other more acute causes may be more dangerous, including airway trauma, the presence of a foreign body, pulmonary embolism, and drug use causing inflammation.[41]

Interventions

In the transport environment, management options are limited. If hemoptysis is significant, on the pulmonary hemorrhage end of the spectrum, efforts are directed at maintaining some kind of airway patency so that oxygenation and ventilation can be maintained until hemostasis is achieved or the bleeding site isolated from the main pulmonary tree.

If the bleeding is deemed life-threatening, it may be necessary to intubate the patient. In the transport setting, the most experienced clinician should prepare to intubate by identifying possible challenges such as decreased visualization due to bleeding and inflammation of the airway. A large-bore endotracheal tube ($\geq$8 mm) should be selected if possible to increase the size of the vessel through which ongoing interventions may be performed. Transport clinicians should have alternate plans for airway management in place should intubation be unsuccessful.

Emergently, application of PEEP may help with lower pressure bleeding and clinicians will consider the nebulization of tranexamic acid. If the patient is coagulopathic, normalization of coagulation is essential. If the bleeding site is past the main bronchial bifurcation, the bleeding site may be excluded from the patent elements of the airway with a double-lumen endotracheal tube or an endobronchial blocker (Fig. 10.4).

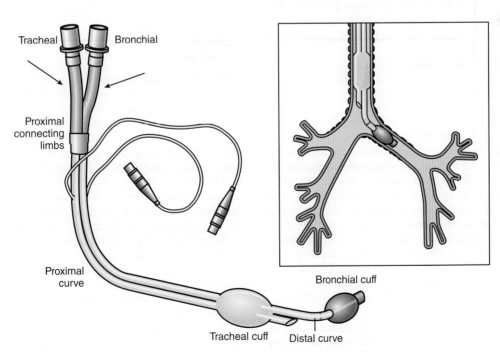

Tracheal Bronchial

Proximal connecting limbs

Proximal curve

Bronchial cuff

Tracheal cuff   Distal curve

• **Fig. 10.4** Double lumen endotracheal tube and placement. (Modified from Pellechi J, DuBois S, Harrison M. Updates to thoracic procedures: perioperative care and anesthetic considerations. *Updates in Anesthesia – The Operating Room and Beyond*. IntechOpen; 2023. Available under a Creative Commons Attribution 3.0 Unported license.)

Pneumonia

Pathophysiology

Pneumonia is a common condition that results in the inflammation of the lung parenchyma caused by either a bacterium or a virus. The severity can vary from mild to life-threatening and is dependent on the specific pathogen and any underlying risk factors the patient may have. Pneumonias can be classified as community-acquired, hospital-acquired (including ventilator-acquired), or from aspiration. In the United States, an estimated 2–4 million cases occur annually, and community-acquired pneumonia is the most common type and one of the primary causes of pneumonia-related mortality and morbidity worldwide. Identifying which classification is most consistent with the patient's symptoms and history can be helpful in determining the most appropriate treatment regimen to initiate. Pneumonias can be caused by and can complicate other underlying disease processes.[42]

Bronchopneumonias occur when areas of normal lung parenchyma are interspersed with affected lung parenchyma. The condition is multilobar and often bilateral, with areas of atelectasis. *Staphylococcus aureus* is the most common infecting organism. Interstitial pneumonia is the result of an inflammatory process that affects the support structures of the lung.

The history of the patient with suspected pneumonia often includes fever and purulent sputum production. Specific testing includes chest x-ray, sputum cultures, blood cultures, Gram stains, and possibly a bronchoscopy.

Interventions

Patients with pneumonia require oxygenation and ventilatory support, as described earlier. Their underlying process is that of infection and sepsis, so resuscitation and management along those guidelines addresses the cause. Accordingly, these patients benefit from early appropriate antibiotic coverage, volume resuscitation, and blood pressure and cardiac output support. Source control by bronchoscopy is sometimes helpful. These patients may progress to an ARDS picture, as described earlier.

Pleural Effusion

Under normal conditions, the parietal pleura forms a small amount of fluid that is then absorbed by the visceral pleura; however, in the presence of a pleural effusion, a collection of excess fluid occurs which overwhelms the absorptive mechanism of the visceral pleura. This can be caused by conditions related to heart failure, liver and renal failure causing decreased capillary oncotic pressure, obstruction or impaired functioning of the lymphatic system, and inflammatory states such as infections.[3] This fluid accumulation causes a burden on the respiratory system and inhibits the lungs from fully expanding. This subsequently causes an impairment in gas exchange and an assortment of associated symptoms. The most common causes are heart failure, pneumonia, malignant disease, and pulmonary embolism.[42]

Some effusions are managed conservatively. Alternatively, the effusion can be drained by aspiration or placement of a thoracostomy tube. The evacuated contents are often sent for laboratory studies to determine the infective agent(s) present and to guide further treatment with medications such as antivirals or antibiotics.

Pneumothorax

In a normal lung environment, the contraction of the diaphragm and ribs creates a negative pressure in the chest cavity, allowing the lungs to remain expanded. There are three ways in which air or gas can enter the pleural space: from an opening in the chest wall, gas-forming bacteria in an empyema in the pleural space, or perforation of the visceral pleura.[43] In the event of a pneumothorax that negative pressure environment is disrupted, and air rushes into the pleural space and accumulates. The lung collapses in varying degrees, and hypoxemia may occur. If the pneumothorax is significant, a tension pneumothorax may occur when the air is trapped in the pleural space under pressure. This may lead to pressure being placed on the great veins, decreased venous return, and, consequently, hemodynamic compromise.[3]

Spontaneous pneumothoraces can be categorized as primary and secondary types. A primary spontaneous pneumothorax occurs in the absence of an underlying lung disease process, and a secondary process occurs in the presence of a condition. Various risk factors include age, gender, genetics, lung disease, smoking, and a history of previous pneumothoraces.

Some patients may be asymptomatic or display only mild signs and symptoms of a small lung collapse; in these cases, a pneumothorax may go undetected until later imaging is performed. When identified, hospitalization for observation may be all that is necessary; however, even in these circumstances it may take weeks for a full recovery. Treatment is driven by symptoms rather than size of the pneumothorax. With involvement of less than 20% of the affected lung, no invasive treatment is usually needed. Conservative approaches like simple bed rest, oxygen, and techniques to re-establish inflation may be all that is necessary.

Symptomatic patients are treated with an evacuation by thoracentesis or placement of a thoracostomy tube. If recurrence continues, chemical pleurodesis is often considered.

Sickle Cell Crisis

Etiology

Sickle cell disease is an inherited disorder of the red blood cells affecting the hemoglobin. A mutation in the beta-globin chain of the hemoglobin molecule causes it to be abnormally shaped, stiff, and sticky. Acute chest syndrome occurs when the abnormal hemoglobin molecules cause occlusion in the pulmonary vasculature. This causes a spiral of deoxygenation and worsening occlusion, ischemia, and endothelial injury. The syndrome can progress quickly, causing a spiral of deoxygenation and worsening occlusion, ischemia, and endothelial injury. Acute chest syndrome is a radiological and clinical diagnosis. Diagnostic criteria are:

1. New pulmonary infiltrates, not atelectasis, on chest imaging (chest x-ray, CT) involving at least one lung segment
2. One of these symptoms:
   - Chest pain
   - Fever above more than 38.5°C
   - Tachypnea, wheezing, rales, coughing, or increased work of breathing
   - Hypoxemia relative to baseline (more than 2% decrease in baseline oxygen saturation or PO_2 less than 60 mmHg

For patients with acute chest syndrome, management is built on pain control, hydration, and antibiotics. The use of a nonsedating analgesic such as acetaminophen or ketorolac is helpful initially. Patients may progress to the need for opiates. Fluid resuscitation is indicated for dehydrated patients, but routine large volume hydration is no longer indicated. All patients with acute chest syndrome should have antibiotic coverage for routine pathogens, atypical pathogens, and with consideration for MRSA.

There is some evidence that blood transfusion for patients with significant or significantly worsening anemia are helpful. Steroids may be helpful, but carry a risk for rebound occlusive crisis and readmission. Supplemental oxygen and bronchodilators are given if clinically indicated.

Pulmonary Embolism and Pulmonary Hypertension

Pulmonary embolism and pulmonary hypertension are diseases of the pulmonary vasculature that predominately affect cardiac function, especially the function of the right ventricle. A pulmonary embolism is the obstruction of the pulmonary artery or one of its branches by material (thrombus, tumor, air, or fat) that originated elsewhere in the body.[44] Pulmonary hypertension is a progressive condition of the arteries of the heart and lungs due to elevated blood pressure in the pulmonary arteries.

Pulmonary Embolism

Acute pulmonary embolism (PE) is a common disease process that has a highly variable clinical presentation, and due to a number of contributing factors, it can be fatal.[45] The incidence of a PE is estimated to be approximately 60–70 per 100,000, and that of venous thrombosis approximately 124 per 100,000 of the general population.[45] PE ranks third among the most common types of cardiovascular diseases closely following coronary artery disease and stroke.[46] Potentiating factors for PE and thrombus formation include conditions of stasis such as prolonged sitting, local pressure, and immobilization. Other forms of stasis are congestive heart failure, shock, and varicose veins. Recent surgeries, trauma, cancer, hypercoagulation disorders, and inherited factors increase the risk for thrombotic events like PE.

When a PE occurs, the pulmonary artery becomes either partially or completely obstructed, compromising the respiratory system or causing hemodynamic alterations. The patient's condition reflects the degree of cross-sectional area involvement. Pulmonary artery pressure increases only if more than 50% of the total cross-sectional area of the pulmonary arterial bed is occluded, and right ventricle failure caused by pressure overload is considered the primary cause of death in severe PE. A PE is considered massive when accompanied by shock or hypotension (either relative or absolute).[47]

The way a patient presents on physical assessment is not always a reliable indicator of a PE or the extent to which a patient may be impacted. Signs and symptoms of PE can mimic other conditions and onset can be variable. These signs and symptoms may include tachycardia, tachypnea, dyspnea, pleuritic pain, cough, wheezes, hemoptysis, lightheadedness, jugular venous distention, orthopnea, dependent edema, and an accentuated S2 heart sound or an S3 noted. A history may show evidence of prolonged travel or immobilization, recent surgeries, oral contraceptive use, congestive heart failure, neoplasms, or family heritable or prothrombotic tendencies.

Laboratory tests are performed to aid in diagnosis and often include D-dimer, and biochemical markers of right ventricular dysfunction such as brain natriuretic peptide (BNP), and troponin.

The diagnostic value that each of these labs carries alone is limited, but in conjunction with a thorough history, assessment, and other diagnostic findings, they can contribute to a timely diagnosis and treatment. PE with elevation of either BNP or troponin carries an increased mortality risk, and PE with elevation of both, showing both myocardial injury and cardiac dysfunction, carries significant risk.

ECG abnormalities can show nonspecific changes. Sensitivity for particular ECG findings is low, so they cannot be used to rule out pulmonary embolism. Specificity is high for the right ventricular strain pattern (simultaneous T-wave inversion in the inferior and precordial leads), P-pulmonale, and S1Q3T3 pattern, but the prevalence of each is low (11.1%, 0.5%, and 3.7%, respectively).[48]

A chest x-ray is often performed in suspected PE patients to aid in understanding the physiology of the acute concern and to provide alternative explanations for the patient's symptoms.[49] Other disease states that can cause similar symptoms include pleural effusions, atelectasis, an elevated hemidiaphragm, and cardiomegaly. Definitive imaging includes CT pulmonary angiography and, less commonly, scanning or other imaging modalities.[44]

This is a condition where ultrasound may be helpful. Even a rudimentary exam can demonstrate right ventricular size and contractility, tricuspid valve function and the relative position of the intraventricular septum. Abnormalities in any of these demonstrate progression down a spiral of synergistically worsening biventricular failure and potential cardiovascular collapse (Fig. 10.5).

Interventions

Some patients are hemodynamically stable on presentation, and attention should be targeted toward supportive measures such as hemodynamic support, anticoagulation, and evaluation of cardiac function for risk stratification and further intervention. For patients with hemodynamic instability, resuscitation is geared toward supporting myocardial perfusion. The right ventricle is

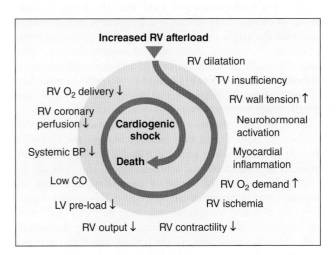

• **Fig. 10.5** Progression of right ventricular failure. *BP*, Blood pressure; *CO*, cardiac output; *LV*, left ventricular; *RV*, right ventricular; *TV*, tricuspid valve. (Modified from Konstantinides SV, Torbicki A, Agnelli G, et al. 2014 ESC Guidelines on the diagnosis and management of acute pulmonary embolism: The Task Force for the Diagnosis and Management of Acute Pulmonary Embolism of the European Society of Cardiology (ESC). *Eur Heart J.* 2014;35(43):3033–3080.)

poorly responsive to volume, and in an unstable PE patient is likely to be easily overdistended. It is best to err on the side of volume restriction and to support blood pressure and cardiac function with an inopressor such as norepinephrine. Vasopressin may be a good second-line agent, as it performs better in acidemic environments, acts as a noncatecholamine agent, and may cause less increase in pulmonary vascular resistance. Inhaled prostacyclins can help to reduce pulmonary vascular resistance, as well.[50] For patients with PE and hypotension, there is a mortality benefit to systemic fibrinolysis.[51]

Pulmonary Hypertension

PH is defined by a mean pulmonary arterial pressure (mPAP) greater than or equal to 25 mmHg at rest and is usually confirmed by a right heart catheterization. Normal pulmonary arterial systolic pressure ranges from 15 to 30 mmHg, diastolic pressure from 4 to 12 mmHg, and normal mPAP is ≤ 20 mmHg.[52] PH has been formerly classified into two separate categories—primary and secondary—according to the existence of causes and risk factors.

The World Health Organization (WHO) established a clinical classification to individualize different categories of PH sharing similar pathologic findings, similar hemodynamic characteristics, and similar management, as PH sometimes carries an unclear etiology and required extensive diagnostic testing and examination of contributing factors.[53] Pulmonary artery hypertension (Group 1) is the narrowing of the vessels to the lungs, adding stress to the right side of the heart. Over time, this added strain and stress on the heart leads to right-sided heart failure. As the condition worsens and progresses, the left side of the heart consequently becomes compromised. Group 1 consists of heritable, drug- and toxin-induced, and connective tissue disorders, among other causes. In Groups 2 to 5, the WHO classification system can be used to understand the pathophysiology and associated similarities and treatment options of the PH. In Group 2, pulmonary hypertension is characterized by left ventricular involvement and valvular disease. This leads to left-sided heart failure and a back-pressure of fluid into the lungs. Group 3 consists of chronic lung disease and hypoxia, which is generally considered the origin for the narrowing of the pulmonary arteries. Group 4 consists of chronic thromboembolism, which causes the vessels to become narrowed and vasoconstrict because of blood clots. Group 5 is PH caused by unspecified multifactorial mechanisms, including hematologic, systemic, and metabolic disorders.[52,53]

The signs and symptoms related to pulmonary hypertension are often generalized and may include, but are not limited to, shortness of breath, chest pain, tachycardia, fatigue, hemoptysis, peripheral dependent edema, lightheadedness, and cyanosis. Due to the rather generalized nature of complaints, the time from symptom onset to diagnosis can be lengthy. This extended period of investigation and recognition can delay diagnosis and prevent early implementation of critical treatments. During the period in which a clinician seeks answers, the patient's condition may exacerbate and PH progresses and advances through worsening and more damaging stages.

The treatment of PH has become increasingly complex and involves a multimodal methodology as a greater number of therapeutic agents continue to become available. Treatment is geared at identifying and remedying the underlying cause(s) with an overarching goal of preventing further escalation of symptoms and to reduce them altogether. An early, aggressive, and goal-directed approach to therapy appears to make PH more manageable and improves patient outcomes.[54] Group 1 interventions are aimed at relaxing the blood vessels in the lungs using calcium channel blockers, prostanoids, phosphodiesterase-5 inhibitors, and endothelin-receptor antagonists. Group 2 consists of left ventricular involvement and valvular disease, thus acute care is directed toward management of preload, afterload, and contractility, keeping in mind the left ventricular function. For Group 3, managing the root of hypoxia is the primary goal. Group 4 may include blood-thinning medications, and Group 5 as a heterogeneous group should again be treated by the underlying cause. Across these groups, the clinician may see that many of the medications overlap, as patients are increasingly being prescribed combination therapies due to research showing clinically important benefits to this approach.[53–55]

Pulmonary arterial hypertension may be treated with a number of pharmacological agents; some of these medications include sildenafil, tadalafil, riociguat, epoprostenol, iloprost, and treprostinil.[29,54] It is important for the transport clinician to be familiar with the variety of medications that may be administered or may be in a patient's regular treatment regimen. Understanding the adverse effect profiles and the patient burden should be considered in PH to guide therapy and maximize tolerability and effectiveness.[54]

Pulmonary Edema

Pulmonary edema is the pulmonary manifestation of a cardiovascular problem, where there ultimately is an abnormal accumulation of fluid collecting in the alveoli. In normal physiology, the interplay of preload, afterload, and contractility, along with autoregulation of body fluid balance, optimize forward flow and fluid volume. Derangements in those elements can ultimately lead to a presentation on the spectrum of acute heart failure syndromes, generally appearing as fluid overload pulmonary edema, sympathetic crashing pulmonary edema, or cardiogenic shock.

The pulmonary management of this edema is best accomplished with early noninvasive ventilation to reduce physiologic shunt and to reduce work of breathing. Noninvasive ventilation also improves left heart performance by increasing preload and reducing afterload, thereby improving left ventricular output. The opposite effects occur on the right side of the heart, so there should be heightened decision-making for the use of positive pressure as the magnitude of right heart failure increases. Noninvasive ventilation clearly reduces intubation, ICU admission, and death rates in heart failure patients.[56]

Pharmacological management for patients with satisfactory blood pressure is afterload reduction, typically with intravenous nitroglycerin. Doses at or above 1 mcg/kg/min are considered to be effective afterload reducers. There is some suggestion that all patients with heart failure and the absence of hypotension should receive intravenous nitrates.[57] For patients with hypotension and pulmonary edema or those with cardiogenic shock, administration of norepinephrine to support blood pressure at a mean of 65 mmHg is appropriate. Patients with normal blood pressure *or* blood pressure supported to normal may benefit from an inotropic agent. The caution is that milrinone and dobutamine both reduce afterload and can cause hypotension. Low-dose epinephrine is an effective inotrope and a mild vasoconstrictor.[58]

References

1. Kacmarek RM, Stoller JK, Heuer AH. *Egan's Fundamentals of Respiratory Care*. 12th ed. St. Louis, MO: Elsevier; 2021.

2. Des Jardins TR. *Cardiopulmonary Anatomy & Physiology*: Essentials of Respiratory Care. 7th ed. New York: Delmar Cengage Learning; 2019.

3. Des Jardins TD, Burton GG. *Clinical Manifestations and Assessment of Respiratory Disease*. 8th ed. St. Louis, MO: Elsevier; 2020.

4. Hess DR, MacIntyre NR, Mishoe SC, Galvin WF. *Respiratory Care*: Principles and Practice. 4th ed. Burlington, MA: Jones and Bartlett; 2021.

5. Brashers VL, Rote NS, Huether SE, McCance KL, eds. *Pathophysiology*: The Biologic Basis for Disease in Adults and Children. St. Louis, MO: Elsevier; 2019.

6. Betts JG, Young KA, Wise JA, et al. Anatomy and Physiology: The lungs. OpenStax. 2013. Available at: https://openstax.org/books/anatomy-and-physiology/pages/22-2-the-lungs.

7. Hallet S, Toro F, Ashurst JV. Physiology: Tidal Volume. In: StatPearls [Internet]. Treasure Island, FL: StatPearls Publishing; 2022. Available at: https://www.ncbi.nlm.nih.gov/books/NBK482502/.

8. Pittman R. *Regulation of Tissue Oxygenation*. 2nd ed. Kentfield, CA: Morgan & Claypool Life Sciences; 2016.

9. Beachey W. *Respiratory Care Anatomy and Physiology*: Foundations for Clinical Practice. 4th ed. Elsevier; 2017.

10. Collins JA, Rudenski A, Gibson J, Howard L, Driscoll R. Relating oxygen partial pressure, saturation and content: the haemoglobin–oxygen dissociation curve. *Breathe*. 2015;11(3):194–201. doi: 10.1183/20734735.001415

11. Turgeman A, McRae HL, Cahill C, Blumberg N, Refaai MA. Impact of RBC transfusion on peripheral capillary oxygen saturation and partial pressure of arterial oxygen. *Am J Clin Pathol*. 2021; 156(1):149–154. doi: 10.1093/ajcp/aqaa219

12. Thomsen T. Needle thoracostomy: Procedure Videos. Elsevier ClinicalKey for Nursing. 2021. Available at: https://www.clinicalkey.com/nursing/#!/content/medical_procedure/19-s2.0-mp_EM-106.

13. Webster JG, ed. *Design of Pulse Oximeters*. CRC Press; 1997

14. Nitzan M, Romem A, Koppel R. Pulse oximetry: fundamentals and technology update. *Medical Devices*. 2014;7:231–239.

15. Bickler PE, Feiner JR, Severinghaus JW. Effects of skin pigmentation on pulse oximeter accuracy at low saturation. *Anesthesiology*. 2005; 102:715–719. doi: 10.1097/00000542-200504000-00004

16. Ward KR, Yealy DM. End-tidal carbon dioxide monitoring in emergency medicine, Part 1: Basic principles. *Acad Emerg Med*. 1998; 5(6):628–636. Available at: https://onlinelibrary.wiley.com/doi/pdf/10.1111/j.1553-2712.1998.tb02473.x

17. Aminiahidashti H, Shafiee S, Kiasari AZ, Sazgar M. Applications of end-tidal carbon dioxide (ETCO$_2$) monitoring in emergency department: a narrative review. *Emerg (Tehran)*. 2018;6(1):e5.

18. Awasthi S, Rani R, Malviya D. Peripheral venous blood gas analysis: an alternative to arterial blood gas analysis for initial assessment and resuscitation in emergency and intensive care unit patients. *Anesth Essays Res*. 2013;7(3):355–358. doi: 10.4103/0259-1162.123234

19. Digby GC, Kukla P, Zhan Z, et al. The value of electrocardiographic abnormalities in the prognosis of pulmonary embolism: a consensus paper. *Ann Noninvas Electrocardiol*. 2015;201520(3), 207–223. doi: 10.1111/anec.12278

20. Seyyedi SR, Sharif-Kashani B, Sadr M, et al. The relationship between electrocardiographic changes and prognostic factors in severely symptomatic pulmonary hypertension. *Tanaffos*. 2019;18(1): 34–40. Available at: https://www.ncbi.nlm.nih.gov/pmc/articles/PMC6690322/.

21. Warnier MJ, Rutten FH, Numans ME, et al. Electrocardiographic characteristics of patients with chronic obstructive pulmonary disease. *COPD J Chron Obstruct Pulmon Dis*. 2013;10(1):62–71. doi: 10.3109/15412555.2012.727918

22. Rogers J. *McCance & Heuther's Pathophysiology*: The Biologic Basis for Disease in Adults and Children. 9th ed. St. Louis, MO: Elsevier; 2022.

23. Hartjes T. *AACN Core Curriculum for Progressive and Critical Care Nursing*. 8th ed. St. Louis, MO: Elsevier; 2022.

24. Randhawa R, Bellingan G. Acute lung injury. *Anaesth Intens Care Med*. 2007;8(11):477–480. doi: 10.1016/j.mpaic.2007.09.003

25. Rozet I, Domino KB. Respiratory care. *Best Pract Res Clin Anaesthesiol*. 2007;21(4):465–482. doi: 10.1016/j.bpa.2007.07.001

26. Hough A. *Hough's Cardiorespiratory Care*. 5th ed. Elsevier; 2018: 69–131.

27. Cottrell JJ. Altitude exposures during aircraft flight. *Chest*. 1998; 93(1):81–84. doi: 10.1378/chest.93.1.81

28. Clinical Overview: Acute Respiratory Distress Syndrome in Adults. Elsevier Point of Care. 2022. Available at: https://www.clinicalkey.com/nursing/#!/content/clinical_overview/67-s2.0-e2872d2d-78ce-47cc-8fbe-7d1ce9e8b9ea

29. Stacy K. *Critical Care Nursing Diagnosis and Management*. 9th ed. Elsevier; 2022:499–533.

30. Deal EN, Hollands JM, Schramm GE, Micek S. Role of corticosteroids in the management of acute respiratory distress syndrome. *Clin Ther*. 2008;30(5):787–799. doi: 10.1016/j.clinthera.2008.05.012

31. Sweet V & Emergency Nurses Association [ENA]. *Emergency Nursing Core Curriculum*. 7th ed. Elsevier; 2017.

32. Seethala RR, Frakes MA, Cocchi MN, et al. Feasibility and safety of prone position transport for severe hypoxemic respiratory failure due to Coronavirus Disease 2019. *Crit Care Explor*. 2020;2(12):e0293. doi: 10.1097/CCE.0000000000000293

33. Guérin C, Reignier J, Richard JC; PROSEVA Study Group. Prone positioning in severe acute respiratory distress syndrome. *N Engl J Med*. 2013;368(23):2159–2168. doi: 10.1056/NEJMoa1214103

34. Nasrullah A, Virk S, Shah A, et al. Acute respiratory distress syndrome and the use of inhaled pulmonary vasodilators in the COVID-19 era: a narrative review. *Life (Basel)*. 2022;12(11):1766. doi: 10.3390/life12111766

35. Torbic H, Saini A, Harnegie MP, Sadana D, Duggal A. Inhaled prostacyclins for acute respiratory distress syndrome: a systematic review and meta-analysis. *Crit Care Explor*. 2023;5(6):e0931. doi: 10.1097/CCE.0000000000000931

36 Combes A, Peek GJ, Hajage D, et al. ECMO for severe ARDS: systematic review and individual patient data meta-analysis. *Intens Care Med*. 2020;46(11):2048–2057. doi: 10.1007/s00134-020-06248-3

37. Krouse JH, Krouse HJ. Asthma: guidelines-based control and management. *Otolaryngol Clin North Am*. 2008;41(2):397–409. doi: 10.1016/j.otc.2007.11.013

38. World Health Organization (WHO). Fact Sheet: Asthma [Internet]. 2022. Available at: https://www.who.int/news-room/fact-sheets/detail/asthma.

39. Kanellakis NI, Jacinto T, Psallidas I. Targeted therapies for lung cancer: how did the game begin? *Breathe*. 2016;12:177–179. doi: 10.1183/20734735.006316

40. Spahn JD, Covar R. Clinical assessment of asthma progression in children and adults. *J Allerg Clin Immunol*. 2008;121(3):548–557. doi: 10.1016/j.jaci.2008.01.012

41. Prey B, Francis A, Williams J, Krishnadasan B. Evaluation and treatment of massive hemoptysis. *Surg Clin North Am*. 2022;102(3), 465–481. doi: 10.1016/j.suc.2021.11.002

42. Flarity K. Environmental emergencies. *Emergency Nursing Core Curriculum*. 7th ed. Elsevier; 2018.

43. Huang T-W, Lee S-C, Cheng Y-L, et al. Contralateral recurrence of primary spontaneous pneumothorax. *Chest J*. 2007;132(4): 1146–1150. doi: 10.1378/chest.06-2772

44. Thompson BT, Kabrhel C. Overview of acute pulmonary embolism in adults. UpToDate. 2022 [updated Dec 2023]. Available at: https://www.uptodate.com/contents/overview-of-acute-pulmonary-embolism-in-adults.

45. Weinberg AS (2022). Treatment, prognosis, and follow-up of acute pulmonary embolism in adults. UpToDate. 2022 [updated Feb 2024]. Avail-

able at: http://www.uptodate.com/contents/overview-of-the-treatment-prognosis-and-follow-up-of-acute-pulmonary-embolism-in-adults.

46. Belohlávek J, Dytrych V, Linhart A. Pulmonary embolism, part I: Epidemiology, risk factors and risk stratification, pathophysiology, clinical presentation, diagnosis and nonthrombotic pulmonary embolism. *Exp Clin Cardiol.* 2013;18(2):129–138.

47. Frakes MA. Shock. In ASTNA; Wolfe AC, Frakes MA, Nayman D, eds. *Principles and Practice of Transport.* 6th ed. St. Louis, MO: Elsevier; 2024.

48. Thomson D, Kourounis G, Trenear R, et al. ECG in suspected pulmonary embolism. *Postgrad Med J.* 2019;95(1119):12–17. doi: 10.1136/postgradmedj-2018-136178

49. Thompson BT, Kabrhel C. Clinical presentation, evaluation, and diagnosis of the adult with suspected acute pulmonary embolism. UpToDate. 2022 [updated Jan 2024]. Available at: http://www.uptodate.com/contents/clinical-presentation-evaluation-and-diagnosis-of-the-adult-with-suspected-acute-pulmonary-embolism.

50. Wilcox SR, Kabrhel C, Channick RN. Pulmonary hypertension and right ventricular failure in emergency medicine. *Ann Emerg Med.* 2015;66(6):619–628. doi: 10.1016/j.annemergmed.2015.07.525

51. Stewart LK, Kline JA. Fibrinolytics for the treatment of pulmonary embolism. *Transl Res.* 2020;225:82–94. doi: 10.1016/j.trsl.2020.05.003

52. Rubin L, Hopkins W. Clinical features and diagnosis of pulmonary hypertension of unclear etiology in adults. UpToDate. 2022 [updated Aug 2023]. Available at: https://tinyurl.com/5n9x9t24.

53. Simonneau G, Gatzoulis MA, Adatia I, et al. Updated clinical classification of pulmonary hypertension. *J Am Coll Cardiol.* 2013;62:D34–D41.

54. Sherman A, Saggar R, Channick R. Update on medical management of pulmonary arterial hypertension. *Cardiol Clin.* 2022;40(1):13–27. doi: 10.1016/j.ccl.2021.08.002

55. Hoeper MM, Granton J. Intensive care unit management of patients with severe pulmonary hypertension and right heart failure. *Am J Respir Crit Care Med.* 2011;184(10):1114–1124. doi: 10.1164/rccm.201104-0662CI

56. Killeen BM, Wolfson AB. Noninvasive positive pressure ventilation for cardiogenic pulmonary edema. *Acad Emerg Med.* 2020;27(12):1358–1359. doi: 10.1111/acem.13986

57. Alzahri MS, Rohra A, Peacock WF. Nitrates as a treatment of acute heart failure. *Card Fail Rev.* 2016;2(1):51–55. doi: 10.15420/cfr.2016:3:3

58. Jentzer JC, Coons JC, Link CB, Schmidhofer M. Pharmacotherapy update on the use of vasopressors and inotropes in the intensive care unit. *J Cardiovasc Pharmacol Ther.* 2015;20(3):249–260. doi: 10.1177/1074248414559838

11

Abdominal Emergencies

JOSEPH HILL

COMPETENCIES

1. Perform a comprehensive assessment of the patient with an abdominal emergency.
2. Identify and differentiate specific abdominal emergencies during transport.
3. Initiate critical interventions for management of abdominal emergencies during transport.

Introduction

Abdominal emergencies encountered by transport teams may include disorders of the esophagus, stomach, intestinal tract, liver, pancreas, gallbladder, or of the abdominal compartment as a whole. A myriad of conditions can arise amongst the several intra-abdominal organs and tracts, to include obstruction, ulceration, hemorrhage, perforation, infection, functional failure, etc. Often these emergencies require critical care transport clinicians to urgently transport the patient to tertiary centers for surgical or advanced medical treatment.

Transport via helicopter or fixed wing aircraft may exacerbate the condition of patients with an abdominal emergency.[1] The physiological effects of patient transport at altitude, particularly from gas laws affecting compartmental pressures, are especially important to patients with pathology of the gastrointestinal (GI) system, which encompasses 26 feet of liquid-producing and gas-producing viscous matter. Patient history, assessment, and pretransport planning are imperative for safe patient transport via air or ground.[2]

The chapter will take a systems-based approach to abdominal emergencies.

Esophagus

The esophagus is a hollow tube of striated and smooth muscle, stretching to approximately 10 inches long by adulthood. Sandwiched between the trachea (anterior) and spine (posterior), the esophagus closely aligns with the left main stem bronchus, exiting the thoracic cavity at the diaphragmatic hiatus. The esophagus provides the primary functions of peristaltic movement of food, prevention of reflux with lower esophageal sphincter activity, and venting for gastric pressure changes.[2,3]

Arterial blood flow to the esophagus is supplied through branches of the descending thoracic aorta. Venous return is supplied via the superior vena cava, azygos system, and portal vein system.

Neurologic intervention is initiated in the medulla and performed by the vagus nerve. Because the esophagus lies in the thoracic cavity, in normal atmospheric conditions, it maintains a subatmospheric pressure of –5 to –10 mmHg, whereas the stomach, which is in the abdominal cavity, rests at an atmospheric pressure of +5 to +10 mmHg. Acute esophageal pathologies include esophageal obstruction, hemorrhage of esophageal varices, and esophageal rupture. Pediatric considerations include tracheoesophageal fistula, esophageal atresia, and foreign body obstruction/trauma (e.g., a button battery).

Esophageal Obstruction

Three areas in the esophagus are narrow and are more likely sites for obstruction and injury. These areas include the cricoid cartilage, the arch of the aorta, and the point at which the esophagus passes through the diaphragm.[1,3]

Esophageal obstruction is common. Often it can be the causative effect of long-standing gastroesophageal reflux disease (GERD), alcohol abuse, or undiagnosed cancer or tumor growth. Strictures, vascular webs, tumors, diverticula, foreign bodies, achalasia, and lower esophageal rings can all reduce or eliminate the venting property and peristaltic movement of the esophagus for the upper GI system. When air medical transport of a patient with esophageal obstruction is undertaken, gradual, stepwise changes in altitude are of great importance. Esophageal obstruction and an expanding gastrum can pose a serious threat if rapid decompression occurs at 35,000 feet. The venting property needs to be established before flight and depends on whether rotor-wing or fixed-wing transport is to be used.[4] Typically this can be accomplished through the use of an orogastric (OG) or nasogastric (NG) tube that is either left open to air or attached to low wall suction to allow for decompression of the gases.

Assessment

The transport team will need to correlate physical assessment findings with interpretation of radiologic and laboratory data to anticipate any potential problems that may occur during the transport process. The transport team should ascertain the patient's chief symptom and medical history, in particular noting a history of varices, tumor formation, or other history of obstruction. Included in these subjective data should be the patient's clinical course since the incident occurred.

Key physical exam findings include:
- The patient's ability to protect their airway
- The patient's ability to clear secretions by swallowing or active suctioning
- The presence and location of pain
- Recognition of abdominal distension

Radiographic studies of the obstruction should accompany the patient. If an esophagoscopy has been performed, a report should be provided to the transport team, so the diagnosis and predicted complications are better understood and continuity of care is ensured at the receiving facility.

Plan and Intervention

Prior to patient transport, several patient factors should be evaluated by the transport team. Depending on mode of transport, and patient condition, considerations for transport altitude (e.g., transporting at sea level altitude) may need to be made in order to prevent exacerbation of pathology. The transport team should evaluate the patient's ability to maintain their airway. Continuous monitoring of respiratory status is also necessary. Even with aircraft pressurization, adequate gastric venting is extremely important if high altitude will be maintained.

Pre-transport medications are often necessary to include: antiemetics, analgesics, sedation, and/or motion sickness preventatives. Vomiting could potentially pose a risk for further compromise or obstruction so pre-treating prophylactically with agents such as ondansetron for nausea or dimenhydrinate for motion sickness would be encouraged. In an obstruction caused by food, glucagon is also used at times to improve relaxation of the lower esophageal smooth muscle and improve passage. When not contraindicated by potential esophageal varices or alterations in coagulopathy, a gastric tube should be inserted and gastric contents emptied before and during transport. If the gastric tube is connected to suction, its flow and contents should be closely monitored during transport. Caution must be exercised when a patient is placed on suction devices during transport as there is potential that the tube can adhere to the stomach lining and create ulcerations. Intermittent disconnection of suction from the gastric tube allows the pressures to equalize and prevents extreme suction against the gastric wall.

Children with a potential esophageal obstruction may benefit from an accompanying parent or other caregiver to decrease anxiety and prevent crying or other movement that may increase the risk of airway compromise. The transport clinician must be prepared to take control of the airway by rapid sequence induction in case foreign body dislodgement causes airway obstruction or airway-compromising emesis.

Esophageal Varices

The most common cause of *esophageal varices* is hepatic congestion, which is present in as many as 50% of patients with cirrhosis. Torturous, fragile, and dilated esophageal veins can bleed from spontaneous rupture, caused by portal hypertension or physical or chemical trauma. Esophageal varices are usually associated with hepatic dysfunction as related to cirrhosis, renal failure,

coagulopathies, and sepsis.[3,5,6] Varices occur frequently at the distal esophagus and hemorrhoidal plexus, and hemorrhagic shock from an esophageal bleed can occur rapidly. Bleeding occurs in 30%–40% of patients who have esophageal varices.[3] Clinically significant bleeding from varices is defined as requiring two or more units of blood within a 24-hour period, a systolic blood pressure below 100 mmHg, a postural systolic change >20 mmHg, and/or a pulse rate >100 beats per minute.[3,6,7]

Assessment

Sequential history of the patient with esophageal varices helps the transport team anticipate patient needs during transport. Patients with preexisting history of coronary artery disease, congestive heart failure, and hepatic disease have a higher rate of mortality and may require advanced intervention prior to or during transport.[5,7,8] Patients with a history of alcoholism may experience withdrawal, which could put them at risk for seizures.[5]

Patients receiving antiplatelet or anticoagulant medications may require reversal therapies, particularly if transport to tertiary care is delayed. Thorough review of the most recent laboratory data (hematocrit and hemoglobin levels, prothrombin time [PT], partial thromboplastin time [PTT], International Normalized Ratio [INR], and electrolyte profile) will allow the transport team to better anticipate the patient's clinical needs during transport.

Plan and Intervention

The transport team's primary priority is to ensure adequacy of the airway before transport. Additionally, the transport team must consider what supplies are needed should an acute hemorrhagic episode occur during transport. Continuous gastric suction can produce large volumes of secretions, and a system to adequately dispose of secretions during transport needs to be ready.

The transport clinician must maintain watchful care of any esophageal balloon tamponade device, such as the Sengstaken–Blakemore,[8] Linton, or Minnesota tubes.[7] These tubes are like a Foley catheter but with a larger balloon. Once inserted, usually via the oral route versus nasogastric, the balloon is inflated and traction is applied to put pressure on the bleeding vessel and control or stop the bleeding at the site. Although infrequently used, traction-dependent or specialized esophageal tubes can pose a problem for transport. Traction maintained with a football helmet can be used during transport (Fig. 11.1). An alternative option is

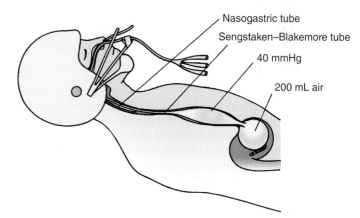

Nasogastric tube

Sengstaken–Blakemore tube

40 mmHg

200 mL air

• **Fig. 11.1** Traction maintained with football helmet for Sengstaken–Blakemore tube. (Modified from Madigan K. Abdominal emergencies. In: ASTNA; Semonin Holleran R, Wolfe, AC, Frakes MA, eds. *Patient Transport: Principles & Practice.* 5th ed. St. Louis, MO: Mosby Elsevier; 2017.)

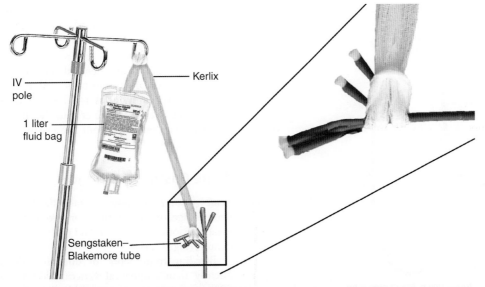

• **Fig. 11.2** Traction using a 1-L bag of intravenous (IV) fluids. (From Bridwell RE, Long B, Ramzy M, et al. Balloon tamponade for the management of gastrointestinal bleeding. *J Emerg Med.* 2022;62(4):545–558. Courtesy of Mark Ramzy, DO.)

to utilize a 1-liter bag of saline as a method of traction but there are risks to any traction method, to include pharyngeal ulcers and mouth ulcers from the localized pressure (Fig. 11.2).[7] With esophageal tubes in place, the transport clinician must anticipate the need for airway management if not addressed prior to insertion (Fig. 11.3).

Airway loss from these particular types of tubes can be from physiologic deterioration or tracheal obstruction. Endotracheal intubation is performed prior to placement of a balloon tamponade device in most situations.[6,9] Pressure changes associated with altitude should be considered by the flight team; saline solution, rather than air, can be used to inflate the balloons in order to prevent expansion during flight.

If an acute hemorrhagic episode occurs, maintenance of airway and circulating volume is the priority.[6] Whole blood and/or blood products (e.g., packed red blood cells and fresh-frozen plasma) may be needed during transport. In patients experiencing acute gastroesophageal bleeding, transfusion should be initiated promptly to maintain hemodynamic stability.[9] Clinician protocols may focus on permissive hypotension strategies because of the deleterious effects of over-resuscitation, such as increased portal vascular pressures and rebleeding.[8,9]

Effective pre-transport planning includes preventing vomiting and aspiration, ensuring adequate venous access, and having airway and transfusion equipment prepared and available. Management of medications such as octreotide, which works by decreasing the inflow of blood to the portal system and constricts the splanchnic arterioles, coagulopathy reversal agents, vasopressin if hypotensive, beta-blockers if hypertensive, and antibiotics should be anticipated during transport. For patients who have undergone angiography, the transport team must secure the cannulization site before any patient movement and monitor the site frequently throughout transport for bleeding and potential for an expanding hematoma.

Esophageal Rupture

Esophageal rupture commonly results from penetrating trauma but may also result from a blunt insult to the thorax. Rupture from invading lesions, tumors, severe vomiting, surgical procedures, or caustic exposure also occurs, but to a lesser extent. If esophageal rupture has occurred, the venting properties and pathways have been altered. During transport, and with possible altitude changes, the distribution and displacement of gases are no longer circumvented by the appropriate course. Complications of gastric pneumonitis, hemopneumothorax, pneumomediastinum, subcutaneous emphysema, shock, leaking of gastric contents into the mediastinum, and alteration in gas exchange may all occur.

Assessment

Evaluation of the causative factors for rupture will inform the transport team's plan of care. Drugs known to have corrosive effects on the esophagus are doxycycline, tetracycline, acetylsalicylic acid, clindamycin, potassium chloride, quinidine, warfarin, and ferrous sulfate. Caustic substances can quickly lead to burning or complete erosion of the tissue. Estimation of the severity of the burn/erosion is extremely difficult and should err on the side of severe. If the rupture is caused by a tumor, hemorrhage and airway control can become quite difficult to manage.

Plan and Intervention

The transport team's priorities are as follows:
- Ascertain adequacy of airway, ventilation, and oxygenation
- Maintain adequate venous access and fluid volume support
- Placement of gastric tube with adequate suctioning, if not contraindicated
- Antibiotics
- Chest thoracostomy if needed

Stomach

The stomach lies beneath the diaphragm and is secured in the peritoneum by the lesser omentum. The stomach is subject to alterations in intra-abdominal pressure (IAP), unlike the esophagus, which maintains a negative pressure. The cardiac sphincter separates the esophagus from the stomach, as the pyloric sphincter separates the stomach from the duodenum and small intestine.

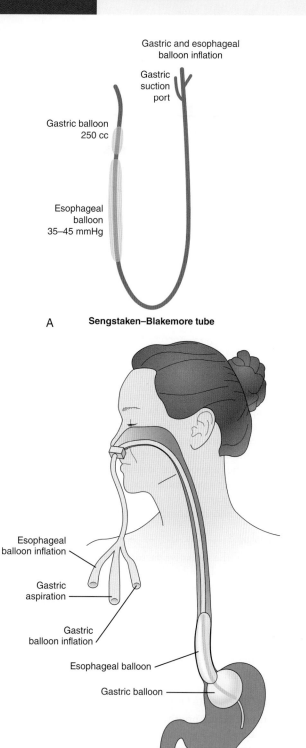

A Sengstaken–Blakemore tube

Gastric and esophageal
balloon inflation

Gastric
suction
port

Gastric balloon
250 cc

Esophageal
balloon
35–45 mmHg

Esophageal
balloon inflation

Gastric
aspiration

Gastric
balloon inflation

Esophageal balloon

Gastric balloon

B

• **Fig. 11.3** Sengstaken–Blakemore tube. **A,** Example. **B,** Placement. The tube is passed to at least the 50-cm mark. The gastric balloon is then inflated with the full recommended volume of air (usually 450–500 mL). A portable chest x-ray should be obtained to check for proper placement. The tube is pulled back gently until resistance is felt against the diaphragm. If bleeding persists from the aspiration port, the esophageal balloon is inflated to the lowest pressure needed to stop bleeding. (A, Modified from Tafoya LA, McGee JC, Kaisler S, et al. Management of acute upper gastrointestinal bleeding in critical care transport. *Air Med J.* 2023;42(2):110–118; B, From Parrillo JE, Dellinger RP. *Critical Care Medicine: Principles of Diagnosis and Management in the Adult.* 5th ed. Philadelphia, PA: Elsevier Saunders; 2019.)

Arterial supply comes from the celiac artery branches, and venous return is through the superior mesenteric, splenic, and portal veins.

The stomach functions as a receptacle of ingested substances and attempts to provide chemical and mechanical breakdown. As the stomach expands, peristaltic action increases. The average time of gastric emptying is 1–8 hours. Chyme is then propelled through the pyloric sphincter into the duodenum. In transport, complications can arise from the expansion and contraction of gases at varying altitudes.

Acute Gastric Occurrences

Acute gastric occurrences can take the form of gastric duodenal hemorrhage, gastric perforation from mechanical or chemical means, pyloric obstruction, and ulceration of the gastrum or duodenum (Fig. 11.4).[3]

Bleeding from peptic or duodenal ulcers occurs more frequently than esophageal variceal bleeding, representing up to 50% of upper gastrointestinal bleeding. Several methods may be used to manage the bleeding, including insertion of gastric tubes, pharmacologic management, endoscopy, and if bleeding is massive and cannot be controlled, surgery. Anticipatory planning and thorough preparation can ensure a safe patient transport.[10,11]

Ulcerative lesions of the stomach or duodenum that lead to bleeding or perforation are in part caused by mucosal membrane erosion. The tissue beneath the mucosa is then subjected to general tissue corrosion. Ulcerations can lead to hemorrhage, perforation, or obstruction and may occur after an attempted repair.

Plan and Intervention

In the event of an acute hemorrhagic episode during transport, transport clinician should perform volume resuscitation, including administration of whole blood, blood products, and medications to manage the bleeding.[4,5,9–11] Complications such as hematemesis, aspiration, and projectile vomiting may arise if the gastric tube becomes obstructed.[11] Gastric dilatation and excessive acid production can cause nausea and vomiting, which may induce hemorrhage. Adequate gastric venting is imperative throughout any altitude changes when the patient is transported via air.

Movement can cause nausea whether via air or ground. The transport team should consider administration of an antiemetic to decrease the risk of vomiting, subsequently decreasing the risk of bleeding and airway compromise during transport. The use of abdominal ultrasound can be key in detecting both initial and ongoing concerns for patients with suspected gastric, intestinal, or vascular disease of the abdomen. The rapid access and portability may also provide input into progression of a diagnosis during transport, particularly in longer transit periods.

Gallbladder and Biliary Tract

The primary function of the gallbladder and biliary tract is to receive approximately 800 mL to 1 liter of bile a day from the liver. Bile, which is stimulated not only by food ingestion but also by stress and acute illness, flows into the duodenum through the common bile duct. This bile—composed of fatty acids, bile salts, phospholipid, cholesterol, conjugated bilirubin, and water—mixes with the chyme to aid digestion. Fluid and electrolyte reabsorption takes place in the gallbladder before the bile enters the duodenum; therefore, with dehydration, an even more concentrated efficacious bile enters the duodenum.

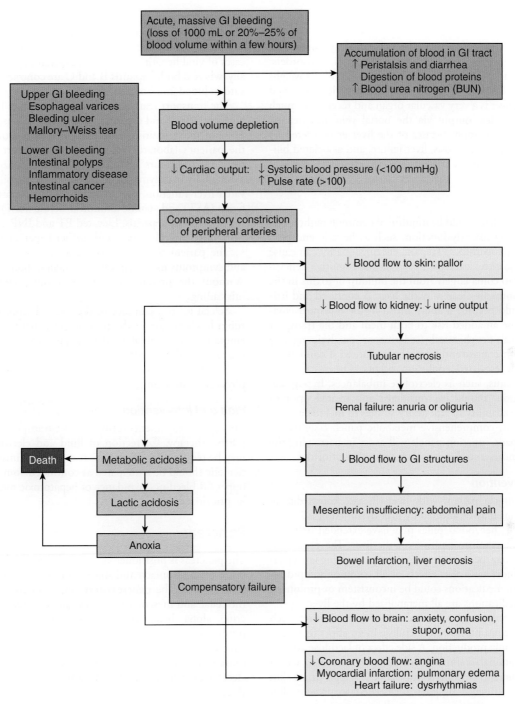

• **Fig. 11.4** Pathophysiology of gastrointestinal bleeding. (From McCance K, Huether S, eds. *The Biologic Basis for Disease in Adults and Children.* 7th ed. St. Louis, MO: Elsevier Mosby; 2014.)

The gallbladder and biliary tracts are stimulated sympathetically by the splanchnic nerve and parasympathetically by the vagus. Vascular supply is provided by the hepatic artery and cystic vein.

The ampulla of Vater and sphincter of Oddi are common sites of disease or injury that dramatically affect the entire tract. Although gallbladder and biliary disorders that necessitate acute medical transport are infrequent, necrotic gangrenous cholecystitis leads to septicemia, acute pancreatitis, gallbladder rupture, and/or hepatic failure because of obstruction of bile flow and production.

Plan and Intervention

Transport of patients with gallbladder and biliary tract disorders includes pre-transport assessment and determination of adequate drainage of gastric and/or cholecystostomy tubes. Careful observation during transport is required for prevention of flow obstruction. Respiratory effort and oxygen saturation should be monitored during transport. Timely, appropriate antibiotic coverage should be evaluated, as well as review of analgesic requirements for the patient.

Liver

The liver is responsible for a number of varied synthetic and metabolic functions, thus may be affected by myriad disorders, diseases, trauma, medications, and toxins.[12] An adult liver weighs approximately 3 lbs. and is supplied by the hepatic artery and portal vein. The liver is a very vascular organ and receives as much as 30% of the cardiac output via the portal vein and hepatic artery.[12] The most common diseases of the liver encountered by transport personnel are cirrhosis, liver failure, and associated biliary atresia; also common are patients who are candidates for liver transplantation.

Assessment

The transport clinician should be mindful of common pathologies that present during liver dysfunction, such as hepatic encephalopathy and coagulopathies.[13] Hepatic encephalopathy can cause confusion, somnolence, asterixis, hyperreflexia, cognitive deficits, and progression to coma largely from the buildup of toxins in the blood that are normally cleared by the liver. A confused and irritable patient could become a safety threat in the transport environment and pose an added risk to both them and the transport team. Mechanical or chemical (sedative or paralytic agents) restraints, or both concurrently, may be warranted if combativeness behavior or escalated confusion occurs. Other causes of altered mental status, such as electrolyte imbalances, hypoglycemia, and ingestion, should be considered and treated prior to transport. The availability of laboratory studies to include a complete blood count, comprehensive metabolic panel, coagulation studies, and hepatic function panels will assist in narrowing the differential diagnoses and direct patient treatment priorities.

Plan and Intervention

When transporting a patient with liver disease, knowledge of which medications may be affected by liver dysfunction is important. For example, benzodiazepines may have extended half-lives because of the metabolism pathway of the liver. The prolonged sedative effects may be misinterpreted as progressing encephalopathy. Also, understand that effects of all commonly rapid sequence induction medications could be inconsistent or prolonged because these medications are all metabolized by the liver.

Hepatic encephalopathy is often treated with medications such as aminoglycoside antibiotics and lactulose in an effort to reduce and absorb ammonia production. A side effect of lactulose administration is abdominal cramping and excessive diarrhea, which may result in fluid and electrolyte imbalances.[11] Appropriate skin barriers and incontinence supplies are needed to prevent skin breakdown from the rectal output as well as to prevent possible contamination of equipment.[9]

Hepatitis

The transport team is very likely to encounter patients with hepatitis and must use appropriate personal protection equipment to protect themselves from disease transmission. Hepatitis is most often caused by viral infection, though it may also be induced as a side effect of medications, heavy alcohol use, sexual contact, or sharing of needles for drug injection. The liver is responsible for much of the body's clotting process so an alteration can affect the body's ability to produce clotting and inhibitor factors. Fresh-frozen plasma, vitamin K, or factor VIIa may be considered to correct this hemorrhagic risk.

Assessment

The most common strains of viral hepatitis include types A, B, C, and delta viruses. These strains are responsible for the most severe cases of viral hepatitis. Hepatitis A is transmitted primarily enterally, whereas both hepatitis B and C are contracted through exposure to blood and body fluids.

The transport team should elicit a thorough history related to both prescribed and recreational drug use because this may be the cause of the hepatitis.[13] The transport team should also evaluate the patient's laboratory data prior to transport, with particular focus on indicators of infections, anemia, coagulopathies, and elevated liver enzymes and bilirubin. Hyperbilirubinemia, elevated liver function tests including serum aspartate aminotransferase (AST) and alanine aminotransferase (ALT) are indicative of the presence of hepatitis. Elevated PT and INR are indicative of a worsening clinical picture and further hepatic failure.

The patient with hepatitis generally describes flu-like signs and symptoms including general malaise, body aches, and fever. Without the presence of jaundice, the presentation may be misleading.

Scleral icterus, jaundice of the sclera, becomes present as bilirubin levels elevate in the presence of hepatitis. On physical examination, abdominal tenderness, palpated hepatomegaly, and increased body temperature are common findings. As bilirubin levels continue to rise, cutaneous jaundice may be appreciated on physical examination.

Plan and Intervention

Anticipated treatment during patient transport is aimed at supportive therapy. Correction of fluid and electrolyte imbalances may be required by the transport team. Administration of an antiemetic should be anticipated as continued vomiting may induce upper GI bleeding. Avoidance of hepatotoxic medications should be prioritized.

Pancreas[3]

The pancreas is positioned horizontally across the abdomen, posterior to the stomach and spleen, and is located in the retroperitoneal space. The pancreas receives its vascular supply through the celiac and mesenteric arteries. The pancreas consists of endocrine, alpha, beta, and delta cells, and is responsible for the production of insulin and glucagon. Pancreatic disorders include pancreatitis, hemorrhagic pancreatitis, cancer, and damage caused by trauma. Devastation of this organ can lead to fluid and electrolyte imbalance, hemodynamic instability, and severe pain (Fig. 11.5).[4]

Assessment

A history of alcohol abuse and dependence is a significant risk factor and one of the primary causes of pancreatitis. Often these patients can have symptoms of alcohol withdrawal which can include confusion, tremors, anxiety, and agitation with severe symptoms including delirium and seizures. Evaluation of fluid and electrolyte status may help the transport team identify additional treatment needs. A gastric tube should be placed before transport. If the patient has already undergone surgery and drains have been placed, the transport team must ensure proper venting of tubes, collection bulbs are emptied and draining, and surgical dressings are intact.

Patients presenting with both acute and chronic pancreatitis often describe constant, severe abdominal pain localized to the epigastrium

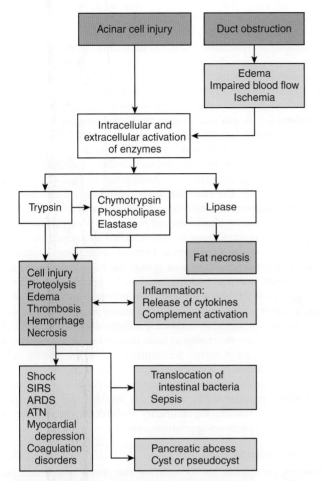

• **Fig. 11.5** Pathophysiology of acute pancreatitis. (From McCance K, Huether S, eds. *The Biologic Basis for Disease in Adults and Children*. 7th ed. St. Louis, MO: Elsevier Mosby; 2014.)

Intestines

The small intestine (duodenum, jejunum, and ileum) is approximately 23 feet long. The primary functions of the intestines are absorption and digestion. The large intestine is composed of the cecum, ascending colon, transverse colon, descending colon, and sigmoid colon. This extensive, enclosed, and gas-producing system can pose many difficulties for transport of a patient who has intestinal pathology.

The intestinal problems most frequently encountered in adults by transport teams are obstructions, ruptures, ruptured diverticula, acute appendicitis, ischemic bowel, intestinal hemorrhage, and mesenteric infarct.[1,14] Many of these patients develop sepsis and septic shock. Bowel necrosis, where part of the bowel becomes ischemic, can also occur, and is often linked to undiagnosed or untreated colon cancer. Intussusception (Fig. 11.6) is one of the most common childhood intestinal surgical emergencies. It occurs when a part of the bowel telescopes into itself. This telescoping not only prevents food and fluids from passing through, but it also cuts off blood flow to the intestinal section.[15] Occurrence in an adult is rare. Malrotation and volvulus are also common pediatric intestinal pathology, where the intestine does not make its appropriate turn (malrotation) and becomes twisted and subsequently obstructed (volvulus). A volvulus also threatens the blood flow to the intestinal section until surgically corrected. Pyloric stenosis occurs in 3 in 1000 births and occurs when there is hypertrophy of the pyloric muscle causing a narrowing of the pyloric sphincter.[15]

Assessment

Many bowel diseases, in particular an obstruction, are slow developing so a more thorough history may be helpful in a patient

or left upper quadrant.[9] The pain is often described as positional, with recumbent positions causing an increase in symptoms.

Elevated vital signs may be indicative of hypovolemia in the patient with pancreatitis but may be confounded by pain. Patients may sequester as much as 6 liters of fluid in their retroperitoneum due to leaky capillary syndrome and vasodilatation.

Evaluation of the patient's laboratory tests for elevated levels of amylase and lipase, along with visualization via computerized tomography, can be helpful in determining the presence of pancreatitis. The white blood cell count, hemoglobin, metabolic panels, and arterial blood gases allow the transport clinician to ascertain clinical severity.[9] Hypocalcemia may also present with cardiac dysfunction and compromise.[9]

Plan and Intervention

Because of the potential for multiorgan involvement, priorities for the patient with pancreatitis include oxygenation, restoration of hemodynamic stability, correction of fluid and electrolyte imbalance, as well as antibiotic administration. Pain management is a challenge for these patients and analgesia should be provided by the transport team before and during transport. It is also important to note that many medications can exacerbate pancreatitis. Additionally, pancreatitis can affect the mechanisms by which medications are absorbed, delaying onset and altering the medication's effect.

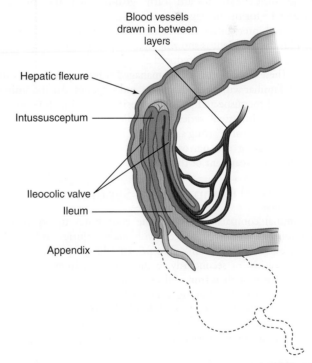

• **Fig. 11.6** Ileocolic intussusception. Dotted outline indicates normal anatomy. (From Djuric CM. Alterations of digestive function in children. In: Rogers JL, ed. *McCance & Huether's Pathophysiology: The Biologic Basis for Disease in Adults and Children*, 9th ed. Elsevier; 2024. Figure 42.6.)

without a definitive diagnosis. A physical examination by the transport clinician should assess for abdominal distension, hyperactive high-pitched bowel sounds, and rectal blood. Also, the transport team should assess the patient for signs and symptoms of peritonitis or sepsis such as fever, nausea and vomiting, tachycardia, and tachypnea.

An infant or toddler with intussusception may present with difficulty feeding, intermittent but severe abdominal pain, inconsolable crying, and typically positioned with the legs drawn upwards toward the abdomen.[15] The abdominal assessment may reveal a sausage-like mass and/or stool with a currant jelly consistency from a mixture of blood, stool, and intestinal mucous. Presentation of children with volvulus is similar to that of intussusception, with abdominal pain, difficulty feeding, vomiting, inconsolable crying, abdominal distension, and bloody stools. Both conditions may present rapidly or insidiously, with vague and gradual symptoms. Pyloric stenosis is typically characterized by increased appetite, weight loss, constipation, and projectile vomiting. There is also often an "olive" mass that may be palpated in the epigastrium to the right of the midline and reverse peristalsis visualized across the abdomen.[15]

Plan and Intervention

The transport team should evaluate venous access and volume needs before transport. The patient in shock may require fluid resuscitation and vasopressors to support hemodynamics. Consideration must be given to aircraft altitude and pressurization to reduce intestinal gas expansion. Gastric tube patency should be assured and continuous gastric tube suctioning provided throughout transport. Of note, some patients may produce an excessive amount of gastric content with prolonged suctioning, so additional suction cannisters may be needed on long-distance transports. Patients with stomas need adequate collection-bag capacity and venting.

If the patient has sepsis or septic shock, the transport team should direct care toward early goal-directed therapy. See Chapter 13 for the management of sepsis.

Surgical intervention may be required for intussusception and volvulus if the patient is showing signs of perforation, bowel ischemia, or is unable to be reduced though nonoperative management. These conditions are best managed at tertiary pediatric care centers familiar with these diagnoses and surgeries. An abdominal ultrasound for suspected pyloric stenosis is often first line but an upper gastrointestinal series with radiopaque material such as barium will reveal a "string sign" which is a fine, elongated pyloric canal indicating the narrowed area.[14] Surgical intervention is indicated for treatment of this finding.

Abdominal Compartment Syndrome

Abdominal compartment syndrome contributes to organ dysfunction and occurs in concert with many injuries and disease processes.[2,16] It may be linked to primary disease processes, such as pancreatitis, or secondarily to the treatment interventions of other diseases, such as from diffuse swelling related to fluid resuscitation and capillary leaking. Increased intra-abdominal pressure results in hypoperfusion of the abdominal organs, increased intrathoracic pressure causing respiratory compromise, and, ultimately, multisystem dysfunction.

Assessment

Patients at risk for abdominal compartment syndrome include those with both traumatic and medical pathologies. Abdominal surgical patients, and those suffering major trauma or thermal burns, are at risk because of aggressive fluid resuscitation, along with leaky capillary syndrome. Medical diagnoses with abdominal compartment syndrome include, but are not limited to, pancreatitis, sepsis, liver dysfunction and cirrhosis, ascites, and intra-abdominal and retroperitoneal tumors. Ascites can represent up to 10 liters of fluid present in the abdominal cavity which can easily compromise other organ systems and create difficulty breathing for the patient. In cases of spontaneous bacterial peritonitis, an acute infection of ascites, the patient may likely present with a fever, chills, abdominal pain, and/or nausea and vomiting.

The patient with an open abdomen following damage control surgery is not precluded from developing abdominal compartment syndrome. The transport team should always consider abdominal compartment syndrome in patients exhibiting early signs of shock, including altered mental status and poor perfusion. An expanding abdomen, along with diminished abdominal wall compliance, are the most common signs of developing abdominal compartment syndrome. Other symptoms include decreased urinary output, hypoxia, and hypercarbia.[14,17] Increased pressure in other parts of the body, including an increased intracranial pressure without a head injury and an increased peak airway pressure without the presence of a thoracic injury, may occur. With all gas-filled cavities, the transport team must take into consideration altitude changes. Gastric decompression with a gastric tube should be completed before transport.

Abdominal compartment syndrome is present when intra-abdominal pressure (IAP) exceeds 20 mmHg. IAP is routinely measured via transducing a urinary catheter in the bladder, in which normal pressures approximate the central venous pressure.[17]

Plan and Intervention

Nonsurgical approaches to reducing the effects of IAP include gastric decompression, sedation, and chemical paralysis. Sedation and chemical paralysis allow for reduction in ventilator asynchrony and a subsequent decrease in intrathoracic pressure. Conservative intravenous fluid use is imperative because volume boluses and aggressive resuscitation can worsen fluid third-spacing and IAP. Avoid placing items on top of the abdomen to prevent increases in pressure.

Abdominal Aortic Emergencies

Patients with acute abdominal aortic pathologies, such as abdominal aortic aneurysms (AAAs), generally require transport to tertiary, specialized care.[8] An AAA is recognized as a bulging or outpouching of the wall of the aorta (Fig. 11.7). Risk factors for AAAs include increasing age, hypertension, hyperlipidemia, family history of abdominal aortic aneurysm, and smoking. New data suggest that one-half of all AAAs occur in woman under 65 years of age and nonsmokers.[12] Once the AAA has ruptured or dissected, operative intervention is emergently indicated. Ruptured abdominal aortic aneurysms (RAAAs) are almost uniformly fatal, though there is data suggesting that hospitals which perform high volumes of RAAA repairs can yield improved mortality results.[17,18]

Assessment

Most patients with AAA or RAAA come from a referral center and have been diagnosed in the emergency department. These patients may present with a range of symptoms, from insidious abdominal pressure to hemodynamic instability and peritoneal signs. The size of the AAA and whether the aneurysm has ruptured often contribute to the manifestation of symptoms. The transport team should

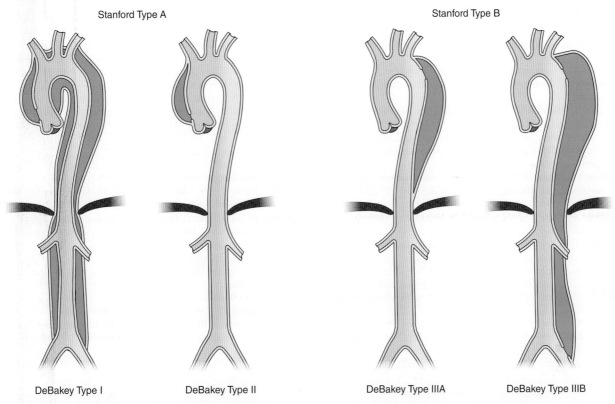

• **Fig. 11.7** DeBakey and Stanford classification of aortic dissection. (Modified from Conrad MF, Cambria RP. Aortic dissections. In: Cronenwett JL, Johnston KW, eds. *Rutherford's Vascular Surgery*, 8th ed. Philadelphia: Elsevier; 2014:2169–2188.)

Stanford Type A

Stanford Type B

DeBakey Type I

DeBakey Type II

DeBakey Type IIIA

DeBakey Type IIIB

focus on critical problems such as hypoxia, hypotension, and bleeding, as well as expediting transport to the receiving surgical center. The traditional physical sign of a palpable, pulsatile abdominal mass is not always identified, as affected by the size of the aneurysm and body habitus. Femoral and pedal pulses may or may not be present, due to the extent of the aneurysm's effect on arterial vasculature.

Plan and Intervention

Rapid transport to an appropriate surgical facility is one of the most important interventions that can be provided by the team.[17] Decreased time to surgical intervention has shown to improve mortality rates.[17] The transport should not be delayed for diagnostic or laboratory data, and a coordinated effort to decrease time to surgical intervention should be the goal. Whole blood or blood products are needed in the event a rupture occurs and the patient develops hemorrhagic shock. The transport team must also be prepared for cardiac arrest during transport. In most cases,

once cardiac arrest has occurred the effort can be futile due to the excessive loss of blood and expansion of the aneurysm preventing occlusion via natural clotting. Because of the high mortality rate associated with RAAA, consider allowing the family to see the patient before transfer or possibly accompany the patient, provided clinical situation and organizational policies allow.

Fluid resuscitation should be administered with caution. Over-resuscitation can lead to increased bleeding from clot dislodgement and dilutional coagulopathy. Maintenance of a relatively low systolic blood pressure of 70–80 mmHg (permissive hypotension[19]) may prevent further tearing of the aorta and limit blood loss and has demonstrated a lower 30-day mortality.[18] Though largely studied in trauma, this practice can be controversial but tends to demonstrate lower death rates amongst that patient population along with a decreased use of blood products utilization, less hemodilution, ischemia, and hypoxia in tissues.[19]

Summary

The clinical team should anticipate the typical clinical course, as well as potential complications, during transport of the patient with an abdominal emergency. Thoughtful planning is necessary, particularly when transporting via air, to prevent physiologic effects of the transport from negatively affecting the patient's condition. Expansion of internal gases with altitude changes is present throughout the GI system; proper venting mechanisms should be placed before flight, and backup devices should be available on the aircraft. The symptoms of many abdominal emergencies are similar and vague until further diagnostics allows for a definitive source

diagnosis. Often treatments such as pain management, nausea relief, antibiotic therapy, and gastric decompression through the use of an OG/NG tube will be standard care for many of these maladies. In more severe cases, correction of hemodynamics with either vasoactive medications or a combination of crystalloid and colloid use may be warranted and necessary.

Clinical changes during transport can be difficult to predict, however, the transport clinician should plan for likely deteriorations and prepare the appropriate equipment and treatment options to be deployed quickly if needed in transport.

References

1. Emergency Nurses Association. *Emergency Nursing Core Curriculum.* 7th ed. ENA: Des Plaines, IL; 2017.

2. Halliwell K. *Transport Professional Advanced Trauma Course: Study Guide.* 7th ed. Aurora, CO: Air & Surface Transport Nurses Association; 2018.

3. McCance K, Huether SE. *The Biologic Basis for Disease in Adults and Children.* 8th ed. St. Louis, MO: Elsevier/Mosby; 2019.

4. Clark DY, Stocking JC, Johnson J, Treadwell D, Corbett P. *Critical Care Transport Core Curriculum.* 2nd ed. Aurora, CO: Air & Surface Transport Nurses Association; 2017.

5. Villanueva C, Escorsell A. Optimizing general management of acute variceal bleeding in cirrhosis. *Curr Hepatol Rep.* 2014;13(3):198–207.

6. Sanyal AJ. Overview of the management of patients with variceal bleeding. *UpToDate.* 2022, May 11. Available at: http://tinyurl.com/4ay5dt65.

7. Murphy EP, O'Brien SM, Regan M. Alternative method of tractioning the Sengstaken–Blakemore tube. *BMJ Case Rep.* 2017 Mar 20:2017:bcr2016218401. doi: 10.1136/bcr-2016-218401

8. Treger R. Sengstaken–Blakemore tube placement. *Medscape.* 2015. Available at: http://emedicine.medscape.com/article/81020-overview#a6.

9. Wolfson A (ed. in chief). *Harwood-Nuss' Clinical Practice of Emergency Medicine.* 6th ed. Philadelphia, PA: Wolters Kluwer; 2020.

10. Barnet J, Messmann H. Management of lower gastrointestinal tract bleeding. *Best Pract Res Clin Gastroenterol.* 2008;22(2):295–312.

11. Marx J, Hockberger R, Walls R, eds. *Rosen's Emergency Medicine.* 10th ed. Philadelphia, PA: Elsevier Saunders: 2022.

12. Knechtle SJ, Galloway JR. Portal hypertensive bleeding: the place of portosystemic shunting. In: Jarnagin WR, ed. *Blumgart's Surgery of the Liver, Biliary Tract and Pancreas,* 2 vols. 6th ed. Elsevier, 2017, pp. 1218–1230.e3.

13. Ferenci P. Hepatic encephalopathy in adults: treatment. *UpToDate.* 2022, Apr 5. Available at: http://tinyurl.com/4b8jw65e.

14. Parillo J, Dellinger RP, eds. *Critical Care Medicine: Principles of Diagnosis and Management in the Adult.* 5th ed. Philadelphia, PA: Elsevier Saunders; 2018.

15. Garzon Maaks DL, ed. *Burns' Pediatric Primary Care,* 7th ed. Philadelphia: Elsevier Health Sciences; 2020.

16. De Waele J, De Laet I, Malbrain M. Understanding abdominal compartment syndrome. *Intens Care Med.* 2015;42(6):1068–1070.

17. Barros A, Haffner F, Duchateau F, et al. Air travel of patients with abdominal aortic aneurysm: urgent evacuation and nonurgent commercial air repatriation. *Air Med J.* 2014;33:109–111.

18. Powell JT, Hinchliffe RJ. Observations from the IMPROVE trial concerning the clinical care of patients with ruptured abdominal aortic aneurysm. *J Vasc Surg.* 2014;59(5):1471. doi: 10.1016/j.jvs.2014.03.265

19. Hamilton H, Constantinou J, Ivancev K. The role of permissive hypotension in the management of ruptured abdominal aortic aneurysms. *J Cardiovasc Surg (Torino).* 2014;55(2):151–159.

12

Metabolic, Endocrine, and Electrolyte Disturbances

CHARLES F. SWEARINGEN

COMPETENCIES

1. Perform a comprehensive assessment of the patient, including past medical and current illness history, detailed physical examination, and laboratory and pertinent radiographic data.
2. Identify key clinical points related to metabolic, endocrine, and electrolyte disturbances that may arise during transport.
3. Describe appropriate interventions, and treatment considerations, for patients with specific metabolic/endocrine imbalances and select electrolyte disorders.

Introduction

Metabolic, endocrine, and electrolyte disturbances are commonly encountered in the transport environment as both standalone conditions and part of a set of conditions in complex cases. Recognition of abnormalities and potential adverse effects is essential for proper diagnosis and effective treatment, as well as prevention of complications. Because of the variety of hormones, electrolytes, and their effects, these emergencies can affect all body systems. Whether one of these abnormalities is the primary reason for the patient's illness or a secondary concern, the transport team should be vigilant in the identification of precipitating events and detection of potential complications. As is the hallmark of quality patient care delivery by the transport team, thorough and frequent reassessment is vital to the survival of these patients.

Endocrine System Physiology

The endocrine system is composed of a collection of glands: the hypothalamus, pituitary, parathyroid, thyroid, adrenals, pancreas, ovaries, and testes. Each of these glands produces hormones that trigger distinct functions, which guide and interact with other physiological functions.[1,2]

Hormone levels that are too high or too low suggest a problem, or multiple problems, with the endocrine system. In an optimally functioning endocrine system, when circulating hormones are at a high level, additional hormone release is not stimulated. Conversely, when circulating hormone levels are low, hormone release is stimulated. This process is often referred to as a feedback loop. Hormone diseases also occur if supporting systems in the body do not respond to hormones in the appropriate ways, such as in type 2 diabetes mellitus. Stress, infection, renal and liver function, and changes in the blood's fluid and electrolyte balance may also influence hormone levels.

Hypothalamus

The hypothalamus is the physiologic centerpiece of the endocrine system. It consolidates information from the autonomic nervous system, environment, cerebrum, and serum hormone levels in the vascular system; and, in turn, directs the pituitary to increase or reduce hormone production. The hormones released by the pituitary travel peripherally to evoke change in most glands of the endocrine system. The physiologic relationship between the hypothalamus and the pituitary is strong enough to term it the hypothalamic-pituitary axis.[1] This axis directly effects functions of the thyroid gland, the gonads, the adrenal glands, and also influences fluid regulation, milk production, and growth. Additionally, the hypothalamus is involved in several non-endocrine functions, such as appetite control, the autonomic nervous system, and temperature regulation.

Pituitary

The pea-sized pituitary gland (Fig. 12.1) is located at the base of the brain, within the sella turcica of the middle cranial fossa. It produces many hormones itself, as well as stimulates other organs to produce hormones. The anterior portion of the pituitary gland produces the following hormones: prolactin, growth hormone, adrenocorticotropin, thyroid-stimulating hormone (TSH), luteinizing hormone, and follicle-stimulating hormone. The posterior portion of the pituitary gland stores and secretes antidiuretic hormone (ADH) and oxytocin (Table 12.1).[1]

Thyroid

The thyroid, a butterfly-shaped gland, sits in the anterior neck below the cricoid cartilage. It partially surrounds the trachea and consists of two lobes connected together in the middle by an

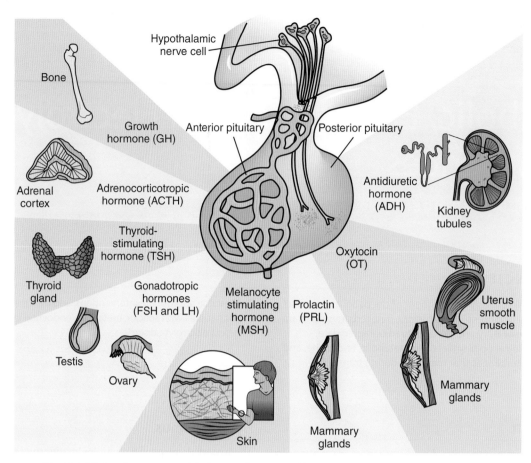

• **Fig. 12.1** Pituitary hormones and their target hormones. (From Patton KT, Thibodeau GA. *Anatomy & Physiology*. 8th ed. St. Louis, MO: Mosby; 2013.)

TABLE 12.1	Pituitary Hormone Functionality
Hormone	**Function**
Anterior Pituitary	
Prolactin	Stimulates milk production and breast development in women; no normal function in men.
Growth hormone (GH)	Stimulates cell growth, reproduction, and regeneration. It increases glucose concentration.
Adrenocorticotropin	Increases the production and release of cortisol, which increases serum glucose, enhances brain uptake of glucose, potentiates vasoconstriction, and increases the availability of substances used to repair tissues
Thyroid-stimulating hormone (TSH)	Stimulates the production of thyroxine (T4) and triiodothyronine (T3), both increase growth and development, metabolism, body temperature, and heart rate.
Luteinizing hormone (LH)	In females, it stimulates ovulation. In males, it stimulates testosterone production
Follicle-stimulating hormone (FSH)	In females, it regulates the development, growth, pubertal maturation, and reproductive processes.
Posterior Pituitary	
Antidiuretic hormone (ADH)	Stimulates water reabsorption in the kidneys to concentrate the urine and control water loss.
Oxytocin	Stimulates uterus to contract and lactation

TABLE 12.2	Thyroid Hormone Ranges
Lab	Normal Range
T3	2.1–4.2 pg/mL
T4	0.8–2.0 pg/mL
TSH	0.1–4.5 μIU/mL

IU, International units; *T3*, triiodothyronine; *T4*, thyroxine; *TSH*, thyroid-stimulating hormone.

isthmus. The thyroid cells secrete thyroxine (T4) and triiodothyronine (T3) when stimulated by TSH via the pituitary. These two hormones increase growth and development, metabolism, body temperature, and heart rate. The parafollicular cells in the thyroid produce calcitonin, which inhibits calcium secretion (Table 12.2).

Parathyroid

On the posterior side of the thyroid gland are four small glands known as the parathyroid. These glands produce parathyroid hormone (PTH), which works to balance calcium levels in the body, allowing the muscular and nervous systems to function effectively. Calcium-sensing receptors release PTH when serum calcium levels decrease below unsafe levels. PTH causes osteoclasts to release calcium, increasing blood calcium levels. PTH also facilitates calcium reabsorption by the kidneys.

Adrenals

The adrenal gland, located above the kidneys in the retroperitoneal area, consists of two layers, an outer cortical layer and an inner medullary layer. Mineralocorticoids (e.g., aldosterone), glucocorticoids (e.g., cortisol), and androgens are produced by the adrenal cortex. Glucocorticoids allow the body to resist stress, and aldosterone helps to maintain internal fluid balance by regulating sodium and potassium. The catecholamines, epinephrine and norepinephrine, are released from the adrenal medulla in response to sympathetic stimulation.

Pancreas

The pancreas lies in the left upper abdomen behind the stomach and between the spleen and duodenum. It functions as both an exocrine and endocrine gland. As an exocrine gland (99%), it produces enzymes and bicarbonate via the pancreatic duct that promote digestion. As an endocrine gland (1%), the pancreas secretes hormones (insulin, glucagon, somatostatin, and pancreatic peptide) directly into the bloodstream, carried to different cells, aiding in glucose balance and metabolism.

Endocrine and Metabolic Emergencies

There is a wide variety of endocrine and metabolic disorders that could potentially present in the transport environment. As a result of ongoing treatments, patients suffering metabolic, endocrine, or electrolyte abnormalities can be some of the most likely to experience a change in clinical status during transport. The importance of continuous monitoring and careful reassessment cannot be overstated. This section focuses on some of the most frequent endocrine and metabolic emergencies encountered in the transport environment.

Hypoglycemia

Hypoglycemia typically occurs when an adult's blood glucose falls <50 mg/dL. The incidence is increased in diabetic patients who utilize insulin, but can vary based on the patient's historic glucose levels. The level of hypoglycemia and the recommended medical treatments depend on the patient's age, a description of their symptoms, and the testing technique. A patient may experience symptoms if their blood glucose level lowers too quickly. The first effects of hypoglycemia are predominantly neurologic, as glucose is the brain's main energy source. Because it is unable to generate glucose on its own or retain it for more than a few minutes, the brain requires a constant supply of glucose from the circulatory system. Any patient exhibiting a change in neurological status or who is not responding should have their glucose assessed.[3]

Hypoglycemia may be an iatrogenic disorder, but can also be brought on by adrenal insufficiencies, sepsis, pancreatic tumors, and congenital metabolic abnormalities. Hypoglycemia can also be precipitated by sulfonylureas, as well as other antiglycemic agents, when used with insulin or in combination. Other factors include pregnancy, alcohol use, nonsteroidal anti-inflammatory drug use, phenytoin, high levels of thyroid hormones, and beta-blockers. Other factors include increased physical stress, liver disease, poor diet, changes in dosages of insulin or other medications, and lack of carbohydrate intake.

Many diabetes patients can identify the signs of hypoglycemia and mitigate the issue on their own. Stimulation of the sympathetic nervous system, such as anxiety, diaphoresis, dry mouth, shakiness, pallor, palpitations, dilated pupils, and hunger, are some of the symptoms of hypoglycemia. However, some individuals might not experience the onset of hypoglycemia as a result of their sympathetic response being suppressed, primarily by beta-blocking agents, although alpha-blocking medications can also minutely contribute to the suppression of this sympathetic response.

When the brain is not receiving enough glucose, symptoms may include irritation, disorientation, difficulty speaking, headaches, ataxia, paresthesias, inappropriate mentation, and stupor. Without treatment, neuroglycopenia can result in seizures, coma, or even death. These symptoms may make it challenging for a patient to seek medical attention.[1]

The use of dextrose-containing intravenous (IV) fluids, or orally administered glucose solutions can be used to establish and maintain fluid and electrolyte balance, as part of evidence-based medical transport protocols. In patients with sufficient hepatic reserves (e.g., nonalcoholic, nonfasting), glucagon may be considered. For patients who misuse sulfonylureas or are at risk for refractory hypoglycemia, octreotide may be indicated.[3] With the appropriate therapy, symptoms should resolve quickly.

Hyperglycemia

Hyperglycemia, or an elevated blood sugar, may be precipitated by multiple factors. These may include physiological stressors such as ischemia or infections, such as urinary tract infections, pneumonia, and skin infections. Medications such as atypical antipsychotics and corticosteroids may also cause hyperglycemia. Abuse of alcohol and cocaine also have the potential to cause hyperglycemia. The most life-threatening causes of hyperglycemia are diabetic ketoacidosis (DKA) and hyperosmolar hyperglycemic state (HHS).[4,5]

Diabetic Ketoacidosis (DKA)[5-7]

DKA is a condition characterized by the presence of ketones and acidosis, and often hyperglycemia. The condition is most often associated with type 1 diabetes mellitus, where insufficient insulin production exists, leading to high blood sugar in the vasculature and a deficiency of glucose within the cells. The body responds by utilizing auxiliary energy production sources by breaking down fats, but proteins may also be broken down. This form of metabolism results in a production of ketones as well as other byproduct acids, giving rise to the condition's namesake. Once the DKA diagnosis is made, it often prompts an initial diagnosis of diabetes. DKA can be initiated by stress, substance abuse, illness, infection, ischemia, or pregnancy in previously undiagnosed patients, as well as failure to maintain a proper insulin regimen in previously diagnosed diabetic patients.

Four acute problems can result from prolonged insulin deficiency: hyperglycemia, dehydration, electrolyte depletion, and metabolic acidosis. Severe hyperglycemia, which occurs from a lack of insulin production, leads to a build-up of serum glucose, which increases osmolality.[8] Hyperosmolarity promotes further insulin resistance, causing increased serum glucose concentrations as well as an increase in osmotic diuresis. This further causes urinary losses of water, sodium, potassium, magnesium, calcium, and phosphorus. Dehydration is brought about by this osmotic diuresis, and results in further increases in osmolality. Next, profound volume depletion can occur; an adult patient typically loses 6 liters of body water. Dramatic changes in body water can lead to electrolyte disorders which will be discussed later in this chapter. The ketones and acids derived by this form of metabolism encourage a pathologic direction towards metabolic acidosis, as energy is derived from fats and muscle proteins causing ketoacidosis. This acidosis may worsen as the hypovolemia can lead to lactatemia as well. More information on anion-gap metabolic acidosis can be found in Chapter 15 of this text.

The disease process begins within a short time-frame, typically 2 or 3 days. Polydipsia, polyuria, weakness, malaise, and weight loss may have been present in the patient's recent past. As the illness progresses, symptoms like nausea, vomiting, loss of appetite, and cramping in the abdomen may be experienced. Additionally, there may be focal or generalized neurologic signs and symptoms, particularly disorientation and unconsciousness. A fruity breath odor may be noted, along with rapid, deep Kussmaul respirations, due to the patient's compensatory respiratory mechanisms for metabolic acidosis. The patient's blood gas results will show a lower PCO_2 level as a result of the physiologically increased respiratory rate. Skin examination will likely reveal heated, dry skin, as well as mucous membranes that appear dry. Hypotension may result from severe dehydration. The most frequent dysrhythmia is sinus tachycardia, however, electrolyte-related dysrhythmias may also be noted. The focus of the management of the DKA patient is the resolution of the ketonic acidosis, which includes the correction of fluid loss with IV fluids; correction of hyperglycemia with insulin; correction of electrolyte disturbances; correction of acid–base balance; and treatment of the potential cause, such as infection. The mechanical ventilator is a powerful weapon in combating acid–base balance; however, it should be used cautiously in patients with DKA. When needed, pre-intubation minute volumes should be maintained after the patient is placed on the ventilator. A failure to maintain adequate minute volume after intubation is likely to result in worsening acidosis and has the potential to cause significant deterioration in

the patient's hemodynamic status. Transport teams must use evidence-based medical protocols to safely manage these patients before and during transport. These protocols should be reviewed on a frequent basis so that team members feel comfortable managing these patients.

Fluid replenishment is crucial in the treatment of DKA since patients with the condition have severe volume depletion. Serum glucose levels will decrease by 20–50 mg/dL per hour with aggressive fluid replacement; replacement of up to 1–2 L in the first hour is recommended.[8] Too-rapid correction of blood sugar can result in a rebound effect linked to increased insulin sensitivity and can result in cerebral edema.[7] Use of 0.9% (normal, isotonic) saline for the first round of IV fluids is usually advised. Normal saline should be given to hypovolemic individuals who are in shock, and shock should thereafter be appropriately controlled. Target 15–20 mL/kg of lean body weight, or around 1 L/hour for adults, is indicated for the hypovolemic patient who is not in shock. With the euvolemic patient, who is more frequently treated with the newer diabetic drugs, normal saline should be infused more slowly; follow evidence-based recommendations and/or consult with medical supervision.[7]

Patients with DKA should get an insulin infusion after an initial fluid bolus. Regular glucose checks are advised, especially following any changes in insulin infusion rate. When treating DKA, only short-acting insulin should be administered, and IV infusion is the preferable method. With pediatrics, insulin infusions are favored over boluses to prevent morbidity, or potentially fatal drops in serum glucose. At a minimum, the patient should have their blood sugar monitored every 15–30 minutes in order to assess the situation and make any required adjustments. When blood sugar reaches 250–300 mg/dL, switch to D5NS or D5½ NS fluids and lower insulin dosage, as per your protocols, guidelines, or medical control. Additionally, if blood sugar levels fall faster than 25 mg/dL every 15 minutes (or >100 mg/dL per hour), you should reduce or stop administering insulin. Cerebral edema may result from blood sugar drops that occur more quickly than this rate (>100 mg/dL).[2,7,8]

As patients are rehydrated and as acidosis is managed, serum potassium might decrease noticeably. Administration of insulin can exacerbate serum hypokalemia. Insulin therapy should be postponed until a potassium level of at least 4 mEq/L is achieved. Additionally, 20–40 mEq/hour of additional potassium should be given when the serum potassium level is below 3.5. It may be safe to begin insulin therapy combined with concurrent potassium replacement if the potassium level is greater than 4 mEq/L but less than 5.2 mEq/L.[7] With serum concentrations higher than 5.2 mEq/L, potassium may be withheld but should be monitored frequently. Due to the fact that serum potassium increases as acidosis increases, providers should anticipate a decrease in serum potassium levels as acidosis is corrected.

The evidence in the literature points to a negative impact of sodium bicarbonate therapy in DKA patients. Only consider administering bicarbonate to DKA patients under specific medical guidance when there is the potential for cardiac dysfunction brought on by severe acidosis (pH ≤6.9), or severe hyperkalemia.[7]

When treating patients for DKA, it is important to remember that the key to treatment is resolving the ketoacidosis, as opposed to resolving the hyperglycemia. This approach may require providers to decrease or cease insulin doses, as discussed earlier, while continuing treatment to address ketones and acidosis.

Hyperosmolar Hyperglycemic State (HHS)[4,8]

HHS is most common in persons over the age of 50, with type 2 diabetes managed by oral medicine and nutrition, or with undiagnosed diabetes.[8] Many patients are also taking additional medications, such as diuretics, which has the potential to worsen the situation. Comorbidities are common in elderly people, and they can hasten the development of this illness. Increased glucose levels often result from disease, surgery, or physical stress. Patients with type 2 diabetes might not create enough insulin to stop hyperglycemia from happening, or the body may be resistant to the small amount of insulin that is produced.

A rise in blood glucose levels leads to severe dehydration. The fluid deficit in these patients can be as much as 10 liters.[4] When patients cannot replenish lost fluids, their condition deteriorates as they can no longer efficiently run their Krebs cycle, and thus contributes to acidosis. If the body starts to break down fat and muscle tissue, levels of fatty acids and amino acids rise. Hepatic gluconeogenesis then worsens the pre-existing hyperglycemia. The glomerular filtration rate will be reduced, and glucose levels rise due to intravascular volume depletion or underlying renal illness. Hyperosmolality occurs when there is a loss of more water than sodium. Especially in cases of insulin resistance, there is not enough insulin available to lower blood glucose levels.

HHS can be triggered by a variety of conditions, including underlying infections, stroke, and myocardial infarction. Other factors that can trigger this disease process include failure to comply with treatment plans, previously undetected diabetes, substance abuse, some prescribed medications, and the presence of other disorders.

HHS symptoms can take days or even weeks to manifest and might be so mild that the patient may be reluctant to seek treatment. Mild abdominal pain, a loss of appetite, polydipsia, and polyuria are some of the early signs. As the illness worsens, headaches, blurred vision, and disorientation start to appear. Additionally, possible signs include tachycardia, dysrhythmias, hypotension, and the potential for seizures or coma. Patients with HHS do not have the fruity ketone odor frequently associated with DKA, albeit their respirations may be faster. The onset of HHS may be so gradual and understated that often, the patient's first medical encounter is due to a change in their mental status late into the disease process.

The initial course of treatment for HHS entails starting IV fluids with saline solution, monitoring intake and output; as HHS patients have a severe volume deficit, fluid resuscitation needs to be carefully managed. Additionally, patients with HHS should receive an insulin infusion following the initial fluid bolus. As previously stated, a quick decrease in serum glucose can be harmful to the patient and put the patient at a significant risk. The standard treatment goal for hyperglycemia is to achieve a reduction in blood glucose that does not exceed 100 mg/dL an hour. Regular glucose and potassium checks are advised, especially following any changes in rate. When blood glucose levels drop to 250–300 mg/dL or drop by more than 100 mg/dL per hour in HHS patients, insulin infusion is routinely slowed.[2,4,8] If seizures have occurred, make sure the patient is transported with padding and in a secure position.

Thyroid Storm

Thyrotoxicosis, often known as a thyroid storm, is brought on by an excessive thyroid hormone release that causes excessive adrenergic activity. Tumors and nodules on the thyroid can promote the overproduction of thyroid hormones. Hyperthyroidism can also be triggered by iodine and iodine-containing medications like amiodarone. In addition, medications such as lithium can increase the uptake of iodine in the thyroid, suppressing the formation and release of T3/T4. Approximately 60%–80% of all cases of hyperthyroidism are caused by the autoimmune condition Graves' disease, in which thyroid-stimulating immunoglobulins enhance thyroid activity.[9] Diagnostic tests will show low levels of TSH and high levels of T3/T4 in patients who are experiencing thyrotoxicosis.[9]

A thyroid storm can develop if hyperthyroidism is not treated effectively.[9,10] Tachydysrhythmias, indications of heart failure, such as pulmonary crackles, and new-onset atrial fibrillation are some of the clinical signs.[9] Neurologic manifestations that may be prominent include agitation, delirium, syncope, tremors, manic behavior, and short-term memory loss. The patient's mental state may deteriorate to a coma in extreme circumstances.

Caution must be exercised in these patients as, without a thorough history and physical exam, the signs of a thyroid storm may easily be mistaken for mania or psychosis.[10] Additionally, acute agitation management must be considered to facilitate safe transport of these patients.

As dehydration develops, symptoms such as skin temperature variations, from warm and diaphoretic to hot and dry, will appear. Diarrhea, nausea, and vomiting can all result from increased stomach motility. Jaundice, hepatic pain, hair thinning, and the development of a goiter (an enlarged thyroid gland) are possible signs. Periorbital edema can form, and the patient may have a heavy eyelid appearance and a gazing stare.

Heart failure, and even death, are possible without prompt and effective management, and mortality rates can reach 25%. Surgery, infection, hospitalization, trauma, emotional stress, childbirth, or an abrupt cessation of antithyroid medications can all cause hormone levels to rise.[11] The patient's medical history, particularly any recent illnesses and medications, is crucial in detecting thyroid storm. It is especially important to determine if the patient has recently discontinued a prescribed medication, specifically an antithyroid medication.

If thyrotoxicosis is suspected, rapid intervention to maintain hemodynamic stability is necessary. The mainstay of treatment for thyrotoxicosis is adrenergic inhibition.[2] Identification and management of the condition causing the thyrotoxicosis are among the treatment's objectives. Priority will be given to treating serious respiratory, circulatory, and airway issues. To control hyperthermia, cooling procedures and antipyretic medications may be necessary. However, salicylates should be avoided since they may cause the displacement of thyroid hormone.

Beta-adrenergic blockers, such as propranolol or esmolol are often administered to treat tachycardia, as well as ventricular arrhythmias. Propylthiouracil or methimazole are two medications that can be utilized to lower thyroid hormone levels. Glucocorticoids are used to treat adrenal insufficiency and decrease peripheral thyroid hormone deiodination. To lower and stabilize thyroid hormone production, potassium iodide saturated solution may be given an hour after the other medications. Lithium may be administered if conventional management is ineffective.

Hyperglycemia and hypercalcemia may be noted in patients experiencing thyrotoxicosis, but should improve with fluid therapy.[4,8,12] The preferred fluid is determined by the patient's electrolyte levels and hemodynamic condition.[12] It is difficult to identify and treat a patient who is experiencing a thyrotoxicosis. To help with the safe management of these patients, it is crucial that evidence-based medical transport protocols or guidelines are followed or the medical director is contacted.

Myxedema Coma[11]

Myxedema coma can develop over time as a result of untreated or undertreated hypothyroidism and often presents in winter, in females over the age of 60. Patients with hypothyroidism transition to myxedema coma upon changes in their level of consciousness (LOC).

Secondary hypothyroidism is caused by pituitary dysfunction. A decrease in TSH release caused by changes in pituitary function lowers thyroid hormone output. Tertiary hypothyroidism happens when the hypothalamus does not release enough thyrotropin-releasing hormone (TRH) or when TRH does not stimulate the pituitary gland.

The condition may also be triggered by GI bleeding, hypoglycemia, hypothermia, burns, infections, DKA, trauma, autoimmune thyroiditis (such as Hashimoto's disease), iodine deficiency, tumors, thyroid ablation therapy, or medication therapies that suppress thyroid activity, such as amiodarone, lithium, beta-blockers, anesthetics, and various anticonvulsants. Additionally, cessation of thyroid replacement therapy may also lead to myxedema coma.

Dyspnea, weight gain, doughy edema, decreases in deep tendon reflex, exhaustion, poor exercise tolerance, and macroglossia (an enlarged tongue) are among the symptoms of hypothyroidism. In the early stages of myxedema coma patients could appear confused and answer questions in a slow manner. Additional clinical manifestations include combativeness, hallucinations, paranoia, sadness, and diminished concern for one's appearance. This collection of symptoms is often referred to as myxedema mania and may pose a risk to the safety of the transport team and the patient during transport.

As a result of their altered LOC and macroglossia, these patients are at a high risk of airway compromise. Alveolar hypoventilation brought on by weakened breathing and diminished respiratory drive can result in hypercarbia, which may worsen the patient's mental state, and long-term alveolar hypoventilation may result in pneumonia. As a result, it is likely that mechanical ventilation may be needed for these patients. Obesity-related sleep apnea has been linked to additional impairment of the respiratory system. In most cases, respiratory failure results in death.

Notable cardiac changes include lower heart rate, cardiac volume, and stroke volume. The average body temperature is less than 96°F (35.5°C), and the skin is often pale and chilly. Reduced renal blood flow, salt reabsorption, and glomerular filtration rates are all observed. Normal fluid excretion from the patient is reduced, and broad nonpitting edema may be apparent. Decreased insulin sensitivity, adrenal insufficiency, and decreased oral intake may lead to the development of hypoglycemia, and system metabolic slowing may also result in constipation.

Diagnostic tests show high levels of TSH and low levels of T3/T4, hemoglobin, and hematocrit, as well as a decreased white blood cell count. As the patient is stabilized, radiographs, scans, and other diagnostic tests might be carried out.

Volume resuscitation, glucocorticoid support, and thyroid hormone replacement, such as thyroxine, are recommended to treat hypotension in these patients.[12,13] Vasopressors should only be used when other treatments are ineffective in treating severe hypotension in this patient population, as they do not function as well in the absence of thyroid hormone, and their administration may raise the risk of arrhythmias and/or angina.

Consider using mechanical ventilation as a strategy to manage respiratory acidosis, weakened respiratory muscles, and elevated oxygen needs. Implement measures to lessen the risk of hypothermia. However, keep in mind that aggressive warming could strain an already stressed system, so opt for passive or moderate warming approaches when reasonable, based on the patient's condition.[12] Before any patient transfer, it is advisable to address gastric decompression as a preventative measure or treatment for paralytic ileus.

Acute Adrenal Insufficiency[2,11–13]

Acute adrenal insufficiency is a rare but serious condition. It can lead to Addisonian crisis or an adrenal crisis, which is the most severe manifestation of adrenal insufficiency. Adrenal mineralocorticoids (primarily aldosterone) and glucocorticoids (primarily cortisol) are depleted with this condition. It can occur when the pituitary gland is damaged, the adrenal glands are injured or removed, when long-term steroid medication is abruptly stopped, or in people with Addison's disease. Trauma, surgery, stress, or infection can all be significant risk factors in people with Addison's disease. Massive bilateral adrenal hemorrhage can be brought on by physiologic pressures that are too severe to manage, like septic shock, complex pregnancies, or myocardial infarction. A malfunctioning adrenal system leads to sodium and water loss from the kidneys and GI tract, which could cause hypovolemia and refractory hypotension. This may eventually result in cardiovascular collapse, coma, or even death. Due to the deficiency in aldosterone, sodium levels drop, and serum potassium levels rise. Hyperkalemia and occasionally deadly dysrhythmias result from this. Cortisol deficiencies result in a failure of gluconeogenesis, ineffective catecholamines, poor glucagon activity, and severely limit the functions of the adrenal medulla.

There are two pathophysiological pathways allowing adrenal insufficiency to manifest: primary and secondary. With primary adrenal insufficiency, also known as Addison's disease, there is an intrinsic failure of the adrenal glands which result in low cortisol and aldosterone levels. This can occur due to adrenal hemorrhage, as with trauma, sepsis, or blood thinners, but also can occur because of infection, medication use, autoimmune causes, and metastases. Secondary adrenal insufficiency results as a failure of pituitary stimulation of the adrenals which results in cortisol deficiency only. This occurs due to abrupt withdrawal of steroid therapy, pituitary disease, or trauma.

Diagnosis of adrenal insufficiency is challenging due to the lack of identifiable symptoms. It is crucial to get a patient's most recent medical history. Fatigue, weight loss, palpitations, headaches, weakness, nausea, abdominal pain, anorexia, and diarrhea are a few examples of complaints. High temperature, dehydration, hypotension, abrupt discomfort in the legs, lower back, or abdomen are all possible symptoms for patients. Loss of consciousness or a change in mental state are possible outcomes of these symptoms.

Orthostatic hypotension, dry mucous membranes, poor skin turgor, lethargy, tachycardia, and delayed capillary refill are a few examples of physical findings. On inspection, hyperpigmentation of the skin and mucous membranes may also be seen in chronic states. In addition to hypoglycemia, patients may also develop hyponatremia, hyperkalemia, and hypercalcemia.

Treatment includes initiating IV fluids with normal saline solution or 5% dextrose in normal saline, administering IV hydrocortisone (to enhance glucagon and catecholamines), plasma (as a volume expander), and monitoring intake and output in order to establish and maintain fluid and electrolyte balance. After achieving a suitable volume replacement, vasopressors may be necessary for refractory hypotension. Additionally, monitoring potassium levels is necessary to prevent hyperkalemia. Anticoagulated patients who continue to have hypotension should be evaluated for the possibility of adrenal hemorrhage. Sedatives should be given as needed for transportation, and steps should be taken to create a setting that is as calm and comfortable as possible.

Diabetes Insipidus[14]

Diabetes insipidus (DI) is brought on by insufficient or impaired ADH secretion as well as inadequate or impaired renal ADH response. When the secretion and release of ADH are compromised, central DI results. This can be brought on by a tumor, surgery, a traumatic brain injury, or genetically produced.

Nephrogenic, neurogenic, dipsogenic, and gestagenic are the four subtypes of DI. Nephrogenic DI results from the kidneys' inability to appropriately concentrate urine; it can be inherited or acquired. Acquired variants of the condition are caused by changes in the kidneys. Most frequently, illnesses, medications, or other disorders like hypokalemia, hypercalcemia, pregnancy, and sickle cell anemia are to blame.

The posterior pituitary gland's decreased production of ADH is the main contributor to neurogenic DI. Among the causes are tumors of the hypothalamus or anterior pituitary gland, infections (such as bacterial meningitis or viral encephalitis), head trauma (such as basilar, sphenoidal, or facial skull fractures), surgeries, granulomas (such as sarcoidosis, histiocytosis), vascular anomalies (such as ischemia, aneurysms, hematomas, and inflammation), and chemical toxins.

Dipsogenic DI, often referred to as primary or psychogenic polydipsia, is brought on by an aberrant thirst mechanism that leads to an excessive consumption of fluids. Granuloma (such as neurosarcoid), infection (such as tuberculous, meningitis), autoimmune conditions (such as multiple sclerosis), and usage of specific drugs are the causes of primary polydipsia. Psychological conditions like schizophrenia, mania, and neurosis can cause psychogenic polydipsia.

Gestagenic DI, which can occur in pregnant women with eclampsia, preeclampsia, multiple gestations, or impaired liver function, is brought on by a brief increase in the breakdown of ADH. Reduced levels of circulating ADH and a sharp rise in vasopressinase activity (i.e., an enzyme produced in the placenta and broken down in the liver) are features of this type of DI. Replacement vasopressin has little effect on these women. Usually, the situation improves after the placenta is delivered.

Laboratory tests that evaluate urine osmolality and urine sodium are used to make diagnoses. When polyuria is present and urine osmolality is less than 200 mOsm/kg, DI is suspected. The water deprivation test can be used to distinguish between nephrogenic and central DI.

Monitoring of the electrolyte levels, electrocardiographic (ECG) rhythm, neurologic status, and fluid status are all necessary for managing a patient with DI. Transport clinicians must differentiate between central and nephrogenic DI, and fluid intake, output, and urine osmolality must all be monitored. Treatment with hormone replacement may be necessary. It is recommended to give isotonic maintenance fluid at a rate that at least corresponds to hourly urine production, and administration of desmopressin acetate or vasopressin may be required.

Syndrome of Inappropriate Antidiuretic Hormone Secretion[1,6,11,12]

ADH, which originates in the hypothalamus and is stored in the pituitary gland, is released in excess by the pituitary gland, resulting in the syndrome of inappropriate antidiuretic hormone (SIADH). SIADH can happen when a condition alters the hypothalamic secretion osmoreceptors or the hypothalamic-pituitary-adrenal axis. Tricyclic antidepressants, opioids, thyroid or pituitary abnormalities, oral hypoglycemic drugs, and carbamazepine are other potential triggers. The patient may have concurrent conditions such as traumatic brain injury, hypothyroid diseases, porphyria, abscesses, or pneumonia.

Due to increased distal renal tubular permeability to water, urine volume is reduced. The serum osmolality and circulatory blood volume are commonly used to calculate ADH. A rise in serum concentration causes the release of ADH to be stimulated. The serum concentration drops as a result of the kidneys responding by absorbing more water. As the circulation capacity increases, urinary output slows. By association, this leads to a fluid overload and dilutional hyponatremia.

The signs and symptoms that patients may experience include diarrhea, nausea, vomiting, weakness, stomach and/or muscle cramps, weight gain, exhaustion, headaches, and decreased urine output. As hyponatremia increases, they could appear disoriented or confused and experience seizures. When severe hyponatremia results in changes in fluid levels, cerebral edema and hyponatremic encephalopathy can happen. Low serum osmolality (less than 280 mOsm/kg) and serum sodium concentrations (less than 125 mEq/L) may be seen in test results.

The severity of the hyponatremia determines how to treat SIADH. Water restriction, starting at 800–1000 mL/day, is frequently sufficient; however, in some circumstances, a 500 mL/day cap may be necessary. Because acute hyponatremia can lead to seizures, cerebral edema, and hyponatremic encephalopathy, close observation is necessary.[12,15] In some situations, a vasopressin antagonist, a vaptan, may be administered.

Select Electrolyte Disturbances[12,15–18]

Electrolytes are crucial for nearly all cellular reactions and functions; they direct acid–base balance, regulate water distribution, transmit nerve impulses, and contribute to blood clotting. Electrolyte abnormalities can manifest in a variety of ways. Electrolyte balance is influenced by normal cell function, fluid intake and output, acid–base balance, and hormone secretion. Normal levels are maintained within very narrow ranges through complex processes within the renal and endocrine systems.

Sodium

Sodium is the body's most abundant solute in extracellular fluid. It assists the regulation of normal extracellular fluid osmolality, maintenance of acid–base balance, activation of nerve and muscle cells, and influences water distribution (with chloride).

Hyponatremia[12,16]

Hyponatremia is defined as a state in which there is a relative deficiency of sodium concentration in relation to the amount of water in the plasma (extracellular compartment). A sodium level of less than 135 mEq/L indicates hyponatremia; a level less than 120 mEq/L is considered a critical value. Causes can be dilutional (i.e., blood becoming too dilute) or the result of direct or indirect sodium loss.

Conditions associated with hyponatremia include the following: congestive heart failure, excessive water intake, cirrhosis, SIADH, acute renal failure with oliguria, renal injury, sepsis, diarrhea, vomiting, excessive sweating, adrenal insufficiency, and renal lesions.

In patients with hyperglycemia, factitious hyponatremia can develop because of intracellular to extracellular fluid shifts. This condition usually corrects itself as the glucose levels are corrected.

Manifestations of hyponatremia vary from patient to patient and are variable depending on how precipitously the patient's sodium level has dropped. If the level drops quickly, the patient is more likely to be symptomatic.

The initial signs and symptoms are primarily neurologic, such as muscle twitching, tremors, and weakness. This can progress to headache, disorientation and changes in LOC.[15,16] When sodium levels fall below 110 mEq/L, severe symptoms, such as delirium, ataxia, psychosis, seizures, or coma, may present, as a result of brain edema.

There are multiple classifications of medications that are largely associated with hyponatremia, such as anticoagulants, anticonvulsants, antidiabetics, diuretics, and sedatives. Medications can cause hyponatremia by potentiating the action of ADH or by causing SIADH. Diuretics may also cause hyponatremia by inhibiting sodium reabsorption in the kidneys.[15,16]

General management depends on the degree of severity. With mild cases, treatment should include limiting free water and consideration of removing or exchanging medications that contribute to hyponatremia. Normal saline could be beneficial in treatment, since it has a sodium concentration of 154 mmol/L. In severe cases, especially in cases of seizures, hypertonic saline should be given; dosing recommendations vary in current literature.[16-18] Hypertonic saline is recommended to be given slowly over 10 minutes, minimally. Sodium replacement should be halted when the serum sodium reaches 120 mEq/dL.

Risks associated with overzealous hyponatremia correction include the possibility of demyelination and "locked-in syndrome." Impaired nerve signal transmission may result from demyelination, which is characterized by damage to the covering that surrounds nerve fibers. A neurological condition known as "locked-in syndrome" causes people to be fully conscious but unable to move anything other than their eyes or eyelids, effectively imprisoning them inside their own bodies. These grave repercussions highlight the need for caution when treating hyponatremia. The key to safely resolving hyponatremia is to replace sodium (Na) gradually and carefully, avoiding any sudden changes that may trigger even more significant and debilitating neurological conditions.[16,18]

Hypernatremia

Hypernatremia is often caused when water losses exceed sodium loss and is defined as a sodium level of greater than 145 mEq/L. Causes may include gastric fluid losses, osmotic diuresis, hypothalamic disorders, such as a lesion-impairing thirst, exercise; seizures, and intake or administration of hypertonic saline solutions.

Neurologic signs are the most critical signs of hypernatremia because fluid shifts have a significant effect on brain cells. Early manifestations to look for include agitation or restlessness, anorexia, weakness, low-grade fever, flushed skin, and nausea and/or vomiting. Severe hypernatremia can lead to seizures, coma, and permanent neurologic damage.[16]

Some medications associated with hypernatremia include antacids with sodium bicarbonate, certain antibiotics, salt tablets, IV sodium chloride preparations, sodium polystyrene sulfonate, and corticosteroids.

Identification and management of the cause, as well as controlled fluid replacement, will generally correct this electrolyte imbalance. Volume depletion should be carefully reversed with normal saline/lactated Ringer's infusion with attention to avoidance of a too-rapid decrease in sodium. Consideration should be exercised with lactated Ringer's over normal saline because of its high sodium concentration (154 mol/L).[12,17,18] The goal for sodium reduction is no more than 0.5–1 mEq/L per hour, and no more than 10 mEq/L per day.[18]

Potassium[12]

Potassium plays a crucial role in many metabolic cell functions and is subject to multiple influences within the body; it is the body's major intracellular ion. An important contributor to potassium balance is acid–base balance. ECG changes are frequently associated with potassium abnormalities, which may or may not correlate with severity.

Hypokalemia

A potassium level of less than 3.5 mEq/L indicates hypokalemia. There exist three main pathways: increased renal and GI potassium loss, intracellular redistribution of potassium, and decreased potassium intake. Excessive diarrhea and vomiting, excessive diuresis, intestinal obstruction, GI suctioning, diuretics, overuse of laxatives or steroids, resin exchange use, and excessive sweating are all associated with hypokalemia, due to renal and GI mechanisms. It also can be a result of intracellular shifting of potassium caused by alkalosis, large doses of beta-agonists, or IV insulin. Finally, starvation and malabsorption leads to low potassium intake.

Hypokalemia may be associated with cardiac conduction abnormalities, which are refractory to therapy until K levels are corrected. Ventricular ectopy is the most common dysrhythmia. The ECG may demonstrate flat or absent T waves, the presence of a U wave, or peaked P waves. IV potassium replacement should never exceed 40 mEq/hour, and typically half that rate is a reasonable target. Oral potassium is well absorbed and safe, although nausea and/or vomiting may occur. Hypomagnesemia should be managed concurrently, as patients with low serum magnesium respond poorly to potassium replacement. With the extracellular shift of potassium in acidotic states, patients who are acidotic and present with hypokalemia should be administered potassium replacement before treatment of acidosis is initiated. Resolution of the acidosis will cause extracellular potassium to be pulled into the cell, thus worsening the underlying hypokalemia.

Hyperkalemia

A potassium level of greater than 5.5 mEq/L indicates hyperkalemia. Causes include renal dysfunction resulting in oliguria, tissue breakdown (i.e., released potassium from lysed or damaged cells), excessive potassium intake, or medications that influence the cellular exchange of potassium, e.g., digoxin, ACE inhibitors, angiotensin-receptor blockers, potassium-sparing diuretics. Various ECG changes correlate well with severity in hyperkalemia. Elevated T waves occur when serum potassium reaches 5.5–6.6 mEq/L, and prolonged PR interval and widened QRS complexes are evident when levels reach 6.5–8.0 mEq/L. Hyperkalemia is also observed frequently in patients with chronic renal disease and renal failure.

Hyperkalemia's primary risks are cardiac, and include refractory ventricular arrhythmias. Treatments as outlined in ACLS (advanced cardiac life support guidelines) include measures to protect the myocardium (calcium chloride/calcium gluconate) and shift potassium into the intracellular space (bicarbonate, insulin/glucose, albuterol), whereas resin exchange, furosemide, or dialysis are instituted to reduce total body potassium. Bicarbonate administration tends to be more effective in patients who are acidotic. Sodium bicarbonate may also benefit these patients in the absence of acidosis, as the large amount of sodium works to balance the sodium and potassium gradient. Additionally, due to the extracellular shift of potassium in acidotic states, patients with severe acidosis, such as DKA, will normally present with hyperkalemia. In these situations the hyperkalemia should not be "treated" as it will resolve with treatment of the acidosis.

Calcium[12]

Calcium is stored primarily in the skeleton, but approximately 2% of the total body calcium is located in the extracellular fluid. Calcium is an essential electrolyte for cardiac and neuromuscular function. Abnormalities in calcium levels are often associated with magnesium and phosphorus abnormalities.

Hypocalcemia

A serum calcium level of less than 8.5 mEq/L indicates hypocalcemia. Causes of hypocalcemia include hypoparathyroidism, malabsorption syndrome, osteomalacia, acute pancreatitis, chronic renal failure, vitamin D or magnesium deficiency, hyperphosphatemia, and increased calcitonin.

Clinical findings are significant for positive Chvostek sign (light facial tap eliciting abnormal facial spasms) and positive Trousseau sign (carpal spasms induced by the inflation of a blood pressure cuff on the upper arm). As a result of increased excitability of brain tissue, seizures are also occasionally observed. Patients may display other symptoms such as numbness or tingling of the fingers, toes, nose, lips, or earlobes; facial grimacing; muscle twitching, hyperactive deep tendon reflexes; and abdominal pain. Critical symptoms include laryngospasms, seizures, bronchospasms, and cardiovascular collapse. ECG signs include potential for prolonged QT interval.

Hypomagnesemia should be managed before treatment for hypocalcemia because patients with low serum magnesium levels respond poorly to calcium replacement. Hypocalcemia can be easily managed with the administration of IV calcium. Most literature favors calcium gluconate over calcium chloride in this case because the chloride version of calcium acts as a greater vesicant than its gluconate version, which can cause tissue necrosis following extravasation. It is for this reason that a central line is preferred when administering calcium chloride. Three grams of calcium chloride is roughly equivalent to 1 gram of calcium gluconate. During administration the patient should be carefully observed to include hemodynamic monitoring, cardiac rhythm, and repeat calcium levels.

Ionized calcium levels may be low in patients receiving blood transfusions despite normal total calcium because of the citrate in banked blood that binds ionized calcium. Additionally, hypocalcemia can occur in hyperventilating patients or patients hyperventilated on the mechanical ventilator due to alkalosis. Consequently, due to the citrate that is included in packaged blood products, which binds to calcium and increases renal pH, it has historically been recommended to administer IV calcium for every 3–4 units of transfused blood products; there is, however, a lack of evidence to support the need or benefit of this additional calcium administration; providers should be sure to follow departmental patient care protocols.

Hypercalcemia

A calcium level of greater than 10.5 mEq/L indicates hypercalcemia. Causes include increased mobilization of calcium from bones, as seen in hyperparathyroidism, prolonged immobilization, thyrotoxicosis, excessive calcium intake, renal tubular acidosis, bone metastasis, and chronic thiazide therapy. Chronic hypercalcemia is associated with renal lithiasis, peptic ulcer disease, and pancreatitis. Patients taking digitalis will have enhanced calcium effects.

Symptoms of hypercalcemia can be vague, including irritability, fatigue, general malaise, nausea, vomiting, constipation, headache, or difficulty concentrating. Primary manifestations are often neurologic. Patients may be confused or have a depressed LOC, as well as delayed deep tendon reflexes. They may also express polyuria, polydipsia, or have an ileus. ECG changes include QT interval shortening.

Treatment of the underlying cause and increasing renal excretion of calcium with IV hydration and loop or osmotic diuretics is the priority in correction of hypercalcemia. Although rare, serum calcium levels of higher than 13.5 mg/dL require urgent attention and sometimes hemodialysis. In patients with hyperparathyroidism, calcitonin may be indicated.

Patient Handoff and Preparation for Transport[15]

History

Obtain a complete past medical and current illness or injury history through subjective and objective review with patient, family, and referring facility/agency providers. A reliable and complete history in patients with metabolic, endocrine, or electrolyte problems can help with identifying the cause of the metabolic or endocrine problem.

1. In some cases, aspects of the history are critical to the diagnosis; for example, previous thyroid surgery, steroid-dependent conditions, and hemodynamic instability after receiving iodinated contrast.
2. Obtain and record patients' past medical history, any surgical history, medications, and any precipitating factors in their current illness. When possible, data should be gathered about patients' social history, alcohol use, use of illicit substances, and family history.
3. Obtain the prior therapies provided and the patient's response to those therapies, paying particular attention to total fluid intake and output, type of fluids administered, labs before and after therapy, basic metabolic panel, lactate, TSH, T3/T4 levels, and urinalysis.

Physical Examination

1. Perform a primary and secondary survey.
2. General inspection of the patient may provide useful clues (e.g., thyroid pathophysiology, thyroidectomy scars, fruity breath in DKA, presence of insulin pump, etc.).
3. Assess the patient's hydration status (e.g., skin and mucous membranes, volume status, intake and output).

4. Although the transport team may be time-limited in some of the very detailed examinations, some findings specific to the clinical circumstance can be quickly performed (e.g., Kussmaul respirations in DKA, abnormally delayed deep tendon reflexes in hypothyroidism, Trousseau sign in hypocalcemia). Consider the lengthier examinations in transport if time and patient access allows.

5. Initial intervention focuses on maintaining airway, breathing (specifically oxygen administration to maintain an oxygen saturation of at least 90%) and circulation, initiating IV access, and assessing pain. Continuous vital sign monitoring should be initiated before and during transport.

Monitoring

1. Monitor for airway patency, ventilation, oxygenation, and perfusion complications via cardiac and hemodynamic monitors including blood pressure (noninvasive or invasive), pulse oximetry monitor, cardiac telemetry, end-tidal CO_2 monitoring, and ventilator data as needed. Be ready to intervene appropriately if needed.

2. Ensure that all medication infusions are running appropriately.

3. Ensure all lines, drains, and tubes are secured, functioning normally and safely, and monitor for changes.

4. Monitor for oxygen consumption to ensure an ample supply during treatment and transport. Remember, serial measurements of oxygen consumption should be routinely conducted as dramatic reductions in available oxygen can occur from leak for a multitude of reasons.

5. Establish and maintain fluid and electrolyte balance by initiating IV fluids with isotonic or other solution, as ordered; insert a urinary catheter as indicated by the patient's condition; and monitor intake and output.

6. If available in transport, consider drawing and running serial labs to further monitor efficacy of therapies.

Vascular Access

1. Ensure adequate peripheral or central vascular access for crystalloid and medication administration.

2. Ensure no infiltration, inflammation, nor obstruction is observed with IV flushing with approximately 10 mL of isotonic crystalloids.

Radiography

1. Radiography (e.g., chest imaging revealing lung mass in SIADH) and ECG (e.g., peaked T waves with hyperkalemia) are infrequently diagnostic but can provide useful clues to the presence and/or explanation of metabolic/endocrine disorders.

Laboratory Data

Laboratory data are of paramount importance in diagnosing and in guiding therapy of metabolic/endocrine/electrolyte disorders.

1. Basic labs (electrolytes, blood urea nitrogen [BUN]/creatinine, glucose, complete blood count, urinalysis) should be assessed in all cases.

2. Blood gas analysis can assist in determining acid–base balance, which is helpful in many patients with significant metabolic/endocrine disorders. Use point-of-care or traditional lab resources, if available, particularly during long transports.

3. Specialized testing (e.g., thyroid panel, hemoglobin A1C) may be performed as clinically indicated; however, it should generally not delay critical care transport.

4. The osmolarity (number of dissolved particles per liter of solution) is frequently important in metabolic/endocrine cases.
   a. Calculated osmolarity: $(2 \times Na) + BUN/2.8 + glucose/18$.
   b. Normal range for osmolarity is 275–295 mOsm/L.
   c. The osmolarity may also be directly measured by the laboratory at most hospitals.
   d. The osmolar gap may be helpful in the differential diagnosis of various conditions. The difference between the calculated and measured osmolarity is called the osmolar gap. The normal osmolar gap is 10–15 mOsm/L; a greater gap suggests the presence of another solute (e.g., lactate, ethanol, methanol, ethylene glycol, isopropyl alcohol).

5. In some instances, laboratory data may be factitiously elevated. To prevent inappropriate treatment, transport teams should be familiar with corrections for at least two common fictitious entities.
   a. Pseudohyponatremia is usually caused by hyperglycemia, hyperlipidemia, or hyperproteinemia. Correction of Na levels for hyperglycemia should be calculated.
   b. Apparent hyperkalemia may be caused by hemolysis, severe leukocytosis such as with chronic lymphocytic leukemia (CLL), significant acidosis, or thrombocytosis.

Medication Administration

1. Medication administration will be guided by clinical circumstances, with medical control orders or using evidence-based medical transport protocols.

2. IV fluid therapy choices are more important in metabolic/endocrine conditions than in most other critical care transports. The specific fluid being administered, the rate of administration, and the rationale for fluid selection should be clear to the transport team.

Patient Stabilization/Planning and Care During Transport

Stabilization and planning for care en route should include specific interventions as dictated by the patient's disease process.

1. Ensure optimal patient positioning. Stressors of transport can exacerbate symptoms in response to pain and changes in vital signs.

2. Continue monitoring the patient during treatment and transport for changes in vital signs, signs of deterioration, development of hypoxia, and evidence of pain and/or discomfort. If seizures have occurred, ensure padding is used to protect the patient during transport.

3. Metabolic/endocrine patients are among those most likely to have a change in status during transport because of ongoing treatment and response. Examples in which transport providers should closely follow patients include ECG rhythm in hyperkalemia, glucose in patients on insulin infusions, and potassium (when possible) in patients being treated for DKA.

4. Explain all aspects of critical care transport to the patient, including plans, interventions, and expectations, both during transport and on arrival at the receiving facility.

5. Ensure that all laboratory results, imaging studies, and the patient care record accompany the patient for interfacility transport.

6. If the patient becomes combative or difficult to control physically, advise the pilot of a need to land immediately or the driver to pull over until the patient can be safely managed in transport.

7. Continual assessment of volume/perfusion status includes monitoring of hemodynamics and urine output, with adjustment of IV infusions, and consideration of medications such as hydrocortisone, in patients who are refractory to traditional therapies, as indicated by the clinical circumstances.

8. Other intra-transport care should follow the disease-specific guidelines as outlined in departmental patient care protocols.

References

1. Brashers V, Jones R, Huether S. Mechanism of hormonal regulation. In: McCance K, Huether S, eds. *The Biologic Basis for Disease in Adults and Children*. 7th ed. St. Louis, MO: Elsevier Mosby; 2014:689–716.

2. Tucci V, Sokari T. The clinical manifestations, diagnosis, and treatment of adrenal emergencies. *Emerg Med Clin North Am*. 2014;32(2):465–484.

3. Llamado R, Czaja A, Stence N, Davidson J. Continuous octreotide for sulfonylurea-induced hypoglycemia in a toddler. *J Emerg Med*. 2013;45(6):e209–e213.

4. Corwell B, Knight B, Olivieri L, Willis G. Current diagnosis and treatment of hyperglycemic emergencies. *Emerg Med Clin North Am*. 2014;32(2):437–452.

5. Hamdy O. Diabetic ketoacidosis treatment and management. Medscape Reference Drugs, Diseases & Procedures. 2016. Available at: http://emedicine.medscape.com/article/118361-treatment.

6. Howard PK, Steinmann RA. *Sheehy's Emergency Nursing Principles and Practice*. 6th ed. St. Louis, MO: Elsevier; 2010.

7. Nyenwe E, Kitabchi A. The evolution of diabetic ketoacidosis: an update of its etiology, pathogenesis and management. *Metabolism*. 2016;65(4):507–521.

8. Kitabchi A, Umpierrez G, Miles J, Fisher J. Hyperglycemic crisis in adults with diabetes. *Diabetes Care*. 2009;32(7):1335–1343.

9. Pokhrel B, Bhusal K. Graves disease. In: StatPearls [Internet]. Treasure Island, FL: StatPearls Publishing; Updated Jun 20, 2023. Available at: https://www.ncbi.nlm.nih.gov/books/NBK448195/.

10. Sharp C, Wilson M, Nordstrom K. Psychiatric emergencies for clinicians: the emergency department management of thyroid storm. *J Emerg Med*. 2016;51(2):155–158.

11. Brashers V, Jones R, Huether S. Alterations of hormone regulation. In: McCance K, Huether S, eds. *The Biologic Basis for Disease in Adults and Children*. 7th ed. Elsevier Mosby; 2014:717–767.

12. Doig A, Huether S. The cellular environment: fluids and electrolytes, acids and bases. In: McCance K, Huether S, eds. *The Biologic Basis for Disease in Adults and Children*. 7th ed. Elsevier Mosby; 2014:103–134.

13. Ramamoorthy S, Cidlowski JA. Corticosteroids: mechanisms of action in health and disease. *Rheum Dis Clin North Am*. 2016;42(1):15–31, vii.

14. Robertson G. Diabetes insipidus: differential diagnosis and management. *Best Pract Res Clin Endocrinol Metabol*. 2016;30(2):205–218.

15. Wolfe AC, Frakes MA, Farmer S, Santiago J, eds. *Critical Care Transport Core Curriculum*. 2nd ed. Air & Surface Transport Nurses Association; 2022.

16. Sterns RH. Treatment of severe hyponatremia. *Clin J Am Soc Nephrol*. 2018;13:641.

17. Mesghali E, Fitter S, Bahjri K, Moussavi K. Safety of peripheral line administration of 3% hypertonic saline and mannitol in the emergency department. *J Emerg Med*. 2019; 56:431.

18. Jones GM, Bode L, Riha H, Erdman MJ. Safety of continuous peripheral infusion of 3% sodium chloride solution in neurocritical care patients. *Am J Crit Care*. 2016;26:37.

13

Infectious and Communicable Diseases

CHAD BOWMAN AND JADE B. FLINN

COMPETENCIES

1. Describe isolation precautions and relate appropriate strategies for ensuring patient and provider safety according to disease/condition.
2. Discuss elements of a transport program infection control plan.
3. Identify assessment strategies and describe clinical findings associated with various infectious and communicable diseases.
4. Describe management strategies for patients with potential infectious or communicable disease.

Introduction

Infectious and communicable diseases are routinely encountered by transport personnel. Patients suffering from the ill effects of infections, and those that are asymptomatic carriers of human pathogens, present challenges to daily practice. In time-critical emergencies, many of the precautions that exist to prevent transmission of infectious agents can become a hindrance to efficient care, however these precautions exist not only to safeguard healthcare worker well-being but to also reduce the risk of further disease spread. Additionally, transporting patients from the scene of motor vehicle collisions or an emergency department may limit the available background information, such as recent community exposures or laboratory culture and sensitivity results to assist decision-making in the implementation of isolation precautions.

In light of the 2020 COVID-19 pandemic and increased public awareness of emerging and re-emerging infectious and communicable diseases, it is prudent to understand infectious diseases and their associated risks and impact on providing safe clinical care. The Air & Surface Transport Nurses Association (ASTNA) updated its position statement on the transport of patients with serious communicable diseases and highlights of this statement are noted in Box 13.1.[1]

This chapter begins with a review of isolation control and prevention including definitions of the types of isolation precautions and descriptions of pillars of basic infection control practices such as hand hygiene. Personal protective equipment (PPE) and decontamination practices are further explored in this chapter by describing various pieces of PPE ensembles and disinfectants and the way in which they safeguard healthcare workers by reducing the risk of disease spread. The chapter is further framed by transmission-based precautions and a description of possible pathogens and their infectious disease process that critical care transport teams may encounter. The section on *Vaccine-Preventable Infections* encompasses a variety of pathogens that include both a

standard precautions approach for blood-borne organisms such as hepatitis B, as well as an approach that may require an additional level of precautionary measures for droplet transmitted organisms such as COVID-19, pneumonia, pertussis or influenza. Pathogens are further differentiated into transmission-based precautions in the *Contact* and *Airborne* sections. The *Special Considerations* section describes infectious processes, including emerging and high consequence pathogens, that may require variations in PPE and isolation practices. It is important to also note the chapter includes infectious disease processes like sepsis and toxic shock syndrome, which are important to discuss in critical care management but may not include a communicable aspect. Regardless of this chapter's transmission-based framework, it is prudent for transport teams to approach every transport with their safety in mind and may default to a conservative approach of implementing transmission-based precautions in a setting when the infectious disease process is unknown or unconfirmed (Table 13.1).

Infection Control and Prevention

Ideally, possible infectious disease patients are identified through routine screening from 911 call takers and emergency medical dispatchers, and that pertinent information is relayed to emergency responders prior to scene arrival.[2] Basic screening information should be acquired using standardized questions to assess for the potential of communicable diseases (both active and non-pathogenic). For prehospital environments, standardized prompting from Emergency Medical Dispatch cards, such as those from the International Academies of Emergency Dispatch (IAED) or similar organizations, can screen for potential infectious disease risks. In response to the 2003 SARS-1, 2009 H1N1, and 2014 Ebola outbreaks, IAED developed and honed the Emergency Infectious Disease Surveillance (EIDS) tool to enable EMS authorities to implement a protocol to not only surveil for early findings

• BOX 13.1   Air & Surface Transport Nurses Association Position Statement

Transport of Patients with Serious Communicable Diseases

"The transport team is likely to be at added risk of exposure due to factors such as environmental conditions and interventions performed, and thus must be aware of the most current information available from infectious disease specialists to make informed practice decisions."

Education and Standards for Infection Control Practices

- Medical teams transporting patients with suspected or confirmed infectious diseases should follow infection control procedures outlined by the World Health Organization (WHO), the Occupational Safety and Health Administration (OHSA), and Center for Disease Control and Prevention (CDC).
- The Commission on Accreditation of Emergency Transport Services (CAMTS), an accreditation body, has developed standards for critical care transport teams, including standards for infection control practices.

Cleaning and Disinfection

- Transport vehicles should be terminally cleaned and decontaminated after transport of patients with highly infectious diseases. The type of vehicle selected for transport may depend on its suitability for effective decontamination before return to service.
- Appropriate Personnel Protective Equipment (PPE) should be donned prior to entering the decontamination area.
- Cleaning agents should be EPA-registered with label claims specific to the suspected organism.

- Emphasis should be on cleaning patient care areas and exposed surfaces, specifically medical equipment and control panels, and flooring, walls, and work surfaces in the transport vehicle. Stretchers and litters, including wheels, brackets, and other areas likely to become contaminated, should receive special attention.
- Only mattresses and pillows with plastic or impermeable covers should be used.
- All soiled supplies and patient-generated waste should be disposed of in accordance with CDC guidelines.

ASTNA Position

ASTNA supports:

- Standards for comprehensive exposure control plans designed to protect team members from exposures to blood and other potentially infectious body fluids, communicable diseases, infectious processes, and other health precautions.
- Use of the most current evidence and practice guidelines for transporting highly infectious patients. These guidelines are based on the most current information collected from OSHA, WHO, and the CDC, and are meant to be baseline knowledge.

Modified from Air & Surface Transport Nurses Association (ASTNA). Air & Surface Transport Nurses Association Position Statement. https://cdn.ymaws.com/www.astna.org/resource/resmgr/newfolder/astna_position_statement_tra.pdf.

TABLE 13.1   Transmission-Based Precautions

Precaution Type	Description of Pathogen Transmission	PPE Recommendation	Example Pathogens
Contact	Direct or indirect contact with the patient or the patient's environment	Gloves, gown	MRSA, VRE, *C. difficile*
Droplet	Close respiratory or mucous membrane contact with respiratory secretions	Masks (surgical and procedure/isolation)	*Bordetella pertussis*, influenza virus, adenovirus, rhinovirus, *Neisseria meningitidis*
Airborne	Remain infectious over long distances when suspended in the air	N95, powered air purifying respirators (PAPR)	*M. tuberculosis*, rubeola virus (measles), varicella-zoster virus (chickenpox), COVID-19 for aerosol-generating procedures

Data from Centers for Disease Control and Prevention (CDC). Infection control. Transmission-Based Precautions. https://www.cdc.gov/infectioncontrol/basics/transmission-based-precautions.html.; and Seigel JD, Rhinehart E, Jackson M, Chiarello L, and the Healthcare Infection Control Practices Advisory Committee. 2007 Guideline for Isolation Precautions: Preventing Transmission of Infectious Agents in Healthcare Settings. [Updates 2014–2023.] https://www.cdc.gov/infectioncontrol/pdf/guidelines/Isolation-guidelines-H.pdf.

of infectious disease spread but also trigger alerts for emergency dispatchers to relay to responders.[3]

Early screening during the pre-arrival preparation is important to identify patients under investigation for contagious/high consequence infectious diseases by asking about recent travel to areas with active disease. These answers can inform the responding crew as to the level of precautions to take. Similarly, for interfacility transports, querying for and recognizing a potentially infectious diagnosis and using precautions in the sending facility is critical to the transporting personnel. Regardless of known information upon dispatch, it is important to note that all transport team members should approach every transport with judicious caution to protect the entire team to the best of their ability, including the pilot or the emergency vehicle operator.

Scene safety begins with personal accountability, consideration of individual risk, and awareness and utility of the resources available to protect oneself and one's team.

Standard Precautions: Vaccines and Hand Hygiene

Standard precautions "combine the major features of universal precautions and body substance isolation and are based on the principle that all blood, body fluids, secretions, excretions except sweat, nonintact skin, and mucous membranes may contain transmissible infectious agents … and constitutes the primary strategy for the prevention of healthcare-associated transmission of infectious agents among patients and healthcare personnel."[4]

By far, the most effective preventive medical countermeasure to combat the spread of infectious diseases has been the development of safe and effective vaccinations associated with large-scale population-based immunization programs, and should be considered the baseline of routine precautions. Vaccine hesitancy has threatened outbreak control success, as demonstrated in the COVID-19 pandemic[5,6] and has also resulted in the re-emergence of previously unseen diseases, including measles and polio.[7,8]

The Commission on Accreditation of Medical Transport Systems (CAMTS), the primary and most widely recognized medical transport accreditation organization, includes specific preventive health measures for employees in its accreditation standards. In addition to routine health care, measures like vaccinations must be implemented to lessen the likelihood of transmission.[9] Based on the Centers for Disease Control and Prevention (CDC), vaccine recommendations for healthcare workers include hepatitis B, influenza, measles, mumps, rubella, varicella, tetanus, diphtheria, pertussis, meningococcal, and COVID-19.[10]

Building upon standard precautions and vaccines, the next effective infection control measure is hand hygiene. Hand hygiene breaks the chain of infection by stopping the progression of pathogens from healthcare workers to surrounding surfaces (fomites) and directly to patients during care contact. Hand hygiene prevents the survival of microorganisms on the skin when performed correctly, and it should be performed frequently throughout patient care, even if gloves are used (Box 13.2).[11] Hand hygiene compliance of medical providers, including emergency medical service personnel, has repeatedly been shown to be very poor.[12,13] Hand hygiene should occur before and after patient contact; however, time pressures typically associated with the transport of emergent, critically ill, or injured patients should theoretically not play a role in preventing this as routine practice. As a direct intervention, hand hygiene is probably one of the most important measures one can take to prevent both self-contamination and cross-contamination.

It is important to recognize situations in which alcohol-based applications are less appropriate than hand washing with soap and water. Indications specifically for washing with soap and water include the following[14]:

- Hands are visibly dirty or contaminated with proteinaceous material or are visibly soiled with blood or other body fluids
- Before eating and after using a restroom

• BOX 13.2 **CDC Healthcare Infection Control Practices Advisory Committee (HICPAC) Recommendations for Hand Hygiene Clinical Indications**

- Immediately before touching a patient
- Before performing an aseptic task (e.g., placing an indwelling device) or handling invasive medical devices
- Before moving from work on a soiled body site to a clean body site on the same patient
- After touching a patient or the patient's immediate environment
- After contact with blood, bodily fluids, or contaminated surfaces
- Immediately after glove removal

From Centers for Disease Control and Prevention (CDC). Hand Hygiene in Healthcare Settings: Hand Hygiene Guidance. https://www.cdc.gov/handhygiene/providers/guideline.html.

- Potential exposure to specific pathogens including norovirus, *Cryptosporidium*, *Clostridium difficile*, *Bacillius anthracis (anthrax)*, and other spore-forming organisms

Personal Protective Equipment (PPE)

Transport personnel should use barrier precautions to prevent potentially infectious substances from contacting their skin, mucous membranes, clothing, and personal items. Personal protective equipment (PPE) is worn to protect the healthcare worker/wearer from unintentional or accidental exposures to pathogens and even chemicals during patient contact.[15] PPE should be routinely provided by the transport program and be readily accessible to the crew members throughout the different phases of a patient encounter. Common PPE pieces utilized in the critical care clinical setting include gloves, face masks, eye shields, respirators (e.g., N95, powered air purifying respirator/PAPR), and clothing coverage (e.g., gowns, aprons, boot covers). Selection of PPE pieces should always consider standard precautions and evaluate risk based on dispatch/screening information, probable clinical tasks required (e.g., airway suctioning, intubation), and clinical syndromes or conditions warranting empiric transmission-based precautions (Table 13.2).[16] The major and common types of transmission-based precautions are described in Table 13.1.[2,4]

Decontamination Practices

Transport vehicles are difficult environments to thoroughly decontaminate and require attention to detail to prevent nosocomial transmission between patients and the transport crew. During cleaning, crew members should wear appropriate PPE and encourage the mechanics to do so as well. Physical cleaning with the appropriate Environmental Protection Agency (EPA)-registered cleaner is necessary for all equipment and surfaces, with special attention to any areas potentially contaminated with bodily fluids. Knowledge and understanding of the potential pathogens can help determine the appropriate cleaning product. All agencies should have dedicated and explicit infection control policies, that include decontamination protocols with varying levels of cleaning and decontamination of the vehicle and durable medical equipment. Ideally, one would provide the fullest level of decontamination between each patient; however, operational realities may preclude this in practice. At a minimum, medical equipment and vehicle surfaces including frequently touched surfaces should be cleaned after every patient contact. The highest level of decontamination and cleaning should be performed on a regularly scheduled basis and after the transport of patients with highly pathogenic conditions.

Following each patient, the vehicle doors and/or windows should be opened, if possible, to allow for air exchange and all equipment should be removed from vehicle storage locations before cleaning. If any visible contamination is present, it should be addressed first before surface disinfection. All surfaces should be wiped or sprayed with an approved disinfecting agent. Following this cleaning, it is necessary to let the vehicle air dry. Medical equipment and transport devices should be inspected and individually decontaminated. Following completion of the decontamination, the team member should remove his or her PPE and dispose of it appropriately. Multiuse cleaning supplies such as mops should be allowed to soak in a bleach and water or disinfecting solution for greater than 30 minutes.

TABLE 13.2 Clinical Syndromes or Conditions Warranting Empiric Transmission-Based Precautions in Addition to Standard Precautions

Disease	Clinical Syndrome/ Condition	Potential Pathogens	Empiric Precautions
Diarrhea	Acute diarrhea with a likely infectious cause in an incontinent or diapered patient	Enteric pathogens	• Contact precautions (pediatrics and adult)
Meningitis		*Neisseria meningitidis*	• Droplet precautions for first 24 hours of antimicrobial therapy; mask and face protection for intubation
		Enteroviruses	• Contact precautions (infants and children)
		M. tuberculosis	• Airborne precautions if pulmonary infiltrate • Airborne + Contact precautions if potential infectious draining body fluid present
Rash or exanthems, generalized, etiology unknown	Vesicular	Varicella-zoster, herpes simplex, variola (smallpox), vaccinia viruses	• Airborne + Contact precautions • Contact precautions only if *Herpes simplex*, localized zoster in an immunocompetent host or vaccinia virus most likely
	Maculopapular with cough, coryza and fever	Rubeola (measles) virus	• Airborne precautions
Respiratory infections	Cough/fever/upper lobe pulmonary infiltrate in an HIV-negative patient or a patient at low risk for HIV infection	*M. tuberculosis*, respiratory viruses, *S. pneumoniae*, *S. aureus* (MSSA, MRSA)	• Airborne + Contact precautions
	Cough/fever/pulmonary infiltrate in any lung location in an HIV-infected patient or a patient at high risk for HIV infection		• Airborne + Contact precautions • Use eye/face protection if an aerosol-generating procedure is performed or contact with respiratory secretions anticipated • Droplet precautions if tuberculosis is unlikely and no airborne infection isolation room (AIIR) and/or respirators are available • Tuberculosis more likely in HIV-infected individual than in HIV-negative individual
Respiratory infections	Cough/fever/pulmonary infiltrate in any lung location in a patient with a history of recent travel (10–21 days) to countries with active outbreaks of SARS, avian influenza	*M. tuberculosis*, SARS/COVID-19, avian influenza	• Airborne + Contact precautions + eye protection • If SARS and tuberculosis unlikely, Droplet precautions instead of Airborne
	Bronchiolitis and pneumonia in infants and children	Respiratory syncytial virus, parainfluenza virus, adenovirus, influenza virus, *Human metapneumovirus*	• Contact + Droplet precautions • Droplet precautions may be discontinued when adenovirus and influenza have been ruled out
Skin/wound infection	Abscess or draining wound that cannot be covered	*Staphylococcus aureus* (MSSA, MRSA), group A streptococcus	• Contact precautions • Add Droplet precautions for the first 24 hours of appropriate therapy if invasive Group A streptococcal disease is suspected

From Centers for Disease Control and Prevention (CDC). Infection Control. Clinical Syndromes or Conditions Warranting Empiric Transmission-Based Precautions in Addition to Standard Precautions. https://www.cdc.gov/infectioncontrol/guidelines/isolation/appendix/transmission-precautions.html.

Precaution-Based Transports for Communicable Infectious Diseases

Vaccine-Preventable Infections

Pertussis

Vaccinations against pertussis have been available since the 1940s. Despite this, pertussis is the least controlled vaccine-preventable disease in the United States.[17] The highest mortality rates with pertussis are for children younger than 1 year of age, in which death is usually caused by complicating pneumonia. Pertussis should be considered in all patients with chronic cough, however, diagnosis can be challenging because of its three poorly defined stages and symptomatic overlap with most other upper respiratory infection syndromes. Pertussis, or "whooping cough," is caused by infection with *Bordetella pertussis* and is easily transmitted by airborne droplets; thus airborne and droplet precautions are necessary to decrease the risk of nosocomial infection. Antibiotics are effective in the early part of the illness to decrease the overall length of infection as well as the duration of infectivity.

Influenza

Influenza is arguably one of the most talked about infectious diseases. Each year influenza impacts roughly 10% of the population worldwide and is responsible for about half a million deaths.[18] One of the most dramatic examples of the power and impact of infectious diseases is the Spanish Influenza pandemic of 1918. The virus swept across the globe in waves, with more than 50 million fatalities worldwide and an estimated 675,000 killed in the United States.[19]

There are three predominant types of influenza: A, B, and C.[20] Type C is not known to cause significant clinical symptoms or outbreaks. Type A influenza is further broken down into subtypes based on their expressed surface proteins (H and N). Type A viruses are found in humans, ducks, chickens, pigs, whales, and seals. Type B virus is only found in humans. Because the virus slowly changes its genome in the host animals (called antigenic drift), the flu vaccine may only be partially effective in raising antibodies in an immunized person. Thus, it is critical to apply appropriate respiratory PPE in addition to annual vaccination when caring for these patients.

Individuals infected with influenza typically present with fever, cough, myalgias, headaches, and sore throat. However, variations on this presentation are the norm. Transmission occurs primarily via airborne droplets from an infected individual's cough or sneeze, or direct contact with surfaces contaminated with respiratory secretions. Droplet precautions and strict hand hygiene are necessary to prevent self-infection regardless of vaccination status. The mortality of influenza often presents as complicating co-infections and usually impacts those at the extremes of age and the immunocompromised. The most common complicating infection is pneumonia, although myocarditis and encephalitis also occur.

Treatment for influenza is primarily supportive. There are several antiviral medications currently approved for treatment in the United States. Generally, only the neuraminidase inhibitors are recommended for the treatment of those at high risk for complications from the disease.[21] The efficacies of these medications are such that they only shorten the length of illness by 1 day and possibly attenuate the severity of illness. They are not recommended for otherwise healthy people unless they are in a high-risk occupation, such as health care, and only when it can be started within the first 48 hours of illness. Because of the limitations in therapy, many healthcare organizations are requiring masks to be worn by all non-immunized healthcare workers to limit the potential spread of infection.

Hepatitis B

The World Health Organization estimates that there are over 296 million carriers of hepatitis B in the world. Although hepatitis B is a vaccine-preventable infection, it is estimated that there are 1.5 million new cases each year, with over 820,000 deaths annually.[22] Infections with hepatitis B virus can range from asymptomatic carriage through fulminant hepatitis and chronic disease.

Acute infection is similar to most other viral infections with nonspecific fatigue and malaise, often accompanied by a low-grade fever. Subsequently, right upper quadrant abdominal pain may develop, associated with mild nausea and vomiting. Jaundice may develop (30% of cases) and may be exacerbated in those with pre-existing hepatitis infections or liver disease. Diagnosis of hepatitis would be suspected by hepatic enzyme elevations (aspartate transaminase and alanine transaminase) and confirmed with serologic testing. Most patients recover uneventfully from acute hepatitis B infection, although a very small percentage (<0.5%) will develop fulminant hepatitis with consequent hepatic failure and significant fatality rate.[23]

Acute hepatitis B progresses to a chronic state and varies by age and ranges from 50% in young children to 5% in adults. Chronic infection may be asymptomatic or progress to cirrhosis and liver failure. Additionally, chronic hepatitis B infection significantly increases the risk of developing hepatocellular carcinoma. There are multiple treatment regimens for hepatitis B, but all carry significant side effect profiles and significant costs.

Hepatitis B is transmitted by percutaneous or mucous membrane exposure to bodily fluids that contain the virus. Percutaneous exposure by needle stick is the most common route for healthcare workers. With successful completion of the hepatitis B vaccine series however, this route of transmission is rare. If the exposed individual does not have these vaccinations or is found to have incomplete immunity, hepatitis B immunoglobulin may be administered following exposure.

COVID-19

The first reported cases of atypical pneumonia believed to be caused by a novel coronavirus were reported in Wuhan, China in December 2019. This novel coronavirus and its associated infection would be called severe acute respiratory syndrome coronavirus 2 (SARS-CoV-2) and coronavirus disease-2019 (COVID-19).[24] This highly transmissible disease quickly spread from Wuhan throughout mainland China and then globally as a result of travel.

The disease is spread with infectious respiratory droplets however, during aerosol-generating procedures like deep suctioning, airborne precautions may be considered. The disease can also be spread by contact with contaminated environmental surfaces where it can remain stable for days and should be considered when decontaminating the transport vehicle. The common presentation of SARS-CoV-2 infection includes fever, cough, upper airway congestion, sputum production, and dyspnea. Headache, hemoptysis, diarrhea, loss of taste, and loss of smell have also been reported with some cases of infection. Case presentations range from mild symptoms to severe refractory hypoxia, acute respiratory distress syndrome (ARDS), and multisystem organ failure.

The treatment of COVID-19 varies depending on the severity of the illness. Cases with mild symptoms are best supported with rest, ensuring adequate hydration, and fever control with antipyretics. Those cases with severe symptoms such as hypoxemia will require respiratory support, which can range from supplemental oxygen to full-ventilatory support and extracorporeal membrane oxygenation (ECMO). Prone position transports have been used as a modality to assist with oxygenation in critically ill patients with reported success.[25] Other treatments which are currently under emergency use authorization, like antivirals and monoclonal antibodies, target high-risk status patients to reduce their likelihood of hospitalization when infected.[26] High-risk status comorbidities include obesity, diabetes, chronic kidney disease, and weakened immune systems. Current FDA-approved therapies initiated upon hospitalization include remdesivir and baricitinib.[27]

Pneumonia

Pneumonia, an infection of the lower respiratory tract, is usually caused by the inhalation of aerosols containing pathogenic microorganisms or by aspiration of oropharyngeal flora. It may also be caused by hematogenous spread from a distant focus of infection.

The causes of community-acquired pneumonia are classified into three categories: typical bacteria, atypical bacteria, and respiratory viruses, with *Streptococcus pneumoniae* and respiratory viruses being the most commonly identified pathogens.[28] In over 60% of cases the pathogen is unknown; however, when a pathogen is identified, the following are common sources: rhinovirus, influenza virus, coronavirus, *Streptococcus pneumoniae*, *Mycoplasma pneumoniae*, *Staphylococcus aureus*, *Legionella pneumophila*, *Haemophilus influenzae*, *Chlamydophila pneumoniae*, and *Moraxella catarrhalis*.[29] The incidences of the other organisms vary throughout different regions of the country and vary significantly when nosocomial infections are considered.

Classic pneumonia presents with abrupt onset of fever, chills, cough, dyspnea, and physical examination findings of fever, tachycardia, rales/crackles, and/or rhonchi. The clinician should have a high level of suspicion for those with advanced age and/or those who are immunocompromised as the clinical presentation may be atypical. Pneumonia is also a leading cause of sepsis, and therefore patients may present with hypotension, altered mental status, and signs of organ dysfunction.

Diagnosis can be suspected clinically and is confirmed or excluded by radiographic findings while in the hospital. Treatment is supportive with prompt administration of *appropriate* antimicrobial therapy based on the most likely pathogen. Many studies have demonstrated increases in mortality when the administration of appropriate antibiotics for hospitalized patients are delayed beyond 4 hours from identification. Ensuring adequate coverage of potential pathogens while weighing the risks of increasing microbial resistance to antibiotics is crucial. Knowledge of local microbiological prevalence and their susceptibility to particular antibiotics is critical for effectively selecting antimicrobial therapy.

Contact Precaution Transports

Scabies

Scabies is a mite infestation of the skin by *Sarcoptes scabiei* that leads to an intensely pruritic reaction.[30] The itching is a type of hypersensitivity reaction to the mite, its feces, and eggs. The mite itself is barely visible with the unaided eye, and its burrowing habits make it usually unobservable to the patient (Fig. 13.1). The distribution of the infestation aids in the clinical diagnosis because it typically affects the web spaces of the digits, wrists, elbows, the area immediately around the nipples in women, the posterior aspect of the feet, and the lower buttocks.

Scabies in and of itself is an unlikely reason for emergent or critical care transport, however, patients may harbor an infestation during transport for an unrelated condition. Because the transmission is from direct contact or contact with heavily infested clothing/linens, knowledge of the infestation can prevent the spreading of this unwanted guest. Strict barrier precautions, including gown and head cover, are essential to prevent the spread to healthcare workers. If possible, the removal of equipment and linen from use for 3 days after exposure will prevent cross-contamination as the mite cannot survive long away from its human host. If this is not possible, linens and clothing should be washed in hot water and placed in a hot dryer or dry cleaned to kill the mites. Transport vehicles should be vacuumed and cleaned thoroughly, and pesticides are not indicated.

Clostridium difficile

C. difficile is a Gram-positive anaerobic bacterium that produces toxins which cause inflammation of the colon and spores that are

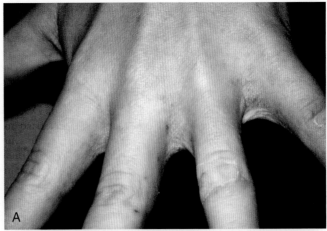

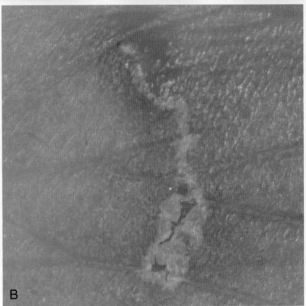

• **Fig. 13.1** Scabies. **A**, In between the fingers is a frequent area for scabies. **B**, The lines indicate burrowing of the organism under the skin. (A, From Micheletti RG, Elston DM, James WD, et al. *Andrews' Diseases of the Skin Clinical Atlas.* 2nd ed. Elsevier; 2023; B, from Rebar CR. Concepts of care for patients with conditions of the skin, hair, and nails. In Heimgartner NM, Ignatavicius DD, Rebar CR, eds. *Medical-Surgical Nursing: Concepts for Clinical Judgment and Collaborative Care.* 11th ed. Elsevier; 2024.)

highly resistant to environmental conditions, affording the active bacteria the ability to survive outside a host. Transmitted via the oral–fecal route, *C. difficile* infection may range from asymptomatic carriage to severe colitis, toxic megacolon with subsequent bowel perforation, and sepsis.[31] Symptoms of infection include diarrhea, fever, stomach tenderness or pain, loss of appetite, and nausea.[32] Standard therapy includes prompt recognition and initiation of vancomycin or fidaxomicin.[31] In severe cases, colectomy may be necessary to provide source control and remove ischemic complications.

Strict contact precautions are necessary to prevent the nosocomial spread of *C. difficile* bacteria and spores. Because of the presence of asymptomatic carriers, it is reasonable to maintain these precautions beyond the duration of diarrhea. The spores can survive on surfaces for several months, so careful attention to decontamination is critical after patient transfer. Given the difficulty in decontaminating some multiuse equipment (such as blood pressure cuffs), the use of disposable supplies may be most appropriate. Environmental cleaning should be performed with products specifically labeled as an EPA-registered sporicidal for *C. difficile* or bleach based, because products that do not carry this label are not effective.

Frequent hand hygiene is a critical step in decreasing transmission as well. Alcohol-based products are *not* sufficient to clean after exposure to *C. difficile* as these are not effective against spores. Vigorous hand washing with soap and water is necessary to remove the spores and is recommended.[33]

Airborne Precaution Transports

Tuberculosis (TB)

Mycobacterium TB can cause infection anywhere in the body, including the kidney, spine, and brain, although predominantly active TB is found in the lung. The bacterium is transmitted by aerosolized respiratory droplets from sneezing, coughing, or during airway interventions (such as intubation or bronchoscopy).[34] Patients without active pulmonary TB also known as latent TB infection, are generally not considered infective. Active pulmonary TB disease symptoms include fever, weight loss, night sweats, malaise, and a minimally productive cough.[35] This presentation may not be different than other respiratory diseases; thus the caregivers must keep TB in their working diagnosis with most respiratory complaints. Certain demographic and historical factors increase the risk for active TB including emigration from an endemic area, prison exposure, homelessness, exposure to others with active TB, active HIV, transplantation, or other immunocompromised states.[36]

Given the airborne droplet transmissibility, all members of the crew should wear submicron, N95 disposable masks during all phases of patient care and throughout the patient encounter. Transport vehicles should maximize fresh air exchange; for example, aircraft with one-direction airflow capabilities should use this during transport to minimize recirculation. Non-intubated patients with active pulmonary TB should be asked to wear a surgical mask, whereas intubated patients should use a high-efficiency particulate arresting (HEPA) filter on the exhalation limb of the vent circuit.

TB is predominantly a treatable condition and potential exposures should be reported to the transport organization and/or public health system as soon as possible. Reporting facilitates close follow-up of the caregiver and definitive diagnostic testing of the potential patient. Most infections remain latent, however, 5%–10% of untreated latent infections will progress to active infections. Treatment for latent TB includes 4, 6, and 9-month regimens which consist of a different combination of medications with variable phases of dosing. Medications included in these regimens for drug-susceptible TB disease are rifapentine, moxifloxacin, isoniazid, pyrazinamide, rifampin, and ethambutol.[37] Drug-resistant TB is increasingly prevalent and can occur when therapy regimens may have previously been misused or mismanaged and the infection has become resistant to isoniazid and rifampin.[38] Extensively drug-resistant (XDR) TB is a very rare disease with resistance to isonazid, rifampin, quinolones, and at least one of the injectable second-line agents.[39]

Measles

Childhood vaccination against measles infection is effective in preventing disease during exposure.[40] Unfortunately, misinforma-tion and vaccine hesitancy has resulted in resurgence of measles outbreaks putting at risk populations, including the very young, elderly, and immunocompromised, who are at greater risk of hospitalization when exposed and infected. The number of reported measles cases between 2018 and 2019 quadrupled from 375 to 1274, the greatest number of cases since 1992.[41]

Clinical manifestations of infection with the measles virus are initially nonspecific upper respiratory illness symptoms typified by fever, cough, runny nose, and conjunctivitis.[42] Following this stage, a rash develops centrally on the body and progresses outward to the face, hands, and feet over the subsequent 3 days. Initially blanchable, the rash develops into non-blanchable spots over the subsequent 4 days (Fig. 13.2). In severe cases, the lesions may become hemorrhagic. The extent of the rash correlates with disease severity. Characteristics of measles infection are Koplik spots, described as small blue–white lesions on the buccal mucosa (Fig. 13.3). Upward of 30% of measles cases develop complications, some of which may be severe.[42] Most commonly, a secondary infection complicates measles because of the immunosuppressive effect

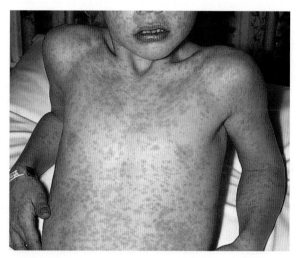

• **Fig. 13.2** Maculopapular rash seen in a child with measles. (From Colledge NR, Walker BR, Ralston SH. *Davidson's Principles and Practice of Medicine.* 21st ed. London: Churchill Livingstone; 2010.)

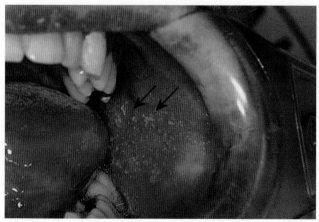

• **Fig. 13.3** Koplik's spots (arrows) seen on buccal mucosa in the early stages of clinical measles. (From Innes JA. *Davidson's Essentials of Medicine.* 3rd ed. Elsevier; 2021. Figure 5.1.)

of the virus. Pulmonary involvement is the leading cause of childhood mortality from measles, followed by diarrhea and central nervous system involvement.

The measles virus is transmitted by respiratory droplets, and aerosolization and precautions against exposure are necessary for at least the first 4 days after the onset of the rash. Measles virus has been found to be suspended in the air up to 2 hours after patient departure. At least a full cabin air exchange should occur before reuse of the transport vehicle.

Varicella

Varicella-zoster virus (VZV) causes two distinct clinical diseases: varicella (chickenpox) and herpes zoster (shingles). Primary infection with VZV causes chickenpox and reactivation of the virus later in life causes shingles. Varicella is usually a mild disease when presenting in childhood, although it can progress to life-threatening when the initial presentation is in adults or in immunocompromised patients.

Following infection with varicella, a prodrome similar to other viral illnesses occurs, including fever and malaise, which is quickly followed by a general vesicular rash within 24 hours.[43] The rash starts as macules and papules that progress to characteristic vesicles, which are extremely pruritic. The vesicles then crust over and form crusted papules (Fig. 13.4). The characteristics of varicella are "crops" of these lesions in different stages of development across the body. New lesions stop appearing usually within 4 days.

Complications of varicella, similar to measles, include primarily superinfection. Central nervous system involvement may occur leading to meningitis or encephalitis. In adults, the development of varicella pneumonia is more common than in children, and it carries a mortality rate of 10%–30%. Those that require mechanical ventilation for pneumonia have mortality rates approaching 50%.[43] Pregnant patients are at risk for maternal varicella, leading to a possible transmission to the neonate with significant mortality. Additionally, primary varicella infection before 20 weeks' gestation puts the fetus at risk for congenital varicella.

VZV is transmitted primarily via aerosolization of nasopharyngeal droplets or by direct contact with fluid found within the vesicles. Patients are contagious until all of the vesicles have crusted over and dried. If possible, non-immune crew members

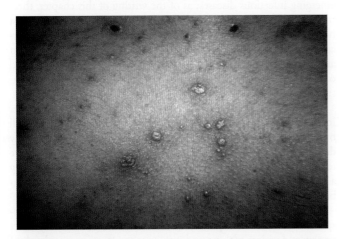

• **Fig. 13.4** Chickenpox lesions on a patient's back, which were displaying the characteristic cropping distribution, manifesting themselves in clusters, each in a different developmental stage. (From Centers for Disease Control and Prevention (CDC). Public Health Image Library (PHIL). https://phil.cdc.gov/Details.aspx?pid=10484.)

who may be pregnant should not be involved with the care of a potentially infected patient or in handling articles potentially contaminated with nasopharyngeal or vesicular discharge. During patient care, crew members should use airborne protection such as an N95 or PAPR and gown and gloves for droplet/contact precautions. This is important even for those crew members who believe they are immune to protect against incomplete immunity and to model behavior for other members of the crew.

Special Considerations for Specific Communicable Infectious Diseases

Meningitis

Bacterial, viral, parasitic, and fungal infections of the central nervous system or its surrounding structures cause inflammation of the membranes called meninges that cover the brain and spinal cord. Typical presentations include fever; headache, neck stiffness, and altered mental status.[44]

Viral meningitis, the most common cause of pathogenic inflammation of the membranes surrounding the brain and spinal cord, generally requires only supportive care with an excellent prognosis in those with normal immune function and vaccines are readily available for the causative viruses like influenza, varicella-zoster, and mumps. Parasitic or amoebic meningitis is relatively rare and can have devastating consequences. Fungal meningitis, usually caused by inhaling spores of these organisms, typically affects those with HIV or poorly controlled diabetes.

Bacterial meningitis, most commonly caused by *Neisseria meningitidis* or *Streptococcus pneumoniae*, requires rapid identification and treatment to impact its high mortality rate.[44] Patients with community-acquired bacterial meningitis are typically quite ill and present quickly after developing symptoms. Aggressive resuscitation with appropriate antibiotics in addition to supportive care is usually necessary. Ideally, a definitive diagnosis should be attempted before initiation of antibiotics; however, if lumbar puncture will be delayed for any reason, blood cultures should at least be gathered because most cases of bacterial meningitis also involve bacteremia.

As the infectious etiology of meningitis is not always known before patient transport, it is important to proceed with precautions to safeguard healthcare worker safety and reduce transmission. It is prudent to initiate airborne precautions in addition to contact/droplet isolation as most meningitis cases are caused by viral sources; however, a definitive diagnosis from a lumbar puncture specimen analysis will be required to confirm and direct appropriate treatment. Close follow-up with the healthcare facility is necessary to ensure that diagnostic culture data are forwarded to the crew members and transport agency.

All members of the transport team, including pilots and emergency vehicle operators, should wear appropriate airborne PPE at a minimum to reduce the risk of exposure to infectious agents. Airflow and air exchanges throughout the cabin and air vehicle should also be considered as an isolation precaution measure and incorporated into decontamination processes (i.e., allow 30–40 minutes of airflow/air exchange before initiating gross decontamination).

Viral Hemorrhagic Fevers

Viral hemorrhagic fevers (VHFs) are a class of diseases characterized by acute febrile illness with bleeding diathesis. Several distinct classes of viruses cause VHF, but they are common in their ability to cause severe multisystem organ dysfunction, including significant damage to the microvascular system of the body. These illnesses cause bleeding, although it is rare for the hemorrhage itself to be life-threatening. All of these viruses depend on animal or insect hosts as reservoirs to propagate infection; however, humans are not the natural host. After transmission from the host, human-to-human transmission is possible. Although there are several known VHFs, this section will concentrate on the Ebola virus because clinical management and personal protection applies to all VHFs.

Ebola infections are severe and often life-threatening in their presentation. A recent significant outbreak from 2014 to 2016 in West Africa affected thousands of people in the region. During the outbreak, citizens from around the globe responded to the region to aid those afflicted by the disease in addition to the travel of local residents out of the affected area. This movement of people in and out of the affected area developed into a situation in which Ebola was being diagnosed and treated outside of the outbreak region. It illustrated the ability for such diseases to be spread easily throughout the world by rapid air travel and ease of transportation. Unfortunately, some of the aid workers who responded to the West African area of need became infected with the Ebola virus, demonstrating the need for coordinated and thoughtful planning to prevent the further spread of the infection.

Symptoms of Ebola (and all VHFs) include the complex of fever, headaches, and myalgias/arthralgias, followed by vomiting and diarrhea with abdominal pain. A few days after symptom onset, maculopapular rashes develop followed by bleeding from ruptured capillaries and microvascular structures. Clinically this bleeding may be from the gastrointestinal tract, ocular mucosa, respiratory tract, and skin. Severe shock and multisystem organ failure then ensue. Treatment is supportive, with a focus on maintaining adequate volume status, supporting oxygenation and hemodynamics, and providing electrolyte repletion.[45] Antiviral medications may shorten the disease course and have been shown to lower 28-day mortality.[46] The use of ring vaccinations to increase immunity within the affected area and for responding healthcare workers has also shown to be effective in reducing disease spread.[47]

Transmission of the virus occurs during contact with an infected animal or (in the case of other VHFs) from bites from infected mosquitoes or ticks. Once a human is infected, transmission can be passed directly through contact or by contact with contaminated objects. There is some concern that Ebola has the ability to be transmitted by airborne droplets during events that may splash bodily fluids such as intubation, venous catheterization, and so forth. Infection control practices are paramount during the transport of these patients and take significant coordination to prevent further nosocomial spread. Unplanned events can alter transport plans and destinations because of security concerns, accidents, and patient clinical events. Dedicated equipment and specifically trained personnel to respond to these high-risk transports are crucial to mitigating these unforeseen events.

Specific instructions in preparing a transport vehicle are beyond the scope of this chapter but are available in several places. Communication and planning with local, regional, and federal health authorities are crucial to a safe transfer and can assist with pretransport planning. Crew members should be well trained and regularly refreshed on the use of appropriate PPE and contingency plans. Box 13.3 lists the CDC recommendations for PPE in caring for potentially infected patients. During patient care, regular and repeated cleansing of gloved hands should be performed using an alcohol-based cleanser. A dedicated monitor should observe and ensure compliance with the appropriate donning and doffing of

---

• BOX 13.3 Recommended Personal Protective Equipment for Ebola Patients

- Single-use impermeable gown (to calf) or coverall
- Powered air-purifying respirator
- N95 is allowed with full face mask and hair covering
- Double-gloved with extended cuffs
- Single-use disposable boots
- Single-use disposable apron

Modified from Centers for Disease Control and Prevention (CDC). Ebola Disease. Guidance on personal protective equipment (PPE) to be used by healthcare workers during management of patients with confirmed Ebola or persons under investigation (PUIs) for Ebola who are clinically unstable or have bleeding, vomiting, or diarrhea in U.S. healthcare settings, including procedures for donning and doffing PPE. https://www.cdc.gov/vhf/ebola/healthcare-us/ppe/guidance.html.

PPE to reduce the risk of self-contamination.[48] Following transport (even with appropriate PPE) of patients with Ebola, personnel should be monitored for fever at least twice daily for 3 weeks postexposure. If the crew member develops a fever greater than 38.3°C, immediate notification of public health authorities is required to evaluate for possible testing and for consideration of high-level isolation.

Emerging Infectious Diseases

Beyond viral hemorrhagic fevers like Ebola, special pathogens and emerging infectious diseases are a national focus and subspecialty of biologic disaster preparedness. Emerging infectious diseases are an umbrella that encompass high consequence infectious diseases that are rare and non-endemic yet may be encountered by healthcare workers in an increasingly globalized society. High-consequence infectious diseases pose a threat to not only healthcare worker safety but also to public health if intense infection control and biocontainment practices are not implemented effectively.

In response to the 2014–2015 US Ebola outbreak, the Administration for Strategic Preparedness and Response (ASPR), designated and continues to fund 10 regional emerging special pathogen treatment centers (RESPTCs), one in each Department of Health and Human Services (HHS) region, to prepare high-level isolation units for the safe care of patients infected with special pathogens and emerging infectious diseases; as of the writing of this chapter, three more have been designated to expand the strategic network.[49] Most notably during the COVID-19 pandemic, the 10 RESPTCs leveraged their expertise to not only support facility-level response but also contributed to regional outreach and coordination, training and educational resource development, and rapid research implementation (Fig. 13.5).[50–52]

ASPR's Health Care Readiness programs (see Fig. 13.5) further include the National Special Pathogen System (NSPS) that will build upon the existing 10 RESPTC infrastructure and newly designated three RESPTCs to improve the US national healthcare readiness to respond to special pathogen encounters by designing a tiered system that coordinates "national expertise, regional capabilities, and state and sub-state healthcare capacity."[53]

It is important for transport teams to be aware of national response strategies and capacities like the RESPTCs as this may affect transport decision-making and influence the frequency or depth of training that may occur based on agency location, proximity, and relationship to RESPTCs.

Transport of special pathogens requires preparation and training to safeguard patients, healthcare workers, and the public as well as

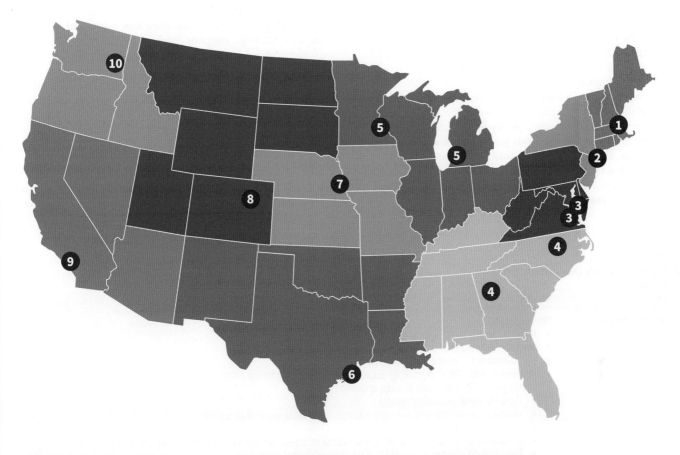

1 CT, ME, MA, NH, RI, VT
- Massachusetts General Hospital

2 NJ, NY, PR, VI
- NYC Health + Hospitals/Bellevue

3 DC, DE, MD, PA, VA, WV
- Johns Hopkins Hospital
- Medstar Washington Hospital Center/
  Children's National

4 AL, FL, GA, KY, MS, NC, SC, TN
- Emory University/
  Children's Healthcare of Atlanta
- University of North Carolina at
  Chapel Hill

5 IL, IN, MI, MN, OH, WI
- University of Minnesota Medical Center
- Corewell Health System

6 AR, LA, NM, OK, TX
- University of Texas Medical Branch

7 IA, KS, MO, NE
- Nebraska Medicine/
  University of Nebraska Medical Center

8 CO, MT, ND, SD, UT, WY
- Denver Health & Hospital Authority

9 AZ, CA, HI, NV, AS, MP, FM, GU, MH, PW
- Cedars Sinai Medical Center

10 AK, ID, OR, WA
- Providence Sacred Heart Medical Center &
  Children's Hospital

• **Fig. 13.5** National distribution of Regional Emerging Special Pathogen Treatment Centers in the United States. (From National Ebola Training and Education Center (NETEC). Annual Report FY2017. NETEC; 2018. https://netec.org/wp-content/uploads/2018/01/NETEC-AR-2017.pdf.)

widescale coordination with local and federal governmental agencies, the receiving facility, and public health. Guidance and resources for this specialty field in transport preparedness continue to grow and best practice support can be found through the National Emerging Special Pathogens Education and Training Center (NETEC) repository in addition to expert support through consultative services for preparedness program development.[54]

Transport of Noncommunicable Infectious Diseases

Toxic Shock Syndrome

Toxic shock syndrome (TSS) is a toxin-mediated illness precipitated by a host response to superantigens and a massive cytokine release.[55] While there are other infections associated with TSS, *Staphylococcus aureus* and *Streptococcus pyogenes* are the most prevalent. Menstrual-related TSS was common in the 1980s in relation to tampon use with a subsequent decline in illnesses after there were changes made in the use and manufacturing of tampons. Non-menstrual staphylococcal TSS is seen postoperatively, postpartum, with soft-tissue injuries, burns, or as a result of pneumonia or influenza infections. Streptococcal TSS is more common with viral infections and local soft-tissue trauma and is associated with high rates of morbidity and mortality.

Symptoms for TSS are similar to many other infectious processes and can include fever, hypotension/shock, myalgias, weakness, and the presence of a skin rash. Skin rash associated with TSS will present a red, macular rash and in some cases involve the mucus membranes. Skin erythema may be more prevalent around surgical sites. Desquamation of the palms and soles about 1–3 weeks after onset is a hallmark sign of TSS but cannot be relied on for diagnosis given the time sensitivity of this disease. Given its similarity to other infectious processes, clinical criteria are listed in Table 13.3, which outlines the Center for Disease Control and Prevention (CDC) TSS Diagnostic Criteria.

Interventions for TSS include shock management, antibiotics, and identification and control of the suspected source. In many cases, there will be a significant capillary leak and fluid resuscitation should be guided by current sepsis guidelines. In addition to fluid resuscitation, vasopressor support may also be needed to support perfusion. Broad spectrum antibiotic coverage is needed and should include coverage for both *S. aureus* and *S. pyogenes*. A thorough assessment for potential sources should also be conducted. This assessment should include a complete skin assessment, removal of foreign bodies (e.g., tampons, packing, intrauterine devices), and exploration and debridement of pre-existing wounds.

Rapid identification of TSS is critical in reducing morbidity and mortality which can be as high as 80%. Box 13.4 outlines common signs and symptoms that should increase suspicion for TSS. If TSS is suspected, the threshold to initiate treatment should be low and not be delayed for definitive diagnosis.

Sepsis

Sepsis is defined as a dysregulated host response to infection which can lead to organ dysfunction and death.[56] Sepsis is a continuum,

TABLE 13.3	CDC TSS Diagnostic Criteria
TSS Type	**Criteria**

Staphylococcal TSS	Clinical Criteria:
	• Fever: > 38.9°C or 102.0°F
	• Rash with diffuse macular erythroderma
	• Desquamation 1–2 weeks after rash onset
	• Hypotension with SBP ≤ 90 mm Hg (adults) or ≤ 5th percentile by age (<16 years old)
	• Multiorgan involvement (three or more systems):
	  • Gastrointestinal (vomiting/diarrhea)
	  • Muscular (severe myalgias or creatine kinase ≥2 times upper limit of normal)
	  • Mucous membrane involvement
	  • Renal (BUN or Cr ≥2 times upper limit of normal or urinary sediment with pyuria with no urinary tract infection)
	  • Hepatic (total bilirubin, ALT or AST ≥2 times upper limit of normal)
	  • Hematologic (platelets ≤100,000/mm³)
	  • Neurologic (alteration in consciousness without focal neurologic signs when fever and hypotension are absent)
	Laboratory Criteria (must be negative if obtained):
	• Blood or cerebrospinal fluid cultures (blood cultures may be positive for *Staphylococcus aureus*)
	• Serologies for Rocky Mountain spotted fever, leptospirosis, or measles
	Classification:
	• Probable: >4 clinical criteria and laboratory criteria met
	• Confirmed: 5 clinical criteria and laboratory criteria met, including desquamation

Streptococcal TSS	Clinical Criteria:
	• Hypotension with SBP ≤90 mmHg (adults) or ≤5th percentile by age (<16 years old)
	• Multiorgan involvement (two or more systems):
	  • Gastrointestinal (vomiting/diarrhea)
	  • Muscular (severe myalgias or creatine kinase ≥2 times upper limit of normal)
	  • Mucous membrane involvement
	  • Renal (Cr ≥2 mL/dL or Cr >2 times upper limit of normal, > twofold elevation from patient baseline)
	  • Hepatic (total bilirubin, ALT, AST ≥2 times upper limit of normal)
	  • Hematologic (platelets ≤100,000/mm³, disseminated intravascular coagulation, or > twofold elevation from patient baseline)
	  • Acute respiratory distress syndrome
	  • Skin (generalized erythematous macular rash that can desquamate)
	  • Soft-tissue necrosis (gangrene, myositis, necrotizing fasciitis)
	Laboratory Criteria:
	• Group A *Streptococcus* isolation from culture
	Classification:
	• Probable: All clinical criteria met and absence of other etiology for illness with isolation of group A *Streptococcus* from nonsterile site
	• Confirmed: All clinical criteria met and isolation of group A *Streptococcus* from sterile site (blood, cerebrospinal fluid, synovial fluid, pleural/pericardial fluid)

ALT, Alanine aminotransferase; *AST*, aspartate aminotransferase; *BUN*, blood urea nitrogen; *Cr*, creatinine; *SBP*, systolic blood pressure; *TSS*, toxic shock syndrome.
Data from Centers for Disease Control and Prevention (CDC). National Notifiable Diseases Surveillance System (NNDSS): Toxic Shock Syndrome (Other Than Streptococcal) (TSS) 2011 Case Definition. https://ndc.services.cdc.gov/case-definitions/toxic-shock-syndrome-2011/; and Centers for Disease Control and Prevention (CDC). Group A Streptococcal (GAS) Disease. Streptococcal Toxic Shock Syndrome. https://www.cdc.gov/groupastrep/diseases-hcp/Streptococcal-Toxic-Shock-Syndrome.html.

• BOX 13.4 Signs or Symptoms Suggestive of TSS

- Diffuse, blanchable erythematous rash with systemic illness
- Young patient with viral-like illness (vomiting, diarrhea, headache, myalgias) and severe septic shock without alternative etiology
- Focal soft-tissue pain that is severe and out of proportion to examination with evidence of systemic toxicity (fever, hypotension, tachycardia)
- Septic shock due to group A streptococcal infection
- Vital signs out of proportion to the degree of infection

TSS, Toxic shock syndrome.

TABLE 13.4 Comparison of qSOFA, NEWS, and SOFA Components

qSOFA	NEWS	SOFA
Respiratory rate greater than or equal to 22 per minute	Respiratory rate	Respiratory support
Altered mentation (GCS)	Oxygen saturation	Coagulation: Platelets
Systolic blood pressure less than or equal to 100 mmHg	Systolic blood pressure	Liver: Bilirubin
	Pulse rate	Blood pressure
	Level of consciousness or new confusion	Glasgow Coma Scale
	Temperature	Kidney: Renal function

composed of three different stages each having specific clinical criteria: *early sepsis*, *sepsis*, and *septic shock*. Identifying patients early in the continuum is critical for reducing mortality associated to sepsis. In 2016, the Society of Critical Care Medicine (SCCM) and the European Society of Intensive Care Medicine (ESICM) introduced the quick Sequential (sepsis-related) Organ Failure Assessment (qSOFA), the National Early Warning Score (NEWS) and the Sequential (sepsis-related) Organ Failure Assessment (SOFA) score. The qSOFA and NEWS scores are used to identify early sepsis, whereas the SOFA score is used to evaluate organ dysfunction.

Early sepsis involves the presence of infection or bacteremia which increases the risk for progression across the sepsis continuum. The use of the qSOFA and NEWS scores allows the clinician to identify patients early with the goal of decreasing sepsis mortality. In Table 13.4 scoring components are listed for these tools. A qSOFA score of two or greater is associated with poor outcomes. If using the aggregate score of qSOFA and NEWS a score of 5–6 is considered a medium risk and 7 or more indicates a high risk of death related to sepsis.

Sepsis differs from early sepsis in that organ system dysfunction is present and there is a known source of infection. An increase in the SOFA score (listed in Table 13.4) by two or more points is indicative of organ dysfunction. While this tool is not diagnostic, it has been proven to be a reliable indicator of those at risk of death from an infection. In addition to scoring, the clinician must take into consideration clinical signs and symptoms of infection as well as radiology and microbiology data to make an official diagnosis.

Beyond early recognition of sepsis, the initial management of the patient should include supporting respiratory needs, establishing venous access with the initiation of fluid resuscitation and early antibiotics, and obtaining a history and patient assessment.[57] The history and patient assessment may afford clues to the source of infection and allow interventions to be made earlier in the continuum. Fluid resuscitation at 30 mL/kg (actual body weight) using a balanced-crystalloid or normal saline should be administered over the first 3 hours. Empirical antibiotics should be initiated within the first hour and target the potential organism or site of infection. Vasopressor support is recommended for those who remain hypotensive after adequate fluid resuscitation.

Summary

As the field of infectious diseases continues to evolve with new outbreaks and the knowledge base of novel and special pathogens like Middle Eastern respiratory syndrome (MERS), SARS, and monkeypox continues to expand, it is prudent for transport teams to approach every transport with awareness and dedication to safety. Lessons learned from the COVID-19 pandemic and ongoing outbreaks remind healthcare workers to utilize the resources available to them, escalate information, and seek guidance early. Transport agencies must devote adequate resources in planning, oversight, and supplies to safely care for and transport these patients. Continuing and frequent education on proper PPE, including its utility, function, and limitations, is crucial to keep crew members safe and ready for the next patient.

References

1. Air & Surface Transport Nurses Association. *Transport of Patients with Serious Communicable Diseases*. Updated 2020. Available at: https://cdn.ymaws.com/www.astna.org/resource/resmgr/newfolder/astna_position_statement_tra.pdf.
2. Administration for Strategic Preparedness and Response; Technical Resources, Assistance Center, and Information Exchange (TRACIE). *EMS Infectious Disease Playbook*. Washington, DC: US Department of Health and Human Service; 2017.
3. AEDR. EIDS tool: the early surveillance system for widespread transmission of infectious disease. *Ann Emerg Dispatch Resp*. October 17, 2020. Available at: https://www.aedrjournal.org/eids-tool-the-early-surveillance-system-for-widespread-transmission-of-infectious-disease.
4. Seigel JD, Rhinehart E, Jackson M, Chiarello L; Healthcare Infection Control Practices Advisory Committee. III: Precautions to prevent transmission of infectious agents. *2007 Guideline for Isolation Precautions: Preventing Transmission of Infectious Agents in Healthcare Settings*. Available at: https://www.cdc.gov/infectioncontrol/guidelines/isolation/precautions.html.

5. Mahmud S, Mohsin M, Hossain S, Islam MM, Muyeed A. The acceptance of COVID-19 vaccine at early stage of development and approval: a global systematic review and meta-analysis. *Heliyon.* 2022;8(9):e10728. doi: 10.1016/j.heliyon.2022.e10728

6. Kattumana T. Trust, vaccine hesitancy, and the COVID-19 pandemic: a phenomenological perspective. *Soc Epistemol.* 2022;0(0):1–15. doi: 10.1080/02691728.2022.2115325

7. Bradshaw AS, Shelton SS, Fitzsimmons A, Treise D. 'From cover-up to catastrophe': how the anti-vaccine propaganda documentary 'Vaxxed' impacted student perceptions and intentions about MMR vaccination. *J Commun Healthc.* 2022;15(3):1–13. doi: 10.1080/17538068.2022.2117527

8. New York declares state of emergency over polio. *BBC News.* September 9, 2022. Available at: https://www.bbc.com/news/world-us-canada-62857112.

9. Commission on Accreditation of Medical Transport Systems. *12th Edition Accreditation Standards.* 2022. Available at: https://www.camts.org/wp-content/uploads/2022/04/12th-Edition-FINAL-draft-03182022.pdf.

10. Advisory Committee on Immunization Practices; Centers for Disease Control and Prevention (CDC). Immunization of healthcare personnel: recommendations of the Advisory Committee on Immunization Practices (ACIP). *MMWR Recomm Rep.* 2011;60(RR-7):1–45.

11. Centers for Disease Control and Prevention. Hand Hygiene Guidance. CDC; 2020. Available at: https://www.cdc.gov/handhygiene/providers/guideline.html.

12. Barr N, Holmes M, Roiko A, Dunn P, Lord B. Self-reported behaviors and perceptions of Australian paramedics in relation to hand hygiene and gloving practices in paramedic-led health care. *Am J Infect Control.* 2017;45(7):771–778. doi: 10.1016/j.ajic.2017.02.020

13. World Health Organization. WHO calls for better hand hygiene and other infection control practices. 2021. Available at: https://www.who.int/news/item/05-05-2021-who-calls-for-better-hand-hygiene-and-other-infection-control-practices.

14. Boyce JM, Pittet D; Healthcare Infection Control Practices Advisory Committee; HICPAC/SHEA/APIC/IDSA Hand Hygiene Task Force. Guideline for hand hygiene in health-care settings. Recommendations of the Healthcare Infection Control Practices Advisory Committee and the HICPAC/SHEA/APIC/IDSA Hand Hygiene Task Force, Society for Healthcare Epidemiology of America/Association for Professionals in Infection Control/Infectious Diseases Society of America. *MMWR Recomm Rep.* 2002;51(RR-16):1–CE4.

15. Occupational Safety and Health Administration. Personal Protective Equipment – Overview. Available at: https://www.osha.gov/personal-protective-equipment.

16. Centers for Disease Control and Prevention. Clinical syndromes or conditions warranting empiric transmission-based precautions in addition to standard precautions. Appendix A: Table 2. Infection Control. CDC; updated February 2017. Available at: https://www.cdc.gov/infectioncontrol/guidelines/isolation/appendix/transmission-precautions.html.

17. Nguyen VTN, Simon L. Pertussis: the whooping cough. *Primary Care: Clin Office Pract.* 2018;45(3):423-431. doi: 10.1016/j.pop.2018.05.003

18. Javanian M, Barary M, Ghebrehewet S, Koppolu V, Vasigala V, Ebrahimpour S. A brief review of influenza virus infection. *J Med Virol.* 2021;93(8):4638–4646. doi: 10.1002/jmv.26990

19. Morens DM, Taubenberger JK, Harvey HA, Memoli MJ. The 1918 influenza pandemic: lessons for 2009 and the future. *Crit Care Med.* 2010;38(suppl 4):e10–e20. doi: 10.1097/CCM.0b013e3181ceb25b

20. Centers for Disease Control and Prevention. Information for Health Professionals. CDC; 2022. Available at: https://www.cdc.gov/flu/professionals/index.htm.

21. Uyeki TM. Influenza. *Ann Intern Med.* 2017;167(5):ITC33–ITC48. doi: 10.7326/AITC201709050

22. World Health Organization. Fact Sheet: Hepatitis B. 2022. Available at: https://www.who.int/news-room/fact-sheets/detail/hepatitis-b.

23. Lok A. Hepatitis B virus: clinical manifestations and natural history. UpToDate. Available at: http://tinyurl.com/bddtcmt8.

24. Tsang HF, Chan LWC, Cho WCS, et al. An update on COVID-19 pandemic: the epidemiology, pathogenesis, prevention and treatment strategies. *Expert Rev Anti Infect Ther.* 2021;19(7):877–888. doi: 10.1080/14787210.2021.1863146

25. Troncoso RD, Garfinkel EM, Leon D, et al. Decision making and interventions during interfacility transport of high-acuity patients with severe acute respiratory syndrome coronavirus 2 infection. *Air Med J.* 2021;40(4):220–224. doi: 10.1016/j.amj.2021.04.001

26. Administration for Strategic Preparedness and Response (ASPR). COVID-19 treatment information for patients. US Department of Health and Human Services. Updated July 2021. Available at: https://aspr.hhs.gov/COVID-19/treatments/Pages/default.aspx.

27. US Food and Drug Administration. Coronavirus (COVID-19) | Drugs. Updated May 2023. Available at: https://www.fda.gov/drugs/emergency-preparedness-drugs/coronavirus-covid-19-drugs.

28. Ramirez JA. Overview of community-acquired pneumonia in adults. UpToDate. Available at: http://tinyurl.com/2z8zs6dy.

29. Rider AC, Frazee BW. Community-acquired pneumonia. *Emerg Med Clin North Am.* 2018;36(4):665–683. doi: 10.1016/j.emc.2018.07.001

30. Centers for Disease Control and Prevention. Parasites – Scabies. CDC; 2021. Available at: https://www.cdc.gov/parasites/scabies/.

31. Smits WK, Lyras D, Lacy DB, Wilcox MH, Kuijper EJ. *Clostridium difficile* infection. *Nat Rev Dis Primers.* 2016;2(1):16020. doi: 10.1038/nrdp.2016.20

32. Centers for Disease Control and Prevention. What is *C. diff*? CDC; review September 7, 2022. Available at: https://www.cdc.gov/cdiff/what-is.html.

33. World Health Organization. Appendix 2: Guide to appropriate hand hygiene in connection with *Clostridium difficile* spread. In: *WHO Guidelines on Hand Hygiene in Health Care: First Global Patient Safety Challenge Clean Care Is Safer Care.* Geneva: World Health Organization; 2009. Available at: https://www.ncbi.nlm.nih.gov/books/NBK144042/.

34. Centers for Disease Control and Prevention. How TB preads. CDC; 2022. Available at: https://www.cdc.gov/tb/topic/basics/howtbspreads.htm.

35. Centers for Disease Control and Prevention. Latent TB Infection and TB Disease. CDC; 2020. Available at: https://www.cdc.gov/tb/topic/basics/tbinfectiondisease.htm.

36. Centers for Disease Control and Prevention. TB Risk Factors. CDC; 2016. Available at: https://www.cdc.gov/tb/topic/basics/risk.htm.

37. Centers for Disease Control and Prevention. Treatment for TB Disease. CDC; 2022. Available at: https://www.cdc.gov/tb/topic/treatment/tbdisease.htm.

38. Centers for Disease Control and Prevention. Drug-Resistant TB. CDC; 2022. Available at: https://www.cdc.gov/tb/topic/drtb/default.htm.

39. Centers for Disease Control and Prevention. Extensively Drug-Resistant Tuberculosis (XDR TB) Fact Sheet. CDC; 2016. Available at: https://tinyurl.com/3kb24kpk.

40. Centers for Disease Control and Prevention. Measles, Mumps, and Rubella (MMR) Vaccination: What Everyone Should Know. CDC; January 2021. Available at: https://www.cdc.gov/vaccines/vpd/mmr/public/index.html.

41. Centers for Disease Control and Prevention. Measles Cases and Outbreaks. CDC; 2022. Available at: https://www.cdc.gov/measles/cases-outbreaks.html.

42. Gans H, Maldonado YA. Measles: clinical manifestations, diagnosis, treatment, and prevention. UpToDate. Available at: https://www.uptodate.com/contents/measles-clinical-manifestations-diagnosis-treatment-and-prevention.

43. Albrecht MA. Clinical features of varicella-zoster virus infection: chickenpox. UpToDate. Available at: https://www.uptodate.com/

contents/clinical-features-of-varicella-zoster-virus-infection-chicken-pox. Accessed October 17, 2022.

44. Mayo Clinic. Meningitis. Available at: https://www.mayoclinic.org/diseases-conditions/meningitis/symptoms-causes/syc-20350508.

45. Bennett JE, Dolin R, Blaser MJ. *Mandell, Douglas, and Bennett's Principles and Practice of Infectious Diseases.* 9th ed. Elsevier; 2020: 2138–2142.

46. Mulangu S, Dodd LE, Davey RT, et al. A randomized, controlled trial of Ebola virus disease therapeutics. *N Engl J Med.* 2019; 381(24):2293–2303. doi: 10.1056/NEJMoa1910993

47. Henao-Restrepo AM, Camacho A, Longini IM, et al. Efficacy and effectiveness of an rVSV-vectored vaccine in preventing Ebola virus disease: final results from the guinea ring vaccination, open-label, cluster-randomised trial (Ebola ça Suffit!). *Lancet.* 2017;389(10068):505–518. doi: 10.1016/S0140-6736(16)32621-6

48. Mumma JM, Durso FT, Ferguson AN, et al. Human factors risk analyses of a doffing protocol for Ebola-level personal protective equipment: mapping errors to contamination. *Clin Infect Dis.* 2018;66(6):950–958. doi: 10.1093/cid/cix957

49. Administration for Strategic Preparedness and Response (ASPR). Press Release: ASPR awards $21 million to health facilities to enhance nation's preparedness for special pathogens. Available at: https://aspr.hhs.gov:443/newsroom/Pages/RESPTC-Prep-Award-24Oct2022.aspx.

50. Garfinkel E, Lopez S, Troncoso R, et al. A critical care transport program's innovative approach to safety during the coronavirus disease 2019 pandemic. *Air Med J.* 2021;40(2):112–114. doi: 10.1016/j.amj.2020.12.002

51. Grein JD, Garland JA, Arguinchona C, et al. Contributions of the regional emerging special pathogen treatment centers to the US COVID-19 pandemic response. *Health Secur.* 2022;20(suppl 1):S-4. doi: 10.1089/hs.2021.0188

52. Flinn JB, Hynes NA, Sauer LM, Maragakis LL, Garibaldi BT. The role of dedicated biocontainment patient care units in preparing for COVID-19 and other infectious disease outbreaks. *Infect Control Hosp Epidemiol.* 2021;42(2):208–211. doi: 10.1017/ice.2020.451

53. Administration for Strategic Preparedness and Response (ASPR). National Special Pathogen System (NSPS): A nationwide, systems-based network approach to special pathogen response. NSPS Fact Sheet, April 2021. Available at: https://aspr.hhs.gov/HealthCareReadiness/COVID-19Resources/Documents/NSPS-FactSheet-April2021-508.pdf.

54. NETEC (National Emerging Special Pathogens Training & Education Center). Consulting for Emergency Medical Services (EMS). Available at: https://netec.org/consulting-services/for-emergency-medical-services/.

55. Gottlieb M, Long B, Koyfman A. The evaluation and management of toxic shock syndrome in the emergency department: a review of the literature. *J Emerg Med.* 2018;54(6):807–814. doi: 10.1016/j.jemermed.2017.12.048

56. Neviere R. Sepsis syndromes in adults: epidemiology, definitions, clinical presentation, diagnosis, and prognosis. UpToDate. Available at: https://www.uptodate.com/contents/sepsis-syndromes-in-adults-epidemiology-definitions-clinical-presentation-diagnosis-and-prognosis.

57. Schmidt GA, Mandel J. Evaluation and management of suspected sepsis and septic shock in adults. UpToDate. Available at: http://tinyurl.com/5dxkva64.

14

Heat- and Cold-Related Emergencies

VAHE ENDER

COMPETENCIES

1. Describe thermoregulation and mechanisms of heat loss.
2. Define mild, moderate, and severe hypothermia.
3. Identify methods to prevent heat loss during patient transport.
4. Identify risk factors that contribute to heat-related illnesses.
5. Identify the different heat-related illnesses, including heat exhaustion and heatstroke.
6. Initiate the appropriate management of a heat-related illness in the transport environment.

Introduction

Regardless of the climate prevalent in their region of clinical practice, transport professionals must be familiar with heat and cold emergencies. Emergency responders working in some of the warmest climates will encounter hypothermia in their clinical practice, just as heat-related illness can be found in patients living in the most frigid environments. Additionally, the resulting loss of thermoregulation seen in critical illness and injury can have a significant impact on the outcomes of patients. As such, it is essential to be aware of these syndromes to maximize the chance of survival of the critically ill patient.

The actual toll of heat- and cold-related illness is unclear, yet as we look back in history, we see evidence of its impact on humanity. However, the toll of temperature extremes is more than just something of the past. As recently as 2003, 52,000 Europeans, predominantly the elderly, were killed by a heatwave; during the peak of this heat, almost 2000 Europeans were dying daily.[1]

Epidemiology

The most vulnerable patient populations are at the highest risk of environmental injury. With age comes the progressive onset of cardiovascular and neurological disorders, which affect one's ability to sense temperature changes. Although the human nervous system is highly sensitive to small changes in temperature, with age comes a loss of sensory acuity. As such, an older person will not sense rising or falling core body temperatures as quickly. Additionally, underlying disease or prescribed medications can suppress intrinsic thermoregulatory mechanisms at a cutaneous and vascular level. People 75 years and older are estimated to have a five times greater chance of death from hypothermia than those younger than 75.[2]

One of the primary sources of body heat originates from skeletal muscle. Sarcopenia, the loss of muscle mass that comes with age, is a fundamental disadvantage in responding to dropping core body temperatures due to impaired shivering. Complicating the matter further is the significant effects of medications routinely prescribed to the elderly, including the subsequent interactions with polypharmacy.

The obese patient is at a greater risk for heat-related illness due to physiologic and anatomic factors. Adipose tissue acts as an effective insulator from the cold. However, the lack of vascularity found in adipose tissue leads to it countering attempts by the human body to cool itself through vasodilatation. Additionally, the weight of adipose tissue against the thorax and diaphragm leads to an impaired ability for the obese patient to match the increased respiratory workload associated with high metabolic states associated with exposure to hot environments.

Infants and neonates are particularly vulnerable to heat- and cold-related illnesses. This is due to a sizeable head-to-body proportion and less tissue insulation compared to adults; as such, a child's body temperature increases 3–5 times faster than an adult's. Additionally, poor motor development leads to infants and newborns being unable to sense and respond to temperature changes and, more importantly, seek protection from the environment.

The challenge of environmental factors resulting in heat- and cold-related injury is also frequently encountered in the homeless population, where due to socioeconomic factors, limited access to water, shelter, and temperature-controlled environments may make them vulnerable during temperature extremes.

Boaters, campers, sailors, hikers, anglers, mountaineers, and others participating in outdoor activities are at risk for environmental injury as they become victims of the environment, physical exhaustion, or carelessness. Outdoor hypothermia is categorized into two groups: immersion and nonimmersion. Examples of nonimmersion hypothermia include exposure to wind, rain, snow, and freezing temperatures. Immersion hypothermia occurs more rapidly than nonimmersion hypothermia; heat loss is 35% higher if the patient swims or treads water rather than stays still.[3,4] A person with immersion hypothermia may drown sooner because the level of consciousness decreases at 30°C (86.0°F).

Methods of Thermal Exchange and Loss

Under normal conditions, 90% of the heat produced by the body is lost to the environment via the skin surface by conduction, radiation, convection, and evaporation. Conduction, together with convection, each account for 15% of heat loss.[4] Conduction occurs when the body directly interacts with a thermal conductor. Examples of good conductors are water, compacted snow, metal, and damp ground. Usually, conduction plays a minor role in heat transfer, but it is an essential factor when the patient has been immersed in cold water, is lying in a snowbank, or is lying on hot asphalt. Heat loss in water is approximately 24 times faster than heat loss in air of the same temperature.[3,4] Immersion in water in temperatures less than 10°C causes hypothermia in only a few minutes, in contrast to more than an hour in air.[5]

Environmental temperature has a direct effect on the patient. The higher the temperature, the more external heat is present. When the environmental temperature is equal to or greater than the body's temperature, passive heat loss through conduction and radiation is decreased. Radiant heat loss, which makes up 45% of total heat loss, occurs when the ambient temperature is lower than the body's temperature; conversely, the body readily absorbs radiant heat from the environment when the surrounding environment is greater than the body temperature.

The primary mechanism for heat dissipation is the evaporation of sweat, which makes up 25% of heat loss. Through vaporization from the body surface, losing 1 mL of sweat reduces body heat load by 1.7 kcal.[1,6–9] Under high ambient temperature and high ambient humidity conditions, the skin cannot provide effective cooling as the evaporation gradient is lost. At 75% humidity, evaporation is significantly reduced; at 90%–95% humidity, evaporation ceases.[6]

Heat-Related Illness

Pathophysiology of Heat-Related Illness

The human body is in a constant state of strict thermoregulation, tightly maintaining a core body temperature of 36–38°C (96.8–100.4°F), all while being exposed to temperatures ranging from the bitter cold of the winter to the scorching summer heat. The hub of thermoregulation is the hypothalamus. Deeply nestled within the brain, this almond-sized structure serves as a control center for the essential parts of the human body, including body core temperature. Input from cutaneous, gastric, and neuronal sensors send stimulus through neurotransmitters and hormones to keep the body within a tight temperature range of ±0.6°C (1.08°F).

Heat Production

Intrinsic heat production is a byproduct of the most fundamental metabolic process in the human body: glycolysis. The muscles of the skeletal system, along with major organs such as the liver, generate significant amounts of total body heat during their essential cellular functions. In an average-sized adult male, approximately 1700 kilocalories are produced daily, though this can increase significantly to nearly twice that with even light to moderate physical activity.[6,10,11] This heat generation can also be increased through intrinsic pathways such as a response to infection or injury.

Fever is an endogenous source of heat caused by an elevation in our thermal "set point," most often as a response to bacteria or viruses which release pyrogens. These stimulate prostaglandin synthesis within the anterior hypothalamus. Fever can also be seen frequently as a response to significant illness and injury, such as post-cardiac arrest syndrome or traumatic head injury where fundamental thermoregulatory mechanisms are disrupted. The mechanism for hyperthermia in heat injury differs from fever, as the human thermal "set point" remains normal in cases of exposure, thus why antipyretics are not an effective means of decreasing core body temperature in heat-injury victims.

This intrinsic heat production can be increased by agents such as illicit drugs, particularly stimulants acting as sympathomimetics, including cocaine, amphetamines, and MDMA. Additionally, with the rising use of novel drugs, such as synthetic cathenones and K2/Spice, Emergency Services are increasingly encountering patients with drug-induced hyperthermia. Additionally, many over-the-counter medications and prescription drugs affect our ability to regulate temperature. Drugs with even mild anticholinergic properties inhibit the activation of sweat glands by sympathetic inhibition, thus impairing one of our primary mechanisms for thermal regulation. Of particular concern are drugs that cause primary hyperthermic syndromes, as seen with psychiatric medications such as lithium, tricyclic antidepressants, and drugs associated with serotonin syndrome (Table 14.1).

The human body is a veritable power plant. If unchecked by environmental heat loss, at rest, core body temperature would rise by 1°C (1.8°F) degree per hour until it would hit the maximal temperature compatible with human life: 43°C (109.4°F). Under maximal exertion, core body temperature would rise by an astonishing 5°C (9°F) per hour without compensatory mechanisms to cool the human body.

TABLE 14.1	Prescription Drugs Associated with Heat Production	
Drug Type	**Example**
Tricyclic antidepressants (TCAs)	Amitriptyline, doxepin
Selective serotonin reuptake inhibitors (SSRI)	Citalopram, fluoxetine, sertraline
Serotonin and noradrenaline reuptake inhibitors (SNRIs)	Venlafaxine
Anticonvulsants	Gabapentin, pregabalin
Antipsychotics – typical and atypical	Haloperidol, risperidone
Antihypertensives – beta-blockers and angiotensin-converting enzyme (ACE) inhibitors	Atenolol, amlodipine, hydrochlorothiazide, valsartan
Diuretics	Furosemide (Lasix), hydrochlorothiazide
Benzodiazepines	Clonazepam, lorazepam, diazepam
Opioids	Morphine, oxycodone, hydromorphone
Medicines with anticholinergic effects	Diphenhydramine, benztropine

From Westaway K, Frank O, Husband O, et al. Medicines can affect thermoregulation and accentuate the risk of dehydration and heat-related illness during hot weather. *J Clin Pharm Ther.* 2015;40(4):363–367.

Heat Loss

Thermal loss due to the environment provides the human body with a fundamental means of offsetting its intrinsic heat generation. Heat loss primarily occurs through the radiation of heat from the warm body to the cooler ambient environment. Thick clothing acts as a barrier for radiating heat away from the body by absorbing the radiated heat and retaining it near the body surface. High environmental humidity also acts as a virtual barrier for this conduction, as it decreases the skin surface-to-air gradient.

Upon exposure to a warm environment, the body will attempt to shift blood towards the periphery to maximize heat exchange, thus promoting heat loss. This hemodynamic change results in decreased systemic vascular resistance and a correlating increase in cardiac output. This increases myocardial workload and oxygen demand. Though this hyperdynamic state can be well tolerated in the young, patients with underlying cardiovascular disease are at increased risk for myocardial injury. It is not uncommon to see rises in cardiac biomarkers in the elderly heatstroke victim as a result of this process. 12-lead ECGs can reveal nonspecific ST-segment changes that are often resolved following supportive care and cooling measures.[12] The respiratory system adapts to this hyperdynamic state by increasing respiratory rates, which increases insensible volume losses through the exhalation of warm, humid gases into the hot air. Metabolically, respiratory alkalosis is caused by hypocarbia.

In severe heat stress, the body loses as much as 1.5 liters per hour, and even 3 L/h in extreme cases.[8,13] This leads to a progressive state of hypovolemia, which, if left uncorrected, leads to a progressive cascade of injury. Hypotension is usually a sign of severe or premorbid heat illness.[8,13]

Ataxia, dysmetria, and dysarthria may be seen early in the onset of heatstroke because the Purkinje's cells of the cerebellum are susceptible to the toxic effects of high temperatures.[14] Because these changes are seen in other neurologic events, such as stroke, heatstroke may not be recognized initially. Cerebral edema and associated diffuse petechial hemorrhage are often found in fatal cases.

When the hyperthermic insult is associated with status epilepticus, the energy requirements of the brain increase. This, in turn, contributes to the spiraling core temperature, increasing up to four times the metabolic rate of the brain. The cerebral vessels dilate maximally; thus, blood flow depends on mean arterial pressure. The added effects of dehydration (hypovolemic source) produce a pathophysiologic state conducive to brain damage and even death.

Kidney function is altered by the loss of sodium and water in sweat. The kidneys retain sodium, causing water retention and the excretion of potassium. Renal dysfunction occurs because of hypovolemia and hypoperfusion. Urinary output drops and acute renal tubular necrosis may ensue. If sodium losses are of sufficient severity, signs of hyponatremia may appear. A risk of hypokalemia may initially develop because of the excretion of potassium in the urine.

The liver, susceptible to temperature damage, is affected in nearly every case.[15,16] Prothrombin times become prolonged.[17,18] Reduced hepatic perfusion caused by shunting of blood to the periphery leads to hypoglycemia in 20% of patients with exertional heatstroke, though its clinical significance is unclear.[19,20] Interestingly, the pancreas is the only organ that does not appear to be damaged by the toxic effects of heat stress.[13]

During heat stress, the gastrointestinal (GI) tract undergoes direct thermotoxicity and relative hypoperfusion because of the shunt of blood to the periphery. Ischemic intestinal ulceration can also occur, which may lead to frank GI bleeding.[13]

Muscle damage is evidenced by rhabdomyolysis. Muscle degeneration and necrosis occur as a direct result of highly elevated temperature. Elevated creatine phosphokinase (CPK) values are a diagnostic hallmark of heatstroke because of this rhabdomyolytic process. The release of destructive lysosomal enzymes occurs due to extensive skeletal muscle damage. The release of lysosomal enzymes into the circulation may cause widespread capillary injury and lead to disseminated intravascular coagulation, acute respiratory distress syndrome, and acute renal tubular necrosis.[20]

Stages of Heat-Related Illness

The most common forms of heat illness, from least to most severe, are heat cramps, heat exhaustion, and heatstroke.

Heat Cramps

Heat cramps involve exquisitely painful sustained muscular contractions, most commonly involving the lower extremity muscles; however, any muscle group in the body can be affected. The patient usually reports heavy exercise in a hot environment, with the onset of cramping after rest. Heat cramps of heavily exercised muscles occur during and after exercise in a hot climate and are an extreme inconvenience to the patient. These cramps usually occur in untrained athletes and non-acclimatized persons. These persons sweat profusely and characteristically replace sweat losses with pure water and inadequate amounts of electrolytes. Hyponatremia ensues, which hinders muscle relaxation mechanisms. Usually, the muscles show fasciculations of fatigue. A slight or moderate rise in CPK enzymes in serum is often observed. These effects have yet to be shown to constitute a significant clinical problem.[7,8,19] No permanent effects have been demonstrated from heat cramps.

Heat Exhaustion

Heat exhaustion is an ill-defined syndrome that can affect anyone. The brain cannot tolerate core temperatures greater than 40.5°C (104.9°F).[7] The typical victim of heat exhaustion is usually not acclimatized to the environment and has worked in the heat for several days. Both infants and elderly bedridden patients are at higher risk of heat exhaustion because of their impaired ability to dissipate heat and communicate thirst.

Heat exhaustion, if allowed to proceed, results in heatstroke. An essential distinction between the two entities is that cerebral function is unimpaired in persons with heat exhaustion, aside from minor irritability and poor judgment. Body temperatures are lower, and the symptoms are less severe in persons with heat exhaustion.

This syndrome results from loss of water, sodium, or both. Pure forms of a single loss of either water or sodium are rare. Water-depletion heat exhaustion, which results from inadequate fluid replacement, is more severe and develops in a few hours. Sodium-depletion heat exhaustion typically develops over the course of several days.

Heat exhaustion is primarily a manifestation of the strain on the cardiovascular system as it attempts to maintain normothermia. With sodium and water loss, the patient becomes dehydrated, tachycardic, and syncopal, with orthostatic hypotension. The patient's temperature is usually less than 38°C to 39°C (100.4°F to 102.2°F) and is often normal. The patient retains the ability to sweat, which gives rise to cool, clammy skin. Headache and euphoria commonly occur because of dehydration and hypoperfusion.

Mental status remains intact, although minor aberrations may be manifested. Flu-like symptoms of nausea, vomiting, and diarrhea with muscle cramps may also be present. Subjective symptoms include intense thirst, vague malaise, myalgia, and dizziness.[21]

Laboratory values show classic signs of dehydration (elevated hematocrit, blood urea nitrogen [BUN], serum protein, and concentrated urine levels) with hyponatremia and hypokalemia, liver function enzymes may also be elevated. These signs, however, may only occur 24–48 hours after the heat injury.[6–8]

Heatstroke

Heatstroke is a life-threatening medical emergency in which the body's physiologic heat-dissipating mechanisms fail, and body temperature rises rapidly and uncontrollably. The central core temperature exceeds 42°C (107.6°F). At 42°C and above, cellular oxygen demands surpass the oxygen supply, and oxidative phosphorylation is disrupted, which causes cell and organ damage throughout the body. The duration of the hyperthermic episode and the temperature reached may be the most critical factors in patient survival and prognosis.

Central nervous system disruption with altered mental status is a crucial diagnostic criterion in heatstroke. Early in the course of heatstroke, some patients may appear confused and show irrational behavior or even frank psychosis; others may become comatose or have seizures. The patient may have hot, flushed skin with or without sweating, vomiting, and diarrhea. Hyperventilation at rates up to 60 is universally seen. Respiratory alkalosis is often present with tetany and hypokalemia. Pulmonary edema is not uncommon.

The cardiovascular system responds by reaching maximal stroke volume. Because vascular shunting through dilated periphery results in impaired forward flow, tachycardia is the only way to increase cardiac output. Heatstroke results in high output failure, with a cardiac output of 20 L or more. As core temperature surpasses 40°C (104°F), progressive heart failure can result in rising central venous pressures. The hyperdynamic state persists even after cooling. The electrocardiographic (ECG) results generally show nonspecific ST-T changes with various atrial and ventricular arrhythmias.[15,22]

Blood studies should include arterial blood gas (ABG), complete blood count (CBC), platelets, prothrombin time/partial thromboplastin time (PT/PTT), electrolytes, blood urea nitrogen (BUN), creatinine, glucose, liver function tests (LFT), creatine phosphokinase (CPK), and lactate dehydrogenase (LDH), and a urinalysis. White blood counts of 30,000 to 50,000 are not uncommon. The platelet count and PT/PTT are monitored for the onset of hypercoagulability. Hypofibrinogenemia and fibrinolysis may occur and progress to frank disseminated intravascular coagulation (DIC).[18]

The muscle enzymes in heatstroke are elevated in the tens of thousands – a diagnostic hallmark. Muscle breakdown occurs from direct thermal injury, clonic muscle activity, or tissue ischemia. In exertional heatstroke, CPK levels up to 1,500,000 IU/L have been reported. CPK levels greater than 20,000 IU/L are ominous and indicative of later DIC, acute kidney failure, and potentially dangerous hyperkalemia.[9,13,15,23]

Reduced renal blood flow from shock and dehydration leads to ischemic kidneys. Acute renal failure is seen in 30% of exertional heatstroke cases and up to 53% of exposure cases resulting in heatstroke; as such, renal function must be closely observed and treated. The urine concentration may lead to the accumulation of uric acid and myoglobin, which can crystallize in renal tubules.

Crystallization may lead to obstructive uropathy and the development of acute tubular necrosis (ATN). BUN levels are frequently elevated. Low serum osmolarity, moderate proteinuria, and dark tea-colored urine (myoglobinuria) often occur in patients with exertional heatstroke.[9,13,16] Additionally, the liver is frequently damaged in heatstroke patients, and frank jaundice may be noted.

Patterns of Heatstroke Presentation

Heatstroke is manifested in three distinct patterns: classic, exertional, and drug-induced. The three essential elements in the diagnosis of heatstroke are exposure to heat stress, internal or external; central nervous system dysfunction; and increased body temperature greater than 40°C (104°F).

Classic heatstroke, which tends to occur in the elderly, the ill, and infants, develops over several days. It often occurs during heatwaves and affects persons who do not have access to a cooler environment or fluids necessary to maintain hydration. In these cases, the patient has hot, red, or flushed skin; has usually ceased sweating; and is significantly dehydrated.

Initial symptoms of classic heatstroke are similar to those of heat exhaustion: dizziness, headache, and malaise, with progression to frank confusion and coma. Fever, tachycardia, and hypotension are additional presenting signs. These patients also hyperventilate, which gives rise to respiratory alkalosis.

Exertional heatstroke usually occurs in young unacclimatized persons, who are often athletes. Physical fitness and conditioning are independent determinants of the risk of heat illness. In a comparison of military recruits where risk was compared across soldiers with varying body mass index (BMI) and conditioning levels, unconditioned normal-BMI soldiers had a twofold risk of heat illness, conditioned but overweight soldiers were at a fourfold risk, and, most striking, poorly conditioned overweight recruits were at an eightfold greater risk of exertional heat illness when compared against conditioned normal-BMI soldiers.[24] As would be expected, environmental factors during exertion matter; hot and humid weather conditions prevent adequate dissipation of generated heat. If the ambient humidity is 100%, the human body cannot use physiologic measures to cool itself in temperatures above 34.4°C (94°F).[25] Of these patients, 50% still sweat profusely from the rapid onset of heat illness; severe dehydration has not yet had time to occur.

Exertional heatstroke produces chills, nausea, throbbing pressure in the head, and piloerection on the chest and upper arms. Concentration wanes, a subjective sense of physical deterioration is noticed, and the person feels increasingly hot, with decreased sweat production. Paresthesia is often noted in the hands and feet.

The onset of irrational behavior occurs. The face turns ashen gray, and the skin may feel relatively cool if sweat is still being produced. This effect is followed by collapse and seizures. Patients with exertional heatstroke often have severe metabolic acidosis from lactate caused by muscle exertion and poor tissue perfusion due to volume depletion. They also have significant rhabdomyolysis.[1,9,26]

Intervention and Treatment

Priorities

The most critical goal and life-saving measure in heat illness is cooling the patient to decrease body temperature rapidly. Immediate treatment, less than 30 minutes after onset, leads to complete recovery.[27] The more rapid the cooling, the lower the risk of mortality. Morbidity and mortality are directly related to the duration and intensity (temperature maximum) of hyperthermia. Performing aggressive cooling before transport is critical to patient survival. The most effective cooling techniques, which require immersion, are often the hardest to continue during transport. A reasonable strategy may be to initiate aggressive measures on scene and to proceed with transport once core temperatures have decreased significantly, with the continuation of cooling by less effective but logistically manageable means.[28]

While the patient is cooled as rapidly as possible, maintenance of the ABCs (airway, breathing, circulation) of emergency care must be remembered. Because the patient may not be able to protect their airway, the transport team must provide effective ventilation and oxygenation, and maintain an adequate circulatory volume with an intact pump while carrying out continuous assessments.

Interventions: Mild to Invasive

Cooling measures for patients with heat-related illness, who are not suspected of suffering from heatstroke, generally follow the progression of:
- Passive external cooling
  - Remove the patient from the hot environment, especially away from hot surfaces, such as concrete and pavement, even if no shaded area is nearby.
- Active external cooling
  - Remove the patient's clothing and place cold packs in vascular areas, such as behind the knees, the axilla, and the groin. Covering the patient with cool fluid and increasing the movement of air over the patient enhance heat loss by increasing the evaporative gradient.
- Passive internal cooling
  - Promoting the patient to breathe in cooled or conditioned air or wall oxygen via blowby or nasal cannula.
- Active internal cooling
  - Cooled intravenous (IV) fluids, gastric lavage[29] with cooled fluids, or other means of invasive temperature management, such as those used to manage post-cardiac arrest patients undergoing targeted temperature management.

Heat cramps constitute a mild form of heat illness. Treatment consists of removal from the source of heat, rest, and fluid and electrolyte replacement. Oral replacement should be started by having the patient drink a balanced electrolyte solution. If oral intake is contraindicated, normal saline solution should be administered intravenously. Mild forms of heat exhaustion are treated similarly. If the patient's body temperature is elevated, the transport team should cool the skin with fans and cool compresses.[26,27]

More severe cases of heat exhaustion necessitate parenteral rehydration. Laboratory values (electrolytes, BUN, and hematocrit) are best used to guide replacement. Fluid is titrated to cardiovascular status. Normal saline solution, half-normal saline solution, and dextrose-half-normal saline solution have all been used; no evidence exists of a clear superiority of any of these fluids.[30] Within 12 hours, patients generally feel well, have typical vital signs, and can be discharged without sequelae.

Heat exhaustion must be regarded on a continuum from the mild case, treated with simple cooling measures, to the severe case, which progresses to full-blown heatstroke. The most important treatment for heat illness is recognition of the hyperthermic insult and rapid initiation of cooling.

When employing aggressive cooling measures, continuous rectal or esophageal thermometry should be used, and cooling measures should be ceased when body core temperature reaches 39°C (102°F) to avoid overshoot. Due to altered thermoregulatory mechanisms, the core temperature will continue to fall to the normal range without further intervention.[16]

Heatstroke necessitates more aggressive methods. Ice-water immersion is a highly effective means of cooling these hyperthermic victims, though performing such a procedure in transport, particularly by aircraft, can be difficult. Considering that less aggressive measures such as fans and ice packs have low cooling efficacy, the benefits of delaying transfer to achieve adequate cooling via cold-water immersion before transport may be beneficial in some cases and should be decided on collaboratively. Alternatively, a modified procedure that does not require complex equipment can be employed prior to and in transport via a conventional body bag, ice, and water to achieve significant gains.[31]

Gastric lavage has been reported to be effective in a controlled canine model.[30] However, evidence is lacking to support its routine use in patients. In severely refractory cases, iced peritoneal lavage, hemodialysis, and cardiopulmonary bypass have been used as "rescue" measures.[8,32,33] These increasingly invasive operative methods require a great resource commitment and have higher risk and complication rates. The value of critical care teams becomes more apparent in their ability to bring these critically ill patients to appropriate centers which might be able to institute these therapies.

Management During Transport

Heatstroke presents a complex patient management picture. If, when the transport team arrives, cooling measures have yet to be implemented or need augmentation, the institution of the previously discussed interventions must be of the highest priority. Therapy is best guided by invasive thermometry, as tympanic and cutaneous thermometers have wide margins of error, especially at the extremes of body temperatures. Placement of an esophageal, urinary catheter or rectal probe with the ability to monitor temperature is essential to the care of these patients. As in any life-threatening case, a secured airway, institution of oxygenation, ventilation, and stabilizing cardiovascular status are critical.

Endotracheal intubation is indicated for any exposure patient with a depressed sensorium because of the risk of emesis, aspiration, and airway obstruction. That being said, resuscitation prior to Rapid Sequence Induction (RSI) may be necessary to decrease the risk of hemodynamic collapse. The combination of volume depletion and the vasoplegic effects of anesthetics require a cautious approach. A systolic blood pressure of 90 mmHg may be a reasonable pre-anesthesia goal, as the literature suggests an associated decreased risk of postintubation cardiac arrest.[34] Induction agents used should be tailored to the patient's hemodynamic state.[21] Following intubation, careful attention should be paid to heatstroke patients requiring mechanical ventilation. Due to their hypermetabolic state, a higher minute ventilation should be maintained to avoid worsening acidosis. Patients with heatstroke are often hypotensive because of dehydration and the physiologic compensation of extreme vasodilatation. In most cases, the hypotension responds to cooling; inotropic agents should be considered once cooling has been performed.

In patients with normotensive conditions or in whom hypotension is readily resolved with cooling, normal saline solution is most often recommended; however, fluid choice should be made in consultation with medical protocols.[33] Vasoactive medications may need to be initiated for vascular support when cooling and fluid resuscitation are ineffective. Because of complications of impaired cardiac function, pulmonary edema, congestive heart failure, adult respiratory distress syndrome, and acute kidney failure, a physical exam should guide fluid replacement and, if available, the use of ultrasound. Field guidelines for fluid replacement recommend an infusion of balanced solution, such as lactated Ringer's, until a systolic blood pressure of 90 mmHg is obtained.[15] Solutions that contain glucose should generally be avoided to maximize absorption.[23]

In the light of the axiom that "the best defense is a good offense," monitoring the patient for multiple organ failure and prompt intervention on the clinical manifestation of such failure are of utmost importance. Placing a gastric tube accomplishes gastric decompression and monitors for the onset of GI bleeding. Protect the GI tract: administer gastric protectants such as proton pump inhibitors or sucralfate, and consider antibiotics to prevent sepsis from bacterial translocation and GI mucosal damage.[23]

An indwelling urinary catheter should be inserted to monitor hourly urinary output and rhabdomyolysis. Because of the possibility of kidney impairment, the transport team must closely monitor and support kidney function. If urine output fails to achieve more than 1 mL/kg after the patient is well hydrated, consider diuretics. After urine flow is initiated, fluid therapy should be continued at two to three times maintenance levels and titrated off.[23]

Liver failure is a frequent complication of heatstroke. When liver failure is combined with kidney failure, the choice of drugs used in treatment becomes difficult. DIC occurs in severe cases; most patients who die of heatstroke have evidence of DIC.[7] Standard treatment measures are instituted.[9] For the prevention of DIC, consider the administration of heparin.[15]

Electrolyte and acid–base imbalances may be manifested. Patients with low serum glucose levels are treated with glucose administration. Both hyperkalemia and hypokalemia are common. Hypokalemia with respiratory alkalosis is transient and needs no treatment; hypokalemia with acidosis necessitates replacement therapy.[1,10] Potassium chloride should be administered for hypokalemia correction.

Hyperkalemia reflects cellular damage and acidosis.[26] Sodium bicarbonate may have to be given for severe metabolic acidosis (pH <6.9). Sodium bicarbonate (0.3 × body weight [kg] × base deficit IV) should be given at 50% of the calculated dose, with subsequent blood gas determinations.[23]

Monitor ECG for arrhythmias. Seizures must be aggressively managed with benzodiazepines followed by second-line antiepileptics such as levetiracetam (Keppra). The neurologic status should be reevaluated constantly. If it deteriorates and increased ICP is suspected, consider mannitol or hypertonic saline.[23]

Summary of Heat-Related Illness

Heat illness presents as a continuum from mild to severe. If untreated, heat exhaustion may proceed to frank heatstroke, a life-threatening medical emergency. Causes of heat illness encompass endogenous, environmental, and drug-related pathologies.

Prompt recognition of the problem and rapid cooling limit the severe sequelae associated with heat toxicity. Various cooling methods are used to limit the duration of exposure to hyperthermia. Research shows that the length of exposure and maximum temperature reached are two critical criteria for the survival and recovery of patients with heatstroke.

Complications of heatstroke affect every organ system and can lead to multiple organ system failure. Liver and kidney failure are

common. Neurologic complications are usually rare, with prompt cooling to achieve euthermia. Cerebellar effects are the residual pathologies most often seen.

The onset of DIC, coma lasting more than 8 hours, cardiac dysfunction, hypotension, and high lactate and CPK levels are ominous signs and are usually predictive of mortality.

Cold-Related Injury

On May 20, 1999, Anna Bågenholm, a Norwegian surgical resident, and a friend set out into the Norwegian mountains for a day of skiing. During a descent, she lost her balance and fell through a sheet of ice head-first, her upper body became trapped under an 8-inch layer of ice, exposed to the frigid glacial waters. Although she was initially able to survive by breathing in an air pocket, she deteriorated into cardiac arrest while rescue teams were attempting to free her from the ice. When she was pulled out of the cold water, she had been trapped for 80 minutes and pulseless for 40 minutes. Resuscitation was started, and she was emergently flown to Tromso University Hospital, an institution that, by chance, was a leading center in the use of cardiopulmonary bypass for hypothermia. Following cannulation and placement onto bypass, she was rewarmed until her heart beat for the first time in over 2 hours. She was stabilized over 9 subsequent hours and survived a complex ICU course. Today, she works as a radiologist at the very same hospital that saved her life. Anna Bågenholm is on record as having one of the lowest body temperatures ever recorded in a survivor of hypothermia: 13.7°C (56.7°F).[35]

Hypothermia, a core body temperature of less than 35°C (95°F), occurs because the body can no longer generate sufficient heat to maintain body functions.[5] *Accidental hypothermia*, in contrast to iatrogenic hypothermia, is the unintentional decrease in core temperature associated with trauma or exposure to the environment.[5,27,36–38] Core body temperature can be measured in the rectum, the esophagus, the bladder, the tympanic membrane, or the bloodstream. Rectal thermometers provide the least reliable measurement of core body temperature. Esophageal thermometry is the most reliable.[4]

Classification

Hypothermia can be both a clinical symptom and a disease. It can be classified as *primary*, with simple environmental exposure in a healthy person, or *secondary*, with hypothermia as a part of a disease process or caused by a predisposing condition.[39] Multiple predisposing factors can place a person at risk of hypothermia. Age, diseases, medications, and type and length of exposure can all contribute to the development of hypothermia. The transport environment can especially place a patient at risk for hypothermia from loss of clothing, wet clothing, lack of environmental protection, medications, diseases and injuries, and lack of environmental control within the transport vehicle itself.[38,40–44]

Hypothermia is classified into four stages. *Mild hypothermia* is defined as a core body temperature greater than 32°C and less than 35°C (89.6°F to 95°F) and is associated with low morbidity and mortality rates. The patient may display symptoms of ataxia, slurred speech, apathy, and even amnesia. Thermoregulatory mechanisms continue to operate.[45] *Moderate hypothermia* occurs when the core body temperature is greater than 28°C but less than 32°C (82–89.6°F). Thermoregulatory actions such as shivering continue but begin to decrease and eventually fail. The patient's level of consciousness continues to decline, and cardiac arrhythmia may develop. *Severe hypothermia* is defined as a core body temperature of 28°C (82°F) or less and is associated with higher morbidity and mortality rates.[29,37,46,47] *Profound hypothermia* occurs at a temperature of 20.0°C to 9.0°C (68.0–48.2°F).[5]

A simplified approach to hypothermia staging has been developed for when core body temperature cannot readily be measured. With an emphasis on clinical symptoms rather than set temperatures, the "Swiss staging system" provides a rapid means of approximating the extent of hypothermia in a victim. This may be helpful as an initial tool in the early stages of managing such a patient before invasive thermometry is placed. These staging criteria and their respective recommended treatments are shown in Table 14.2.

Physiologic Response to Hypothermia[5,29,37,47–52]

The hypothalamus is sensitive to temperature changes as small as 0.5°C (0.9°F).[5] Stimuli sent from the hypothalamus to the sympathetic nervous system increase heart rate and dilate blood vessels in the musculature to increase heat production. In addition, shivering generates heat by increasing muscular activity. At the same time, cutaneous vasoconstriction reduces heat loss by shunting blood from the periphery to the core.[53–60]

The ability to shiver is affected by hypoglycemia, hypoxia, fatigue, alcohol, and drugs. Shivering is the body's primary mechanism of heat production and its strongest defense against hypothermia. However, shivering requires increased blood flow to peripheral muscles. Pre-shivering increases heat production by 50%–100%. Visible shivering increases heat production by up to 500%.[5] An average 70-kg person produces about 100 kcal/h of heat under basal conditions and up to 500 kcal/h when shivering.[5] This degree of heat production, however, cannot be sustained for long because the patient becomes fatigued once glycogen stores are depleted. Maximal shivering occurs at 35°C (95°F) and stops below 32°C (89.6°F). Cessation of shivering when paired with unconsciousness is a sign that the patient has made the transition from moderate to severe hypothermia.[61]

Hypothermia results when the thermoregulation system becomes overwhelmed or damaged centrally at the hypothalamic level or systemically by decreased heat production or increased heat loss. Thermoregulation is disrupted at the hypothalamic level by head trauma, cerebral neoplasm, cerebrovascular accident, acute poisoning, acid–base imbalance, Parkinson's disease, and Wernicke's encephalopathy. An acute spinal injury can eliminate vasoconstrictive control by the hypothalamus. Heat production is decreased by malnutrition, hypothyroidism, hypopituitarism, and rheumatoid arthritis. Typically, 90% of the heat produced by the body is lost to the environment through radiation, conduction, convection, and evaporation.

Metabolic Derangements

Complications of hypothermia result mainly from the sequelae of metabolic derangements. Initially, metabolism increases to generate heat. Optimal metabolism begins to decrease at 35°C (95°F). Symptoms of mild hypothermia consequently include shivering, hypoglycemia, and increased respiratory rate, heart rate, and cardiac output. A dramatic decrease in metabolic rate occurs between 30°C and 33°C (86.0–91.4°F) as the patient transitions from moderate to severe hypothermia. Every 10°C (18°F) decrease in temperature decreases metabolism by half.[5] At 28°C (82.4 °F), all thermoregulation ceases. The liver's metabolic functions also begin to falter at temperatures below 33°C (91.4°F). The liver no longer efficiently metabolizes fats, proteins, and carbohydrates, or drugs, alcohol, and lactic acid. Symptoms of severe hypothermia

---

TABLE 14.2 Hypothermia: Clinical Signs and Recommended Treatment

Hypothermic Stage	Swiss Stage	Core Body Temperature	PRESENCE OF CLINICAL SIGNS			Recommended Treatment
			Shivering	Vital Signs	Consciousness	
Mild	1	33–35°C	Yes	Yes	Yes	Prevent further heat loss Gentle rewarming measures (passive or active if appropriate): changing wet clothes for dry clothes; applying a blanket; drinking warm, sweet liquid Additional *gentle* active rewarming may be appropriate for some patients (i.e., patient exercise/movement)
Moderate	2	28–32°C	No	Yes	Impaired	Rewarming measures: changing wet clothes for dry clothes; carefully insulate/shelter patient from external temperatures; apply external heat source to armpit, groin, trunk Some patients may tolerate active rewarming assistance under direct supervision Transport to tertiary care as soon as possible
Severe	3	21–27°C	No	Yes	No	Prevent further heat loss (i.e., insulation from external temperature) Rewarming measures: apply external heat sources; do NOT give drink/food Careful cardiac monitoring If possible, transport to facility with available cardiac care
Profound	4	<21°C	No	No	No	Prevent further heat loss (very gently) Initiate external rewarming (very gently) Initiate CPR when appropriate (i.e., when it can be continued; do not start and stop) Must be transported to facility with available cardiac care

include the absence of shivering, hyperglycemia, and decreased respiratory rate, heart rate, and cardiac output. Bowel sounds are decreased, if not absent, due to decreased gastric motility and dilatation.[47]

Hypoglycemia is associated with chronic mild hypothermia, whereas hyperglycemia is associated with acute severe hypothermia. Long-term shivering depletes glucose, and glucose stored in the form of glycogen. Shivering can stop at temperatures greater than 33°C (91.4°F) if glucose or glycogen stores are depleted, or insulin is no longer available. Shivering begins again when the core body temperature increases to 32°C (89.6°F) if depleted glucose is replaced. Hyperglycemia occurs below 30°C (86°F) because insulin no longer promotes glucose transport into cells once metabolism significantly decreases.[7,11] Hyperglycemia does not occur if glucose and glycogen stores have been previously depleted but not replaced.

Oxygenation and Acid–Base Disorders

Respiratory rate initially increases after sudden exposure to cold but decreases as body temperature and metabolism decrease.[39] Ventilation is usually adequate at temperatures above 32°C (89.6°F). At 30°C (86°F), respirations are shallow and difficult to observe. Apnea and respiratory arrest commonly occur between 21°C and 24°C (69.8–75.2°F). Although carbon dioxide production also decreases to about half the basal level with each 8°C (14.4°F) drop in temperature, the reduced respiratory rate is inadequate to effectively excrete CO_2 at a temperature below 33°C (91.4°F).[44] Consequently, respiratory acidosis develops in the hypothermia victim.

Cellular respiration is impaired by the decrease in metabolism, drop in cardiac output, and left shift on the oxyhemoglobin dissociation curve. Hypothermia decreases cardiac output by reducing heart rate and circulating blood volume and increasing blood viscosity and peripheral vascular resistance. Blood shifting to the core results in perceived overhydration, and the body responds by removing the extra volume through diuresis. Prolonged hypothermia also causes plasma to leak from the capillaries, thereby increasing blood viscosity by 2% for every 1°C (1.8°F) decline.[39,44]

Hypothermia shifts the oxyhemoglobin dissociation curve to the left at 34°C (93.2°F). Oxygen then binds tenaciously with hemoglobin, reducing tissue oxygen delivery. In addition, Biddle has noted that oxygen consumption was half of normal at 27°C (80.6°F) and, at 17°C (62.6°F), had fallen to one-quarter the normal value.[39,62] Anaerobic metabolism and lactic acid production increase from decreased cardiac output, oxygen delivery, and oxygen consumption. The increase in lactic acid leads to cardiac arrhythmia and death.

The cardiovascular system is more sensitive to the effects of acid–base disturbances than any other body system. Acidosis is commonly associated with asystole, and alkalosis is associated with ventricular fibrillation.[39,63–65] Hypoventilation and lactic acid production lead to respiratory and metabolic acidosis. Acidosis usually corrects itself once the patient is rewarmed. Hyperkalemia is associated with metabolic acidosis, muscle damage, and kidney failure, which may all be present in the rewarmed hypothermic patient. Iatrogenic respiratory and metabolic alkalosis is challenging to treat and should be avoided.

Central Nervous System

The central nervous system (CNS) displays some of the most impressive sequelae in hypothermia patients. Complete recovery is possible even after prolonged cardiac arrest. Hypothermia protects CNS integrity and may allow the brain to withstand long periods of anoxia. Cerebral blood flow decreases 6%–7% for every 1°C (1.8°F) decline until 25°C (77°F) is reached.[39,62] Cerebral oxygen requirements decrease to 50% of normal at 28°C (82.4°F), to 25% of normal at 22°C (71.6°F),[37,64] and to 12.5% of normal at 16°C (60.8°F).[55] The brain can survive without perfusion for about 10 minutes at 30°C (86°F),[66] whereas it can survive for up to 25–30 minutes at 20°C (68°F).[55] Remarkably, Steinmann et al.[57] noted that at 16°C (60.8°F) the brain can survive without oxygen for up to 32–48 minutes.[57,58]

Patients with mild hypothermia are clumsy, apathetic, withdrawn, and irritable. Reflexes are hyperactive at temperatures above 32°C (89.6°F). Below this temperature, the level of consciousness begins to decrease markedly, and patients become lethargic or disoriented and begin to hallucinate. Hypothermia victims may remove jackets, gloves, shoes, and other protective clothing. This reaction is *paradoxical undressing* and is often one of the first signs that patients are becoming severely hypothermic as they can no longer process their temperature.

The cough reflex is absent at decreased temperatures, and aspiration of stomach contents can occur. Coma develops between 28°C and 30°C (82.4–86°F). The pupils dilate and become nonreactive at temperatures below 30°C (86°F). In addition, corneal and deep-tendon reflexes may be absent. At temperatures below 20°C (68°F), the electroencephalographic results, if they are available, would be expected to be flat.[57,58]

Cardiac Arrhythmia

The effects of hypothermia on heart rhythm were noted as early as 1912. Hypothermia was found to produce bradycardia that progressed to asystole.[39,62,67] In 1923, subjects reportedly showed T-wave changes on electrocardiograms (ECGs) after drinking 600 mL of ice water.[68,69] Up to 90% of all patients with hypothermia are believed to have some electrocardiographic abnormality, including atrial fibrillation, sinus bradycardia, and junctional rhythms.[45,70–74]

The heart initially responds to mild hypothermia with an increase in heart rate due to sympathetic stimulation; this response is short-lived. The heart rate then decreases to 50–60 beats per minute (bpm) at 33°C (91.4°F) and to 20 bpm at lower temperatures.[45] Atrial fibrillation with a slow ventricular rate is common at temperatures below 29°C (84.2°F). Studies have found that atrial fibrillation was unusual in mild hypothermia (temperature greater than 32°C [89.6°F]) and was often observed in moderate (32°C to 26°C [89.6–78.8°F]) and moderately deep (less than 26°C [78.8°F]) hypothermia.[75] About half of the cases studied in moderately deep hypothermia remained in sinus, atrial, or junctional rhythm. The atrial fibrillation found in hypothermia patients has been found to spontaneously convert to sinus rhythm after return to normothermia.[63,74]

Changes in the conduction system begin at 27°C (80.6°F) and may be observed as a widened QRS interval and prolonged PR and QT intervals. The Osborne, or J, wave is seen clearly at 25°C (77°F). The J wave is described as an extra deflection at the junction of the QRS and ST segments (Fig. 14.1). The origin of the J wave is unknown. However, the prolongation of the Q-T interval and the presence of J waves are directly related to the severity of the hypothermia.[74] Large J waves (see Fig. 14.1) are seen at less than 30°C (86°F), whereas small J waves are seen at higher temperatures.

Several theories have been offered for the presence of J waves in hypothermia. The J wave may represent hypothermia-induced

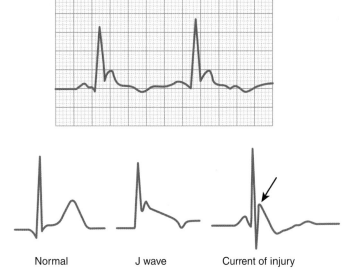

| Normal | J wave | Current of injury |

• **Fig. 14.1** ECG tracing showing the characteristic J, or Osbourne, wave of hypothermia. (From Ender V, Semonin Holleran R. Heat- and cold-related emergencies. In: ASTNA; Semonin Holleran R, Wolfe AC, Frakes MA, eds. *Patient Transport: Principles and Practice.* 5th ed. St. Louis, MO: Mosby Elsevier; 2017. Figure 14.1.)

ion fluxes that cause delayed depolarization or early repolarization of the left ventricle. The J wave is not entirely pathognomonic; it may also be a hypothalamic or neurogenic factor. J waves may also be seen in patients with central nervous system lesions or cardiac ischemia, in patients who are septic, or even in young, healthy people.[76]

Ventricular irritability, which occurs at temperatures less than 30°C (86°F), is commonly associated with alkalosis and is the most lethal cardiovascular response to hypothermia. At 28°C (82.4°F), rough handling or careless intubation can irritate the heart. Ventricular fibrillation can occur spontaneously at 25°C (77°F). Unfortunately, arrhythmia at temperatures below 30°C (86°F) becomes increasingly refractory to drugs and defibrillation because of decreased perfusion and metabolism.

Asystole occurs at 20°C (68°F) but has a surprisingly good prognosis if the patient is rewarmed quickly. Asystole is associated with acidosis and appears to be the primary arrhythmia in accidental hypothermia.[77] One study found that in a review of 73 ECGs of hypothermic patients, atrial fibrillation and junctional bradycardia were associated with poor outcomes.[76]

Circum-Rescue Collapse

Some years ago, physiologists postulated that the collapse that often occurred after victims were removed from hypothermic situations to warm environments was caused by an after drop in core temperature. However, research has shown this belief to be incorrect; the main problem appears to be sudden circulatory changes. This condition is now referred to as *circum-rescue collapse*; it most commonly occurs after rescue from immersion in water but can also be seen in crevasse rescue.[78]

In the water, an increased hydrostatic pressure around the victim's legs and trunk results in an increase in venous return and hence an increase in cardiac output. This increase in central volume is sensed as hypervolemia by the body, and thus, a diuresis and subsequent sodium loss (natriuresis) occur. Peripheral vasoconstriction occurs because of the relatively cold temperature of the water, even in temperate climates, which results in a further increase in venous return and exacerbation of this response.[79]

One suggested mechanism that leads to circulatory collapse is the stress on the myocardium from increased venous and arterial pressures that result in increased catecholamine release. Coupled with hypoxia, the increase in circulating catecholamines may provoke cardiac dysrhythmias. A second part of the theory is that vertical removal from the water causes a sudden release in the hydrostatic pressure around the abdomen and legs and a consequent positional venous pooling in the lower limbs and reduced venous return to the heart. The acute decrease in coronary perfusion may provoke ventricular fibrillation or acute myocardial ischemia, causing death.[78–80]

Frostnip and Frostbite[71,81]

Frostnip, a superficial form of frostbite usually found on the face, nose, and ears, is manifested by numbness and pallor of the exposed skin. Management consists of warming the area with a warm hand or wrapping or covering the area for protection.

Frostbite results from cooling body tissue to the point of ice crystal formation[82] and most often involves the distal extremities. Destruction of the skin produces a more severe injury than frostnip. Although frostbite is commonly associated with below-freezing temperatures, it can be produced at above-freezing temperatures by wind, altitude, humidity, and prolonged exposure. It can be exacerbated by impaired vascular integrity and decreased cardiac output.[54,70]

The injury caused by frostbite has been divided into four phases: the pre-freeze phase, the freeze–thaw phase, the vascular stasis phase, and the late ischemic phase. This pathophysiology results in cell dehydration and shrinkage, abnormal intracellular electrolyte imbalances, thermal shock, and denaturation of the lipid-protein complexes.[71]

Blood cells "sludge" in the vessels and, eventually, circulation to the tissue ceases.[71] Frostbite is classified as first, second, or third-degree. First-degree injury, superficial freezing without blistering or peeling, is characterized by hyperemia and edema. The tissue becomes mottled, cyanotic, and painful after rewarming. Second-degree frostbite produces blistering or peeling of the skin and is characterized by hyperemia and vesicle or bleb formation. When rewarmed, the skin is deep red, hot, and dry to the touch. Third-degree frostbite is characterized by the death of the dermis and even deeper tissue, such as muscle and bone.[81]

Prehospital care focuses on protecting the affected area from trauma and partial thawing.[83] A superficial skin injury can be treated by removing wet clothing and placing warm, dry coverings on the injured area. The affected area should be kept frozen if any possibility of refreezing exists; the site must never be massaged.[83] The patient should not be allowed to walk if the legs are involved unless it is a matter of survival.

Patients should be given ibuprofen, fluids, and pain management with an appropriate analgesic.[27,71,83,84] The affected part needs to be carefully immobilized and protected from additional injury. Patients should be transported to a center familiar with the care of frostbite.

Rewarming Techniques[81,85–88]

Expert consensus is that the patient should be rewarmed as quickly as possible because the myocardium is refractory to therapy below 30°C (86°F). The three techniques for rewarming are passive external, active external, and active internal. Only passive external, active external, and limited forms of active internal rewarming may be able to be initiated in the transport setting. Consequently, rapid transportation to a facility that can provide more extensive rewarming techniques is imperative. Transport personnel must be aware of the existence of these facilities in their service areas.

Passive External Rewarming

Passive external rewarming is simple, inexpensive, and easily instituted. The patient is placed in a warm environment, covered with blankets, and allowed to rewarm naturally. Careful attention should be paid to removing wet clothing and linens from the patient, as it can significantly undermine attempts at rewarming. Passive external rewarming is available in any transport vehicle with a blanket, including foil layers to promote radiant warmth, and a heater. Passive external rewarming increases core body temperature by 1°C (1.8°F) per hour.[62]

Active External Rewarming

Active external rewarming involves the placement of heat on the external surface of the body. Heated blankets, chemical warming pads, and forced air devices such as the Bair Hugger are examples of active rewarming. Devices are also available that circulate warm water around the patient's body. Large electric or chemical heat pads should be placed to contact the axilla, chest, and back where the highest amount of conductive heat transfer occurs.[61,89] It is imperative that precautions be taken when using active rewarming tools to avoid thermal burns; all heat pads should be wrapped in some barrier material such as towels or sheets.

Afterdrop is a phenomenon that can occur in the initial stages of passive and active external rewarming. Afterdrop is defined as a decline of 1–2°C (1.8–3.6°F) in the core body temperature when cool blood from the extremities moves to the core.[49,60] Any action that moves blood rapidly from the extremities to the heart, including moving the patient or injudiciously applying heat to the periphery, can cause this phenomenon. As such, active rewarming of the extremities should be avoided especially considering its lack of efficacy. One study suggests a possible explanation for the afterdrop phenomenon is that the myocardial irritability of afterdrop is caused by a blood chemical shift and not necessarily from a blood temperature shift.[90] There is limited evidence, however, that the physiologic effects of afterdrop are clinically significant.

Active Internal Rewarming

Active internal rewarming delivers heat directly to the body core, thereby avoiding the risk of afterdrop. The heart, lungs, and brain are warmed first and, in turn, rewarm the rest of the body. Heated oxygen, IV fluids, hemodialysis and/or peritoneal dialysis, mediastinal lavage (after chest tube placement), extracorporeal membrane oxygenation (ECMO), and cardiopulmonary bypass are all examples of active internal rewarming. The least invasive method of active internal rewarming is used when the patient has severe hypothermia but a stable cardiovascular condition. On the other hand, the most rapid active internal rewarming methods, such as ECMO and cardiopulmonary bypass, provide the most effective forms of rewarming, are increasingly used by centers to manage profoundly hypothermic patients with hemodynamic instability, and are considered the "gold standard" if the patient has severe hypothermia and an unstable condition with cardiovascular collapse unresponsive to drugs and defibrillation, or cardiac arrest. A patient can be placed onto mechanical circulatory support with a warming unit providing rapid correction of hypothermia through the percutaneous placement of large arterial and venous cannulas.

Management During Transport

Management of hypothermia has been controversial since Napoleon's chief surgeon, Baron Larrey, noted that hypothermic soldiers closest to the fire were the ones who died.[11] Hypothermia experiments in human subjects can be safely performed to only 35°C (95°F), and those in animals are not equivalent because the physiologic response of animals to hypothermia is different from that of humans. Consequently, current medical management of hypothermia patients is based mainly on anecdotal reports in the literature.

All patients with hypothermia should be transported, regardless of cardiopulmonary status. Using the adage "A patient is not dead until warm and dead,"[13,45,46] *warm* is defined as 32°C (89.6°F). Severe hypothermia takes priority over any other problem except obstructed airway or significant trauma with rapid exsanguination.

Preparation for the transport of a patient who is hypothermic should include the following:

1. Gentle removal of all wet clothing and application of dry clothing or insulation system.
2. Keeping the patient supine and avoiding massaging of extremities.
3. Stabilization of all injuries, including applying splints and covering any open wounds.
4. Initiation of intravenous fluids and administration of a fluid challenge.
5. Active rewarming during transport, which should include heated oxygen and truncal heat. Any heating pack used should be adequately insulated to avoid causing burns to the patient. Covering the head with a hat or towels may help rewarming efforts.
6. Wrapping the patient in layers with access available to the airway, breathing, and monitoring equipment. Ideally, the outermost layer should be windproof to decrease exposure to winds encountered during aeromedical evacuation.[63]

Management of the patient with mild hypothermia is relatively uncomplicated; covering the patient with blankets prevents further heat loss and allows the patient to warm naturally. Management of the patient with severe hypothermia is more complicated and tests the expertise and knowledge of medical providers.

Gentle Handling

The patient must be handled gently during transport, minimizing stimulation. Any movement, particularly vertical lifting, has been shown to precipitate ventricular fibrillation. As such, patients should be kept supine. Rubbing or massaging the patient is contraindicated. Medical personnel should always cut clothing rather than pull it off.

Prevention of Further Heat Loss

Prevention of further heat loss is paramount in the management of the patient with hypothermia. Limited exposure during assessment prevents heat loss during the examination. The patient's wet clothing should be removed immediately to prevent conductive and evaporative heat loss. The patient should be removed or protected from any wind source, including helicopter turbulence, which can produce wind up to 100 mph. Insulated and windproofed blankets should be placed under and over the patient, with the face exposed and the patient's head protected with a wool hat. The cold railings of the stretcher conduct heat and should not be allowed to touch the patient during transport. The interior of transport vehicles should be warmed, ideally to 24°C (75.2°F).

Warm oral fluids should be considered for the conscious patient only after an active gag reflex has been confirmed. Aspiration can be a problem, especially if the size of the transport vehicle does not permit the patient to sit upright or at least at a 45-degree angle. Beverages containing alcohol are contraindicated.

Active Internal Rewarming

The respiratory tract is a major area of heat exchange and evaporative loss. Administration of warm, humidified oxygen effectively rewarms the heart, lungs, and brain through bronchial circulation. In addition, the cilia become more active during rewarming and humidification, and can assist in decreasing and mobilizing secretions. Warm humidified oxygen is easy to administer, safe, relatively effective, noninvasive, and largely available in the air medical setting. Mask or bag-valve apparatus at 42°C (107.2°F) to 46°C (114.8°F) should administer 100% warm humidified oxygen. A high flow rate is essential for this method to be effective. Core temperature increases an additional 0.3°C (0.54°F)/h by increasing the ventilatory rate by 10 L/min.

Rehydration of the patient with hypothermia using warm IV fluids increases blood flow to the heart and decreases blood viscosity, vasoconstriction, the potential of afterdrop, and the likelihood of cardiac arrhythmias.[62] Patients with hypothermia appear to have a better chance of survival when a bolus of warm IV normal saline solution is given before the patient is moved or externally rewarmed.[62] The transport team should establish an IV line in the largest vein available. A small amount of heat may be applied to the area to facilitate venous access if needed. The fluid of choice is normal saline, as the liver does not fully metabolize Ringer's solution in severe hypothermia.[62] An adult patient may be infused with at least 200 mL/h, and the pediatric patient with at least 4 mL/kg/h, with adjustment if the patient needs additional fluid resuscitation. Pulmonary edema, jugular vein distention, and other problems associated with fluid overload should be monitored. IV fluids should be administered at 40°C (104°F) to avoid worsening hypothermia. Fluids can be warmed en route by wrapping them in an electric blanket or other commercial warming devices. Fluids can additionally be warmed during administration through the use of commercially available devices.

Monitoring Vital Signs

The patient's temperature, heart rate, and respirations should be monitored carefully and regularly. A special thermometer capable of registering to 20°C (68°F) is necessary for the patient with profound hypothermia. The most accurate means of thermometry is an esophageal thermometer inserted into the lower third of the esophagus, approximately 24 cm for the average adult. The placement of an esophageal probe also avoids the repeated exposure of the patient to obtain temperatures by other means. Both temporal artery and tympanic thermometers frequently used in other healthcare settings are unreliable for measuring temperature in hypothermia and should not be used. Readings from rectal temperature probes lag behind actual core temperature and are influenced by leg temperature and placement of the rectal probe.[62]

Inaccurate assessment of the patient's respirations can lead to improper management and can precipitate life-threatening arrhythmias. The patient must be observed carefully for at least 1 full minute for the presence of respirations to be determined. A spontaneous respiratory rate of 4–6 breaths per minute is adequate in hypothermia. An effective cardiac rhythm may be assumed if the patient is breathing spontaneously. Cardiac monitoring may be difficult because of muscle tremors. Baseline oscillations on the

ECG may be the only sign that the patient is shivering. Blood pressure may not be obtainable or may be inaccurate because of vasoconstriction.

Cardiac Resuscitation

Cardiac resuscitation in the patient with hypothermia is a controversial topic. The main concern is that chest compressions could be initiated on a patient with a slow but viable rhythm. As such, pulse checks should be performed for a full minute. External cardiac massage on a hypothermic bradycardic heart can precipitate ventricular fibrillation. Established ventricular fibrillation or asystole on the heart monitor is the only indication for prehospital CPR of a patient with severe hypothermia.[65] Maximal amplification should be used on the cardiac monitor to detect QRS complexes.

Cardiac compressions should be started according to ACLS guidelines once ventricular fibrillation or asystole is established. If spontaneous respirations are present at any rate, a viable rhythm may be assumed, and CPR may be deferred. In cases of avalanche rescue, it is reasonable to withhold resuscitative measures for victims who have spent more than 35 minutes with an airway obstructed by snow or whose serum potassium is greater than 10–12 mmol/L.[91] Mechanical CPR devices may play a role in transporting cases of hypothermic cardiac arrest, as these devices offer a safer means of providing compressions during transport while minimizing interruptions encountered during litter carries and patient loading procedures. An ultrasound may be useful in assessing the presence of cardiac activity and guiding in the resuscitation of the hypothermic patient. The use of end-tidal capnography can also be an adjunct to guide rescuers in resuscitative efforts.

Though defibrillation may not be as effective in profound hypothermia, some studies suggest the efficacy of defibrillation is higher than previously thought. Although defibrillation is generally more successful at 30°C (86°F) and above, there are case reports of successful defibrillation at temperatures as low as 26°C (78.8°F). It is reasonable to defibrillate ventricular tachycardia/ventricular fibrillation in hypothermia while performing rewarming measures. If core body temperature is below 30°C (86°F), deliver a single shock until rewarming has increased core body temperature. Once 30°C (86°F) has been achieved, standard AHA defibrillation guidelines should be followed.[61]

Pharmacologic Therapy

Little clinical evidence to confirm or rule out the effectiveness or complications of pharmacologic therapy has been noted.[62] Medications should be used with extreme caution. Decreased circulation pools medications in the extremities; a toxic reaction can occur when the patient is rewarmed and medication flows to the core. Considering this possibility, several authors have suggested withholding all medications from hypothermia patients.[62] However, there is limited evidence currently available to contradict the reasonableness of administering epinephrine during resuscitation once core temperature has reached 30°C (86°F). Overzealous resuscitation can precipitate ventricular fibrillation, so dosing intervals should be increased to twice-normal intervals.[91]

Pharmacologic manipulation of pulse, blood pressure, and respiratory rate should be avoided.[62] Medications given during hypothermia can have a prolonged mechanism of action due to decreased metabolic rates; dosing should be adjusted accordingly. Medications given for anesthesia, including anesthetics and paralytics, should have their doses decreased to the lowest-reasonable dose. Medications should not be given orally or intramuscularly because of decreased absorption rates. Other medications should be deferred until the core temperature is 30°C (86°F). The administration of vasopressors and other advanced treatments should never undermine rewarming and resuscitative efforts.

Special Considerations

In the management of cold-related emergencies, transport personnel should consider the following principles:

1. Treat major trauma as the first priority and hypothermia as the second.
2. Remove all wet clothing and apply dry blankets as quickly as possible.
3. Notify the receiving facility as early as possible to allow time for the activation of appropriate resources.
4. Consider transport to an ECMO/CPB-capable center.
5. Monitor temperature via esophageal thermometry when feasible.
6. Avoid vasopressors. Consider them only if hypotension during rewarming is unresponsive to fluids.
7. Follow ACLS guidelines and continue CPR until the patient is rewarmed to 32°C (89.6°F).

Summary

The toll of temperature extremes is most felt by the vulnerable, including children and the elderly. These patients pose a particular challenge to transport teams, but fundamentally, the care of these patients is focused on correcting core body temperature through escalating levels of intervention. The transport team must have the appropriate equipment to care for the victims of environmental exposure. This includes the equipment necessary to warm or cool the patient while providing protection from the environment. Teams should anticipate multiorgan involvement and provide the appropriate supportive care. A collaborative approach to caring for these patients is paramount. Early notification to receiving hospitals to mobilize therapies can help provide the best chance of survival for victims of extreme heat or cold.

References

1. Earth Policy Institute. Setting the record straight: more than 52,000 Europeans died from heat in summer 2003. Plan B Updates. July 28, 2006. Available at: https://www.earth-policy.org/plan_b_updates/2006/update56#.
2. McCauley RL, Killyon GW, Smith DJ, et al. Frostbite. In: Auerbach P, ed. *Wilderness Medicine*. 6th ed. St. Louis, MO: Mosby Elsevier; 2011.
3. Auerbach P. Injuries and illness due to cold. In: Auerbach P, ed. *Medicine for the Outdoors*. 5th ed. St. Louis, MO: Mosby Elsevier; 2009.
4. Giesbrecht G, Steinman A. Immersion in cold water. In: Auerbach P, ed. *Wilderness Medicine*, 6th ed. St. Louis, MO: Mosby Elsevier; 2011.
5. Crawshaw LL, Wallace H, Dasgupta S. Thermoregulation. In: Auerbach P, ed. *Wilderness Medicine*, 5th ed. St. Louis, MO: Mosby; 2007.
6. Epstein Y, Hadad E, Shapiro Y. Pathological factors underlying hyperthermia. *J Thermal Biol*. 2004;29:487–494.
7. Huether SE, Defriez CB. Pain, temperature regulation, sleep and sensory function. In: McCance KL, Huether SE, eds. *Pathophysiology*, 5th ed. St. Louis, MO: Elsevier Mosby; 2007.
8. Platt M, Vicario S. Heat illness. In: Marx J, ed. *Rosen's Emergency Medicine Concepts and Clinical Practice*, 8th ed. St. Louis, MO: Mosby Elsevier; 2013.
9. Sidman RD, Gallagher EJ. Exertional heat stroke in a young woman: gender differences in response to thermal stress. *Acad Emerg Med*. 1995;2(4):315.
10. Hoffman JL. Heat-related illness in children. *Clin Pediatr Emerg Med*. 2001;2:203–210.
11. Kavner L. Bonnaroo festival reports tenth death since 2002. Huffington Post, June 14, 2001. Available at: https://www.huffingtonpost.co.uk/entry/bonnaroo-festival-reports-tenth-death_n_877005.
12. Schlader ZJ, Davis MS, Bouchama A. Biomarkers of heatstroke-induced organ injury and repair. *Exp Physiol*. 2022;107(10):1159–1171.
13. Gaffin SL, Hubbard R. Experimental approaches to therapy and prophylaxis for heat stress and heatstroke. *Wilder Environ Med*. 1996;4:312.
14. Sardana V, Sharma SK, Saxena S. Heat hyperpyrexia-induced cerebellar degeneration and anterior horn cell degeneration: a rare manifestation. *Ann Indian Acad Neurol*. 2019;22(2):244–245.
15. Gaffin SL, Moran DS. Pathophysiology of heat-related illnesses. In: Auerbach P, ed. *Wilderness Medicine*, 6th ed. St. Louis, MO: Mosby Elsevier; 2011.
16. Huether SE, Defriez CB. Pain, temperature regulation, sleep and sensory function. In: Rodway GW, Huether SE, Belden J, eds. *Pathophysiology*, 7th ed. St Louis, MO: Elsevier Mosby; 2016.
17. Bledsoe BE, Benner RW. *Critical Care Paramedic*. Upper Saddle River, NJ: Pearson Prentice Hall; 2006.
18. Iba T, Connors JM, Levi M, Levy JH. Heatstroke-induced coagulopathy: biomarkers, mechanistic insights, and patient management. *EClinicalMedicine*. 2022;44:101276.
19. Centers for Disease Control and Prevention. Heat-related illnesses and deaths – United States, 1994–1995. *MMWR* 1995;44(25):465.
20. Pouton TJ, Walker RA. Helicopter cooling of heat stroke victims. *Aviation Space Environ Med*. 1987;58:358.
21. Westaway K, Frank O, Husband O, et al. Medicines can affect thermoregulation and accentuate the risk of dehydration and heat-related illness during hot weather. *J Clin Pharm Ther*. 2015;40(4):363–367.
22. Wagner C, Boyd K. Pediatric heatstroke. *Air Med J*. 2008;27(3):118–122.
23. Hubbard RW, Armstrong LE. Hyperthermia; new thoughts on an old problem. *Phys Sportsmed*. 1989;17(6):97–113.
24. Bedno SA, Urban N, Boivin MR, Cowan DN. Fitness, obesity and risk of heat illness among army trainees. *Occup Med (Lond)*. 2014; 64(6):461–467.
25. Yousef H, Ramezanpour Ahangar E, Varacallo M. Physiology: thermal regulation. In: StatPearls [Internet]. Treasure Island, FL: StatPearls Publishing; 2023 Jan [update May 8, 2022].
26. Harker J, Gibson P. Heat stroke: a review of rapid cooling techniques. *Intens Crit Care Nurs*. 1995;11(4):198.
27. Cauchy E, Chetaille E, Marchand V, et al. Retrospective study of 70 cases of severe frostbite lesions: a proposed new classification scheme. *Wilder Environ Med*. 2001;12:248.
28. Belval LN, Casa DJ, Adams WM, et al. Consensus Statement: Prehospital care of exertional heat stroke. *Prehosp Emerg Care*. 2018; 22(3):392–397.
29. Proehl J. Environmental emergencies. In: Kitt S, ed. *Emergency Nursing*. Philadelphia, PA: Saunders; 1995.
30. Syverud SA, Barker WJ, Amsterdam JT, et al. Iced gastric lavage for treatment of heat stroke: efficacy in a canine model. *Ann Emerg Med*. 1985;14: 424.
31. Kim DA, Lindquist BD, Shen SH, Wagner AM, Lipman GS. A body bag can save your life: a novel method of cold water immersion for heat stroke treatment. *J Am Coll Emerg Physicians Open*. 2020; 1(1):49–52.

32. Tek D, Olshaker JS. Heat illness. *Emerg Med Clin North Am.* 1992; 10(2):299.

33. Tomarken JL, Britt BA. Malignant hyperthermia. *Ann Emerg Med.* 1987;16:1253.

34. Kim WY, Kwak MK, Ko BS, et al. Factors associated with the occurrence of cardiac arrest after emergency tracheal intubation in the emergency department. *PLoS ONE.* 9(11): e112779.

35. McDonald A, Stubbs R, Lartey P, Kokot S. Environmental injuries: hyperthermia and hypothermia. MacEwan University Student EJournal, 2020; 4(1). Available at: https://doi.org/10.31542/muse.v4i1.1854

36. Antretter H, Muller LC, Cottogni M, et al. Successful resuscitation in severe hypothermia following near drowning. *Dtsch Med Wochenschr.* 1994;119(23):837–840.

37. Ehrmantraut WR, Ticktin HE, Fazekras JF. Cerebral hemodynamics and metabolism in accidental hypothermia. *Arch Intern Med.* 1957;99:57.

38. Frakes M, Duquette L. Body temperature preservation in patients transported by air medical helicopter. *Air Med J.* 2008;27(1):37–39.

39. Collins KJ. *Hypothermia: The Facts.* New York: Oxford University Press; 1983.

40. Gordon AS. Cerebral blood flow and temperature during deep hypothermia for cardiovascular surgery. *J Cardiovasc Surg.* 1962;3:299.

41. Gregory J, Flanbaum I, Townsend M. Incidence and timing of hypothermia in trauma patients. *J Trauma* 1991;31:795.

42. Gregory RT, Patton JF. Treatment after exposure to cold. *Lancet.* 1972;1:377.

43. Hattfield ML, Lang AM, Han ZQ, et al. The effect of helicopter transport on adult patient's body temperature. *Air Med J.* 1999; 18(3):103–106.

44. Hauty M, Esrig B, Long W. Prognostic factors in severe accidental hypothermia: experience from the Mt. Hood tragedy. *J Trauma.* 1987;27;1107.

45. Giesbrecht G, Steinman A. Immersion in cold water. In: Auerbach P, ed. *Wilderness Medicine,* 5th ed. St. Louis: Mosby Elsevier; 2007.

46. Arthurs Z, Cuadrado D, Beekley A, et al. The impact of hypothermia on trauma care at the 31st combat support hospital. *Am J Surg.* 2006;191:610–614.

47. Purdue GF, Hunt JL. Cold injury: a collective review. *J Burn Care Rehabil.* 1986;(4):331.

48. Reuler JB. Hypothermia: pathophysiology, clinical settings and management. *Ann Intern Med.* 1978;89:519.

49. Vaughn PB. Local cold injury-menace to military operations: a review. *Milit Med.* 1980;145:305.

50. Weast RC. *Handbook of Chemistry and Physics,* 55th ed. Cleveland; CRC Press; 1974.

51. Wilson FN, Finch R. The effect of drinking iced water upon the form of the T deflection of the electrocardiogram. *Heart.* 1923;10:275.

52. York-Clark D, Stocking J, Johnson J. *Flight and Ground Transport Nursing Core Curriculum,* 2nd ed. Denver, CO: Air and Surface Transport Nurses Association; 2006.

53. Slovis CM, Bachvarov HL. Heated inhalation treatment of hypothermia. *Am J Emerg Med.* 1984;2:533.

54. Smith DS. Accidental hypothermia: giving "dead" victims the benefit of the doubt. *Postgrad Med.* 1987;81(3):38.

55. Smith DS. The cold water connection. First International Hypothermia Conference, Kingston, Jamaica. January 23–27, 1980.

56. Steinman AM. The hypothermic code: CPR controversy revisited. *JEMS.* 1983;8(10):32.

57. Steinmann S, Shackford S, Davis J. Implications of admission hypothermia in trauma patients. *J Trauma.* 1990;30:200.

58. Tek D, Mackey S. Non-freezing cold injury in a marine infantry battalion. *J Wilderness Med.* 1993;4:353.

59. Tolman KG, Cohen A. Accidental hypothermia. *Can Med Assoc J.* 1970;103:1357.

60. Wilkerson JA, Bangs CC, Hayward JS. *Hypothermia, Frostbite and Other Cold Injuries.* Seattle, WA: Mountaineers Books; 1986.

61. Zafren K, Giesbrecht GG, Danzl DF, et al. Wilderness Medical Society practice guidelines for the out-of-hospital evaluation and treatment of accidental hypothermia: 2014 update. *Wilder Environ Med.* 2014;25:425–445.

62. Danzl DF, Pozos RS, 1987 Multicenter hypothermia survey. *Ann Emerg Med.* 1987;16(9):1042.

63. Danzl D. Accidental hypothermia. In: Auerbach P, ed. *Wilderness Medicine,* 5th ed. St. Louis: Mosby Elsevier; 2007.

64. Okada M. The cardiac rhythm in accidental hypothermia. *J Electrocardiol.* 1984;17:123.

65. O'Keefe KM. Accidental hypothermia: a review of 62 cases. *JACEP.* 1977;6:491.

66. Caroline NL. *Emergency Care in the Streets,* 2nd ed. Boston, MA: Little, Brown; 1983.

67. Knowlton FP, Starling EH. The influence of variations in temperatures and blood pressure on the performance of the isolated mammalian heart. J Physiol. 1912;44:206.

68. Rango N. Exposure-related hypothermia mortality in the United States, 1970–1979. *Am J Public Health.* 1984;74:1159.

69. Rango N. Old and cold: hypothermia in the elderly. *Geriatrics.* 1980;35(11):93.

70. Lunardi N. Case review: ED management of hypothermia in an elderly woman. *Austral Emerg Nurs J.* 2006;8:165–171.

71. McAniff JJ. The incidence of hypothermia in scuba-diving fatalities. First International Hypothermia Conference, Kingston, Jamaica, January 23–27, 1980.

72. McCauley RL, Killyon GW, Smith DJ, et al. Frostbite. In: Auerbach P, ed. *Wilderness Medicine,* 5th ed. St. Louis: Mosby Elsevier; 2007.

73. Miller JW, Danzl DF, Thomas DM. Urban accidental hypothermia: 135 cases. *Ann Emerg Med.* 1980;9:456.

74. White JD. Hypothermia: the Bellevue experience. *Ann Emerg Med.* 1982;11:417.

75. Okada M, Nishimura F, Yoshiro H. The J-wave in accidental hypothermia. *J Electrocardiol.* 1983;16:23.

76. Graham CA, McNaughton GW, Wyatt J. The electrocardiogram in hypothermia. *Wilder Environ Med.* 2001;12:232–235.

77. Rankin AC, Rae AP. Cardiac arrhythmias during rewarming of patients with accidental hypothermia. *Br Med J.* 1984;289:874.

78. Golden FS, Hervey GR, Tipton Jr ML. Circum-rescue collapse: collapse, sometimes fatal, associated with rescue of immersion victims. *Nav Med Serv.* 1999;77(3);139–149.

79. Golden F, Tipton M. *Essentials of Sea Survival.* Champaign, IL: Humana; 2002.

80. Golden FS, Tipton MJ, Scott RC. Immersion, near-drowning and drowning. *Br J Anaesth.* 1997;79:214–225.

81. Mills WJ, Whaley R. Frostbite: experience with rapid rewarming and ultrasonic therapy. Reprinted in Lessons from History. *Wilder Environ Med.* 1998;9:226.

82. Lloyd EL. Accidental hypothermia treated by central rewarming through the airway. *Br J Anaesth.* 1973;45:41.

83. Giesbrecht GG. Prehospital treatment of hypothermia. *Wilder Environ Med.* 2001;12:24–31.

84. Butler FK, Zafren F. Tactical management of wilderness casualties in special operations. *Wilder Environ Med.* 1998;9:64.

85. Davies DM, Miller EJ, Miller IA. Accidental hypothermia treated by extracorporeal blood-warming. *Lancet* 1967;1(7498):1036–1037.

86. Dobson JAR, Burgess JJ. Resuscitation of severe hypothermia by extracorporeal rewarming in a child. *J Trauma.* 1996;40(3):483–485.

87. Lloyd EL, Frankland JC. Accidental hypothermia: central rewarming in the field (Correspondence). *Br Med J.* 1974;4:717.

88. Morrison JB, Conn ML, Hayward JS. Thermal increment provided by inhalation rewarming from hypothermia. *J Appl Physiol.* 1979;46:1061.

89. Hayward JS, Collis M, Eckerson JD. Thermographic evaluation of relative heat loss areas of man during cold water immersion. *Aerosp Med.* 1973;44:708–711.

90. Savard GK, Cooper KE, Veale WL, Malkinson TJ. 1985 Peripheral blood flow during rewarming from mild hypothermia in humans. *J Appl Physiol.* 1985;58(1):4–13.

91. Brugger H, Durrer B, Elsensohn F, et al. Resuscitation of avalanche victims: evidence-based guidelines of the International Commission for Mountain Emergency Medicine: intended for physicians and other advanced life support personnel. *Resuscitation.* 2012;84:539–546.

15

Toxicologic Emergencies

MICHAEL D. GOOCH

COMPETENCIES

1. Identify the common sources of poisoning.
2. Describe the care of the poisoned patient during critical care transport.

3. Name three antidotes for specific poisons.

Introduction

The human environment contains natural and manufactured toxins from plants, animals, chemicals, drugs, and chemotherapeutic agents. A phenomenon that has been increasing over the last several decades is the abuse of prescriptive medications, which has led to an increase in poisonings from medications including sedatives, opioids, and stimulants.[1]

Each year, more than two million human poison exposures are reported to the American Association of Poison Control Centers, which compiles the Toxic Exposure Surveillance System, the largest database of information about toxic exposures in the United States. Over half of these exposures involve medications, and more than 90% of all exposures occur in the victim's home. Others occur in locations such as the workplace, schools, public areas, and numerous other locations. Almost half of the poisonings occur in children less than 6 years of age. Almost 80% of poisonings continue to be unintentional, with over 80% being by ingestion. Sources of unintentional exposure include therapeutic error (too much medication taken/given), bites and stings, environmental exposures, and food poisoning. Intentional poison exposures usually result from suicide attempts, abuse, and intentional misuse of medications.[2]

Safety must be the number one concern when transporting a potentially poisoned patient. Some toxins can cause injury to caregivers, so appropriate decontamination must be accomplished before transport (decontamination is addressed in Chapter 13). Additionally, the team must consider the risks from a patient's current or potential future aggressive behavior related to the poisoning. Clinically, the vast majority of care for a poisoned patient is supportive.[3,4]

The purpose of this chapter is to discuss the general management of the poisoned patient, identify the pathophysiology of selected substances, and describe the management of the poisoned patient during critical care transport.

General Management of the Poisoned Patient

Once team safety is ensured, the initial approach to patient management for a poisoned patient is the same as for any other patient: primary assessment and stabilization, history and physical examination, and laboratory and other clinical studies. Clinical care is always directed at ensuring physiologic safety (patients with inadequate oxygenation or ventilation are supported as described in Chapters 9 and 10). Patients with shock are managed as described in that section of this text. It is on this standard clinical foundation that considerations for specific antidotes and therapies are overlaid.[4-6] Box 15.1 summarizes the care for the poisoned patient.

A patient's medical history and any known history of the events around a toxic exposure provide important information that can help identify a toxin. It is important to have a high index of suspicion; a poisoning should be suspected in any patient whose history suggests the possibility or in any patient whose clinical symptoms are not well explained by other sources. Poisoning or an overdose should be suspected in patients with mental status changes, seizures, altered body temperatures, metabolic and electrolyte derangements, and cardiac arrhythmias. The converse is also true. Pathologic causes of body system alterations must be excluded before attributing them to a toxicologic cause. Any patient rescued from a fire, particularly from a fire in an enclosed space, should be considered as a possible poisoning.[4-6]

The patient may be exposed to a toxin by absorption, inhalation, ingestion, or injection. In the case of a known poisoning, the history should include the type of substance or suspected substance that was taken, the exposure route, the time of the exposure, and the size or dosage of the exposure.[4-6]

If a thorough history cannot be obtained, the environment in which the patient was found should be explored for clues to the

BOX 15.1   Care of the Poisoned Patient by the Transport Team

1. Provide basic and advanced life support after ensuring that the environment is safe for the transport team.
2. Remove the patient from the toxic environment.
3. When indicated, decontaminate the patient by removing clothing and washing off toxin.
4. Administer appropriate antidote when indicated.
5. Assess respiratory, neurologic, and cardiovascular status frequently.
6. Document or obtain baseline data.
7. Ensure the patient and transport team's safety in transport with the use of chemical or physical restraints. With use of chemical restraints, provide adequate analgesia and sedation.
8. Explain to the patient and family the plan of care, along with the patient's destination.
9. Transfer appropriate records and specimens.
10. Consult an expert when patient management questions arise.

TABLE 15.1   Odors Associated with Poisonings

Odor	Possible Poison
Bitter almond	Cyanide
Freshly mowed grass/hay	Phosgene
Fruity or sweet	Isopropyl alcohol ingestion, acetone
Garlic	Arsenic, organophosphates
Wintergreen	Methyl salicylate

Adapted from Erickson TB, Thompson TM, Lu JJ. The approach to the patient with an unknown overdose. *Emerg Med Clin North Am.* 2007;25(2):249–281.

cause of the poisoning; however, this should not delay treatment. Prescription medications, even those prescribed for someone other than the patient; nonprescription medications; and substances in the environment can suggest the etiology of a poisoning. This may be particularly true for pediatric patients. Bottles, containers, or other items may provide additional information about a suspected or unknown toxic substance. These items should be transported with the patient provided there is no risk of harm to the transport team. Identification of witnesses to the event can add more information concerning what may have caused the poisoning or toxic exposure.[4–6]

Medical history, including allergies, previous surgeries, and past hospitalizations, should be noted. When possible, assessment of whether the patient has attempted suicide in the past is important.

In the care of the pediatric or elderly patient, the possibility of abuse or neglect must be kept in mind. A referral may be necessary to outside agencies, including law enforcement, so that the patient's environment may be evaluated to see whether it is appropriate and safe.[4,6]

The physical examination of a poisoned patient should be as orderly and complete as the physical examination of any patient with illness or injury. Obtain a full set of vital signs including a core temperature, if possible. As always, baseline assessment data are particularly important to illuminate changes in the patient's condition during transport.

Some elements of the physical examination can be particularly helpful in identifying a poisoned patient or the nature of a poisoning[4–6]:

- *Neurologic*: Seizure-like activity, abnormal motor movements or behaviors, mental status, pupil size, shape, reactivity, and eye movements, hallucinations, or psychotic symptoms.
- *Respiratory*: Rate, depth, breathing pattern, and adventitious lung sounds. Breath and other odors may suggest a particular poisoning or help rule out another cause. For example, the smell of oil of wintergreen can indicate salicylate poisoning. Table 15.1 lists odors associated with certain poisonings.[5]
- *Cardiovascular*: A full 12-lead electrocardiogram (ECG), ECG rhythm abnormalities, and conduction intervals, especially the QRS duration and corrected QT interval (QTc).
- *Cutaneous*: Skin color, temperature, moisture, and the presence of abnormal rashes, erythema, cutaneous bullae, petechiae, or the presence of injection or burn marks.

Assessment findings rather than laboratory results alone should guide the management. The single most important laboratory study is a rapid glucose assessment in any patient with a mental status change or presumed poisoning. Other baseline studies, such as the metabolic panels, complete blood count, coagulation studies, and a blood gas, can be helpful. Evaluation of the anion gap can be helpful in developing differentials in patients who are acidotic and suspected of a toxic poisoning. The anion gap can be calculated by using this formula: $(Na^+ \pm K^+) - (Cl^- + HCO_3^-)$. A normal serum gap is often considered to be 12 ± 4 mEq/L. Transport providers should be concerned about toxic exposures in any patient with an anion gap metabolic acidosis.[4–6] Table 15.2 lists common causes of a gap acidosis using the mnemonic MUDPILES.

Serum levels of therapeutic drugs and "tox screens" can be difficult to interpret because the level of specific toxins may be incongruous with clinical manifestations. Most drug screens evaluate for the metabolites of commonly abused drugs; if the patient has not been exposed to those substances or has received them as part of a treatment regimen, then these screens are not necessarily helpful. The timing is also important. If the specimen is collected too late or early, it may affect the results. Some substances or screens may yield false-positive and false-negative results. Presence of a positive result on a drug screen also does not necessarily imply toxicity.[4–6] Some regular screening, however, is important. Any patient with a presumed or possible ingestion

TABLE 15.2   Causes of Anion Gap Metabolic Acidosis

M	Methanol
U	Uremia (renal failure)
D	Diabetic ketoacidosis
P	Propylene glycol (preservative in some intravenous medications)
I	Ingestion, iron, isoniazid
L	Lactic acidosis
E	Ethylene glycol
S	Salicylates (aspirin)

Modified from Erickson TB, Thompson TM, Lu JJ. The approach to the patient with an unknown overdose. *Emerg Med Clin North Am.* 2007;25(2):249–281; Murray L, Daly F, Little M, Cadogan M. *Toxicology Handbook.* 2nd ed. Sydney, NSW: Churchill Livingstone; 2011.

should have aspirin and acetaminophen levels tested. In particular, the history does not suggest ingestion in up to 2.2% of patients with toxic acetaminophen levels. Female patients of childbearing years should have a pregnancy test.[5,7–9]

Although multiple substances and various sources of toxins and poisons exist, only a limited number of specific antidotes are available. Again, supportive, standard critical care is the foundation of toxicologic management. Table 15.3 lists most of the available antidotes that may be useful in the management of a poisoned patient.

Drug removal can also be helpful. The most common method of gastrointestinal (GI) decontamination is accomplished with the administration of activated charcoal. Charcoal is effective in limiting the absorption of most ingested substances but must be given within the first few hours, or less, of the ingestion to have a significant benefit. Table 15.4 lists agents that are not amenable to activated charcoal, which can be remembered by the mnemonic PHAILS. Activated charcoal should be used cautiously in those with altered mental status or those at risk for altered airway reflexes. Whole bowel irrigation with an osmotic agent such as polyethylene glycol solution may be an effective option for some toxins as well.[4–6] Enhanced elimination can also be accomplished with the alkalinization of the poisoned patient's urine, which causes an ion-trapping diuresis to facilitate elimination of some acids. For alkalinization of urine, sodium bicarbonate is added to intravenous (IV) fluids, which are administered to yield a urine pH of 7.5. The patient must be monitored closely for complications from fluid and electrolyte imbalances, especially hypokalemia.[4–6] Some poisons are amenable to removal by dialysis.

Pharmacologic Properties of Drugs

Therapeutic dose responses are affected by multiple variables including the rate of absorption, distribution, binding or localization in tissues, inactivation, and excretion. The *rate of absorption* is defined as the time needed for ingested substances to cross the enterovascular barriers and circulate in the cardiovascular system. Agents dissolved in solution are absorbed more rapidly than those in solid forms. Timed-release or enteric-coated products are engineered to greatly decrease the absorption rate. Medications given in higher concentrations are absorbed more rapidly.

Most drugs are administered orally. Sites of absorption include the oral mucous membranes, stomach, and small intestine. Sublingual or buccal administration usually promotes quick absorption and rapid distribution. Absorption in the stomach is a passive process mediated by dissolution and diffusion. The nonionized form of a dissolved medication passes the mucosal barriers and enters the vascular compartment. Most drugs are either weak bases or weak acids. Gastric pH and contents affect both dissolution and diffusion. Weak acids, such as salicylates and barbiturates, are predominantly nonionized in a strongly acidic environment; therefore they are readily absorbed. Weak bases are in an ionized form in the stomach and are poorly absorbed. The intestinal pH is approximately 6.0 and much less acidic than the stomach pH of 1.5–3.0. Weak bases are readily absorbed, but weak acids cross the mucosal barrier less readily. In addition, the gastric mucosa is a lipid membrane, which absorbs lipid-soluble substances, such as alcohol, rapidly. Factors that change gastric emptying time also alter the rate of absorption of a drug. IV injection achieves the most immediate and is the most immediate and consistent blood concentration for any drug. After injection, a redistribution phase may significantly decrease the blood level of the drug. Absorption of

TABLE 15.3	Toxin Antidotes and Reversals
Toxic Agent	**Antidote-Reversal Agents**
Acetaminophen	N-Acetylcysteine (Mucomyst, Acedote)
Acetylcholinesterase inhibitors (cholinergic agents, e.g., organophosphates, nerve agents, carbamates)	Atropine and pralidoxime (2-PAM)
Anticholinergics (e.g., antihistamines, antispasmodics, some antiparkinsonism, antipsychotics, some antidepressants, phenothiazines)	Physostigmine, rarely used
Benzodiazepines	Flumazenil (Romazicon), rarely used
Beta-blockers and calcium channel blockers	Glucagon, calcium, high-dose insulin therapy, intravenous lipid emulsion therapy
Carbon monoxide	High-flow oxygen
Cyanide	Hydroxocobalamin (Cyanokit)
Digoxin	Digoxin Fab antibodies
Heavy metals (e.g., lead, mercury, arsenic)	Edetate calcium disodium (EDTA), dimercaprol (BAL), succimer (DMSA), or d-penicillamine
Heparin	Protamine
Iron	Deferoxamine
Methemoglobinemic agents (e.g., nitrates, topical anesthetics)	Methylene blue
R: Reserpine O: Opioids C: Clonidine L: Diphenoxylate/atropine (Lomotil) A: Methyldopa (Aldomet) V: Valproate A: Angiotensin-converting enzyme inhibitors and angiotensin-receptor blockers X: Tizanidine (Zanaflex)	Naloxone (Narcan) Opioids: 0.4 mg and titrate to effect All others: 10 mg
Selective serotonin reuptake inhibitors (serotonin syndrome)	Cyproheptadine, benzodiazepines
Sulfonylureas (e.g., glimepiride, glyburide, glipizide)	Octreotide
Sympathomimetics (e.g., cocaine, amphetamines, 3,4-methylenedioxymethamphetamine [MDMA]) Hallucinogenics (e.g., phencyclidine [PCP])	Benzodiazepines
Toxic alcohols (e.g., ethylene glycol, methanol)	Fomepizole (Antizol) or ethanol
Tricyclic antidepressants and aspirin	Bicarbonate infusion therapy
Warfarin (Coumadin)	Vitamin K ± plasma or prothrombin complex concentrate

Modified from Murray L, Daly F, Little M, Cadogan M. *Toxicology Handbook.* 2nd ed. Sydney, NSW: Churchill Livingstone; 2011; Mazor SS. Poisoning antidotes. In: Schaider JL, Barkin RM, Hayden SR, Wolfe RE, Barkin AZ, Shayne P, eds. *Rosen & Barkin's 5-Minute Emergency Medicine Consult.* 6th ed. Philadelphia, PA: Lippincott Williams & Wilkins; 2020:898–899.

TABLE 15.4	**Substances not Amenable to Activated Charcoal**
P	Pesticides and potassium
H	Hydrocarbons
A	Acids, alkalis, alcohols
I	Iron, insecticides
L	Lithium (as well as most metals)
S	Solvents

Modified from Erickson TB, Thompson TM, Lu JJ. The approach to the patient with an unknown overdose. *Emerg Med Clin North Am.* 2007;25(2):249–281; Murray L, Daly F, Little M, Cadogan M. *Toxicology Handbook.* 2nd ed. Syndey, NSW: Churchill Livingstone; 2011.

medications given subcutaneously or intramuscularly depends on the site of injection, the solubility of the drug, and the vascularity of the injection area.

Once the drug is absorbed into the cardiovascular compartment, distribution occurs throughout the body. Agents enter or pass through the various body-fluid compartments (plasma, interstitial, and cellular fluids). Medications are restricted in distribution by their ability to pass through cellular membranes and the blood–brain barrier.

Drugs may accumulate in storage depots because of protein binding, fat accumulation, and active transport. Medications are stored in equilibrium and released as plasma concentrations are reduced. Storage depots permit maintenance of plasma levels for long periods, prolonging pharmacologic effects. Anatomic components that act as storage depots include plasma proteins, connective tissue, adipose tissue, and transcellular fluids.

The mechanism responsible for drug transport across cell membranes may be an active or passive process. Passive transfer is diffusion driven by concentration gradients. Active transport is mediated by a carrier and requires expenditure of energy. The ultimate fate of a drug is metabolism and excretion. Biotransformation involves chemical reactions, classified as either nonsynthetic or synthetic. The nonsynthetic class involves oxidation, reduction, and hydrolysis. The parent drug is changed to a more active, a less active, or an inactive metabolite. However, there are some medications that undergo little or no hepatic biotransformation. Hepatocytic enzymes mediate most nonsynthetic reactions. Exceptions include nonenzymatic hydrolysis in the plasma, plasma cholinesterase and pseudocholinesterase, and synaptic metabolism of neurotransmitter analogs.

Synthetic reactions or conjugation occur in the liver or kidney. The process couples the parent drug or its metabolites to endogenous substrates (usually carbohydrates, amino acids, or inorganic sulfates). Conjugated drugs form inactive, highly ionized, and water-soluble substances that are excreted in the urine. Conjugation is an active process that requires energy expenditure.

Active parent drugs and metabolites are excreted in the urine as a primary route of disposal. Drugs are also eliminated through excretion of feces. Metabolites are dissolved in bile, secreted into the alimentary tract, and passed through the GI tract. In addition, the unabsorbed parent drug is removed with fecal passage.

This discussion has focused on the incidence of poisoning; general considerations in the care of the poisoned patient; general management of the poisoned patient; signs and symptoms of toxicity; physical examination of the poisoned patient; useful laboratory studies; removal, elimination, or disruption of the poison; supportive and emotional care of the poisoned patient; transport nursing care of the poisoned patient; and the pharmacologic properties of drugs. The next part of this chapter focuses on the toxicity and treatment of toxicity of specific substances. Information about each of these drugs is presented for quick reference.

Toxicity and Treatment of Poisoning by Specific Substances

Acetylsalicylic Acid

Aspirin is one of the oldest nonprescription pharmaceutical agents. Its therapeutic popularity is mainly a result of its antipyretic, anti-inflammatory, antiplatelet, and analgesic effects. Aspirin can be taken orally, topically, or rectally. The most common route of toxicity is via ingestion. Many over-the-counter medications contain aspirin, and multiple sources of poisoning may be involved.

An ingestion of greater than 150 mg/kg is considered toxic. Salicylate toxicity ultimately can lead to a severe anion-gap metabolic acidosis. The absence of acidosis should not be falsely reassuring: salicylates directly stimulate the respiratory center, so the first acid–base abnormality is a respiratory alkalosis. Clinical manifestations of mild intoxication include headache, vertigo, tinnitus, mental confusion, sweating, thirst, hyperventilation, nausea, vomiting, and drowsiness. Severe intoxication produces similar symptoms combined with acid–base and electrolyte imbalances. Patients are agitated, restless, and uncommunicative and may have seizures or become comatose. Noncardiac pulmonary edema and hyperthermia are observed in severe poisoning, whereas bleeding diatheses are less common.[6,10]

Initial treatment of salicylate poisoning may involve administration of activated charcoal, if given within the first few hours of the ingestion, and alkaline diuresis. Alkaline diuresis is performed to increase the pH of the patient's urine to improve salicylate excretion. Supportive care and maintenance of vital functions are mainstays of treatment in this type of poisoning. If intubation is required, it is important to maintain a controlled hyperventilation to match the patient's pre-intubation minute ventilation, which will maintain the patient's respiratory alkalosis during initial management.[6,10,11]

The patient with severe poisoning may need hemodialysis. Hemodialysis not only enhances the removal of the toxic levels of the salicylate, but it can also correct the fluid, electrolyte, and acid–base imbalances that occur with salicylate toxicity.[6,10,11]

Acetaminophen

Acetaminophen, similar to aspirin, has antipyretic and analgesic properties. It is not chemically related to the salicylates. Acetaminophen has become a useful alternative to aspirin because it does not cause the GI and bleeding complications that can occur with aspirin use. Like aspirin, acetaminophen is contained in many over-the-counter drugs and may be administered orally, IV, or rectally. The main site of absorption is the small intestine, and the drug is uniformly distributed throughout most body fluids.[6,12,13]

Acetaminophen toxicity is increased by the liver because of metabolites that attach to the hepatic cell membrane and injure the lipid bilayer if they are not neutralized by the antioxidant glutathione. When hepatic glutathione stores are depleted because of an overdose of acetaminophen, the metabolites are not neutralized and cause injury and death of the hepatic cells.[6,12,13]

The classic clinical course of an acute acetaminophen poisoning occurs in four stages. The initial stage of toxicity occurs within the first 24 hours after ingestion and produces anorexia, nausea, vomiting, malaise, pallor, and diaphoresis.

The second stage begins 24–72 hours after ingestion. Right upper quadrant pain and tenderness may result from liver enlargement. The levels of liver enzymes, serum bilirubin, and prothrombin time begin to increase 36 hours after ingestion. Oliguria may result from acute tubular necrosis.

The third stage begins 72–96 hours after ingestion and is the time of peak liver function abnormalities. Anorexia, nausea, vomiting, and malaise return and jaundice become apparent. Fatalities from acetaminophen poisoning usually occur during this stage and result from fulminant hepatic necrosis.

The fourth stage, or resolution period, occurs 4 days to 2 weeks after poisoning. Patients are asymptomatic, and liver function parameters return to baseline values.[4,6,13]

Ingestions of more than 150 mg/kg are considered toxic. Activated charcoal may be helpful but must be administered within a few hours of the ingestion. The serum level of acetaminophen should be measured 4 hours after ingestion in any person who has ingested a potentially toxic dose of acetaminophen. If the acetaminophen level is still toxic at 4 hours after ingestion or if the level cannot be assayed after 8 hours have passed since ingestion and the history or evaluation of the hepatic transaminases suggests a toxic ingestion, N-acetylcysteine (NAC) should be administered. In the case of unknown time of exposure or >24 hours, treatment with NAC is indicated if there is a measurable acetaminophen level or elevated transaminases. NAC replaces glutathione and is administered IV or orally at an initial dose of 150 mg/kg or 140 mg/kg, respectively. Administration is continued over a prescribed period. To have the most benefit, administration should occur within 8 hours of ingestion; there is little benefit after 24 hours post ingestion.[6,11–13]

Anticholinergics

There are several medications (e.g., antihistamines, antipsychotics, antispasmodics, tricyclic antidepressants [TCAs]) and natural substances (e.g., jimson weed, mushrooms, deadly nightshade) that have anticholinergic properties.[14–16] These substances block the action of acetylcholine at central and peripheral muscarinic receptors. Since they have no effect on nicotinic receptors, they are better referred to as antimuscarinics. Inhibition leads to mydriasis, dry mouth, urinary retention, hyperthermia, tachycardia, altered mental status, agitation, and seizures. This is sometimes summarized by the mnemonic blind as a bat, red as a beet, dry as a bone, mad as a hatter, hotter than hades, and sick like a seizure.[14,16] Anticholinergic toxicity should be considered in any patient who presents with unexplained tachycardia, hyperthermia, and altered mental status.

Management is supportive, hypotension should initially be managed with IV normal saline solution, and a norepinephrine infusion may be needed in some patients. Agitation and seizures are best managed with benzodiazepines. If the patient is hyperthermic, cooling measures are warranted. If QRS widening is encountered, IV sodium bicarbonate therapy is preferred, as described in a later section. The use of cholinergic agents such as physostigmine may be indicated in managing severe agitation

refractory to benzodiazepines, but should be used cautiously and is not commonly recommended.[14–16]

Benzodiazepines

Benzodiazepines became available in the United States in 1960 for control of anxiety. These drugs are now used to decrease anxiety and as sedative-hypnotics, muscle relaxants, and anticonvulsants. Generally, to be lethal, the blood level of benzodiazepines must be quite high; however, benzodiazepines are often taken in combination with other substances, such as alcohol or opioids, which can cause death.[6,17,18]

The syndrome of benzodiazepine toxicity is nonspecific. The clinical picture is usually mild compared with that of other sedative-hypnotic poisonings. Most oral poisonings result in drowsiness, and sometimes respiratory depression and even coma.

Transport team members must keep in mind that other depressant medications and alcohol can place the patient at risk of toxicity with the administration of medications such as midazolam or lorazepam to manage a patient during transport.

The treatment of benzodiazepine poisoning begins with management of the patient's ABCs. Flumazenil can be administered to reverse the sedative, anxiolytic, and muscle-relaxant effects of toxic benzodiazepine ingestion. However, this drug must be administered in small doses with caution because many patients with overdoses take a combination of drugs, some of which may cause seizures at toxic levels, such as TCAs. Flumazenil reverses the anticonvulsant effects of benzodiazepines and may lead to withdrawal seizures, especially in chronic users, which also leaves patients with polysubstance overdoses at risk for lack of effective seizure management. Additionally, most benzodiazepine overdoses can be managed successfully with supportive care alone. Therefore, flumazenil is generally not recommended.[6,17,18] Patients with rapidly reversed overdoses may also present with aggressive behavior as their mental status suddenly improves.

Carbon Monoxide

Carbon monoxide (CO) is a colorless, odorless, tasteless gas yielded by the incomplete combustion of carbon containing materials. Sources include automobile or machine exhaust; flame-type heaters, furnaces, and ovens; defective fireplace flues; poorly ventilated charcoal and gas grills; and fires of all types. There is an increased incidence of accidental exposures during prolonged power outages caused by weather events when people attempt to stay warm from nonconventional sources and obtain electrical power from portable generators without proper ventilation.[6,19,20]

CO poisoning should be suspected in any patients with unexplained or vague symptoms, such as a headache or confusion, who may have been exposed to machinery running in an enclosed poorly ventilated space; exposed to a furnace that is new or run for the first time when the weather changes; or exposed to smoke in an enclosed space. It should be suspected with unexplained symptoms in multiple people in the same living or workspace. Animals are more sensitive than humans to CO poisoning and may have been ill long before their human owners.

CO combines with the hemoglobin molecule in the red blood cell. The affinity of hemoglobin for CO is greater than 200 times that for oxygen. Not only does CO compete with oxygen for hemoglobin, but the presence of carboxyhemoglobin also greatly impedes the dissociation of oxygen from hemoglobin. This leads to a decreased partial pressure of oxygen in the blood and diminished gradient for oxygen diffusion from the red blood cell to the tissues, which results in tissue hypoxia. Arterial hypoxemia results from any of the following conditions: pulmonary venous admixture from an uneven ventilation/perfusion relationship; marked inhibition of the circulatory system; direct effect of CO on the pulmonary tissue, which results in increased capillary permeability and decreased production of surfactant; and shifting of the oxygen–hemoglobin dissociation curve to the left. Patients can develop lactic acidosis, cardiac dysrhythmias and ischemia, and seizures as the cellular hypoxia worsens.[6,19,20]

The concentration of CO in the blood has been found to relate poorly to the clinical features observed in the person who has been exposed. Table 15.5 describes the symptomatology of CO poisoning related to CO saturation in the blood.[6]

The treatment of acute CO exposure is high-flow oxygen delivery, including intubation if warranted, despite pulse oximetry readings. An important aspect of management is recalling that pulse oximetry is not reliable because it cannot differentiate between carboxyhemoglobin and oxyhemoglobin. Noninvasive CO oximetry devices exist and perform reliably within their published specifications. The available literature still does not fully support broad use of such devices to replace clinical judgment, a high index of suspicion, and blood testing in at-risk patients.[21] Carboxyhemoglobin dissociates and converts to oxyhemoglobin if high concentrations of oxygen are provided. Hyperbaric oxygen therapy has also been found to be effective in some patients, especially those who are pregnant or have levels greater than 25%.[6,19,20]

Cardiotoxic Medications

Beta-Blockers and Calcium Channel Blockers

Beta-blockers and calcium channel blockers have numerous benefits in managing patients with cardiovascular disease. Beta-blockers and calcium channel blockers exert negative chronotropic and inotropic effects on the heart. Beta-blockers and nondihydropyridine calcium channel blockers also exert negative dromotropic effects. Calcium channel blockers also cause smooth muscle relaxation in the myocardium and vascular smooth muscle. However, in an overdose scenario, these effects are exaggerated and can be lethal. Patients may experience bradycardia, atrioventricular heart blocks, and hypotension, which lead to poor tissue perfusion, and impaired glucose utilization is also common. Beta-blockers may cause respiratory distress caused by the blockade of beta-2 receptors in the lungs.

TABLE 15.5	Signs and Symptoms of Various Blood Levels of Carboxyhemoglobin (COHb)
Level (%)	**Clinical Manifestations**
<10	Typical smoker
10	Maybe asymptomatic to slight headache
20	Dizziness, nausea, worsening headache
30	Vertigo, ataxia, visual disturbances
40	Confusion, coma, seizures
50	Cardiovascular and respiratory failure, seizures, death

Modified from Murray L, Daly F, Little M, Cadogan M. *Toxicology Handbook*. 2nd ed. Syndey, NSW: Churchill Livingstone; 2011.

First-line treatments include the administration of IV fluids and the use of norepinephrine and epinephrine to support heart rate, blood pressure, and contractility. The administration of IV calcium can also be beneficial in beta-blocker overdoses as well as with calcium channel blocker overdoses. High-dose insulin (HDI) therapy has been shown to be effective in overcoming the cardiotoxic effects of beta-blockers and calcium channel blockers, as well, and is considered a first-line therapy. Sometimes referred to as hyperinsulinemia/euglycemia, this therapy increases glucose uptake in the cardiac cells and has positive inotropic effects, similar to glucagon. Careful monitoring of the patient's glucose and potassium are critically important.[6,11,22–27]

If the patient does not improve with the previously mentioned therapies, pacing, incremental increases in the HDI, and IV lipid emulsion (ILE) therapy may be beneficial. Lipids are a great source of energy for the myocardial cells, and this therapy is also theorized to create a "lipid sink," which pulls lipophilic medications out of the cardiac cells, removing the blockade and allowing for more effective contractility and conduction. With the administration of HDI and ILE therapy, vasoactive and inotropic agents may need to be adjusted to prevent overcorrection of the toxic effects. Both HDI and ILE therapies are new and consultation with toxicology may be helpful in managing these patients.[6,22,23,25,27,28]

IV glucagon can also be administered as a 3- to 5-mg bolus, followed by an infusion. Glucagon exerts positive inotropic and chronotropic effects despite blockade of the beta receptors or calcium channels. To avoid the common side effect of vomiting, glucagon should be administered slowly; premedicating with an antiemetic is sometimes helpful. Glucagon's benefit is dependent on adequate calcium stores, in the setting of hypocalcemia or a calcium channel blocker overdose, and the administration of IV calcium may improve the effect.[6,11,22–26] In some guidelines, glucagon is now considered a second-line therapy because of inconsistent clinical responses, the occurrence of side effects, and the availability of more effective therapies.[27]

Digitalis

The term cardiac glycoside is used to describe a group of drugs prescribed to treat heart failure and atrial arrhythmias. These drugs have been used throughout history, with early mention of the compound found in ancient writings in the year 1500 BCE. *Digitalis* has become the most familiar of the group. It is derived from the dried leaf of the foxglove plant *Digitalis purpurea*. Several factors contribute to digitalis poisoning, including patient age; heart and renal disease; electrolyte imbalances (especially hypokalemia); and drug therapy, such as the use of diuretics.[29,30]

Clinical manifestations of digitalis toxicity are classified as cardiac and noncardiac. Cardiac manifestations including bradydysrhythmias are the result of depression through the sinoatrial and atrioventricular nodes and alteration of impulse formation and the development of hyperkalemia. Noncardiac signs and symptoms include fatigue, anorexia, nausea, vomiting, diarrhea, confusion, restlessness, insomnia, drowsiness, hallucinations, frank psychosis, blurred vision, photophobia, and yellow-halo visual effects.[6,29,30]

Treatment of digitalis toxicity includes support of vital functions and correction of the hyperkalemia. Digoxin-specific antibody fragments (Fab) are indicated in any life-threatening dysrhythmias and hyperkalemia in the setting of digitalis toxicity. Fab fragments bind to digoxin, and the Fab-digoxin complex is excreted in the urine. If Fab is not readily available, lidocaine or phenytoin are the preferred agents to treat ventricular dysrhythmias. Hyperkalemia can then be managed with standard care with careful monitoring to avoid hypokalemia. In the past, the use of calcium was controversial, however, most now consider calcium to be appropriate in the management of digoxin-induced hyperkalemia if Fab is not available. Bradyarrythmias can be treated with atropine.[6,29,30]

Tricyclic Antidepressants and Other Sodium-Channel Blocking Agents

TCAs are indicated in the treatment of refractory depression, chronic pain syndromes, and insomnia. Overdose statistics show that TCAs are one of the deadliest types of poisoning, with a high degree of morbidity and mortality in significant overdoses. Many TCAs are available in the United States.[6,31,32]

TCAs are well absorbed in the GI tract. The parent compound and active metabolites are quickly bound to plasma proteins. They exert their effects by inhibiting the amine pump mechanism responsible for the reuptake of norepinephrine and serotonin in adrenergic and serotonergic neurons. These antidepressants also block cholinergic receptors in the parasympathetic nervous system and have anticholinergic properties.[6,31,32]

The TCA agents, along with other sodium-channel blocking drugs, block the fast sodium channels responsible for the rapid depolarization (phase 0) of the cardiac action potential. In the management of patients with poisoning, it is important to understand that the list of medications that exert sodium-channel blocking effects is long and, in addition to the TCAs, includes the class I antiarrhythmics, cocaine, and some of the calcium and beta-blocking drugs. Accordingly, an evaluation of the ECG and consideration of the potential for sodium-channel poisoning is important in the management of any patient with possible ingestion.

The clinical manifestations of TCA poisoning include anticholinergic symptoms such as mydriasis, tachycardia, dry mucous membranes, urinary retention, and decreased peristalsis. Central nervous system (CNS) signs include confusion, agitation, hallucinations, seizures, and coma. Twitching, jerking, and myoclonic movements have also been reported. Generalized tonic–clonic seizures are reported in up to 20% of TCA poisoning cases and are often associated with QRS widening. Respiratory depression is common.

Cardiac toxicity comes from the sodium channel blockade and enhanced adrenergic stimulation of the myocardium. Sinus tachycardia and mild hypertension occur early in poisoning, coupled with a quinidine-like cardiac action that depresses conduction velocity, widens the QRS interval, and produces a rightward axis deviation and right bundle branch block as well as wide complex tachyarrhythmias. A terminal R wave over 3 mm in height in lead aVR is also consistent with sodium channel poisoning. Acidemia occurs because of cardiac and respiratory depression.[6,31,32]

In TCA and other sodium-channel blocker poisonings, support of vital functions is essential. Hypotension is initially managed with an IV infusion of saline solution. Vasopressor support with norepinephrine may be indicated if IV fluids are ineffective in correcting hypotension. Sodium bicarbonate therapy is indicated in any toxicologic patient with a widened QRS over 100 ms and should be given until the QRS duration normalizes. If sodium bicarbonate is not available or there is concern for the pH effect of a tremendous amount of sodium bicarbonate, hypertonic saline can be used. Seizures should be managed with benzodiazepines.[6,31,32]

Cyanide

Cyanide poisoning is rare but often fatal if not quickly identified and managed. Poisoning may result from inhalation of toxic gases from a fire involving wool, plastics, or rubber; exposure to agents used in metal refining, electroplating, and photography; or prolonged infusions of high-dose nitroprusside.[33,34] Cyanide is often associated with the smell of bitter almonds, but this is not always the case. Cyanide inhibits oxygen transport, oxidative phosphorylation, and the production of adenosine triphosphate. This leads to severe tissue hypoxia, anaerobic metabolism, and a severe anion gap metabolic acidosis. The patient often displays symptoms of otherwise inexplicable metabolic acidosis and hypoxia including altered mental status, headache, GI upset, tachypnea and tachycardia, and eventually bradycardia and hypotension. Cyanide interferes with oxygen extraction, so oxygen saturation measurements are not clinically reliable in patients with cyanide poisoning.[33,34]

Management starts with the airway and administration of 100% oxygen. If available, hydroxocobalamin (Cyanokit) should be quickly administered.[33,34] Hydroxocobalamin binds with cyanide to form cyanocobalamin (a form of vitamin B_{12}), which is then excreted in the urine. This reaction may cause a reddish discoloration to the patient's skin and urine and can alter the results of some blood analyses.

Ethanol

Ethanol is the most widely used and abused drug in the United States. It is often involved in poison emergencies because it is frequently used with other drugs. Ethanol alcohol is rapidly absorbed from the GI tract. Food reduces the rate of absorption by 2–6 hours. Once ethanol is ingested, equilibration is rapid, and distribution uniformly occurs throughout all bodily tissues and fluids. Passage across the placenta has been documented.[6,35,36]

Ethanol metabolism occurs mainly in the liver. Acute intoxication produces psychomotor retardation; reflex slowing; lethargy; sleep; and ultimately, coma and death. Initially, respirations are stimulated as a result of the production of carbon dioxide. However, with increasing concentrations of alcohol, respirations can be dangerously depressed. Ethanol enhances cutaneous blood flow, which causes heat loss through vasodilatation. Excessive amounts depress the central thermoregulatory mechanism, adding to the hypothermia effects. Ethanol stimulates gastric secretions, which causes an irritation of the gastric mucosa. In addition, ethanol causes diuresis mediated through inhibition of antidiuretic hormone (ADH), which decreases renal tubular reabsorption of water.[6,35,36]

Patients respond differently to alcohol poisoning. Table 15.6 correlates signs and symptoms of alcohol intoxication with blood alcohol levels, though each patient is different.[6]

Care of the alcohol-poisoned patient consists of supportive care. Such patients may become combative, and precautions should be taken for appropriate restraint before transport.

Hallucinogens

In addition to toxic exposures to anticholinergics, two drugs that cause hallucinations are phencyclidine (PCP) and lysergic acid diethylamide (LSD). The use of both has declined over the last few decades. Marijuana is sometimes laced with PCP and is known as "whacko tobacco." Both can have effects that last hours

TABLE 15.6	Assessing Severity of Alcohol Intoxication by Blood Alcohol Level	

| Serum Ethanol Concentration | | Clinical Features (Dependent on Use History and Tolerance) |
mg/dL	%	
50	0.05	Disinhibition and euphoria
100	0.1	Mild CNS depression, slurred speech
200	0.2	Increased CNS depression: nausea and vomiting, possible coma
400	0.4	Severe CNS depression: coma, respiratory depression, hypotension

CNS, Central nervous system.

Modified from Murray L, Daly F, Little M, Cadogan M. *Toxicology Handbook*. 2nd ed. Syndey, NSW: Churchill Livingstone; 2011.

after use. PCP was initially developed as a general anesthetic in 1958 and has similar properties to ketamine. However, because of the postanesthetic reactions that occurred with its use, it has not been used legally since 1965, though it remains a schedule II controlled substance.[37]

PCP is often smoked, but can also be snorted or ingested and is distributed to all tissue compartments, metabolized by the liver, and excreted through the kidneys. The drug can produce bizarre and dangerous behavioral manifestations, as well as tachycardia, hypertension, and hyperthermia. In larger doses, it can cause psychosis, hostility, seizures, and coma. A common neurologic sign of PCP intoxication is nystagmus.[31,37–40]

LSD is one of the most potent hallucinogens known. Psychiatrists initially used the drug in the 1950s as an aid in clinical psychotherapy. Abuse became popular in the 1960s during the "psychedelic movement," and it was listed as a schedule I controlled substance in 1966. LSD is usually taken orally. Doses as low as 25 mcg will produce clinical effects, and the intensity of its effect is dose-dependent. Doses greater than 100 mcg are often needed for the full effect but also cause sympathomimetic effects similar to PCP and other stimulants. Absorption of the drug is rapid, and LSD is distributed to all tissues, including the brain. Initial effects occur in 30–45 minutes and may last for 10–12 hours. LSD is metabolized in the liver, and small amounts are excreted unchanged in the urine.[41]

Psychologic effects are generally pleasurable, and may include euphoria, dreams, and pseudo-hallucinations. The user may have enhanced color perception and experience transforming visual imagery of their surroundings and their body. Occasionally, a person may have an intense panic reaction ("bad trip") that includes frightening hallucinations and mood swings or a "flashback." Such a person may become confused, aggressive, suicidal, or violent.[38,41]

Treatment consists of supportive care. During air medical transport, patients who have taken any hallucinogen demand close observation. Patients may become hostile, belligerent, and destructive. Be observant for signs of sympathetic stimulation including hypertension, tachycardia, and hyperthermia-induced rhabdomyolysis. Use of ear protection, sedation, and prophylactic chemical and/or physical restraints may be necessary before transport.[31,38,40,41]

Organophosphates

Insecticides, pesticides, and nerve agents (e.g., soman, sarin, VX) are examples of organophosphates (Ops). This toxicity may be seen in purposeful ingestions, occupational or pharmaceutical exposures, and chemical exposures during a terroristic event. Some may report the associated smell of garlic with these toxins. These chemicals cause a cholinergic crisis by inhibiting acetylcholinesterase and preventing the breakdown of acetylcholine, which leads to the buildup of acetylcholine and prolonged stimulation of muscarinic and nicotinic receptors in both the central and peripheral nervous system.[42,43] Overstimulation of muscarinic receptors leads to the classic SLUDGEM presentation: salivation, lacrimation, urination, defecation, GI, expectoration and emesis, and miosis. This overstimulation can also causes bronchorrhea, bradycardia, and hypotension. Nicotinic stimulation leads to tachycardia, hypertension, mydriasis, muscle fasciculations, seizures, and eventually paralysis, including the diaphragm.[42,43]

Safety is of the upmost priority with Ops, and the patient must be decontaminated before transport. Providers should don proper protective equipment to ensure they do not contact the substance because it is easily inhaled or absorbed through the skin.[42,43] Once the patient is safe for transport personnel, the head of the bed should be elevated because of the massive amounts of airway secretions. Atropine is administered to block the overstimulation of muscarinic receptors with the goal of drying up pulmonary secretions and stabilizing the airway. The patient may require multiple large doses as there is no maximum dose of atropine for these patients.[42,43] If the patient requires intubation, then succinylcholine should be avoided because Ops prevent its breakdown and prolonged paralysis may occur. Once available, pralidoxime (2-PAM) is administered to stop the overstimulation of the receptors and reverse paralysis. 2-PAM binds to and inactivates the Ops, freeing up acetylcholinesterase. Some Ops irreversibly bind to acetylcholinesterase over time, often referred to as aging, which results in prolonged receptor stimulation. The sooner 2-PAM can be administered, the less likely this aging will occur. Patients will benefit from an initial bolus and continuous infusion. Benzodiazepines remain the agent of choice for managing seizures.[42,43]

Sympathomimetics

Cocaine, amphetamines, methamphetamines, 3,4-methylenedioxymethamphetamine (MDMA) or ecstasy (E or X), and the newer street drugs including synthetic cannabinoids, bath salts, and Molly's plant food, are commonly abused substances with sympathomimetic properties. These substances may be insufflated, smoked, ingested, injected, and now vaped. Most of these substances are metabolized by the liver and excreted by the kidney. They stimulate both the peripheral and central sympathetic nervous systems, and both alpha- and beta-receptors. They can produce mild-to-moderate CNS stimulation manifested by euphoria, decreased fatigue, and excitement, which can progress to anxiety, paranoia, hostility, hyperthermia, and seizures. They can have significant cardiovascular effects, including tachycardia, arrhythmias, hypertension, and vasospasms, which can lead to a myocardial infarction, stroke, and even death.[6,11,31,44,45]

Synthetic cannabinoids, bath salts, and Molly's plant food are newer illicit substances, which are often encountered because of their popularity. They can be obtained illegally online and at retail shops. Most are labeled "not for human consumption" and contain various chemicals. They are highly addictive and users often experience a rapid tolerance requiring more with each use to achieve the desired effect. Because these substances are synthetic, they are not detectable in the routine urine drug screen, hence, their popularity.[11,46–49]

Synthetic cannabinoids (e.g., K2 and Spice) are herbal incenses that have been treated with psychoactive chemicals, which stimulate cannabinoid receptors similar to delta-9-tetrahydrocannabinol (THC). These chemicals are more potent than THC and lead to a stronger effect, including euphoria and activation of the sympathetic nervous system and inhibition of the parasympathetic system. Some patients may experience tachycardia, hypertension, paranoia, agitation, and GI distress. Bath salts (e.g., Bliss, Ivory Wave, Vanilla Sky) and second-generation bath salts (e.g., "gravel" or "flakka") are synthetic amphetamines that mimic cathinone, a naturally occurring psychostimulant found in the khat plant. These substances alter the reuptake of norepinephrine, dopamine, and serotonin, which leads to an overstimulation of the sympathetic nervous system. Bath salts have been associated with suicidal and homicidal ideations and actions.[11,46–51]

Molly's plant food or Molly, which is short for molecule, is "marketed" as pure MDMA and is usually in a powder form, unlike MDMA, which is usually a pill. Molly may or may not contain MDMA, as well as many other chemicals. However, both increase serotonin levels more than the other neurotransmitters and increase the release of oxytocin and ADH. Serotonin and oxytocin have empathogenic effects and have earned MDMA the nicknames of the "hug drug" and the "love drug." The increased release of ADH can suppress the thirst response, and users often increase their water intake knowing this effect, along with the concern for overheating. This may cause some users to develop hyponatremia that leads to seizures. Both have been associated with risky sexual behaviors, infection transmission, and sexual assaults.[6,11,52,53]

The main objectives in the treatment of acute sympathomimetic exposures are to control the hyperactivity and hypertension, suppress malignant cardiac arrhythmias, correct metabolic acidosis, reduce hyperthermia, and minimize seizure activity. Benzodiazepines, such as midazolam (Versed), are the first-line intervention for patients experiencing hyperactivity, tachyarrhythmias, hypertension, hyperthermia, and seizures associated with these substances. A continuous infusion may be warranted in some patients. If the hypertension is not controlled with benzodiazepines, then vasodilators (e.g., nitroglycerin) or alpha/beta-blockade (e.g., labetalol) may be needed. However, pure beta-blockers should not be used alone because this would leave alpha receptors unopposed and could worsen the patient's condition. Sympathomimetic substances may cause sodium channel blockade, which can cause QRS widening and wide complex dysrhythmias. These rhythm changes should be managed with sodium bicarbonate and/or lidocaine if not resolved with initial therapy. Cooling measures will be needed when there is severe hyperthermia with a core temperature greater than 40°C (104°F). Patients with prolonged hyperthermia are at an increased risk for rhabdomyolysis and acute renal failure.[6,11,31,45–48,50]

Toxic Alcohols

Ethylene glycol is an odorless water-soluble solvent most commonly used in antifreeze and coolants. Ingestion usually occurs in the inquisitive toddler, as an ethanol substitute, or suicide attempt. Ethylene glycol is rapidly absorbed and reaches peak blood levels in 1–4 hours after ingestion. Large doses result in an inebriated patient without the odor of alcohol. Ethylene glycol approximates ethanol in CNS toxicity; however, its metabolites produce profound systemic effects, especially cardiac and renal.[6,11,54,55]

Ingestion of greater than 1 mL/kg of ethylene glycol is often lethal. It is hepatically metabolized to several metabolites, including glycolic and oxalic acid. Calcium oxalate crystals are formed and deposited systemically, especially in the heart and kidneys and often lead to acute renal failure. Ethylene glycol ingestion leads to intoxication similar to ethanol ingestion. A profound anion gap metabolic acidosis is a hallmark of this poisoning, but it only occurs after metabolism has begun. Severe hypocalcemia from chelation of calcium may produce tetany and cardiac compromise.[6,11,54–56]

Methanol, a wood alcohol, is found in some fuels, windshield washing fluids, and solvents. Ingestion of greater than 0.5 mL/kg is often lethal in most patients. Initial presentation is also similar to an acute ethanol ingestion. Methanol is metabolized to formaldehyde and then formic acid. A severe gap metabolic acidosis and blindness will develop and eventually death if not treated.[6,11,54–56]

Serum levels can guide treatment for toxic alcohol ingestions; however, treatment should not be delayed while awaiting results if there is a concern for or known toxic ingestion. Fomepizole (Antizol) should be administered to inhibit alcohol dehydrogenase, the enzyme which metabolizes alcohols. Inhibition prevents the buildup of the toxic metabolites and may prevent or limit the development of acidosis and renal failure. If fomepizole is not available, ethanol can be given orally or infused, if available. (Ethanol is not an FDA-approved treatment.) Ethanol has a higher affinity to hepatic enzymes compared to other alcohols and blocks the conversion of ethylene glycol and methanol to their toxic metabolites and can slow the development of acidosis and toxicity. Dialysis may be needed to remove the toxins and stabilize any imbalances. If fomepizole is administered early enough, dialysis may not be needed in some patients.[6,11,54–56]

Snakebites

Responding to the needs of a victim of a snakebite may not be one of the most common flights encountered by the transport nurse; however, knowledge of how to care for such patients can decrease complications and save lives. Many thousands of snakebites are reported in the United States each year. Venomous snakes inflict about 7000–8000 of those bites. Death does occur but is rare.[57,58]

Venom is a special category of poison that must be injected by one organism into another to produce a harmful effect. It is secreted by special epithelial cells in certain organisms and is stored in the lumina or exocrine glands. The venom is comprised of multiple chemicals and enzymes, and some of them toxic. The toxins may affect particular body systems such as the neurologic, hematologic, and cardiovascular systems.[57,58]

The effects of venom are dependent on the pharmacologic complexity of the venom and the action that the venom exerts on the tissues. The location of the venom injection also affects the spread of the venom. The closer the bite is to the trunk, the higher the risk for systemic effects. However, any bite in the area of a blood vessel could potentially spread the venom more quickly.[57–61]

The most prevalent venomous snakes in the United States are the pit vipers, which include rattlesnakes, copperheads, and water moccasins (cottonmouths). These snakes produce a hemotoxin and are native to all states except Maine, Alaska, and Hawaii. The

Mojave rattlesnake is unique in that its venom also contains neurotoxins. Coral snakes only account for 5% of envenomations and can be found in the southwestern states, gulf coastal states, and the Carolinas. In addition to the venomous snakes native to the United States, venomous snakes have been collected from all over the world. A bite from any one of these snakes may be fraught with complications or may even be instantly fatal.[57–60]

The following subsections describe the indigenous venomous snakes, the initial treatment of snakebites, transport nursing care of patients with snake bites, and the role of the transport team in the care of these victims.

Recognition of Venomous Bites

Figure 15.1 compares pit viper and non-pit viper snakes. Pit vipers belong to the *Crotalidae* family (as shown in Fig. 15.1) and have a pit midway between the eye and nostril on each side of the head. This pit is a heat-sensing organ that helps the snake locate its prey. This particular characteristic, unlike others in Fig. 15.1, is a 100% consistent characteristic in the identification of pit vipers.

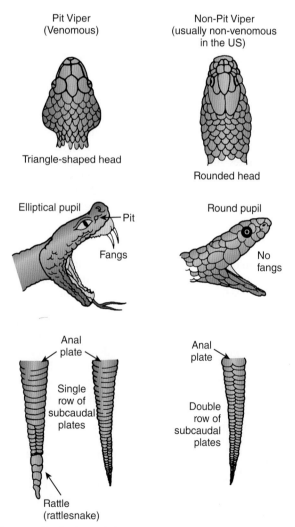

• **Fig. 15.1** Comparison of pit viper (venomous) and non-pit viper (usually non-venomous in the United States) snakes. (Modified from Otten M. Venomous animal injuries. In: Marx JA, et al., eds. *Rosen's Emergency Medicine: Concepts and Clinical Practice.* 6th ed. St. Louis, MO: Mosby; 2006.)

Envenomation by a pit viper usually results in one or two distinct puncture wounds with symptoms of localized pain, swelling, and edema in the bitten area. Other symptoms include diaphoresis and chills, paresthesias, nausea, hypotension, faintness, weakness, muscle fasciculations, local ecchymosis, and coagulopathies.[57–61]

The second largest family of snakes in the world is the *Elapidae*, which contains some deadly species including cobras, mambas, sea snakes, and coral snakes. One of the distinguishing characteristics of the coral snakes found in the United States is their color pattern, which helps differentiate them from the scarlet kingsnake. These differences are sometimes summarized with the mnemonic "Red on Yellow Kills a Fellow, Red on Black Venom Lack." Envenomation by a coral snake may result in a neurotoxic course. Systemic manifestations include drowsiness, euphoria, weakness, nausea, vomiting, fasciculations, dysphagia, salivation, extraocular muscle paresis, hypotension, and cardiopulmonary failure.[57–59]

Initial Management of Snakebites

Envenomation does not always occur with a snake bite. Estimates are that 20%–30% of crotalid bites and 50% of elapid bites do not result in envenomation; such bites are called dry bites.[57–60] In the following discussion of the general management of patients with snakebite, it is important to emphasize that experts should be consulted when questions arise about the care of a patient with a snakebite. Identification of the snake is important so that appropriate treatment can be initiated and unnecessary care limited.

If the snake has not been secured, the patient should be moved to a safe environment. The patient must be kept calm and the affected part immobilized. These two interventions decrease the circulation of venom throughout the patient's system. The wound should be cleansed, any constrictive clothing removed, the extremity immobilized at the level of the heart, and the patient transported. With coral snake bites, the application of a compression dressing or pressure immobilization to the affected area may slow systemic absorption; however, this is controversial and should never be performed with pit viper bites.[57–61]

The airway, ventilatory, and circulatory status of the patient should be constantly evaluated. Two large-bore IV lines should be started, preferably in an area away from the bite. The patient must be observed closely for progression of symptoms from a localized reaction at the wound site to a systemic reaction and development of a compartment syndrome in the affected extremity.

When possible, blood samples for baseline laboratory work should be drawn before transport. These tests may include a complete blood count, coagulation studies, a metabolic panel, creatine kinase, and urinalysis. Included in the coagulation studies should be fibrin split products and fibrinogen levels.[57–61]

If the patient shows signs of severe envenomation, such as worsening edema, shock, renal failure, coagulopathy, or paralysis, administration of antivenin should be started. Antivenin facilitates removal of the venom from the body but does not reverse any tissue damage. The size of the patient needs to be considered in relation to the amount of venom that the person may be able to tolerate. A child or small adult may be more severely affected.[57–61]

Snake antivenin is prepared from the serum of animals that were hyperimmunized against a specific venom or venoms. Unlike other drugs, the dosage of antivenin should be based on clinical findings rather than on the age and weight of the patient. For several years, Crotalidae Polyvalent Immune Fab

---

(Ovine) (FabAV, Crofab) was the only pit viper antivenin available in the United States. In 2019, Crotalidae Immune F(ab')2 (Equine) (Fab2AV, Anavip) was approved for use in the United States. The dosing varies between the two available pit viper antivenins. Unlike the older equine antivenin, these two have less risk of allergic reactions. Skin testing and pretreatment before administration is no longer recommended although clinicians should be prepared in case there is a reaction. Epinephrine and antihistamines remain the medications of choice for antivenin induced anaphylaxis.[57–61]

North American Coral Snake Antivenin (Equine) is no longer manufactured but is usually available in those previously mentioned geographic areas of the country. Given the shortage of this antivenin, the Food and Drug Administration has extended its printed expiration date and reevaluates this on a yearly basis. This antivenin should be used cautiously in those with previous reactions to equine serum. Skin testing to observe for a reaction and pretreatment is usually recommended before administration of US coral snake antivenin. When any antivenin is given, the package instructions should be followed and resuscitation equipment should be readily available. In 2023, the results of a clinical trial evaluating a new antivenin for US coral snake bites were released, and it is now approved as an investigational drug by the FDA.[57–61]

Serum sickness may develop after antivenin administration. The incidence rate of serum sickness varies in patients given antivenin therapy. The symptoms of serum sickness have occurred up to 3 weeks after antivenin administration. They include fever, joint pain, rash, nausea, vomiting, and neurologic symptoms. Treatment of serum sickness includes corticosteroids.[57,60,61]

Transport Care of Patients with Snakebite

The transport team may become involved in the care of the patient with a snakebite by directly responding to the scene of the injury or by transporting the patient to more definitive care. Experts in the care of snakebites note that rapid transport of these patients to a facility that can manage the injury is imperative in saving lives and preventing complications.[57] Box 15.2 summarizes care to be provided for the patient bitten by a snake.

Summary

The transport of the poisoned patient generally involves support of the patient's airway, breathing, and circulation. Few antidotes are available for the poisoned patient, and generally the transport team may have limited resources to determine the cause of the poisoning. However, the patient management can be interesting in the detective work used to uncover cues to ingestion and, when indicated, novel therapies for specific poisonings. The transport team should always ensure safety before transport begins so they do not become victims of the poison or the patient's behavior, as well.

References

1. McCabe SE, Cranford JA, West BT. Trends in prescription drug abuse and dependence, co-occurrence with other substance use disorders, and treatment utilization: results from two national surveys. *Addict Behav.* 2008;33(10):1297–1305. doi: 10.1016/j.addbeh.2008.06.005
2. Gummin DD, Mowry JB, Beuhler MC, et al. 2020 Annual Report of the American Association of Poison Control Centers' national poison data system (NPDS): 38th annual report. *Clin Toxicol.* 2021;59(12):1282–1501. doi: 10.1080/15563650.2021.1989785
3. Air & Surface Transport Nurses Association. Position Statement: Critical care transport nurse safety in the transport environment. 2018. Available at: https://cdn.ymaws.com/www.astna.org/resource/collection/4392B20B-D0DB-4E76-959C-6989214920E9/ASTNA_Safety_Position_Paper_2018_FINAL.pdf.
4. Mycyk MB. Poisoning. In: Schaider JL, Barkin RM, Hayden SR, Wolfe RE, Barkin AZ, Shayne P, eds. *Rosen & Barkin's 5-Minute Emergency Medicine Consult.* 6th ed. Philadelphia, PA: Lippincott Williams & Wilkins; 2020:896–897.
5. Erickson TB, Thompson TM, Lu JJ. The approach to the patient with an unknown overdose. *Emerg Med Clin North Am.* 2007;25(2):249–281. doi: 10.1016/j.emc.2007.02.004
6. Murray L, Daly F, Little M, Cadogan M. *Toxicology Handbook.* 2nd ed. Sydney, NSW: Churchill Livingstone; 2011.
7. Ashbourne JF, Olson KR, Khayam-Bashi H. Value of rapid screening for acetaminophen in all patients with intentional drug overdose. *Ann Emerg Med.* 1989;18(10):1035–1038.
8. Lucanie R, Chiang WK, Reilly R. Utility of acetaminophen screening in unsuspected suicidal ingestions. *Vet Hum Toxicol.* 2002;44(3):171–173.
9. Sporer KA, Khayam-Bashi H. Acetaminophen and salicylate serum levels in patients with suicidal ingestion or altered mental status. *Emerg Med Am J.* 1996;14(5):443–446.
10. Zell-Kanter M. Salicylate antidotes. In: Schaider JL, Barkin RM, Hayden SR, Wolfe RE, Barkin AZ, Shayne P, eds. *Rosen & Barkin's 5-Minute Emergency Medicine Consult.* 6th ed. Philadelphia, PA: Lippincott Williams & Wilkins; 2020:1002–1003.
11. Roberts E, Gooch MD. Pharmacologic strategies for treatment of poisonings. *Nurs Clin North Am.* 2016;51(1):57–68. doi: 10.1016/j.cnur.2015.11.003
12. Mycyk MB. Acetaminophen poisoning. In: Schaider JL, Barkin RM, Hayden SR, Wolfe RE, Barkin AZ, Shayne P, eds. *Rosen & Barkin's 5-Minute Emergency Medicine Consult.* 6th ed. Philadelphia, PA: Lippincott Williams & Wilkins; 2020:20–21.
13. Olson KR. Acetaminophen. In: Olson KR, Anderson IB, Benowitz NL, et al., eds. *Poisoning & Drug Overdose.* 7th ed. New York: McGraw-Hill; 2018.

14. Garlich Horner FM. Anticholinergic agents. In: Wolfson AB, ed. *Harwood-Nuss' Clinical Practice of Emergency Medicine.* 7th ed. Philadelphia, PA: Lippincott Williams & Wilkins; 2021:1530–1533.

15. Manning BH. Anticholinergics. In: Olson KR, Anderson IB, Benowitz NL, et al., eds. *Poisoning & Drug Overdose.* 7th ed. New York: McGraw–Hill; 2018.

16. Whiteley PM. Anticholinergic poisoning. In: Schaider JL, Barkin RM, Hayden SR, Wolfe RE, Barkin AZ, Shayne P, eds. *Rosen & Barkin's 5-Minute Emergency Medicine Consult,* 6th ed. Philadelphia, PA: Lippincott Williams & Wilkins; 2020:72–73.

17. Nelson ME. Benzodiazepine poisoning. In: Schaider JL, Barkin RM, Hayden SR, Wolfe RE, Barkin AZ, Shayne P, eds. *Rosen & Barkin's 5-Minute Emergency Medicine Consult.* 6th ed. Philadelphia, PA: Lippincott Williams & Wilkins; 2020:134–135.

18. Tsutaoka B. Benzodiazepines. In: Olson KR, Anderson IB, Benowitz NL, et al., eds. *Poisoning & Drug Overdose.* 7th ed. New York: McGraw–Hill; 2018.

19. Hampson NB, Piantadosi CA, Thom SR, Weaver LK. Practice recommendations in the diagnosis, management, and prevention of carbon monoxide poisoning. *Am J Respir Crit Care Med.* 2012; 186(11):1095–1101. doi: 10.1164/rccm.201207-1284CI

20. Thompson TN. Carbon monoxide poisoning. In: Schaider JL, Barkin RM, Hayden SR, Wolfe RE, Barkin AZ, Shayne P. eds. *Rosen & Barkin's 5-Minute Emergency Medicine Consult.* 6th ed. Philadelphia, PA: Lippincott Williams & Wilkins; 2020:180–181.

21. Wilcox SR, Richards JB. Noninvasive carbon monoxide detection: insufficient evidence for broad clinical use. *Respir Care.* 2013;58(2): 376–379. doi: 10.4187/respcare.02288

22. Barton CA, Johnson NB, Mah ND, et al. Successful treatment of a massive metoprolol overdose using intravenous lipid emulsion and hyperinsulinemia/euglycemia therapy. *Pharmacotherapy.* 2015;35(5): e56–e60. doi: 10.1002/phar.1579

23. Doepker B, Healy W, Cortez E, Adkins E. High-dose insulin and intravenous lipid emulsion therapy for cardiogenic shock induced by intentional calcium-channel blocker and beta-blocker overdose: a case series. *J Emerg Med.* 2014;46(4):486–490. doi: 10.1016/j.jemermed.2013.08.135

24. Engebretsen KM, Kaczmarek KM, Morgan J, Holger JS. High-dose insulin therapy in beta-blocker and calcium channel-blocker poisoning. *Clin Toxicol.* 2011;49(4):277–283. doi:10.3109/15563650.2011.582471

25. Dzeba M, Aks SE. Beta-blocker poisoning. In: Schaider JL, Barkin RM, Hayden SR, Wolfe RE, Barkin AZ, Shayne P, eds. *Rosen & Barkin's 5-Minute Emergency Medicine Consult.* 6th ed. Philadelphia, PA: Lippincott Williams & Wilkins; 2020:136–137.

26. Lim CS, Aks SE. Calcium channel blocker poisoning. In: Schaider JL, Barkin RM, Hayden SR, Wolfe RE, Barkin AZ, Shayne P, eds. *Rosen & Barkin's 5-Minute Emergency Medicine Consult.* 6th ed. Philadelphia, PA: Lippincott Williams & Wilkins; 2020:172–173.

27. St-Onge M, Anseeuw K, Cantrell FL, et al. Experts consensus recommendations for the management of calcium channel blocker poisoning in adults. *Crit Care Med.* 2017;45(3):e306–e315. doi: 10.1097/CCM.0000000000002087

28. Schultz AE, Lewis T, Reed BS, et al. That's a phat antidote: intravenous fat emulsions and toxicological emergencies. *Adv Emerg Nurs J.* 2015;37(3):162–175. doi: 10.1097/TME.0000000000000067

29. Benowitz NL. Digoxin and other cardiac glycosides. In: Olson KR, Anderson IB, Benowitz NL, et al., eds. *Poisoning & Drug Overdose.* 7th ed. New York: McGraw–Hill; 2018.

30. Troendle MM, Cumpston KL. Digoxin poisoning. In: Schaider JL, Barkin RM, Hayden SR, Wolfe RE, Barkin AZ, Shayne P, eds. *Rosen & Barkin's 5-Minute Emergency Medicine Consult.* 6th ed. Philadelphia, PA: Lippincott Williams & Wilkins; 2020:322–323.

31. Rasin A, Aks SE. Tricyclic poisoning. In: Schaider JL, Barkin RM, Hayden SR, Wolfe RE, Barkin AZ, Shayne P, eds. *Rosen & Barkin's 5-Minute Emergency Medicine Consult.* 6th ed. Philadelphia, PA: Lippincott Williams & Wilkins; 2020:1168–1169.

32. Benowitz NL. Antidepressants, tricyclic. In: Olson KR, Anderson IB, Benowitz NL et al., eds. *Poisoning & Drug Overdose.* 7th ed. New York: McGraw–Hill; 2018.

33. Blanc PD. Cyanide. In: Olson KR, Anderson IB, Benowitz NL, et al., eds. *Poisoning & Drug Overdose.* 7th ed. New York: McGraw–Hill; 2018.

34. Long H. Cyanide. In: Wolfson AB. Ed. *Harwood-Nuss' Clinical Practice of Emergency Medicine.* 7th ed. Philadelphia, PA: Lippincott Williams & Wilkins; 2021:1451–1453.

35. Kreshak A. Ethanol. In: Olson KR, Anderson IB, Benowitz NL, et al., eds. *Poisoning & Drug Overdose.* 7th ed. New York: McGraw–Hill; 2018.

36. Meehan TJ. Alcohol poisoning. In: Schaider JL, Barkin RM, Hayden SR, Wolfe RE, Barkin AZ, Shayne P, eds. *Rosen & Barkin's 5-Minute Emergency Medicine Consult.* 6th ed. Philadelphia, PA: Lippincott Williams & Wilkins; 2020:42–43.

37. Bey T, Patel A. Phencyclidine intoxication and adverse effects: a clinical and pharmacological review of an illicit drug. *Cal J Emerg Med.* 2007;8(1):9–14.

38. Routsolias JC. Hallucinogen poisoning. In: Schaider JL, Barkin RM, Hayden SR, Wolfe RE, Barkin AZ, Shayne P, eds. *Rosen & Barkin's 5-Minute Emergency Medicine Consult.* 6th ed. Philadelphia, PA: Lippincott Williams & Wilkins; 2020:478–479.

39. Armenian P. Lysergic acid diethylamide (LSD) and other hallucinogens. In: Olson KR, Anderson IB, Benowitz NL, et al., eds. *Poisoning & Drug Overdose.* 7th ed. New York: McGraw–Hill; 2018.

40. Aks SE. Phencyclidine poisoning. In: Schaider JL, Barkin RM, Hayden SR, Wolfe RE, Barkin AZ, Shayne P, eds. *Rosen & Barkin's 5-Minute Emergency Medicine Consult.* 6th ed. Philadelphia, PA: Lippincott Williams & Wilkins; 2020:868–869.

41. Passie T, Halpern JH, Stichtenoth DO, Emrich HM, Hintzen A. The pharmacology of lysergic acid diethylamide: a review. *CNS Neurosci Ther.* 2008;14(4):295–314.

42. Holstege CP. Organophosphate and carbamate insecticides. In: Wolfson AB, ed. *Harwood-Nuss' Clinical Practice of Emergency Medicine,* 7th ed. Philadelphia, PA: Lippincott Williams & Wilkins; 2021:1425–1429.

43. Vohra R. Organophosphorus and carbamate insecticides. In: Olson KR, Anderson IB, Benowitz NL, et al., eds. *Poisoning & Drug Overdose.* 7th ed. New York: McGraw–Hill; 2018.

44. Nordt SP. Sympathomimetic poisoning. In: Schaider JL, Barkin RM, Hayden SR, Wolfe RE, Barkin AZ, Shayne P, eds. *Rosen & Barkin's 5-Minute Emergency Medicine Consult.* 6th ed. Philadelphia, PA: Lippincott Williams & Wilkins; 2020:1098–1099.

45. Aks SE. Cocaine poisoning. In: Schaider JL, Barkin RM, Hayden SR, Wolfe RE, Barkin AZ, Shayne P, eds. *Rosen & Barkin's 5-Minute Emergency Medicine Consult.* 6th ed. Philadelphia, PA: Lippincott Williams & Wilkins; 2020:246–247.

46. McGraw M, McGraw L. Bath salts: not as harmless as they sound. *J Emerg Nurs.* 2012;38(6):582-588. doi: 10.1016/j.jen.2012.07.025

47. Mills B, Yepes A, Nugent K. Synthetic cannabinoids. *Am J Med Sci.* 2015;350(1):59–62. doi: 10.1097/MAJ.0000000000000466

48. Miotto K, Striebel J, Cho AK, Wang C. Clinical and pharmacological aspects of bath salt use: a review of the literature and case reports. *Drug Alcohol Depend.* 2013;132(1-2):1–12. doi: 10.1016/j.drugalcdep.2013.06.016

49. Terry SM. Bath salt abuse: more than just hot water. *J Emerg Nurs.* 2014;40(1):88–91. doi: 10.1016/j.jen.2013.05.013

50. Ruby AJM, Lu JJ. Bath salts–synthetic cathinones poisoning. In: Schaider JL, Barkin RM, Hayden SR, Wolfe RE, Barkin AZ, Shayne P, eds. *Rosen & Barkin's 5-Minute Emergency Medicine Consult.* 6th ed. Philadelphia, PA: Lippincott Williams & Wilkins; 2020: 130–131.

51. Salani DA, Zdanowicz MM. Synthetic cannabinoids: the dangers of spicing it up. *J Psychol Nurs.* 2015;53(5):36–43. doi: 10.3928/02793695-20150422-01

52. White CM. How MDMA's pharmacology and pharmacokinetics drive desired effects and harm. *J Clin Pharmacol.* 2014;54(3): 245–252. doi: 10.1002/jcph.266

53. Mycyk MB. MDMA poisoning. In: Schaider JL, Barkin RM, Hayden SR, Wolfe RE, Barkin AZ, Shayne P, eds. *Rosen & Barkin's*

5-Minute Emergency Medicine Consult. 6th ed. Philadelphia, PA: Lippincott Williams & Wilkins; 2020:694–695.

54. McMahon DM, Winstead S, Weant KA. Toxic alcohol ingestions: focus on ethylene glycol and methanol. *Adv Emerg Nurs J.* 2009; 31(3):206–213. doi: 10.1097/TME.0b013e3181ad8be8

55. Cumpston KL. Ethylene glycol poisoning. In: Schaider JL, Barkin RM, Hayden SR, Wolfe RE, Barkin AZ, Shayne P, eds. *Rosen & Barkin's 5-Minute Emergency Medicine Consult.* 6th ed. Philadelphia, PA: Lippincott Williams & Wilkins; 2020:392–393.

56. Rietjens SJ, de Lange DW, Meulenbelt J. Ethylene glycol or methanol intoxication: which antidote should be used, fomepizole or ethanol? *Neth J Med.* 2014;72(2):73–79.

57. Norris RL, Bush SP, Cardwell MD. Bites by venomous reptiles in Canada, the United States, and Mexico. In: Auerbach PS, Cushing TA, Harris NS, eds. *Auerbach's Wilderness Medicine*, 7th ed. Philadelphia, PA: Elsevier; 2017:729–760.

58. Weinstein SA, Dart RC, Staples A, White J. Envenomations: an overview of clinical toxinology for the primary care physician. *Am Fam Physician.* 2009;80(8):793–802.

59. Clark RF. Snakebite. In: Olson KR, Anderson IB, Benowitz NL, et al., eds. *Poisoning & Drug Overdose.* 7th ed. New York: McGraw–Hill; 2018.

60. Lank PM, Erickson TB. Snake envenomation. In: Schaider JL, Barkin RM, Hayden SR, Wolfe RE, Barkin AZ, Shayne P, eds. *Rosen & Barkin's 5-Minute Emergency Medicine Consult.* 6th ed. Philadelphia, PA: Lippincott Williams & Wilkins; 2020:10481049.

61. Dart RC, White J. Snakebite. In: Tintinalli JE, Ma OJ, Yealey DM, et al., eds. *Tintinalli's Emergency Medicine: A Comprehensive Study Guide.* 9th ed. New York: McGraw–Hill; 2020.

16

Gynecologic and Obstetric Emergencies

BROOKE TURNER AND MICHAEL A. FRAKES

COMPETENCIES

1. Perform a focused assessment of the pregnant patient, which includes subjective and objective data related to the patient's pregnancy.
2. Identify normal physiologic changes that occur during pregnancy.
3. Perform a focused assessment of the fetus before and during transport.
4. Initiate and perform appropriate interventions for the patient in preterm labor.
5. Describe and discuss common indications for transport of the high-risk obstetric case.
6. Discuss common gynecologic emergencies.

Care of the pregnant patient brings the added stressor of caring for not just one, but two or more patients. The competing concerns for the pregnant patient and the fetus, as well as the physiological changes of pregnancy, could complicate patient management priorities. Generally, resuscitation of the mother optimizes fetal outcomes. Transport team must be aware of maternal and fetal therapies that can improve survivability and decrease morbidity of the fetus as well as the mother.

Determination of Team Composition for Transport of the Pregnant Patient

Perinatal transport team models are variable. Some patients are cared for by specialized teams, while many pregnant patients are transported by teams composed of personnel who transport a variety of patients. There is no demonstrated benefit to any particular model. The challenge for non-specialty teams is how to provide adequate training to assure proficiency in the assessment and care of the obstetrical patient.

The transport team should allow access to both the mother and the child if there is the possibility of delivery during transport. Each transport program should have a procedure in place that addresses when transport of a pregnant patient is and is not appropriate and what team members should provide care during transport. In some cases, the alternative of waiting for delivery and utilizing a different team to transport the newborn is appropriate.

Normal Physiologic Changes in Pregnancy

Understanding the normal physiologic changes that occur during pregnancy can assist the transport clinician in understanding normal variations, identifying important concerns, and in avoiding preventable complications with the pregnancy. The information gained with the general obstetric assessment (Box 16.1) aids the transport team in setting priorities for care during the transport. This review of systems is brief and highlights key areas of normal physiological change associated with pregnancy.[1–8]

Airway: The mucosa in the pharynx of the pregnant patient is hyperemic and more edematous. The trachea of the term pregnant patient tends to be anterior, and the epiglottis is reported to be friable. The risk for difficult or failed oral intubation is higher in the pregnant patient than in the nonpregnant patient – about 2% for obstetrical patients, compared with 0.12% of non-obstetrical patients. Interestingly, the risk factors for difficult intubation are similar to those for nonpregnant patients. Risk factors for difficult intubation include increased body mass index, Mallampati score III or IV, small hyoid-to-mentum distance, limited jaw protrusion, limited mouth opening, and cervical spine limitations.[3,4,6–8]

Hematologic: By term, the maternal blood volume has increased by 40%–50%. Plasma volume increases more than does the volume of red blood cells and platelets, so a dilutional anemia is normal in pregnancy. In cases of maternal blood loss, maternal hypotension is often not noted until the patient has lost approximately 30% of the blood volume because of the extra volume created during the pregnancy. During pregnancy, procoagulant activity from factors VII, VIII, X, and fibrinogen increases, while anticoagulant from fibrinolysis and protein S activity decreases, making pregnant patients hypercoagulable.[3,4,6,7]

Respiratory: Tidal volume increases by about 40%, and respiratory rate slightly increases; thus pregnant women normally have a mild compensated respiratory alkalosis. Alveolar ventilation increases by up to 50%. Importantly, the functional residual capacity decreases by about 20% and chest wall, but not lung, compliance worsens during pregnancy.[3,4,6,7]

Cardiac: Cardiac output increases by about 50%, related to the increased blood volume, and heart rate slightly increases, by about

• BOX 16.1 General Obstetric Assessment

1. Age of patient: Age (for women less than 18 or greater than 35 years of age) predisposes the obstetric patient to many complications.
2. Gravida/para: Gravid is the number of times pregnant, regardless of outcome. Parity is broken down into four sections. The first assessment is the number of term deliveries (after 36 weeks' gestation), and the next section is the number of deliveries before 36 weeks' gestation but less than 20 weeks. The next section is the number of abortions and miscarriages. The final section is the number of now living children. This more specific assessment of parity provides a tremendous amount of obstetric history. For example, a woman has been pregnant six times. She has two term deliveries, one preterm delivery, two abortions, and one baby who died of sudden infant death syndrome. Her G/P is: G6 P 2122.
3. Estimated date of confinement (EDC): The EDC can be estimated from the first day of the last menstrual period (LMP) by using Nägele's rule, which is to count back 3 months from the LMP and then add 7 days. The due date is accurate within 2 weeks. Applications (Apps) for mobile devices operating programs have free versions for calculating LMP/EDC and gestational age.
4. Ultrasound scan: Has the patient had an ultrasound scan? How many? When was the first ultrasound? In the event of an uncertain or unknown LMP or irregular menses, an ultrasound scan performed between 12 and 30 weeks is reliable for dating the pregnancy within 2 weeks. An ultrasound scan can confirm the EDC estimated by the LMP. Early ultrasound scans performed before 12 weeks are accurate for dating within 1 week. An ultrasound scan is invaluable with any question about placental location, amount of amniotic fluid present, fetal presentation, expected fetal growth, or anomalies.
5. In addition to the inquiry into medical history and allergies, obstetric history is of significance. The following information may be of some predictive value for the outcome of the current pregnancy:
   a. Did the patient deliver vaginally or by cesarean section? Has she had a vaginal birth after a cesarean section? Observe for the location and extent of any abdominal scars.
   b. Did she or the baby experience any delivery complications?
   c. Did she experience any complications associated with any past pregnancies?
   d. Has she had any preterm deliveries? At what gestation did she deliver, and what was the outcome?
   e. Has she had either spontaneous or elective abortions? Was a dilatation and curettage required?
   f. How many living children does she have? What were the birth weights and genders of each child?
   g. Has less than 1 year elapsed between the last delivery and commencement of the current pregnancy?
   h. What was the length of her last labor?
6. Pertaining to the current pregnancy:
   a. Is the patient having contractions? If so, when did the contractions begin? Has there been a change in the intensity or frequency of contractions? Is there accompanying backache or pelvic or rectal pressure? How strong do the contractions palpate and how do they compare with patient reporting? What are the frequency, duration, and regularity of the contractions?
   b. Is any vaginal bleeding or bloody show present? Is there active, frank bleeding? Attempt to help the patient quantify the bleeding by the number of towels, pads, or amount of clothing soaked before arrival and observe for evidence of dried blood on the perineum, legs, and soles of the feet. Was the bleeding painless or associated with contractions or abdominal pain? Was the blood bright red or dark? Was mucus combined with the blood (bloody show)? When did the bleeding begin? Was there any previous activity that may have precipitated the bleeding?
   c. Does the patient report leaking fluid vaginally? Does the patient believe her "bag of waters" has ruptured? Was there a gush or an intermittent trickle? A small leakage of clear fluid may be confused with urinary incontinence. Leakage of amniotic fluid is uncontrollable. What time did it happen? What color was the fluid: meconium-stained, dark (presence of blood in the fluid), or clear? Was an odor present? Is the Chux pad under the patient wet or pooling with fluid?

d. Does the patient smoke? If so, how much? Is there any evidence of alcohol or substance abuse? Attempt to ascertain from the patient the frequency and time of last usage.
   e. Has the patient had an adequate weight gain? Does she appear malnourished or obese?
   f. Has the patient had consistent prenatal care, no prenatal care, or limited prenatal care (three or fewer visits)? Obtain prenatal record if available because it provides a tremendous amount of obstetric information including history, ultrasound scan reports, laboratory reports, vital signs, and so forth.
   g. Has there been any change in fetal activity in the past several days?
   h. Is the patient currently taking any medications? If so, what is she taking and when was the last dosage?
   i. Is the patient having any current medical problems or problems with this pregnancy?
   j. Have any diagnostic tests been done?
7. Assess initial vital signs, including temperature: The blood pressure (BP), pulse, and respirations should be assessed every 15 minutes or as indicated. The obstetric patient should be positioned in the left lateral recumbent position before the BP is taken. When the patient is in the supine position, the gravid uterus may cause obstruction of the inferior vena cava, diminishing venous return to the heart, which may lead to supine hypotension. Consequently, uteroplacental blood flow is decreased, placing the fetus at risk for compromise.
8. Fetal heart tones (FHTs): If the patient is currently being monitored with electronic fetal monitoring (EFM), evaluate the baseline fetal heart rate (FHR) and baseline variability, observing for accelerations and decelerations. FHR should be assessed with Doppler if EFM is unavailable. FHR auscultation should be assessed every 15 minutes or more frequently if any irregularities are noted. For strip interpretation, refer to the discussion in this chapter on fetal monitoring.
9. Fundal height (FH): FH should be measured in centimeters from the symphysis to the fundus. The fundal height roughly correlates to the gestation of the pregnancy in weeks. In the presence of polyhydramnios, multiple gestations, a large-for-gestation fetus, or a fetus with intrauterine growth restriction, the fundal height may not correlate with the gestation, signaling the possibility of complications. If no tape measure is available or the patient is unable to provide information, such as in the case of a trauma, assess the fundus in relation to the umbilicus. If the fundus is above the umbilicus, it is estimated the pregnancy is at least 20–24 weeks' gestation.
10. Lightly palpate the fundus for strength, frequency, and duration of contractions: The fingertips can indent the fundus freely with mild contractions and slightly with moderate contractions; firm tension is noted with strong contractions. Between contractions, palpate the abdomen for localized or generalized tenderness and observe the patient's coping response to the contractions. Gestures, posture, and facial expressions in response to contractions and verbal description should be noted. If the patient is in labor, observe for indications of advancing labor such as apprehension, restlessness, increasing difficulty coping with the contractions, screaming, nausea and vomiting, bearing-down effort, increase in bloody show, or a bulging perineum.
11. Determine the fetal position with abdominal palpation: With the fingertips and palms, lightly palpate the fundus for the head or buttocks, moving down the sides to identify the fetal spine and small parts, and palpate the lower uterine segment for the presenting part. If the fetal position remains unclear, the fetus may be in a transverse lie. The FHT is heard most clearly over the fetal spine.
12. Assess cervical status as indicated by the presence of contractions: If the amniotic membranes are intact, cervical status just before departure should be documented. If the membranes are ruptured, a sterile vaginal examination (SVE) should never be attempted unless delivery is deemed imminent. In the presence of hemorrhage, an SVE should never be attempted unless a placenta previa has been ruled out with ultrasound scan. During transport, an SVE is not indicated unless signs of advancing labor are noted.
13. Observe for the presence of other risk factors that predispose the obstetric patient to complications.

From Seidel HM, et al. *Mosby's Physical Examination Handbook*. St. Louis, MO: Mosby; 2011.

10 beats at term. Blood pressure is modestly decreased until near the end of pregnancy.[3,4,6,7]

Gastrointestinal: Slowing of peristalsis and resulting constipation occur. The stomach empties slowly, and the pregnant patient is at a high risk of aspiration with altered levels of consciousness. Because of this effect, a pregnant woman is always considered to have a full stomach no matter when her last meal was. Increased salivation is common, and frequent suctioning may be needed in the case of oral intubation. An increased incidence of cholelithiasis is found during pregnancy.[3,4,6–8]

Renal: Increased renal filtration of glucose and sodium occurs during pregnancy. Blood urea nitrogen (BUN) and creatinine (CR) levels are both lower during pregnancy. This is important and easy to overlook – a creatinine over 0.75 mg/dL (66 μmol/L) is elevated in a pregnant patient, but would be unremarkable in nonpregnant patients.[5]

Uterus: The uterus becomes the largest intra-abdominal organ. Uterine and placental perfusion increases to 600–800 mL of blood per minute at term. A very high risk of maternal hemorrhage is found in the presence of uterine or placental injury.[3,4,6,7]

Musculoskeletal: The abdominal viscera become stretched and distended because of the growing uterus. These distorted viscera may cause abdominal pain to be referred. The effects of the hormone relaxin also cause the symphysis pubis cartilage to slightly separate, increasing pelvic instability. The gravid uterus causes the patient's center of gravity to be altered, and an increase in falls may be noted. The thoracic cavity also expands during pregnancy to allow greater lung expansion because the lungs have less distance to elongate because of the gravid uterus.[3,4,6,7]

Liver: The liver is the only organ to not increase efficiency during pregnancy. Hepatic function values remain the same as nonpregnant values.[3,4,6,7]

Metabolic: All metabolic functions increase to provide for the demands of the fetus, placenta, and uterus as well as for the mother's increased basal metabolic rate and oxygen consumption. Protein metabolism increases for maternal and fetal growth. The pancreas cannot supply the increased demand. After delivery, the mother will become hypoglycemic because insulin levels are still high. The infant's blood sugar should also be checked because there still may be a large amount of insulin in its body after delivery. Use particular caution in infants of diabetic mothers.[3,4,6,7]

Obstetrical Assessment and Preparation

As with all patients, assessment begins with a primary assessment to identify life threats before proceeding to the secondary assessment. The secondary assessment is where the obstetric assessment will take place. The assessment of an obstetrical patient is built on the foundation of the same good complete examination and review of systems that every patient receives. Some assessments are then geared specifically to the obstetrical patient (see Box 16.1).[1–4,6,7]

The obstetrical patient who is greater than 20 weeks' gestation should be positioned in a lateral position. Although patients are traditionally positioned left lateral, displacement either direction is sufficient to displace the uterus from the inferior vena cava (IVC) in order to optimize venous return to the heart. If the patient must be supine, such as for resuscitative procedures, displace the uterus manually.[1–4,6,7]

Assess for infection. Observe for symptoms of urinary tract infection, pyelonephritis, vaginitis, chorioamnionitis, or signs of viral infection. These signs may include uterine tenderness, vaginal discharge, an elevated white count, uterine contractions, fetal tachycardia, maternal fever, and maternal tachycardia.[1–4,6,7]

Determine status of amniotic membranes and assess for fluid leakage. Note and quantify any bleeding or fluid from the vagina. Note the color and odor of the fluid. Volume loss should be assessed as objectively as possible. Use pad counts, weighing of blue Chux pads, or actual description on the pad (i.e., a 1 × 4-inch stain). Clots can be measured in a graduated cylinder or suction canister. Assess whether blood loss is associated with any pain or contractions. Premature or prolonged rupture of the amniotic membrane is associated with preterm labor and increased risk for infection, respectively.[1–4,6,7]

Determine the contraction pattern. Contractions initiate in the uterine fundus and diminish as they progress toward the cervix, so contractions are always palpated at the fundus. Patients do not always perceive contractions, particularly when the uterus is smaller. If at the peak of the contraction the fundus palpates similar to the consistency of a nose, then the contraction is considered mild. If the contraction palpates as firm as the chin, then it is considered a moderately strong contraction. If it palpates as firm as a forehead, then it is considered a strong contraction.[3,6]

Determine cervical status and fetal station. Cervical dilation patterns vary from primiparas to multiparas. Primiparas tend to have effacement (cervical thinning) before dilation occurs, while the multiparous patient often has dilation before significant effacement occurs. Because of predictable dilation and effacement patterns, the primipara shows more signs of active labor (Fig. 16.1). Cervical status is always reported as dilation-effacement-station (e.g., 3/90/−1). Dilation is the number of centimeters the cervix is open. The cervix is considered completely dilated when it is approximately 10 cm. An important transport consideration is that with premature gestations the fetus is small and may fit though a cervix that is not completely dilated. For example, a 500-g, 23-week fetus may fit through a cervix that is only 6–7 cm dilated. Effacement is thinning of the cervix.[3,6]

Station is location of the presenting fetal part in relation to the ischial spines, which are protruding bones on the lower pelvis. These spines can be palpated through the vaginal basement, and the presenting part is compared with the location of these protrusions. Station is the number of centimeters above or below those spines. The head begins to crown at +3 station and is delivered at +4.[3,6]

Assess fetal well-being. Fetal well-being is evaluated by looking at the fetal heart rate, pattern, and asking about fetal movement compared with historical patterns. Fetal monitoring may be accomplished with intermittent Doppler auscultation, intermittent point of care ultrasound, and with continuous external fetal monitoring, where an external ultrasound scan device records fetal heart tones and a tocodynamometer detects subjective uterine activity.[9,10] Fetal heart tones are best auscultated through the fetal back, which can be found by palpating for the most rigid part of the fundus. The maternal pulse should be compared with the fetal heart rate (FHR) tracing to confirm that the maternal signal is not being traced instead of the fetal heart rate.

The mode of FHR assessment is program- and institution-dependent, and the American Congress of Obstetricians and Gynecologists (ACOG) does not make a statement on which method of fetal monitoring is recommended. Intermittent Doppler or ultrasound auscultation does not allow for assessment of variability but can assess for FHR and responses to contractions if auscultation is performed during and after contractions. ACOG does recommend that FHR assessment should be done a minimum of every 15 minutes during transport.[9] Continuous fetal monitoring with cardiotocography is not associated with differences in

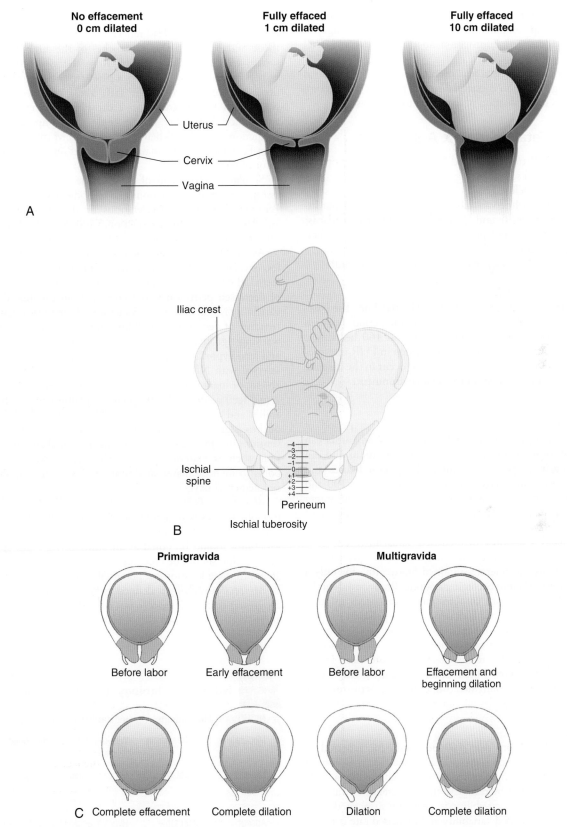

• **Fig. 16.1** Cervical status and fetal station. **A**, Cervical effacement and dilation in various stages of labor. **B**, Fetal station height of presenting part in relation to maternal ischial spines. **C**, Cervical dilation and effacement. (A, B, Copyright © Shutterstock.com; C, from McKinney E, et al. *Maternal-Child Nursing.* 4th ed. Philadelphia, PA: Saunders; 2013.)

cerebral palsy, infant mortality or other standard measures of neonatal well-being compared with intermittent monitoring, but does provide additional information about maternal and fetal condition.[11]

For teams that use external fetal monitoring, appropriate initial and continuing education is essential to safe practice. The section below describes the evaluation of fetal monitor tracings.[9,10]

Continuous Fetal Heart Rate Assessment

Assessment of FHR tracings should follow a systematic approach with these sequential steps:

1. Assessment of baseline FHR
2. Assessment of baseline variability with NICHD (National Institute of Child Health and Human Development) standards
3. Assessment of periodic/episodic changes, including accelerations or decelerations
4. Assessment for the presence of tachycardia or bradycardia

Baseline

The first parameter to be assessed is the FHR baseline. The baseline is the average of the FHR over a 10-minute period, between contractions, and is typically between 110 and 160 beats/min. Evaluation of the FHR baseline is a critical step in FHR interpretations. It allows interpretation of trends that occur in the baseline and can reflect subtle changes in the fetal environment.

Bradycardia

A baseline FHR of less than 110 beats/min for a period of 10 minutes or longer is defined as bradycardia. Bradycardia can occur as result of numerous acute or chronic conditions and can be hypoxic or nonhypoxic in nature. Many term fetuses and those past maturity may have a stable baseline between 100 and 120 beats/min, reflecting a more mature fetal neurologic system that is more parasympathetically controlled. In the absence of hypoxia, adequate variability and accelerations are also noted.

Bradycardia is a response of increased parasympathetic tone and is reflected by a decrease in fetal CO in the presence of hypoxia. The fetus can tolerate sustained bradycardia for only a short length of time before becoming acidotic. Bradycardia can be acute because of severe cord compression. It can occur minutes before delivery when the cord is drawn into the pelvis in the second stage or with a cord prolapse. Bradycardia can also occur with hypertonic or tetanic contractions as seen with placenta abruptio and any event that causes maternal hypotension. In the presence of chronic hypoxia, bradycardia is usually a late occurrence. Evaluation of variability determines how the fetus tolerates the stress.

Tachycardia

A baseline FHR of more than 160 beats/min for a period of 10 minutes or longer is considered tachycardia. Tachycardia is a response of increased sympathetic tone and is reflected by a compensatory mechanism to increase CO in the presence of transient hypoxia. A decrease in variability is generally associated with tachycardia. This decreased variability and increased rate is reflective of the fetus returning to a more primitive or sympathetic response. Fetal tachycardia may be maternal or fetal in origin. Factors that contribute to tachycardia include smoking, maternal fever, use of beta-sympathomimetic agents, fetal anemia, fetal hypovolemia, fetal tachydysrhythmias, chorioamnionitis, and maternal hyperthyroidism.

Variability[9,10]

Fluctuations in the FHR reflect interplay between the sympathetic and parasympathetic branches of the autonomic nervous system (ANS). A constant pull from the sympathetic nervous system increases the HR, and a push from the parasympathetic nervous system decreases the HR. These normal variations between each fetal heartbeat give the FHR tracing its "squiggly" appearance. Variability is the single most important factor in prediction of fetal well-being, based on EFM monitor interpretation. Fetal movement remains the number one non-monitor indicator of fetal well-being.

Similar to assessment of the baseline, variability can only be assessed between contractions and episodic and periodic changes. Periodic changes are accelerations or decelerations, which are associated with uterine contraction, while episodic changes are accelerations/decelerations not associated with uterine contractions.

As blood flow decreases across the placenta or umbilical cord, less oxygen is available for the fetus. If the hypoxic events are corrected, the fetus usually tolerates them well. However, if the cause of decreased perfusion is not corrected, an eventual decrease in variability is noted. Careful evaluation of the FHR tracing reflects trending of decreasing variability (minimal or absent), which is a warning sign that the fetus is losing compensatory mechanisms and fetal hypoxia and acidosis are increasing. Variability should be assessed with NICHD terminology such as moderate, minimal, absent, or marked (Table 16.1) Interestingly, the incidence rate of actual fetal acidemia in the presence of minimal or absent variability and decelerations are only 23%.[10] However, the presence of these signs remains an indicator for intervention. These interventions include measures to increase placental and uterine perfusion, such as maternal position change, intravenous (IV) fluid bolus to increase maternal volume/perfusion, and application of supplemental oxygen.

Absent variability occurs when the amplitude range is undetectable. Causes may include fetal metabolic acidosis, neurologic abnormality, marked prematurity, and cardiac arrhythmia. Absent variability should be noted as an ominous sign and appropriate intervention should be taken immediately with rapid transport to an appropriate location for potential delivery.

Minimal variability is defined as fluctuations in the FHR that are greater than undetectable but less than 5 beats/min. This variability is often associated with fetal hypoxia and acidosis. However,

TABLE 16.1	**NICHD Terminology for FHR Variability**	
NICHD	**Fluctuations**	**Indications**
Moderate	6–25 beats/min	Well-oxygenated, nonacidotic, intact/mature CNS
Minimal	≤5 beats/min	Hypoxia, acidosis, sleep patterns, maternal drug use, cardiac or CNS insult, prematurity
Absent	Undetectable from baseline	Hypoxia, acidosis, sleep pattern, maternal drug use, cardiac or CNS insult
Marked	>25 beats/min	Fetal movement or early hypoxia

CNS, Central nervous system; *NICHD*, National Institute of Child Health and Human Development.

benign or expected minimal variability can occur in certain clinical situations including fetal sleep and sedation if, for example, the mother has received narcotics. Narcotics are a central nervous system (CNS) depressant, and anything that decreases the maternal CNS can decrease fetal CNS as it passes through the placenta. As the maternal drug is metabolized and excreted, the effects on the fetus should also be seen to diminish. The most common reason for benign minimal variability is the fetal sleep pattern. The fetus has frequent sleep periods that range from 20 to 40 minutes. A key assessment pearl is that although fetal sleep patterns are common, they are transient in nature and rarely last longer than 40 minutes. In addition, moderate variability should be documented before and after the sleep pattern. Another common reason for minimal variability is immaturity in gestational age, which is associated with CNS immaturity. Fetuses that are less than 32 weeks' gestation show less variability because the ANS may not yet be fully developed. Fetal arrhythmias and cardiac or CNS anomalies may also be responsible for minimal or absent variability. These causes show variability changes from the time monitoring is initiated.

Moderate variability is indicative of an adequately oxygenated, normal pH, mature and intact ANS. Moderate variability is defined as fluctuations in the FHR that range between 6 and 25 beats/min. The presence of moderate variability is reassuring because it indicates that the fetus is tolerating blood flow changes within the uterus.

Marked variability of more than 25 beats of fluctuation may be one of the earliest signs of hypoxia. Although it may also be an indication of increased fetal activity, constant assessment and reevaluation are necessary. If continuous EFM is used during transport, the clinician should keep in mind that a greater degree of variability may be recorded than is actually present because of vibrations from the vehicle.

Periodic Changes/Episodic Changes

Periodic changes are changes that occur in the FHR tracing related to uterine contractions. Episodic changes are changes in the FHR tracing that are not associated with uterine contractions and are often related to fetal movement. The FHR may accelerate, decelerate, or not respond.

Acceleration

Accelerations above the baseline are usually associated with fetal movement but may occur during contractions (Fig. 16.2). Because the hypoxic fetus with metabolic acidosis is unable to accelerate its HR, accelerations are viewed as a sign of fetal well-being. The true definition of acceleration is a transient increase above the baseline greater than 15 beats/min for 15 seconds or longer and typically lasting less than 2 minutes in duration for fetuses that are greater than 32 weeks' gestation. The definition of acceleration for a fetus younger than 32 weeks is a transient increase over baseline of greater than 10 beats/min for at least 10 seconds and typically less than 2 minutes. Uniform accelerations are accelerations that occur with each contraction and are uniform in shape and size. This acceleration pattern may be associated with breech presentation or early and mild cord compression. In very early labor, the contractions are not strong and the fundus or top of the uterus gently compresses the breech during contractions, which causes a sympathetic response and accelerations are noted. Later, as the contractions increase in strength and the head of the fetus is pushed down into the pelvis, uniform decelerations are seen (see the section Early Decelerations).

Although the presence of accelerations and moderate variability are excellent monitor signs of fetal well-being, fetal movement remains the best non-monitor indicator of fetal well-being. Only well-oxygenated fetuses with normal pH levels have consistent fetal movement patterns. Certainly, all fetuses have different movement patterns that are unique to themselves. During transport, the clinician should assess the current movement pattern compared with the usual movement pattern. For example, a fetus that is known to have movements of at least 15 times an hour that is now reported to have only moved once in the past 2 hours shows a significant deviation from normal patterns and

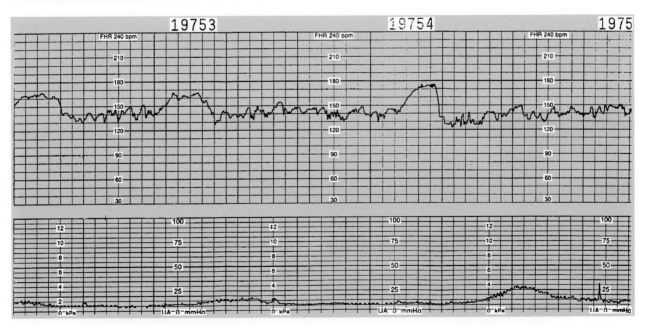

• **Fig. 16.2** Accelerations. (From Wade K, Greenwood T. Gynecologic and obstetric emergencies. In: ASTNA; Semonin Holleran R, Wolfe AC, Frakes MA, eds. *Patient Transport: Principles and Practice.* 5th ed. St. Louis, MO: Mosby Elsevier; 2017.)

further assessment and documentation are necessary. The transport team should take note of fetal movements and whether the mother, the greatest assessor of fetal movement, has noticed a decrease, increase, or no change in fetal movement. Decreased fetal movement may be indicative of hypoxia. Although a decrease in fetal movement may be anticipated, such as in the event of maternal trauma and blood loss, the transport team is expected to inform the maternal fetal medicine physicians of this change in fetal status.

Variable Deceleration

Variable decelerations can occur at any time during a contraction (Fig. 16.3). The shape may also vary and is frequently V-shaped or W-shaped. The decelerations are known as variable because of the varied shape and timing. Cord compression is typically responsible for these decelerations, though may also occur from head compression because of vagal stimulation in the second stage of labor (pushing). Physiologically, as the cord is compressed, blood flow through the umbilical cord is decreased. Baroreceptors cause a brief increase in the FHR to compensate. The blood flow is further impeded, and a sharp decrease occurs in the FHR. As the umbilical cord compression is relieved, the FHR responds with a quick increase above the baseline in an attempt to increase oxygenation status. After a short period of time, typically less than 5–10 seconds, the FHR returns to baseline with moderate variability. Initially, variables may have a characteristic appearance; frequently, a short acceleration is observed, followed by a rapid deceleration for some seconds and then a rapid rise and a short acceleration before a return to the FHR baseline.

Late Decelerations

Late decelerations begin at or after the apex (peak) of the contraction. They gradually decelerate in a uniformed "U" shape and return to the FHR baseline well after the contraction is over (Fig. 16.4). By definition, late decelerations must be recurrent, which means they occur in greater than 50% of all uterine contractions (NICHD).[1] Physiologically, during a normal contraction, a decreased amount of oxygen crosses the placenta. A healthy fetus can tolerate this decrease in oxygen via its oxygen reserves. A compromised fetus that has experienced prolonged or chronic hypoxia does not have oxygen reserves available; therefore it cannot tolerate the decreased oxygen availability found during contractions. Not until the contraction is over, and the maternal–fetal exchange can resume, does the FHR return to baseline. Late decelerations always mean uteroplacental insufficiency: either the placenta, the fetus, or the uterus presents with conditions that interfere with normal exchange of oxygen between the mother and fetus. One analogy is a child being dunked in a pool. The child tolerates the dunking early on, but if it continues, the child becomes fatigued, loses O_2 reserve, and ends up gasping every time it surfaces. When a contraction is stronger, the insufficiency is greater and the deceleration is proportional. However, "size does not matter." With severe hypoxia, the myocardial depression may be such that the heart is unable to decelerate in response to the stress of the contraction, and very subtle late decelerations are seen accompanied by a flat FHR baseline. Simply stated, the fetus becomes so hypoxic and acidotic that it cannot render a response to the impeded blood flow. The fetus is too sick to "wave the white flag." A FHR tracing that is tachycardia with minimal or absent variability and subtle late decelerations is considered ominous and interventions must be made to improve fetal oxygenation. These interventions include measures to increase placental perfusion, such as maternal position change, supplemental O_2 via a nonrebreather mask, IV fluid (IVF) boluses, and possible delivery, if improvement is not noted.

Uteroplacental insufficiency may result from numerous maternal and fetal conditions, such as hypertensive disorders of pregnancy, diabetes mellitus (DM), cardiovascular or kidney disease, chorioamnionitis, smoking, a fetus that is past maturity, and fetal hydrops. Uteroplacental insufficiency may also result from decreased placental perfusion in placental abruption or previa, uterine hypertonus as a result of oxytocin stimulation, and hypotension. As with variable decelerations, evaluation of late decelerations with respect to FHR baseline, variability, and changes noted over time is necessary in determining the

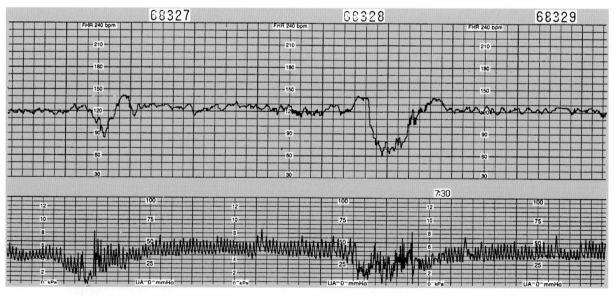

• **Fig. 16.3** Variable decelerations. (From Wade K, Greenwood T. Gynecologic and obstetric emergencies. In: ASTNA; Semonin Holleran R, Wolfe AC, Frakes MA, eds. *Patient Transport: Principles and Practice.* 5th ed. St. Louis, MO: Elsevier; 2017.)

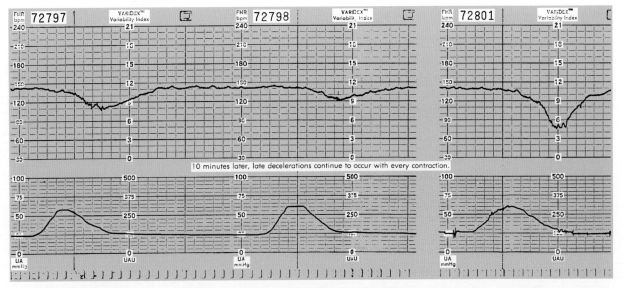

• **Fig. 16.4** Late decelerations. Also note minimal variability. (From Wade K, Greenwood T. Gynecologic and obstetric emergencies. In: ASTNA; Semonin Holleran R, Wolfe AC, Frakes MA, eds. *Patient Transport: Principles and Practice.* 5th ed. St. Louis, MO: Elsevier; 2017.)

well-being of the fetus. Even an otherwise healthy well-oxygenated fetus can experience late decelerations in the presence of acute hypotension and hypoxia. An example of this is a mother that is obtunded and was laid flat on her back on a backboard. This position alone can cause inferior vena cava syndrome (IVCS) and rapid decrease in maternal venous blood return, which then causes maternal hypotension that leads to profound fetal hypotension and results in late decelerations. Once the maternal position is tilted to the right lateral position (RLP) or left lateral position (LLP), the blood flow improves, and the late decelerations resolve.

Early Deceleration

Early decelerations are innocuous decelerations that begin close to the beginning of the contraction and end close to the end of the contraction. These decelerations appear to mirror the contractions. As the head is compressed, the vagus nerve is stimulated and causes a parasympathetic response that leads to a deceleration. The deceleration ends as the contraction ends because the vagus nerve (head) is no longer compressed. Early decelerations are usually associated with moderate variability and are considered benign in nature. These decelerations frequently occur in active labor when the cervix has dilated 4–7 cm, as the head is compressed into the pelvic cavity with contractions. A transport consideration is that a sterile vaginal examination (SVE) or sterile speculum examination should be performed before transport to rule out advanced cervical dilation when early decelerations are noted. In FHR interpretation, late decelerations should not be confused with early decelerations. Also, consider other reassuring attributes such as moderate variability and the presence of accelerations or fetal movement to help discern early from late decelerations.

Sinusoidal

Sinusoidal is a rare FHR pattern in which a uniform sine wave pattern occurs. This FHR remains within normal baselines but has an obvious unusual appearance. It is often described as an undulating pattern that is saw-toothed in appearance. Possible causes of this pattern are fetal hypovolemia or anemia; it may occur in cases of erythroblastosis fetalis, accidental tap of the umbilical cord during amniocentesis, fetomaternal transfusion, placental abruption, or another type of accident. Neither variability nor accelerations/decelerations can be assessed. When this pattern is recognized, rapid delivery is usually recommended unless the underlying pathology can be corrected. For example, in the case of severe fetal anemia, a blood transfusion can be administered to the fetus via a percutaneous umbilical cord sampling procedure. Once the anemia is resolved, the sinusoidal pattern is resolved. However, a more commonly observed FHR pattern is a pseudosinusoidal or undulating pattern that is not pathologic (Fig. 16.5). This pattern is linked to maternal drug administration, both prescribed and illicit.

Complications of Pregnancy and Delivery

Supine Hypotension

The inferior vena cava (IVC) is responsible for transporting venous blood from the lower part of the body back to the right atrium in which it can travel through its normal cardiac flow and then be returned to the central circulation as oxygenated blood. The IVC was once described by a cardiovascular surgeon as having the consistency of a wet paper towel roll. With this description, imagine the weight of the fetus, amniotic fluid, placenta, and uterus compressing the IVC. When a gravid (pregnant) patient lies supine, she quite effectively compresses the IVC. Venous blood return is dramatically decreased, which causes a logical decrease in cardiac output (CO). If blood is not brought to the heart, the heart does not have volume to pump out.

For awake and alert patients, IVCS is rarely a problem because they cannot tolerate lying supine if the weight of the gravid uterus is enough to compress the IVC. The patients experience nausea and naturally turn themselves to their sides. Position gravid patients, greater than 20 weeks' gestational age, in either left or right lateral position on the stretcher. If the patient cannot be turned, the uterus can be manually displaced.[3,4,6]

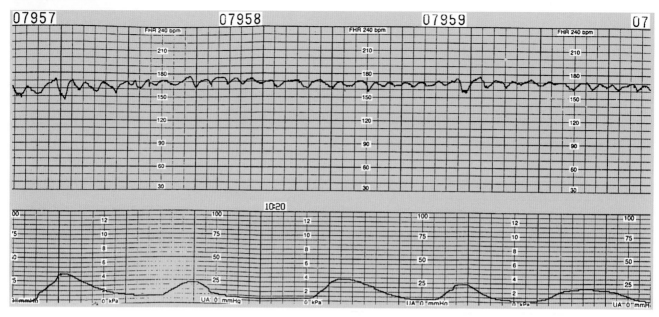

• **Fig. 16.5** Sinusoidal pattern. (From Wade K, Greenwood T. Gynecologic and obstetric emergencies. In: ASTNA; Semonin Holleran R, Wolfe AC, Frakes MA, eds. *Patient Transport: Principles and Practice.* 5th ed. St. Louis, MO: Elsevier; 2017.)

Diabetes in Pregnancy

The obstetric patient with a pregnancy complicated by diabetes mellitus (DM) is at an increased risk compared with the remainder of the pregnant population for development of gestational hypertension and related disorders; polyhydramnios; and infections such as vaginitis, urinary tract infections, and pyelonephritis. Delivery via cesarean section and preterm delivery also occur with increased frequency because of macrosomia or changes in fetal status and well-being.

Macrosomia is a fetus that is large for gestational age with increased fat deposition and an enlarged spleen and liver. Macrosomia is seen more commonly when the mother has gestational DM or DM without vasculopathy. As commonly found with patients with diabetes, vascular changes can affect perfusion. The placentas of women with diabetes tend to have decreased perfusion and more calcification. This in turn leads to decreased fetal perfusion and higher risks of intrauterine growth restriction (IUGR) and changes in fetal status and well-being.

The fetus of a mother with diabetes is at increased risk as well. Complications associated with the fetus include congenital anomalies, IUGR, macrosomia, delivery trauma, fetal distress, hypoglycemia, hypocalcemia, hyperbilirubinemia, respiratory distress, and intrauterine death. Congenital anomalies are seen more frequently when pregnant women with diabetes are in poor control of their diabetes.[3,4,6]

Gestational Hypertension

Hypertension is the most common medical problem encountered during pregnancy, complicating 2% to 8% of pregnancies, and accounting for 16% of maternal deaths.[12–17]

Gestational hypertension refers to a group of hypertensive disorders that have their onset during pregnancy and resolve after pregnancy. Persistent hypertension not associated with pregnancy

that develops before 20 weeks' gestation is considered to be chronic and is called essential or primary hypertension.

Gestational hypertension is a rise in systolic pressure of 30 mmHg or a rise in diastolic pressure of 15 mmHg based on previously known pressures. Diastolic pressure tends to be a more reliable predictor of the disease process. The blood pressure is ideally taken with the patient in the left lateral recumbent position. Blood pressure associated with gestational hypertension is labile and may change in the time it takes to retake the blood pressure.[14,15]

The absolute cause of gestational hypertension is unknown. Primarily, gestational hypertension is a disease of the primigravida, the teenaged primigravida, or the primigravida over 35 years of age. The patient with DM, preexisting cardiovascular or kidney disease, polyhydramnios, family history of gestational hypertension, or no prenatal care is also at risk. Other predisposing factors include pregnancy that is exposed to a superabundance of chorionic villi, such as with multiple gestation, hydatidiform mole, or fetal hydrops, or poor nutritional status, large fetus, or Rh incompatibility.[14–16]

Preeclampsia and Eclampsia

Background

The diagnostic criteria for preeclampsia and eclampsia continue to evolve. The most current definition for preeclampsia is new onset hypertension (systolic >140 mmHg and diastolic >90 mmHg) between 20 weeks' gestation and 6 weeks postpartum and accompanied by one or more other features: proteinuria, other maternal organ dysfunction (including liver, kidney, neurological), or hematological involvement, and/or uteroplacental dysfunction, such as fetal growth restriction and/or abnormal Doppler ultrasound findings of uteroplacental blood flow. Preeclampsia is considered to have severe features when accompanied by significant hypertension (systolic blood pressure ≥160 mmHg or diastolic blood pressure ≥110 mmHg), persistent headaches, changes in vision, epigastric or right upper quadrant pain, pulmonary edema, or organ dysfunction such as increased creatinine, transaminitis, oliguria, or thrombocytopenia.[14–17]

Importantly, the risk for gestational hypertensive disease persists after delivery: the reported prevalence of postpartum hypertension and postpartum preeclampsia is up to 28% of cases, usually within 48 hours after birth, although the syndrome can occur up to 6 weeks after childbirth. Nearly half of eclampsia cases present after delivery, and 10% of maternal deaths from hypertension occur during the postpartum period.[18]

There are multisystem effects from preeclampsia. In patients with gestational hypertension, an increased sensitivity to angiotensin II develops and vasospasm, particularly arteriolar vasospasm, occurs, initiating vasoconstriction. Compromised uterine and placental blood flow leads to placental degeneration. With chronic decreased perfusion, fetal intrauterine growth restriction can result.[12,14–17]

Decreased renal blood flow decreases glomerular filtration rate. Changes in the glomerular endothelium cause proteinuria. Plasma uric acid and creatinine are elevated because of decreased renal clearance. With decreased kidney function, sodium and water are retained. In conjunction with a decreased circulating albumin and a decrease in colloid osmotic pressure, fluid is shifted from the intravascular space to the extracellular space, causing the characteristic edema of preeclamptic patients.[12,14–17]

The normal hypervolemia of pregnancy is decreased or nearly absent when preeclampsia is present. The pregnant patient still has a tremendous amount of volume in her body; it just is no longer in the intravascular compartment where it belongs. Also observed is intravascular platelet and fibrin deposition, which occurs in response to vessel wall damage as the disease progresses.[12,14–17]

Reduction in blood flow to the liver impairs liver function. Swelling of the capsule (the fibrous sheath that completely covers the liver) and subcapsular hemorrhage may occur. Epigastric pain (right upper and mid-upper quadrant pain) is associated with hepatic swelling. This epigastric pain is caused by hepatic swelling but is often misdiagnosed as heartburn, an accepted symptom associated with pregnancy.[12,14–17]

Although cerebral perfusion is not initially impaired, osmotic changes and vasospasm give rise to cerebral edema, hemorrhage, and CNS irritability, evidenced by hyperreflexia, headaches, visual disturbances, clonus, nausea and vomiting, decreasing LOC, and clonic and tonic seizures. Retinal arteriolar spasms, ischemia, and edema because of decreased perfusion are the sources of the visual disturbances seen in preeclampsia. Blurring, scotoma (blind or twinkling spots in the vision), and diplopia (double vision) may occur. Retinal detachment is a rare occurrence. Questions related to blurred vision or visual changes are key in assessment of patients with preeclampsia.[12,14–17]

The rhythmic, oscillating stretch reflex of clonus is an indicator of neuromuscular irritability in patients with preeclampsia. It is classically evaluated at the ankles: the examiner supports the leg in knee flexion and, with the other hand, briskly dorsiflexes the foot while feeling and watching for rhythmic contractions[2,6] (Table 16.2).

Eclampsia is seizures superimposed on obstetrical patients with hypertensive disease. Eclampsia can occur before labor, during labor, or in the postpartum period. Eclamptic seizures are generally tonic–clonic and may begin around the mouth in the form of facial twitching. Eclampsia is the development of convulsions in a preexisting preeclampsia or it may appear unexpectedly in a patient with minimally elevated blood pressure and no proteinuria.

TABLE 16.2	Assessment of Edema and Hyperreflexia	
Evaluation of Edema Score		**Score**
Minimal edema of lower extremities		+1
Marked edema of lower extremities		+2
Edema of lower extremities, face, and hands		+3
Generalized massive edema, including abdomen and sacrum		+4
Evaluation of Hyperreflexia		**Grade**
None elicited		0
Sluggish or dull		+1
Active, normal		+2
Brisk		+3
Brisk with transient clonus		+4
Brisk with sustained clonus		+5

Note: Assessment of hyperreflexia is usually accomplished with eliciting patellar deep tendon reflexes. Clonus can be assessed at the same time with swift dorsiflexion of the foot. Clonus indicates neuromuscular irritability, and each beat should be counted.
Data from Seidel HM, Ball JW, Dains JE, Benedict GW. *Mosby's Physical Examination Handbook*. 3rd ed. St. Louis, MO: Mosby; 1999.

Eclamptic seizures are generally self-limiting and self-terminating. If an eclamptic seizure persists for more than 5 minutes, evaluate for an additional neurological insult. Traditional intervention with short- or long-acting anticonvulsants is not indicated for the self-limiting seizures.[7,12,14–17]

Management

The critical initial step in decreasing maternal morbidity and mortality is to administer antihypertensive medications within 60 minutes of documentation of persistent hypertension. Among women with stroke in one key study, all had systolic blood pressure greater than 155 mmHg and nearly one-quarter had diastolic blood pressure over 105 mmHg.[12–14]

Various agents are used as antihypertensives: labetalol, hydralazine, and nicardipine are common intravenous agents. Labetalol is given at a 20 mg dose initially, followed by doses of 40 mg in 10–14, 15 minutes and 80 mg in 10–14, 15 minutes if hypertension persists. Hydralazine is typically dosed at 5–10 mg up to maximum of 20–30 mg, and nicardipine as an infusion between 5 and 30 mg/h.[7,14–16]

Magnesium sulfate is the other therapeutic cornerstone for preeclampsia and eclampsia. Conceptually, magnesium prevents the next seizure. Accordingly, the preeclamptic patient is loaded with magnesium and the patient who has an eclamptic seizure receives additional magnesium. Physiologically, it slows impulse transmission at the neuromuscular junction by displacing calcium to interfere with the release of acetylcholine. Patients are typically loaded with 4–6 grams of magnesium sulfate, followed by an infusion of 1–2 grams/hour and given an additional 1–2 grams if seizures occur.[7,14–16]

Adverse, but not toxic, reactions to magnesium include transient hypotension, flushing, sweating, nausea and vomiting, and drowsiness. A decrease in FHR variability may be observed because magnesium is a known CNS depressant. Magnesium sulfate is primarily excreted in the urine, and toxicity may develop rather rapidly in the patient with significantly impaired kidney function. Recall that pregnant patients should have a lower-than-normal baseline creatinine, so urine output should exceed 30 mL/h while the patient is receiving the infusion. Magnesium should be used cautiously in patients with renal or cardiac disease.[5,7,14–16]

Patients on magnesium should have regular assessment of reflexes, mental status, and respiratory strength. When therapeutic magnesium levels are achieved, generalized weakness and lethargy are common, and deep tendon reflexes (DTRs) may be depressed. While neuromuscular depression carries some risk for respiratory depression, it is uncommon, occurring in just over 1% of all treated obstetrical patients. The generalized weakness and lethargy which is common with magnesium therapy occurs at serum magnesium levels 50%–75% lower than those which cause respiratory depression.[6,7,14–16]

The antidote for magnesium toxicity is calcium, usually administered as calcium gluconate. Calcium stimulates the release of acetylcholine, stimulating nerve transmission to the muscle, and acts as a counterbalance to the magnesium level. The recommended dosage of calcium gluconate is 1 gram solution administered intravenously over at least 3 minutes. If one ampule is not enough to reverse the side effects of hypoventilation, the dose may be repeated. The goal is the return of adequate ventilation and reflexes.[6,7,14–16]

HELLP Syndrome

The HELLP syndrome was first identified and described as a serious complication of preeclampsia by Weinstein in 1982.

H stands for hemolysis, which is confirmed with the evidence of red cell fragments and irregularly shaped red cells on peripheral blood smears. The belief is that as red cells pass through the constricted vessels that have sustained wall damage with platelet and fibrin deposition, red cell integrity is altered, and many cells are lysed. As a result, hyperbilirubinemia is frequently seen. Hemorrhagic necrosis is a serious complication of HELLP. Hepatic infarction may occur because of gross ischemia and obstruction of blood flow from the fibrin deposits.

EL stands for elevated liver enzyme levels. Elevated serum glutamic oxaloacetic transaminase and serum glutamic-pyruvic transaminase values are observed.

LP stands for low platelet count. Consumptive thrombocytopenia (a platelet count lower than 100,000/mm^3) unaccompanied by any other coagulation factor abnormalities is characteristic of the HELLP syndrome.

Management of HELLP syndrome is primarily supportive and includes control of hypertension; bed rest; frequent fetal evaluation; and careful assessment of hepatic, glucose, and coagulation studies. Disseminated intravascular coagulation (DIC) is a significant potential complication of HELLP.[6,7,13–16]

Fetal Distress

When fetal heart rates, monitor tracings, or movement patterns suggest distress, identify and address possible causes of fetal hypoperfusion. A mnemonic for response is LOCK.[3,4,6]

L – Place the patient in the left lateral or right lateral recumbent position. Change the position of the mother. If the LLP does not relieve the cord compression as indicated by continued variable decelerations, then reposition the mother to the right side; to the hands and knees; or last, to the knee–chest position. A transport consideration is the inability to restrain the maternal patient in the knee-to-chest position in some vehicles, especially small helicopters.

O – Provide supplemental oxygen.

C – Correct or improve contributing factors.

- Hypotension: Initiate a 500-mL IVF bolus, depending on the condition of the patient. If the patient has no comorbidities that promote pulmonary edema, the maternal patient can receive 2 L of crystalloids to improve maternal and placental perfusion. Correct for supine hypotension with a change to the LLP or RLP, uterine displacement, or a towel roll under the backboard.
- Rule out cord prolapse. A SVE is used to confirm the presence of a cord. Lift the presenting part off the cord to relieve the cord compression and reposition the patient, following the recommendations provided in this chapter.
- Assess for placental abruption or other complications that may affect the FHR.
- Assess for signs of maternal hemorrhage. Changes in FHR, including tachycardia and loss of variability, are often the first signs of maternal blood loss. The maternal patient has 40%–50% more blood volume at term; therefore she can mask signs of hypovolemia. In addition, the maternal patient shunts blood to her vital organs, and the uterus is *not* considered a vital organ.

K – Keep reassessing the FHR and intervene when indicated.

Preterm Labor

Regular and rhythmic contractions that produce progressive cervical changes after week 20 of gestation and before week 37 are considered to be preterm labor. Many patients with preterm labor do not feel or perceive these contractions. Preterm delivery occurs in 6%–12% of all deliveries. Preterm labor should be suspected if the patient has a history of contractions 10 minutes apart or less for a period of 1 hour or longer. Another definition is more than six contractions in a 1-hour period. The transport team should assess for factors associated with preterm labor.[3,4,6]

Background

In any situation in which uterine blood flow is reduced or impaired, an increase in uterine irritability can be noted and may result in the onset of labor. Viral infections with symptoms of fever, nausea, vomiting, or diarrhea may predispose to preterm labor primarily because of dehydration, which reduces uterine blood flow. Other similar conditions in which uteroplacental perfusion is compromised include gestational hypertension, diabetes, cardiovascular or kidney disease, overdistension of the uterus, heavy smoking, placental abruption, or placenta previa.[3,4,10]

Hormonal influence contributes to increased uterine activity and the onset of labor. Prostaglandin release is associated with PROM, bacterial infections, abdominal trauma, and overdistension of the uterus. In at least half the patients who have PROM, labor begins in 48 hours. Meconium-stained amniotic fluid contains high levels of oxytocin, which can initiate labor. The fetus is also believed to play a role in the activation of preterm labor, but little is known of this contribution.

When a patient has cervical incompetence, the cervix is unable to support and maintain the growing pregnancy to term and often dilates without perceptible contractions. Cervical incompetence is characterized by premature, painless, bloodless cervical dilation in which the membranes can bulge and rupture. Obstetric history of numerous second trimester losses or "painless" preterm labors and deliveries is suspect. Another concerning presentation is the patient with vaginal fullness or pressure, which is often caused by the presenting fetal part causing lower uterine segment pressure.

For cases of known or suspected cervical incompetence, a cervical cerclage may be placed at 12–14 weeks' gestation. A cervical cerclage is a purse-string suture that is applied through the cervix or transabdominally and then tied off. It is intended to maintain cervical integrity so the cervix is not prematurely opened. Any patient with a cervical cerclage that has preterm labor is at risk of cervical dilation and tearing of the cervix. Maternal fetal medicine physicians or the receiving physician should be consulted, and decisions regarding aggressive tocolysis or removal of the cerclage and delivery by the referring facility are made before transport.

The lower the fetus, the more pressure on the cervix and the more likely preterm delivery will occur. Even vague symptoms need to be evaluated. Advanced cervical dilation and rupture of the amniotic fluid lead to certain delivery.

Management

After an effective primary survey, secondary survey, and general obstetric assessment, the transport team should first assure maternal hydration and an empty bladder. Both dehydration and a full bladder can be contributors to an irritable uterus. IV fluids are a low cost, easy first step in treating preterm labor.[3,4,6]

Tocolytics are used to decrease or stop contractions. The medications used most frequently in suppressing labor are indomethacin (for patients under 32 weeks' gestational age), magnesium sulfate, and nifedipine.[3,4,6]

Tocolytics have not been shown to be successful in maintaining a pregnancy, but they can be useful in delaying delivery to improve maternal and fetal preparation for delivery.[3,4,6,7] Both betamethasone and dexamethasone decrease the incidence and severity of respiratory distress syndrome, intraventricular hemorrhage, necrotizing enterocolitis, and death in babies born between 23 and 36 weeks' gestation. The greatest efficacy is achieved when given 2–7 days prior to delivery. Betamethasone is most frequently used in the United States, and is given in two doses of 12 mg intramuscularly (IM) 24 hours apart. Alternatively, dexamethasone 6 mg IM can be given, but requires four doses, 12 hours apart. Even a single dose of steroids prior to preterm delivery can be helpful, and should be considered for any baby who is at risk for early delivery between 23 and 36 weeks' gestation. Benefits are noted even when only one dose can be given prior to delivery.[18]

Magnesium sulfate, in addition to having transient effects on slowing uterine contraction, has neurological protective features for the fetus. Although not well explained, studies show a significant decrease in the incidence of cerebral palsy in babies born at 34 or fewer weeks' gestational age when they have prenatal magnesium exposure.[19]

Placental Abruption

Placental abruption is the premature detachment of a normally implanted placenta from the uterine wall. The separation may occur over a small area with little evidence or can separate totally with devastating results. The incidence of abruption varies widely, depending on the source.

The primary cause of placental abruption is unknown. Hypertension, whether chronic or gestational hypertension, and previous abruption are two factors that are known to greatly increase the risk of placental abruption. Other factors that place the obstetric patient at risk include abdominal trauma, an unusually short umbilical cord, amniocentesis, multiparity, age over 35 years, uterine anomalies or tumors, and sudden uterine decompression (such as when a twin is

delivered and the other twin remains in utero, or when a hypertensive crisis is acutely resolved). Other risk factors include cigarette smoking and substance abuse, especially abuse of cocaine.[3,4,6,20]

Hemorrhage occurs from the arterioles that supply the decidua (lining of uterus), causing a retroplacental hematoma. As the hemorrhage continues, more vessels are disrupted, which leads to increased hemorrhage and further separation. Placental separation can be an avalanche that continues to total separation or suddenly stops for reasons unknown. Sometimes a clot blocks the hemorrhage. The decidua is rich in thromboplastin, and clotting occurs rapidly. When vaginal bleeding is observed, the blood is usually dark because of the rapid clotting and the distance it takes to reach the vagina and be seen externally. If separation occurs at the margin of the placenta or if the amniotic membranes are dissected from the decidua because of the hemorrhage, vaginal bleeding is observed. No vaginal bleeding is observed if the hemorrhage is completely concealed behind the placenta. Use the mental imagery of a fried egg: the yellow yolk is the abruption, and the white egg is the attached placenta. Bleeding is certainly associated with the abruption; it is just occult and cannot escape vaginally to be seen.[3,4,6,20]

Symptoms of placental abruption may range from slight abdominal tenderness and lower back discomfort with a mild abruption to severe, unceasing abdominal pain in a large abruption. Sudden, severe pain without vaginal bleeding may be indicative of retroplacental hemorrhage into the myometrium. However, most presentations of placenta abruptio include dark red vaginal bleeding. A classic presentation of placenta abruptio is profound abdominal pain that appears disproportionate to the contractions palpated. With moderate to large abruption, labor tends to progress rapidly and the risks for precipitous delivery and fetal distress are greater. Preparation must be taken for immediate vaginal delivery, or in the case of extensive hemorrhage, cesarean delivery.[3,4,6,20]

The intensity, frequency, and duration of contractions may vary from contractions with a slight increase in uterine tone to hypertonic or tetanic contractions. Tetanic contractions are very strong contractions that typically last longer than 90 seconds and have minimal resting tone in between. Assessment should include palpation of the uterus for the frequency, duration, intensity, and resting tone. The uterus is often described as board-like, primarily because of the tetanic contractions and the accumulation of blood within the uterus.[3,4,6,20]

Early signs of maternal bleeding are reflected in the FHR with an increasing baseline and loss of variability noted. Fetal distress because of placental separation or placenta previa occurs primarily from placental insufficiency (hypertonic uterus, maternal hemorrhage, or decreased placental perfusion) or fetal hemorrhage because of placental separation. Before any change in maternal vital signs, shunting away from the placenta to the vital organs occurs, and a FHR indicative of placental insufficiency is seen. FHR changes often include increasing or tachycardia baseline and loss of variability.[3,4,6,20]

As blood loss progresses, maternal tachycardia is then noted. Approximately one-third of the maternal blood volume is lost before significant changes are seen in the maternal blood pressure. The bleeding from placenta abruptio is often unpredictable, and may continue until delivery of the placenta, or stop spontaneously.[3,4,6,10,20]

Placenta Previa[3,4,6,20]

Placenta previa occurs when the placenta becomes implanted in the lower uterine segment and as a result covers or partially covers the internal cervical os. A marginal or low-lying previa extends to or close to the internal os but does not cover any part of it. Placenta previa occurs approximately once in every 200–400 deliveries. The incidence of placenta previa is higher preterm. As the pregnancy progresses, the fundus grows and the lower uterine segment elongates, which allows the placenta to migrate away from the internal os toward the fundus. In reality, the placenta does not move; it is merely carried up toward the fundus as the uterus grows.

Although the exact cause is unknown, a higher incidence of placenta previa is seen with uterine scarring. A previous cesarean section, dilatation and curettage (D&C), increased parity, multiparity with short intervals, and a previous occurrence of placenta previa can scar the uterus. Other factors that place the obstetric patient at risk for placenta previa include previous chorioamnionitis, multiple gestation (for which a larger surface area is covered by the placenta), fetal erythroblastosis, maternal age over age 35 years, substance abuse, previous myomectomy, and uterine tumors. Normal placental implantation usually occurs in the fundus or body segment of the uterus. Defective perfusion of the decidua has been suggested to favor implantation of the placenta in the lower uterine segment. Because less vascularization exists in the lower uterine segment, the placenta compensates and tends to grow thinner and larger, covering a larger area and increasing perfusion.

In cases of vaginal bleeding after 20 weeks' gestation, placenta previa should be considered. Before the onset of labor, the cervix begins to soften, efface, and dilate. These cervical changes disrupt the placental attachment, tearing the vessels, and hemorrhage results. Bright red vaginal bleeding is observed; it is initially painless and is not initially associated with contractions. The primary episode usually involves less than 250 mL of blood and tends to cease spontaneously as clot formation rapidly occurs. Recurrence is unpredictable. Generally, the greater the extent to which the internal os is covered, the sooner the initial episode occurs. In addition, subsequent bleeds are often larger.

Potential complications of placenta previa include complications similar to those of placental abruption, such as DIC, hypovolemic shock, kidney damage (from hypoperfusion), anemia, postpartum infection, postpartum hemorrhage, and fetal distress or death. A common complication of placenta previa and the resulting bleeds is preterm labor. As with other areas in the body, blood is an irritant, and as with abruptions, bleeding leads to uterine irritability and contractions, and contractions lead to more bleeding. Because hemorrhage may occur at any time without warning or precipitating events, the risk is increased with premature delivery. Furthermore, placenta accreta is a rare complication of placenta previa. With placenta accreta, the placenta (chorionic villi) attaches to the myometrium vs. its normal placental attachment to the endometrium. Placenta accreta may advance to placenta increta or placenta percreta. Patients with anticipated accreta, or other morbidly adherent placentas, should be transported to an appropriate level of care, capable of massive blood transfusion.

Contractions may or may not be present with placenta previa. The onset usually occurs during or after the hemorrhage because of increased uterine irritability, following the irritating exposure to blood. An ultrasound scan can confirm the location of the placenta. If an ultrasound scan is not available, a previa cannot be ruled out. A SVE may stimulate profuse bleeding by dislodging a clot and should never be done. With cervical changes that accompany active labor, occasionally an increase in bloody show is noted and may appear excessive, which may lead the transport professional to believe that a placenta previa is present. If unsure, do not attempt a vaginal examination, but relay concerns to the receiving facility for proper preparation. Blood loss can be more accurately estimated with placenta previa, for which only external hemorrhage is observed.[3,4,6,20]

For patients with abruption or previa, transport care is directed at maternal resuscitation, accurate evaluation of external bleeding and contraction patterns, and fetal surveillance.[3,4,6,20]

Postpartum Hemorrhage

Postpartum hemorrhage, defined as a cumulative blood loss of greater than or equal to 1000 mL or blood loss accompanied by signs or symptoms of hypovolemia within 24 hours after the birth process, is a leading cause of worldwide maternal mortality. Postpartum hemorrhage causes approximately 11% of maternal deaths in the United States and is the leading cause of death that occurs on the day of birth. Importantly, 54%–93% of maternal deaths due to obstetric hemorrhage may be preventable.[21,22]

Background[4,7,21,22]

Uterine atony is the most common cause of postpartum hemorrhage. Normally, bleeding from the placental site is controlled when the interlacing muscle fibers of the uterus contract and retract in conjunction with platelet aggregation and clot formation in the vessels of the decidua. This occurs immediately after delivery of the placenta as the uterus contracts to spontaneously clamp off uterine blood vessels that once perfused the placenta. Factors that predispose to uterine atony and prevent compression of the vessels at the implantation site predispose to postpartum hemorrhage. Uterine atony can occur after a prolonged or tumultuous labor or after general anesthetic is used. The uterus that is overdistended because of multiple gestation, uterine tumors, polyhydramnios, or a large fetus is more likely to be hypotonic after delivery. Multiparity, chorioamnionitis (*intra-amniotic infection*), previous postpartum hemorrhage, placenta previa, and use of labor stimulants place the obstetric patient at increased risk for uterine atony and postpartum hemorrhage. There is some synergistic effect, as well – as the uterus fills with clots, it is increasingly unable to contract and retract normally, compounding the problem of hemorrhage.

If some or all of the placenta or membranes are retained, the same circumstances are created. Retained products of conception is the second most common cause of postpartum hemorrhage. Normally, the placenta separates spontaneously approximately 5–20 minutes after delivery of the fetus. When the placenta is partially retained effective uterine contraction and hemostais are precluded. Ultrasound examination can be helpful in identifying retained products of conception.

The third common cause of postpartum hemorrhage is laceration, particularly of the cervix, vagina, or lower uterine segment. An instrumented delivery with forceps may be associated with laceration and hemorrhage. Lacerations should be suspected when hemorrhaging occurs in the presence of a firmly contracted uterus and may require a speculum exam for detection.

Coagulopathy associated with DIC, placental abruption, congenital coagulopathies, acquired coagulopathy from resuscitation, and gestational hypertension is the fourth common cause of postpartum hemorrhage.

Management

The transport team should carefully evaluate uterine tone and the patient's vital signs. Estimates of blood loss must be accurate. Some studies have shown that estimated blood loss was approximately half the amount actually lost. Techniques used to improve objective blood loss measurement are pad counts, weighing of

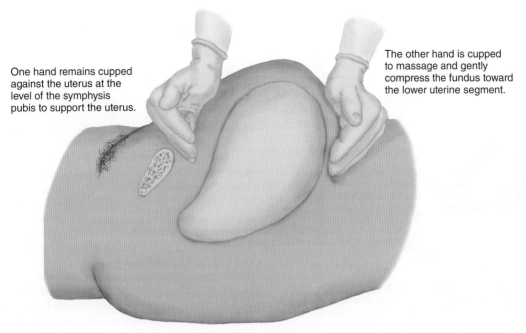

One hand remains cupped against the uterus at the level of the symphysis pubis to support the uterus.

The other hand is cupped to massage and gently compress the fundus toward the lower uterine segment.

• **Fig. 16.6** Fundal massage. (From Weiler Ashwill J, Carroll Ashwill J, Nelson KA, et al. *Maternal-Child Nursing.* 6th ed. Elsevier; 2022.)

Chux pads, or collection of blood clots in a graduated cylinder or suction canister.[21]

Management of postpartum hemorrhage begins with optimizing uterine tone. Manual fundal massage is very effective. To perform effective massage, one hand should cup the fundus while the other provides support to the lower uterine segment, supporting the bladder, just above the symphysis pubis (Fig. 16.6). When the uterus is firm, it palpates like a small grapefruit and vaginal bleeding is greatly decreased. Fundal massage can be painful for patients and pain relief medications should be offered and titrated to relieve pain. Often, clots are expressed, and frequent massage alone may be all the stimulation that is needed for the uterus to adequately contract and retract. Fundal massage should be performed at least every 5–15 minutes, and the location of the fundus in relation to the level of the umbilicus, the degree of firmness, and the vaginal flow should be noted.[4,7,21,22]

A full bladder is often the reason that the uterus remains boggy and cannot involute. The puffy full bladder lies directly beneath the uterus and interferes with its ability to contract. Simply having the patient void or inserting a Foley catheter for the transport tremendously decreases uterine bleeding.[4,7,21,22]

Uterotonic medications augment uterine contraction and tone. Oxytocin, a hormone produced by the hypothalamus and secreted by the posterior pituitary gland, stimulates uterine contraction and is ubiquitous in the active management of labor. An infusion of 10–40 units in a liter of crystalloid IV fluid is generally prepared and infused "to effect" for uterine tone.[4,7,21,22] If fundal massage, oxytocin infusion, and bladder drainage do not achieve adequate uterine tone, prostaglandin F2-alpha, methylergonovine, and misprostol are nonintravenous uterotonics available for use. There is no evidence that any single agent is preferable. The combination of oxytocin (Pitocin), fundal massage, bladder drainage, and additional uterotonic agent abates postpartum hemorrhage in about 95% of cases. The uterotonic agents are summarized in Table 16.3.[4,7,21,22]

TABLE 16.3	Comparison of Uterotonic Medications	
Drug	**Dose/Route/Frequency**	**Contraindications**
Oxytocin	10–40 units in 1000 mL of crystalloid infused to effect	Hypersensitivity
Methylergonovine	0.2 mg IM, repeated in 2–4 hours	Hypertension, cardiovascular disease, hypersensitivity
Prostaglandin F2-alpha	0.25 mg IM, repeated in 15–90 minutes to 8 doses maximum	Asthma, relative contraindication for hypertension
Misoprostol	600–1000 mcg PR	Hypersensitivity

IM, Intramuscular; *PR,* per rectum.
Reproduced with permission Baldisseri MR, Plante LA, eds. *Fundamental Critical Care Support: Obstetrics.* Society of Critical Care Medicine; 2017.

For cases resistant to initial interventions, add an additional uterotonic medication, begin resuscitation, and begin to plan for massive transfusion and intervention in surgery or interventional radiology. Intrauterine tamponade devices are also available. The Bakri balloon is placed in the uterus and inflated, providing counterpressure for an atonic uterus. There is a drainage port on top of the balloon and a collection bag on the distal end (Fig. 16.7). The Jada system is an intrauterine suction device that removes debris and aids in reducing intrauterine volume to support hemostasis (Fig. 16.8).

Patients with ongoing hemorrhage should be resuscitated for hypovolemic hemorrhagic shock using packed red blood cells and other components. Resuscitation of hypovolemic hemorrhagic

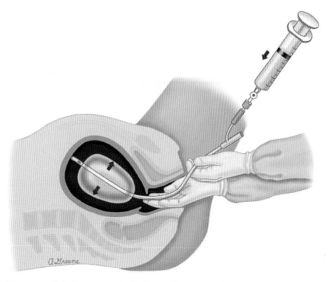

• **Fig. 16.7** Bakri tamponade balloon. (Courtesy Cook Women's Health. From Francois KE, Foley MR. Antepartum and postpartum hemorrhage. In Landon MB, Galan HL, Jauniaux ERM, et al., eds. *Gabbe's Obstetrics: Normal and Problem Pregnancies.* 8th ed. Philadelphia, PA: Elsevier; 2021.

shock is well discussed in other chapters of this textbook. Tranexamic acid may have a role in postpartum hemorrhage.[23]

Trauma in Pregnancy[21,24–26]

Minor accidental injuries are common during pregnancy. The gravid uterus, loosened joints, altered center of gravity, shortness of breath, dizziness, increased fatigue, and edema all contribute to minor accidents, including falls. Up to 9% of pregnant women experience intimate partner violence during the pregnancy.

Serious injuries during pregnancy place not only the obstetric patient but also the fetus at risk. The most common etiologies of serious obstetric trauma are motor vehicle crashes, falls, stabbings, burns, and domestic violence. The fetus is well protected in the confines of the uterus because it is surrounded by amniotic fluid, which serves as an excellent shock absorber. Physical trauma to a fetus is extremely rare, except from direct penetrating wounds or extensive blunt trauma. The fetus is at greatest risk for fetal distress and intrauterine death because of hypoperfusion from maternal trauma and death.

There is also the risk of placental injury. About 6% of pregnant trauma patients and a quarter of pregnant patients with major trauma have some degree of placental abruption. It is an essential element of the differential diagnosis for all pregnant patients and should be part of the patient evaluation.

The obstetric patient is more vulnerable to hemorrhage because of the increased vascularity surrounding the gravid uterus. Early signs and symptoms of hypovolemia may be masked by the normal physiologic changes of pregnancy. Thus blood is shunted away from nonvital organs, including the uterus, which threatens the well-being of the fetus. In dealing with a trauma patient who is pregnant, the best interest of the fetus is served by prompt assessment and interventions on behalf of the mother. Maternal shock resuscitation will improve fetal viability.

The pregnant trauma patient needs to be appropriately immobilized for transport with the same guidelines as nonpregnant patients. They should be maintained in a lateral position. Stretcher straps should be placed low and tight over the pelvis. The pregnant trauma patient is at high risk of aspiration because of the hormones of pregnancy. No contraindications for rapid sequence intubation (RSI) exist during pregnancy; however, the baby is also paralyzed until neuromuscular blocking agents wear off. This is not a concern if the fetus remains in the uterus because it is oxygenated via the placenta and umbilical cord, however would be important in the event of an immediate cesarean delivery.

Consideration should be made to transport pregnant patients even in the presence of injuries that may be incompatible with life, particularly when a pulse remains. If proper resuscitation occurs on the mother, the fetus may maintain viability and be delivered with minimal complications.

Anaphylactic Syndrome of Pregnancy[7,27]

Amniotic fluid embolism is now known as *anaphylactic syndrome of pregnancy.* Previously, it was thought that amniotic fluid gained access to the maternal circulation during labor or delivery or immediately after delivery, resulting in obstruction of the pulmonary

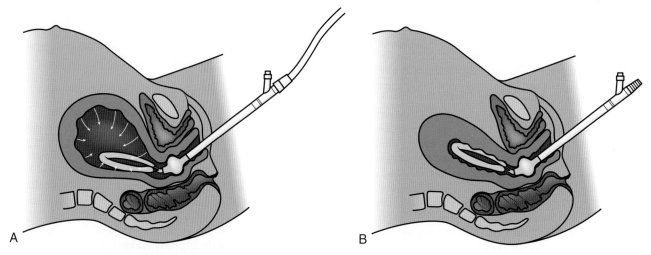

• **Fig. 16.8** Jada system. **A,** Jada with vacuum being applied. **B,** Jada with uterus collapse. (From D'Alton ME, Rood KM, Smid MC, et al. Intrauterine vacuum-induced hemorrhage-control device for rapid treatment of postpartum hemorrhage. *Obstet Gynecol.* 2020;136(5):882-891.)

vasculature. In addition, particulate matter in the amniotic fluid, such as meconium, lanugo hairs, fetal squamous cells, bile, fat, and mucin, was also thought to form emboli. The belief now is that the process is more likely to be an anaphylactic reaction to the amniotic fluid and the fetal cells it contains. In the United States amniotic fluid embolism causes 10% of maternal deaths. The complication is very rare and is frequently fatal, with a maternal mortality rate nearing 90%. Anaphylactoid syndrome of pregnancy is often initially misdiagnosed as a result of the vague clinical picture. Unfortunately, the rapid progression of this syndrome is associated with a high maternal mortality that is often not diagnosed until postmortem.

The route by which amniotic fluid enters the circulatory system of the mother is not clear. The most frequently suggested sites of entry are lacerations in the endocervical veins during cervical dilation and lacerations in the lower uterine segment, the placental site on separation and delivery of the placenta, and uterine veins at sites of uterine trauma. Under the pressure of uterine contractions, amniotic fluid gains access to the circulatory system of the mother and travels quickly to the pulmonary vasculature, where embolization and anaphylactic reaction quickly ensue.

Factors that place the patient at risk include uterine rupture, cesarean section, and the use of uterine stimulants to induce labor, a large fetus, placenta previa, placental abruption, intrauterine fetal death, meconium in the amniotic fluid, multiparity, precipitous delivery, knee–chest position, and maternal age of more than 30 years.

Sudden acute dyspnea is the most characteristic symptom, followed by profound cyanosis and sudden shock. Other symptoms may include chest pain, restlessness, anxiety, coughing, vomiting, pulmonary edema with pink frothy sputum, seizures that are frequently confused with eclamptic seizures, and coma. If the patient has delivered, the transport team should watch for symptoms of postpartum hemorrhage caused by uterine atony (and coagulation disorders, such as DIC that often follow).

Because of the extremely rare occurrence of anaphylactoid syndrome of pregnancy and the rapidity of onset of symptoms with deterioration, the transport team may be unsure of the clinical picture. Treatment focuses on supportive care. This syndrome most commonly occurs postpartum, but if the patient is still gravid, the fetal heart tones (FHTs) should be monitored for signs of severe distress.

Normal and Abnormal Deliveries

The steps for normal vertex vaginal delivery are shown in Table 16.4 and the movement of the fetus through and out of the vagina is presented in Fig. 16.9. The goal is to prevent the

TABLE 16.4	Vaginal Delivery
Stage of Delivery	**Provider Action**
Preparation	• Assure adequate resources. • Assess for fetal and maternal risks such as multiple gestation, prematurity, congenital anomalies, maternal coagulopathy, and maternal hypertension. • Position the mother with hips raised, flexed, and abducted.
Delivery of the head	• Place one hand on the crowning portion of the fetal head and apply light pressure to maintain the head in a flexed position. Use the other hand to ease the perineum over the fetal face (the most common fetal position at expulsion is facing the mother's back). • Do not pull on the head; let the mother gradually push it into your hands. • If the membranes still cover the baby's head, use a clamp, fingers, or forceps to rupture them.
Restitution of the head and nuchal cord	• After the infant's head has delivered, it will usually rotate to the side. • Feel for a loop of umbilical cord around the baby's neck, called nuchal cord. If present, gently slip it over the head. If it resists, it may be possible to slip it caudally over the shoulders and deliver the body through the loop. • If these maneuvers are unsuccessful and leaving the cord alone is not feasible, doubly clamp and cut the cord. • It is important not to rupture or avulse the cord because serious fetal/neonatal bleeding can occur.
Delivery of the shoulders	• With the next push, guide the head slightly downward so that the anterior shoulder slips under the symphysis pubis and delivers, then guide the head slightly upward to deliver the posterior shoulder over, rather than through, the perineum. • If the shoulders do not deliver easily, have your assistant or the mother sharply flex her thighs back against her abdomen. This opens the pelvis to its maximum dimension. • Do not pull on the head in an attempt to extract the baby if it does not slide out of the vagina easily. Advanced maneuvers for management of shoulder dystocia are described in detail separately.
Delivery of the body	• Once both shoulders have delivered, the rest of the baby usually immediately follows. • Document the time of expulsion. Use your hands to hold onto the back of the head and buttocks of the baby securely as it delivers. • The baby can then be cradled against your body, with the back of its head in your cupped hand and its body supported by your forearm.
Post-delivery management	• Manage the baby as described in neonatal references. • Double clamp the umbilical cord and cut between the clamps. • Dry the baby and maintain warmth with blankets, skin-to-skin contact with the mother, ambient temperature, and external means, if necessary.
Placental delivery	• The placenta classically delivers between 5 and 30 minutes of delivery. The typical progression is umbilical cord lengthening, a gush of blood from the vagina, and a change in uterine height and tone. • If the placental is not expelled naturally, ask the mother to bear down and apply mild traction on the umbilical cord. With this maneuver, place a hand on the abdomen to secure the uterine fundus.

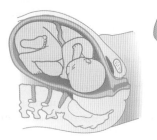 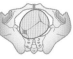

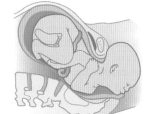 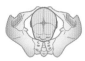

1. Head floating, before engagement

5. Complete extension

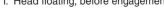

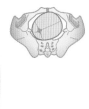 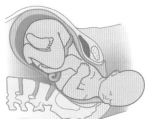

2. Engagement, flexion, descent

6. Restitution, external rotation

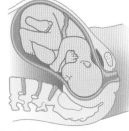 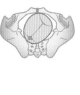

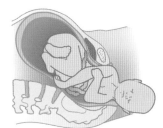

3. Further descent, internal rotation

7. Delivery of anterior shoulder

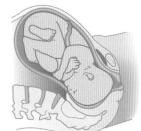 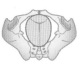

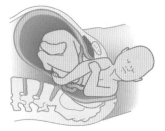

4. Complete rotation, beginning extension

8. Delivery of posterior shoulder

• **Fig. 16.9** Mechanisms of normal labor in a left occipitoanterior vertex position. *1*, Head floating before engagement. *2*, Engagement, flexion, and descent occur as the head moves toward the pelvic inlet; descent continues. *3*, Descent and internal rotation to occiput anterior (OA) position. *4*, Complete rotation and beginning extension as the head reaches the pelvic floor. *5*, The head is born by complete extension. *6*, Restitution and external rotation, returning to left OA (LOA) position and alignment with the shoulders. *7*, Delivery of the anterior shoulder. *8*, With delivery of the posterior shoulder, expulsion occurs as the body of the baby is rapidly born. (From Matteson P. *Women's Health During the Childbearing Years: A Community-Based Approach.* St. Louis, MO: Mosby; 2001.)

fetal head from delivering rapidly and tearing through the maternal introitus and perineum. Delivery complications can be predicted in some situations and may be quite unforeseen in others.

Multiple Gestation

A pregnancy with more than one fetus is a multiple gestation. Twins occur in approximately 3% of all live births and are the predominate form of multiple gestation.[3,6]

Background

Embryologically, twins may result from multiple ovulations, in which two distinct ova are fertilized (dizygotic, or fraternal), or from one ovum that subsequently divides into two (monozygotic, or identical). The same processes can also result in larger numbers of multiples. The incidence of dizygotic twins is influenced by heredity, maternal age, race, and treatment for infertility, whereas the frequency of monozygotic twins is relatively constant. In vitro fertilization and fertility medications also contribute to the incidence of multiple fetuses. Previous delivery of twins, maternal family history of fraternal twins, advanced maternal age, infertility treatment, and multiparity all increase the chance of multiple gestations.

The number of placentas (chorionicity) and amniotic sacs is important with multiple gestations. This disorder highlights the importance of determining the chorionicity (number of placentas) and amnionicity (number of amniotic sacs) for all twin gestations. Dizygotic twins have separate placentas and amniotic sacs. Monozygotic twins have a shared placenta and can have shared or separate amniotic sacs (Fig. 16.10). When there is a shared placenta, there is risk for twin-to-twin transfusion, which will complicate the management of the neonate.[3,6]

Pathophysiology is related to the complications associated with multiple gestations. The large area of the uterine surface covered by the placenta is suspected in several complications. Portions are more likely to implant in the lower uterine segment where less vascularity is found, increasing the chances of IUGR, or at or near the cervical os, increasing the chances of placenta previa. The superabundance of chorionic villi appears to predispose the obstetric patient to hypertensive disorders of pregnancy, especially in a first pregnancy.[3,6]

Other complications may be caused by uterine overdistension and hemodynamic and endocrinologic changes associated with multiple gestations. The mother is placed at risk for anemia, glucose intolerance, polyhydramnios, dysfunctional labor associated with uterine overdistension, and dystocia. In addition, multiple gestations predispose to premature rupture of membranes (PROM), preterm labor and delivery, placental abruption, cesarean section, uterine atony and resulting postpartum hemorrhage, and malpresentations.[3,6]

The greatest threat to multiple gestations is premature labor and delivery. One theory for this is overdistension of the uterus caused by multiple fetuses. The average gestational age for onset of labor is about 36 weeks for pregnancies that have spontaneous multiple gestations. Multiple gestation pregnancies because of infertility often deliver before 36 weeks' gestation.[3,6]

Management

The transport team must be aware that any multiple gestation is a pregnancy at risk and must assess for additional risk factors associated with a multiple gestation.

Fetal monitoring of multiple gestations during transport is extremely difficult but might be accomplished with continuous or intermittent FHR assessment via Doppler or ultrasound, dependent on availability and transport protocols. Of special note is that multiple gestations should be identified as A, B, C, etc., and not as 1, 2, and 3. Numbering indicates birth order, which is not determined until the actual delivery. In addition, location should also be described in relationship to the quadrants of the uterus. For example, a triplet pregnancy may have a fetus in the left lower quadrant (LLQ), the right upper quadrant (RUQ), and the right lower quadrant (RLQ). The babies are labeled as A: RLQ, B: RUQ, and C: LLQ. This distinction avoids confusion for monitoring purposes so the fetuses do not get mixed up. Caution must be taken to monitor each fetus separately.[3,6]

Because of close fetal lie, a single fetus may be inadvertently monitored in more than one location. For example, triplet A may be monitored in the RUQ and may also be picked up in the LLQ. Clinicians think they are monitoring two separate fetuses, but they are actually monitoring one fetus, twice. Ultrasound scan may help to guide monitoring of separate fetuses. When the babies are actually delivered, the first fetus delivered is 1, the second is 2, and so forth.[3,6]

Breech Presentation

Background

Breech presentation involves a fetus in a longitudinal lie with the feet or buttocks closest to the cervix. The body often can be felt through the cervix on vaginal examination. With a breech presentation, the buttocks may descend first, with the legs flexed on the fetal abdomen and the feet alongside the buttocks (complete breech); the legs may also be extended upward (frank breech), or one or both feet or knees may be present (footling or incomplete breech). At or near term, the incidence rate of breech is 3%–4%. Because of the effects of gravity, most fetuses are cephalic or vertex. However, before 34 weeks' gestation, the incidence is considerably higher.[3,6,28]

Breech presentation is more likely to occur in situations with uterine abnormalities, such as a septum that extends part or all of the way from the fundus to the cervix (septate uterus) or a

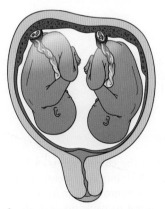
A Monochorionic/monoamniotic

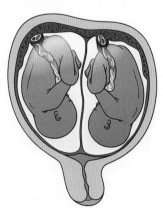
Monochorionic/diamniotic

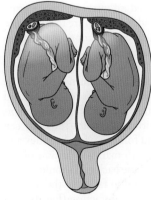
Dichorionic/diamniotic

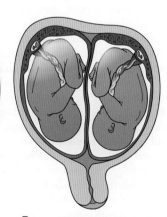
B   Fraternal twins

Identical twins

• **Fig. 16.10** Multiple pregnancies. **A**, Monozygotic (identical) twins develop from one ovum and one sperm. **B**, Dizygotic (fraternal) twins develop from two ova and two sperm. (From Cooper K, Gosnell K. Care of the high-risk mother, newborn, and family with special needs. In: *Foundations of Nursing*. 9th ed. Elsevier; 2023.)

Y-shaped uterus (bicornuate uterus). The belief is that as the pregnancy progresses, the uterine cavity provides the most room for the fetus' bulkier and more movable parts, with the extremities in the fundus of the uterus and the cephalic presenting. Before 34 weeks' gestation, the head of the fetus is disproportionately larger than the body, favoring the breech presentation. For the same reason, the hydrocephalic fetus has a high incidence of breech presentation.[3,6,28]

Other factors that appear to predispose to the breech presentation are grand multiparity, a previous breech delivery, multiple gestations, polyhydramnios, oligohydramnios, placenta previa, uterine tumors, and congenital anomalies.

Complications associated with breech presentation are inherent because of the position of the fetus. With the buttocks and lower extremities presenting, cord prolapse, cord entanglement around the extremities, and cord compression are more likely to occur. When delivery is managed too forcefully, birth trauma may result. Trauma to the fetal cervical spine and brachial plexus and fractures of the humerus, clavicle, skull, and neck may occur. A common concern with breech presentation is that the body of the neonate can be delivered but the head is too large to fit through the pelvis.[3,6,28]

The fetus in breech presentation is at higher risk for birth asphyxia (hypoxia, hypercapnia, and metabolic acidosis) compared with the fetus that has a vertex presentation. Head entrapment is a complication that occurs when the buttocks and lower extremities of the premature fetus pass through a cervix that is not completely dilated and is inadequate for the head to be delivered without trauma, asphyxiation, or both for the infant.

Management[3,6,28]

Essentially, the fetus in a breech presentation should not be touched until the umbilicus has spontaneously delivered. However, the risk of hypothermia is great for these babies, and a dry warm towel should be wrapped around the torso to prevent heat loss and allow for greater control when handling a slippery baby. The team should disengage the legs if one or both have not delivered spontaneously. This maneuver can be accomplished by hooking a finger on the leg by the groin and gently reducing the leg so it is extended outside the mother's body. Caution must be taken to avoid palpating the exposed umbilical cord. At one time, it was taught to palpate the cord to assess the FHR. However, this palpation could cause venospasm and the umbilical cord could clot off. The cord should be covered to prevent temperature and moisture loss from convection. Adding moisture to gauze and application of this gauze may result in cool or room temp fluids being applied to these vessels, leading to vasoconstriction.

At this point, the arms can usually be delivered by hooking the index finger over each of the baby's shoulders in turn (Fig. 16.11). After the shoulders have been delivered, the baby's trunk is rotated so that the back is anterior (facing up), and gentle steady downward traction is applied until the hairline is visible. The body can now rest on the palm of one hand and forearm with the index and middle fingers applied in the mouth, to maintain flexion of the head. With the other hand supporting the back and shoulders, the body can then gently be brought upward to facilitate the delivery of the head with a minimal amount of neck traction (Fig. 16.12).

Care must be taken to achieve slow and controlled delivery of the head, allowing the chin, face, and brow to sweep over the perineum. As soon as the infant is delivered, the airway should be cleared with a bulb syringe. These deliveries can be traumatic for the neonate. Preparation for resuscitation should be initiated before delivery.

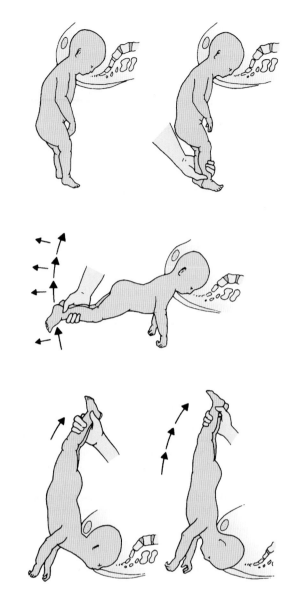

• **Fig. 16.11** Breech extraction. Upward traction to effect delivery of the posterior shoulder and freeing the posterior arm. (Modified from Hickman M. *Midwifery*. 2nd ed. Oxford: Blackwell Scientific; 1985.)

Because breech delivery is a rare occurrence for the transport team, the tendency may be to act in haste when this situation arises. The team should guard against haste because it increases the risk for birth trauma.

Umbilical Cord Prolapse

Overt cord prolapse occurs when the cord slips down into the vagina or appears externally after the amniotic membranes have ruptured. When the cord slips down into or near the pelvis, adjacent to the presenting part, it is not palpable on vaginal examination (occult prolapse). The cord may also have slipped down to a position in which it is palpable through the cervix but in intact membranes (forelying prolapse). Varying degrees of prolapse may occur. The weight of the presenting fetal part causes compression of the umbilical cord. The amount of change in the fetal status and well-being is directly related to the degree or compression.[3,6]

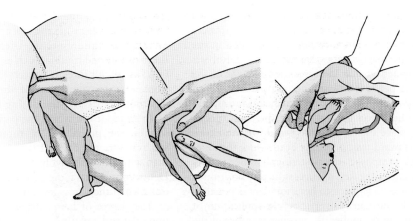

• **Fig. 16.12** Delivery of the head. Note that flexion is maintained with suprapubic pressure by an assistant and simultaneous pressure on the maxilla by the operator as traction is applied. (Modified from Hickman M. *Midwifery*. 2nd ed. Oxford: Blackwell Scientific; 1985.)

Background

Circumstances that cause maladaptation of the presenting part to the lower uterine segment or prevent descent of the presenting part into the pelvis predispose the obstetric patient to cord prolapse. These factors include breech presentation, transverse lie, premature rupture of membranes (PROM), a contracted pelvis, unengaged large fetus multiparity, polyhydramnios, multiple gestations, a long cord, and preterm labor. Complications include severe changes in fetal status and well-being, and fetal death.

Cord prolapse occurs suddenly and requires quick identification of the problem and quick action. Identification of the obstetric patient who is vulnerable to cord prolapse is of primary importance. Clinical signs of prolapse include sudden fetal bradycardia and recurrent variable decelerations that do not respond to a change in maternal position, administration of oxygen, or hydration. Compression of the cord between the presenting part and the pelvic tissues causes the FHR patterns that are observed.[3,6]

Management

Actions necessary in the event of cord prolapse include elevating the presenting part off the cord with a hand in the vagina that must remain there during the entire transport to prevent further cord compression. The mother should be positioned in a Trendelenburg or knee–chest position as safety allows to further reduce pressure on the cord. The cord may spontaneously retract, depending on the degree of prolapse, but should never be manually replaced because severe compression may occur. Tocolysis may be considered.[3,6]

Intervention to elevate the presenting part off the cord must be maintained during the transport and through delivery. The cord should not be palpated because of the risk for vasospasm, and the cord should be covered to prevent temperature and moisture loss from convection. Adding moisture to gauze and application of this gauze may result in cool or room temperature fluids being applied to these vessels, leading to vasoconstriction.[3,6]

If cord prolapse occurs when the patient is en route, the receiving facility should be alerted to prepare for an emergency cesarean section.

Shoulder Dystocia

After delivery of the head, the anterior shoulder pushes against the pubic symphysis bone on the anterior aspect of the pelvis, creating a situation commonly referred to as shoulder dystocia. In most circumstances, the head is the largest diameter of the fetus. Occasionally, the shoulders have a larger diameter. The obvious concern is that the head will fit through the pelvic bones and the shoulders will be unable to. The condition becomes apparent when gentle downward traction is applied to the fetal head and the anterior shoulder does not deliver. Or may be seen with the "turtle sign," when the head/face extends out during a contraction and then "retracts back" against the perineum after the contraction because the shoulders prevent further progression.[3,6]

Background

Several predisposing factors have been linked to shoulder dystocia. However, shoulder dystocia can occur quite unexpectedly without obvious associated factors. The complication occurs more frequently with the presence of a large fetus or with a macrosomic fetus such as those found with gestational diabetes. Other risk factors include patients with a contracted pelvis, maternal obesity, or a prolonged second stage of labor, including deliveries that require instruments for delivery. First-time mothers, primigravidas, particularly those with limited or no previous prenatal care, should be considered high risk for shoulder dystocia due to a historically unproven pelvic outlet.

Possible complications of shoulder dystocia include brachial plexus damage and fractured fetal clavicle. Fetal hypoxia can occur when the cord is drawn into the pelvis and compressed.

In any situation of imminent delivery, unless the fetus is expected to weigh 2500 g or less, shoulder dystocia is a possibility. However, any fetus greater than 4000 g is at a considerably higher risk. After the head has been delivered and inspection for a nuchal cord has been performed, the delivery of the anterior shoulder should be attempted. If the anterior shoulder is unable to be delivered, consider the possibility of shoulder dystocia. Careful considerations for preparation for a difficult delivery, anticipated neonatal resuscitation, and possible diversion should be initiated.[3,6]

Management

Unnecessary haste and overly aggressive force should be avoided because of the increased possibility of birth trauma to the fetus. Excessive lateral flexion of the neck and overly vigorous traction of the head and neck increase the risk of damage to the brachial plexus.

Once the team member is aware of the situation, the head may be observed to retract against the perineum. Fundal pressure aggravates the shoulder impaction and should be avoided in the evidence of shoulder dystocia or any delivery. The McRoberts maneuver, a simple maneuver that increases the diameter of the pelvis by stretching the pelvic joints, should be tried next. With the patient's legs flexed at the knees, the maternal clinician should help the patient draw her knees up and toward the chest (dorsal knee–chest position), place the head of the bed down, and continue, with gentle downward traction of the head. Once the anterior shoulder clears the symphysis, the posterior shoulder usually delivers without resistance. The key to success in this position is to have the mother's knees as far back to her shoulders as possible. If this is ineffective, the next maneuver is gentle application of suprapubic pressure. It can be applied by another member of the medical crew (the shoulder may be palpated above the pubis). Gentle downward traction of the head should be applied concurrent with gentle suprapubic pressure. Suprapubic pressure should never be excessive because it can lead to uterine rupture and bladder trauma. The team should not persist if the shoulder does not slip under the symphysis.[3,6]

Delivery of the posterior shoulder can also be attempted with rotation of the posterior shoulder downward and into the left posterior quadrant. With release of the posterior arm and shoulder, the anterior shoulder follows. Internal rotation of the fetal shoulders may also be considered. As a last resort, the infant's clavicle may be deliberately broken; however, when this is done, the chance of damage to the brachial plexus is increased. Vaginal delivery increases the risk for perinatal mortality and morbidity by 3%.[3,6]

Uterine Rupture[3,6,20]

A spontaneous or traumatic disruption of the uterine wall, known as *uterine rupture,* can occur. If the laceration is extensive and comes in direct contact with the peritoneal cavity, it is a complete rupture. The rupture most frequently occurs in a weak area of the myometrium, usually at the site of a previous incision. Examples of previous incisions include a previous cesarean section scar, a scar from a myomectomy, or a scar from the result of rapid deceleration forces (such as may occur with a fall or in a motor vehicle collision).

Background

Before further discussion of uterine rupture, differentiation between rupture and dehiscence of a scar is necessary. *Rupture* refers to the separation of an old incision and possibly an extension into previously uninvolved myometrium, with rupture of membranes. Fetal parts may extend through the rupture into the peritoneal cavity. Hemorrhage is usually present from the edges of the separation and may be massive. A *dehiscence* does not involve the fetal membranes and may not even involve the entire previous scar. Bleeding may be minimal or bloodless. Dehiscence occurs gradually, whereas rupture occurs as a sudden event. A dehiscence may become a rupture with labor or trauma.

Factors that predispose to uterine rupture include previous surgery involving the myometrium, previous cesarean section with a higher incidence of a "classic" vertical scar being involved, use of labor stimulants, trauma, and previous rupture, overdistension of the uterus because of multiple gestation or polyhydramnios, and grand multiparity. Uterine rupture usually occurs during labor but can occur before the onset of labor. It can be seen with an unscarred uterus resulting from blunt

trauma. This trauma is most likely a rapid deceleration injury in which pressures inside the uterus are too high because of sudden impact and rupture occurs. Uterine rupture may also occur because of internal trauma, such as perforation with an instrument (e.g., a difficult forceps delivery); from external pressure, such as from an external version of the breech fetus; or from overly vigorous fundal pressure during delivery attempts.

In situations in which the patient has had a previous cesarean section, the probability of rupture is much greater when the scar traverses the body of the uterus vertically (classical incision) than when the scar involves the lower uterine section transversely. Dehiscence occurs more frequently without subsequent complications when the scar is low and transverse.

The degree of hemorrhage and extent of possible complications depend on the location and extent of the rupture. If the rupture does not involve the large arteries, the hemorrhage is less severe. If the rupture is complete, the mortality rate for the fetus is high. Potential complications are postpartum infection, injury to the bladder, potential for hysterectomy for uncontrolled bleeding, hypovolemic shock, kidney failure, DIC, and death.

Signs and symptoms of uterine rupture include severe sudden continual abdominal pain and signs of hypovolemic shock. Contractions may cease or may increase in intensity and frequency. Shoulder or chest pain may result from the collection of blood under the diaphragm (Kehr's sign). Generalized tenderness with rebound pain or vaginal bleeding is likely when the rupture occurs in the lower uterine segment. However, many of these patients are obtunded from blood loss and are unable to report pain. Most bleeding is intra-abdominal, and the abdomen may be distended. Frequent assessment of fundal height may be an indication that the uterus is filling with blood. Use a marker to mark the top of the fundus with ink, and frequently reassess the fundal height. Palpation of the uterus also reveals a firm or hardening uterus, which is reflective of accumulating blood. Remember the maternal patient carries 40%–50% more blood at term and can compensate for a longer period of time before maternal vital sign changes are noted. Another textbook description of uterine rupture is that the clinician is able to palpate fetal parts as the uterine wall integrity is lost. Although this may or may not be true, this is a *secondary* assessment, and because of tremendous blood volume losses, it is unlikely the clinician has moved beyond the primary survey.

Management

Rapid recognition of the signs and symptoms of uterine rupture often mean the difference between life and death for the obstetric patient. Surgical intervention is necessary, and care is supportive. Oxytocin (Pitocin), 20 to 40 units in a 1000-mL solution administered IV, may incite uterine contraction with vessel constriction and reduce the bleeding after delivery of the fetus, and should be considered with consultation of transport guidelines/policies. Serial abdominal measurements can be made to further assess intra-abdominal bleeding. Acute fetal distress with increasingly severe variable decelerations, late decelerations, minimal to absent variability, or absent FHT is observed.[3,6,20]

A history of previous cesarean sections and observation of abdominal scar is of primary importance. Although the scar noted may be low and transverse, documentation is needed to determine the location of the scar on the uterus. For the patient in labor who has had a previous cesarean section, the first sign of placental abruption may actually be rupture. Tocolytics may be considered for patients with a previous classical incision that is at risk for contracting or is currently contracting. Appropriate medical staff must be contacted for direction and management.[3,6,20]

Resuscitative Hysterotomy[29–31]

Resuscitative hysterotomy (RH) is the new term for what was previously called perimortem caesarean delivery (PMCD). The new nomenclature is being adopted to highlight the importance of the procedure to a successful resuscitation during maternal cardiopulmonary arrest (MCPA). It is defined as the procedure of delivering a fetus from a gravid mother through an incision in the abdomen during or after MCPA. The goal of the procedure is to improve the survival of the mother and the neonate.

There are physiologic changes that occur during pregnancy which reduce the probability of return of spontaneous circulation (ROSC) during cardiac arrest. Physiologic anemia of pregnancy reduces the oxygen carrying capacity of blood and results in decreased delivery of oxygen during resuscitation. The large gravid uterus elevates the diaphragm and reduces the lung's functional reserve capacity (FRC), which when combined with increased oxygen demand from the fetus results in decreased oxygen reserves and resultant risk for rapid oxygen desaturations. The size of a gravid uterus at 20 weeks results in aortocaval compression which reduces the amount of venous return from the inferior vena cava and reduces cardiac output during resuscitation. The theory behind resuscitative hysterotomy is to increase the probability of ROSC by reducing the impact of aortocaval compression.

For any resuscitation of a pregnant patient with a gravid abdomen, the patient should remain in supine position with manual uterine displacement to reduce compression of the great vessels. If chest compressions are not required, the patient can be placed in a lateral position. High-quality CPR is the cornerstone of any successful attempt at cardiac arrest resuscitation.

Resuscitative hysterotomy is a consideration in pregnant patients with cardiac arrest whose fundal height is above the level of the umbilicus – this estimates a gestational age over 20 weeks. Best outcomes are achieved with delivery in 5 minutes or less. There are maternal and fetal benefits with delivery after that timeframe; time-to-delivery clearly is linked with better outcomes. To achieve delivery in this time frame, decision for procedure usually has to be made at about 3 minutes into the arrest. The procedure should be performed at the site of resuscitation without delay to prep the incision site or gather instruments, as long as a scalpel and scissors are available.

Gynecologic Emergencies

Ovarian Torsion

Ovarian torsion is a condition associated with reduced venous return from the ovary as a result of edema, internal hemorrhage, hyperstimulation, or a mass. An ovary and fallopian tube are typically involved.

Torsion of a normal ovary is most common among young girls with excessively long fallopian tubes or absent mesosalpinx. Few ovarian torsion cases in pediatric patients have involved cysts, teratomas, or other masses. Women with pathologically enlarged ovaries can develop unilateral ovarian torsion. The irregularity of the ovary likely creates a fulcrum around which the oviduct revolves. The process affects both the ovary and the oviduct (adnexal torsion). Approximately 60% of torsions occur on the right side.[20,32]

During the physiologic changes in early pregnancy, which cause the presence of an enlarged corpus luteum, a cyst likely predisposes the ovary to torsion. Physiologic changes may also affect the weight and the size of the ovary, which could alter the position of the fallopian tube and allow twisting to occur. Approximately 20% of cases occur during pregnancy. Women receiving infertility treatment carry an even greater risk, in that numerous theca lutein cysts significantly expand the ovarian volume. Patients with a history of tubal ligation are at increased risk for torsion, probably because of adhesions that provide a site around which the ovarian pedicle may twist. Fifty percent to 60% of ovarian cases of torsion are associated with ovarian tumors. Ovarian torsion is the fifth most common gynecologic surgical emergency, accounting for 2.7% of cases of acute abdominal pain in the female patient. With early diagnosis and treatment, the prognosis of ovarian torsion is good.[20,32]

The classic presentation of adnexal torsion is sudden onset of unilateral lower abdominal pain, which is initially vague in character and may be accompanied by nausea and vomiting. It may radiate to the groin or flank. Patients may describe several episodes of pain over the course of hours, days, or even weeks, if the ovary has been experiencing intermittent torsion.[7]

Common complications associated with an ovarian torsion included infection, peritonitis, sepsis, adhesions, chronic pain, and, rarely, infertility. Early recognition of this emergency can help decrease the risk of or limit the impact of these complications.[20,32]

Surgical intervention is critical and the patient should be transported to an appropriate facility as quickly and safely as possible.[7] The patient should be closely monitored for signs of shock and appropriate management for shock should be initiated. The patient should be placed in a safe position of comfort for transport. Pain should be managed using medications per transport protocols.[20,32]

Ectopic Pregnancy

An ectopic pregnancy is a complication of pregnancy in which the embryo attaches outside the uterus. Ninety-five percent to 98% of tubal pregnancies implant in the fallopian tube. Nontubal ectopic pregnancies are rare and may occur in the ovaries, broad ligaments, and abdominal cavity. Heterotopic pregnancy, which is a rare case of an ectopic pregnancy, is one in which there may be two fertilized eggs: one embryo inside the uterus and one outside the uterus.

This can occur in the fallopian tubes, in the interstitial portion of the tube, in the horn of the uterus, in the cervix, in the abdomen, or in the ovary. One of every 100–200 pregnancies are ectopic and of those 95% occur somewhere within the fallopian tubes. In the United States 1 of 819 women will die of complications from an ectopic pregnancy, such as a rupture.[4,19]

In most ectopic pregnancies, there exists some abnormality or constriction in the fallopian tube resulting in the delay or prevention of the fertilized ovum from reaching the uterus. The fertilized ovum then implants itself within the fallopian tube. Causes of fallopian tube narrowing or constriction can include previous pelvic inflammatory disease (causing scarring), previous inflammatory processes (from infections), endometriosis, developmental abnormalities, adhesions from previous abdominal or tubal surgeries, tubal sterilization, and use of low-dose progesterone oral contraceptives. Other causes include smoking and IUD use. If the fetus dies at an early gestation, there is no harm to the fallopian tube. However, if the fetus continues to grow within the fallopian tube, it can rupture the wall of the fallopian tube, causing significant bleeding. Slow blood loss will cause pain and lower abdominal pressure.

Rapid bleeding will cause a sudden drop in blood pressure and may lead to severe hemorrhage, shock, and even death.[4,19]

There is a clinical triad of symptoms referred to as the 3 As: amenorrhea, abdominal pain, and abnormal vaginal bleeding. The abdominal pain is usually in the lower abdomen and described as sharp. It may only occur on one side of the body. The patient may also have a positive Kehr's sign, which is acute pain in the shoulder on the side of the rupture due to blood in the peritoneal cavity. Because of bleeding, the patient may present in hemorrhagic shock.[4,19]

If the patient is suffering from hemorrhagic shock, the shock should be managed before, during, and after transport. If the patient does not present in shock, she should be monitored closely for signs of shock. The patient should be safely transported in a position of comfort. Pain management should be started and continued during transport. The patient should be transported as quickly as possible to an appropriate facility for evaluation and surgical management, if indicated.

Summary

The transport of the patient with an obstetric or gynecologic emergency requires experience and skills so that both the mother and fetus may benefit. If the mother does not receive appropriate care, the fetus suffers; but at times, the condition of the patient or fetus may warrant personnel with specific abilities not generally obtained by a general transport service. Each transport service must ensure that they are competent and capable of providing care for both the mother and fetus as well as for a patient with a gynecologic emergency.

References

1. American Academy of Pediatrics and American College of Obstetricians and Gynecologists. *Guidelines for Perinatal Care.* 7th ed. Elk Grove, IL: American Academy of Pediatrics/American College of Obstetricians and Gynecologists; 2012.

2. Bickley LS. *Bate's Guide to Physical Examination and History Taking.* 10th ed. Philadelphia, PA: Walters Kluwer/Lippincott Williams & Wilkins; 2009.

3. Gilbert E. *The Manual of High Risk Pregnancy and Delivery.* 5th ed. St. Louis, MO: Mosby Elsevier; 2011.

4. Lam K. Gynecological and obstetric emergencies. In: Salyer S, ed. *Emergency Medicine for the Healthcare Provider.* Philadelphia, PA: Saunders; 2007:183–190.

5. Lopes van Balen VA, van Gansewinkel TAG, de Haas S, et al. Maternal kidney function during pregnancy: systematic review and meta-analysis. *Ultrasound Obstet Gynecol,* 2019;54:297–307. doi: 10.1002/uog.20137

6. Simpson KR, Creehan PA. *Perinatal Nursing.* 4th ed. Philadelphia, PA: Wolters Kluwer Lippincott Williams and Wilkins; 2011.

7. Society of Critical Care Medicine. *Fundamental Critical Care Support – Obstetrics.* Mount Prospect, IL: SCCM; 2017.

8. Reale SC, Bauer ME, Klumpner TT, et al., Multicenter Perioperative Outcomes Group Collaborators. Frequency and risk factors for difficult intubation in women undergoing general anesthesia for cesarean delivery: a multicenter retrospective cohort analysis. *Anesthesiology.* 2022;136:697–708. doi: 10.1097/ALN.0000000000004173

9. ACOG Practice Bulletin No. 106: Intrapartum fetal heart rate monitoring: nomenclature, interpretation, and general management principles. *Obstet Gynecol.* 2009;114(1):192–202. doi: 10.1097/AOG.0b013e3181aef106

10. Menihan CA, Kopel E. *Electronic Fetal Monitoring: Concepts and Applications.* Philadelphia, PA: Wolters Kluwer/Lippincott Williams and Wilkins; 2008.

11. Alfirevic Z, Devane D, Gyte GM, Cuthbert A. Continuous cardiotocography (CTG) as a form of electronic fetal monitoring (EFM) for fetal assessment during labour. *Cochrane Database Syst Rev.* 2017;2(2):CD006066. doi: 10.1002/14651858.CD006066.pub3

12. Pettit F, Mangos G, Davis G, Henry A. Pre-eclampsia causes adverse maternal outcomes across the gestational spectrum. *Pregnancy Hypertens.* 2015;5(2):198–204.

13. Mammaro A, Carrara S, et al. Hypertensive disorders in pregnancy. *J Prenat Med.* 2009;3(1):1–5.

14. ACOG Practice Bulletin, Number 222: Gestational hypertension and preeclampsia. *Obstet Gynecol.* 2020;135(6):e237–e190. doi: 10.1097/AOG.0000000000003891

15. Brown MA, Magee LA, Kenny LC, et al.; International Society for the Study of Hypertension in Pregnancy (ISSHP). Hypertensive disorders of pregnancy: ISSHP classification, diagnosis, and management recommendations for international practice. *Hypertension.* 2018;72(1):24–43. doi: 10.1161/HYPERTENSIONAHA.117.10803

16. Poon LC, Magee LA, Verlohren S, et al. A literature review and best practice advice for second and third trimester risk stratification, monitoring, and management of pre-eclampsia: compiled by the Pregnancy and Non-Communicable Diseases Committee of FIGO (the International Federation of Gynecology and Obstetrics). *Int J Gynaecol Obstet.* 2021;154 Suppl 1(Suppl 1):3–31. doi: 10.1002/ijgo.13763

17. Yoselevsky E, McElrath T, Little S. Readmission for postpartum eclampsia in the United States. *J Matern Fetal Neonatal Med.* 2002;35(25):10082–10085. doi: 10.1080/14767058.2022.2089552

18. Gyamfi-Bannerman C, Thom EA, Blackwell SC; NICHD Maternal–Fetal Medicine Units Network. Antenatal betamethasone for women at risk for late preterm delivery. *N Engl J Med.* 2016;374(14):1311–1320. doi: 10.1056/NEJMoa1516783

19. Doyle LW, Crowther CA, Middleton P, Marret S, Rouse D. Magnesium sulphate for women at risk of preterm birth for neuroprotection of the fetus. *Cochrane Database Syst Rev.* 2009;(1):CD004661. doi: 10.1002/14651858.CD004661.pub3

20. Hill CC, Pickinpaugh J. Trauma and surgical emergencies in the obstetric patient. *Surg Clin North Am.* 2008;88(2):421–440.

21. Quantitative Blood Loss in Obstetric Hemorrhage: ACOG Committee Opinion Summary, Number 794. *Obstet Gynecol.* 2019;134(6):1368–1369. doi: 10.1097/AOG.0000000000003565

22. ACOG Practice Bulletin, Number 183: Postpartum hemorrhage. *Obstet Gynecol.* 2017;130(4):e168–e186. doi: 10.1097/AOG.0000000000002351

23. Sentilhes L, Winer N, Azria E, et al.; Groupe de Recherche en Obstétrique et Gynécologie. Tranexamic acid for the prevention of blood loss after vaginal delivery. *N Engl J Med.* 2018;379(8):731–742. doi: 10.1056/NEJMoa1800942

24. Campbell J. *International Trauma Life Support for Prehospital Care Providers.* 8th ed. Boston, MA: Pearson; 2016.

25. Petrone P, Marini C. Trauma in pregnant patients. *Curr Probl Surg.* 2015;52(8):330–351.

26. Jain V, Chari R, Maslovitz S, et al. Guidelines for the management of a pregnant trauma patient. *J Obstet Gynaecol Can.* 2015;37(6): 553–574. doi: 10.1016/s1701-2163(15)30232-2

27. Barnhart ML, Rosenbaum K. Anaphylactoid syndrome of pregnancy. *Nurs Womens Health.* 2019;23(1):38–48. doi: 10.1016/j. nwh.2018.11.006

28. Mirza E, Chandraharan E. Breech delivery. In Chandraharan E, Arulkumaran S, eds. *Obstetric and Intrapartum Emergencies: A Practical Guide to Management* (pp. 56–65). Cambridge: Cambridge University Press; 2021.

29. Einav S, Kaufman N, Sela HY. Maternal cardiac arrest and perimortem caesarean delivery: evidence or expert-based? *Resuscitation.* 2012;83(10):1191–1200. doi: 10.1016/j.resuscitation.2012.05.005

30. Jeejeebhoy FM, Zelop CM, Lipman S, et al. Cardiac arrest in pregnancy: a scientific statement from the American Heart Association. *Circulation.* 2015;132(18):1747–1773. doi: 10.1161/CIR.0000000000000300

31. Eldridge AJ, Ford R. Perimortem caesarean deliveries. *Int J Obstet Anesth.* 2016;27:46–54.

32. Acmi S. Acute ovarian torsion in young girls. *J Acute Dis.* 2016;4(1): 59–61.

17

Care and Transport of the Newborn

MICHAEL A. FRAKES AND JAMIE R. EASTMAN

COMPETENCIES

1. Understand the anatomic and physiologic aspects of neonates.
2. Identify and prioritize components of peripartum management in the neonatal patient.
3. Discuss assessment and management goals for neonatal patients post delivery.
4. Describe management strategies for neonatal respiration and perfusion.
5. Identify cardiopulmonary pathologies in neonatal patients and discuss goals for management, strategies for intervention, and techniques for assessment.

6. Identify gastrointestinal pathologies in neonatal patients and discuss goals for management, strategies for intervention, and techniques for assessment.
7. Identify infectious pathologies in neonatal patients and discuss goals for management, strategies for intervention, and techniques for assessment.
8. Identify neurologic pathologies in neonatal patients and discuss goals for management, strategies for intervention, and tools and techniques for assessment.

The neonatal patient is an infant less than 28 chronologic days of age or under 28 days beyond the due date, for preterm infants. A term pregnancy is 38–42 weeks. Premature infants are defined as infants born before 37 weeks' gestation, with very preterm being 28 to less than 32 weeks, and extremely preterm if under 28 weeks' gestation. Even late preterm babies, those between 34 and 36 weeks' gestational age, have a threefold higher infant mortality rate compared with term babies.[1] Post-term infants are born later than 42 weeks' gestation. Further subgrouping is defined by birth weight: low birth weight (LBW) is less than 2500 g, very low birth weight (VLBW) is less than 1500 g, and extremely low birth weight (ELBW) is less than 1000 g.

Neonates have a unique anatomy, physiology, and pathophysiology that requires advanced knowledge and understanding to deliver appropriate care. Interfacility transport of neonates requires an emphasis on maintaining an equal or higher level of care during stabilization and transport to the receiving hospital. Teams that transport neonatal patients are expected to be specialists that can provide critical care interventions with progressive and goal-directed therapies. Specialized teams have been associated with improved outcomes compared with nonspecialized teams.[2]

The American Academy of Pediatrics (AAP) offers specific criteria for the composition, education, and operations of a neonatal transport team, and the Commission on Accreditation of Medical Transport Systems publishes industry-established standards for medical transport that can also be helpful.[3,4]

Fetal Circulation and Transition

In utero, the placenta and fetus are nourished by an umbilical vein that carries highly oxygenated blood to the right atrium via the ductus venosus and the inferior vena cava.[5] Most of this blood is directed across the foramen ovale to the left atrium, then the left ventricle, and into the ascending aorta to perfuse the coronary arteries and the brain with the most highly oxygenated blood in fetal circulation. Some of the blood from the umbilical vein, along with blood returning from the superior vena cava, flows through the tricuspid valve to the right ventricle and out through the pulmonary valve. Most of the blood flow from the right ventricle shunts from the pulmonary artery through the ductus arteriosus and into the descending aorta as a result of the high pressure of the pulmonary vascular system. The shunted blood mixes with the remainder of the blood coming from the left side of the heart (Fig. 17.1).

The transition to extrauterine life begins the moment the neonate takes its first breath. The expansion of the lungs and exposure to oxygen at birth causes the pulmonary vascular resistance (PVR) to fall and allows a rapid increase in pulmonary blood flow and a consequent decrease in flow across the ductus arteriosus. Simultaneously, as the umbilical cord is clamped, the low-resistance placental circuit is removed and an increase in systemic resistance occurs. This increase in afterload, and the increased return to the left atrium from the pulmonary circuit, helps to close the flap-like foramen ovale.

In the normal infant, once the transition to extrauterine life is complete, the ductus venosus, foramen ovale, and ductus arteriosus close, and there is not a communication between the systemic and pulmonary systems. However, if there is an abnormal connection between these two systems, shunting can take place at atrial, ventricular, or arterial levels. Blood will shunt from a higher to a lower resistance circulation, and the clinical presentation will vary by the size and location of the shunt. Shunts that occur left to

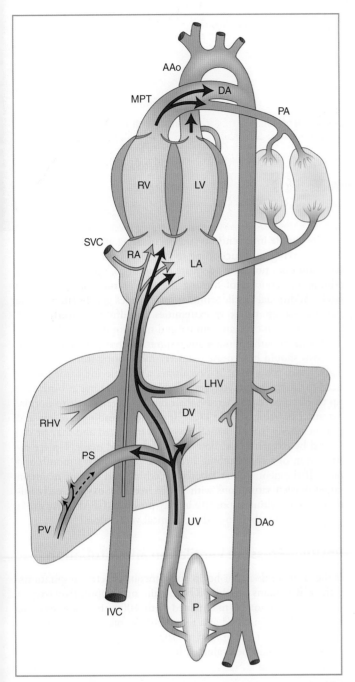

• **Fig. 17.1** Diagrammatic representation of the normal fetal circulation and major fetal blood flow patterns. *AAo,* Ascending aorta; *DA,* ductus arteriosus; *DAo,* descending aorta; *DV,* ductus venosus; *IVC,* inferior vena cava; *LA,* left atrium; *LHV,* left hepatic vein; *LV,* left ventricle; *MPT,* main pulmonary trunk; *P,* placenta; *PA,* main branch pulmonary arteries; *PS,* portal sinus; *PV,* portal vein; *RA,* right atrium; *RHV,* right hepatic vein; *RV,* right ventricle; *SVC,* superior vena cava; *UV,* umbilical vein. (From Fineman JR, Maltepe E. Fetal cardiovascular physiology. In: *Creasy & Resnik's Maternal-Fetal Medicine: Principles and Practice.* 9th ed. Elsevier; 2023.)

right, or systemic to pulmonary, tend to be acyanotic because oxygen-rich blood is mixing with the oxygen-poor side of the heart. Abnormalities that cause blood to shunt from the right to the left side of the heart, or pulmonary to systemic, will cause the infant to appear cyanotic. Some defects require a shunt for the infant to maintain either pulmonary or systemic circulation.

Careful ongoing assessment and early intervention are critical during this time period. Neonatal hypoxia, hypoglycemia, hypothermia, sepsis, stress, and acidosis can all interfere with the normal progression of this transition, and the baby may exhibit abnormal findings such as intermittent grunting, mild retracting, tachypnea, and poor feeding.[5] The infant must be observed and monitored closely until all these symptoms have been addressed or resolved. Subtle, persistent abnormalities can indicate undiagnosed congenital cardiac diseases.

Initial Priorities: Peripartum Management

Preparation for Delivery

Preparation is the key to a successful neonatal resuscitation. Approximately 4%–10% of term and late term newborns will require some form of resuscitation.[5] In the transport setting and when available, the information to consider when preparing for delivery includes antepartum risk factors such as preeclampsia and multiple gestations, and intrapartum risk factors including maternal anesthesia and placental abruption. The clinician will want to know the gestational age, whether the amniotic fluid is clear, the number of births anticipated, if there are any other risk factors, and the umbilical cord management plan.[5] Transport teams attending the delivery of an infant in an uncontrolled, austere environment will want to make sure they have the ability to provide the following:

- Warmth
  - Increase ambulance temperature
  - Use a radiant warmer or provide a thermal mattress
  - Remove wet garments, dry the baby, and apply fresh, warm linens
  - Provide skin-to-skin contact with mother (except during transport), or wrap body in plastic wrap to prevent heat loss
- Suction, with both bulb syringe and catheter
- Positive-pressure ventilation (PPV) with self-inflating bag, flow-inflating bag, or T-piece resuscitator. Mask sizes 00, 0, and 1. Airway adjuncts such as laryngeal mask.
- Supplies for endotracheal intubation
- Supplemental oxygen with a blender
- Emergency medications, especially epinephrine for intravenous (IV) push and infusion
- Surfactant administration kit
- IV supplies
  - For standard IV access
  - Umbilical catheterization, if trained to do so
  - Intraosseous (IO) access equipment

Assessment

The initial assessment should be brief and focused on identification and treatment of life-threatening issues related to airway, breathing, or circulation. Evaluation of color, respiratory effort, heart rate (HR), body tone, and responsiveness to stimuli all provide an immediate snapshot of how the transition to extrauterine life is progressing at that particular moment in time and guides resuscitation.[6] The Apgar score, presented to the public in 1953 by Dr. Virginia Apgar, is a basic, rapid evaluation of the infant's overall status regarding adaptation to extrauterine life. It is not used to make real-time resuscitation decisions (Table 17.1).[7]

TABLE 17.1	Apgar Score			
		SCORE		
Sign	**0**	**1**	**2**	
Appearance, color	Blue, pale	Centrally pink	Completely pink	
Pulse, heart rate	None	Less than 100 beats/min	Greater than 100 beats/min	
Grimace, reflex	No response	Grimace	Cough, gag, cry	
Activity/attitude	Flaccid/limp muscle tone	Some flexion	Well-flexed/active motion	
Respiratory, effort	None, irritability	Weak/irregular	Good, crying	

Provide Warmth

The temperature of the newly delivered neonate without asphyxia should be maintained between 36.5°C and 37.5°C.[8,9] If possible, provide prewarmed towels or blankets for the resuscitation. As soon as possible after delivery, the infant should be dried, wet linens removed, and an external heat source provided, such as radiant warmers. Adjuncts to the radiant warmers include plastic wrap, thermal mattresses, and heated and humidified gases. If an external heat source is not immediately available, particular attention must be paid to ambient temperature. Unintended neonatal hypothermia increases the risk of intraventricular hemorrhage (IVH), respiratory problems, hypoglycemia, and late-onset sepsis.[9] A transport isolette should have double-lined walls, continuous temperature monitoring, and provide a temperature-controlled environment. Continuous assessment and documentation should include the set temperature of the isolette.

Clearing the Airway

The infant should be positioned with the neck in a neutral position, which allows for proper positioning of the airway in a sniffing position. If the airway needs to be cleared, this can be done by wiping the nose and mouth or using a bulb syringe or suction catheter with mechanical suction. The oropharynx should normally be cleared before suctioning of the nares because stimulation may cause the infant to gasp and aspirate secretions present in the oropharynx. Stimulation of the vagus nerve from suctioning too vigorously and too deeply may result in severe bradycardia; therefore suctioning after the initial clearing of the airway should be done on an as-needed basis. The Neonatal Resuscitation Program (NRP) recommends that no greater than 100 mmHg of negative pressure should be used to avoid injury to the neonate.[5]

Aspiration of meconium-stained fluid into distal airways may significantly contribute to morbidity and mortality. It has been common practice to routinely intubate nonvigorous meconium-stained infants presenting with inadequate respirations, poor tone, or a heart rate (HR) less than 100 beats/min before there are many respirations. This practice is no longer supported by the American Heart Association or AAP because of insufficient evidence of benefit.[10] If an infant delivered through meconium is nonvigorous, initiate the initial steps of neonatal resuscitation as described previously.[9]

Initiation of Breathing

Most neonates initiate spontaneous breathing without intervention. Neonates that do not initiate breathing on their own may require simple interventions such as opening and positioning the airway, drying, and suctioning to stimulate breathing. If the neonate still does not have adequate respirations, appropriate tactile stimulation consists of flicking the feet or rubbing the infant's back. Additional tactile stimulation includes gently rubbing the newborn's back, trunk, or extremities. Mindful that overly vigorous stimulation can cause injury and may not be helpful.

Neonates with spontaneous respirations but persistent central cyanosis should have pulse oximetry monitoring initiated on the right hand. Skin color is not always a reliable indicator for the need for supplemental oxygen.[5] Babies transitioning at birth take up to 10 minutes to increase their blood oxygen levels to normal extrauterine values (Table 17.2). If oximeter readings are low and not increasing, supplemental oxygen is indicated and may be delivered by oxygen mask, flow-inflating bag and mask, T-piece resuscitator, or oxygen tubing held close to the baby's mouth and nose. If the neonate has labored breathing and cannot maintain target oxygen saturations with 100% free-flow oxygen, early initiation of continuous positive airway pressure (CPAP) may avoid the need for intubation and mechanical ventilation.[5,11,12]

Positive-Pressure Ventilation and Intubation

If the neonate does not begin spontaneous effective respirations, if the HR remains below 100 beats/min, or if appropriate oxygen saturations cannot be maintained with 100% free-flow oxygen, PPV should be initiated at a rate of 40–60 breaths/min with the minimal amount of oxygen to support oxygenation. Effective ventilation should be evaluated by auscultation of breath sounds

TABLE 17.2	Normal Neonatal Preductal Oxygen (Right Hand) Oxygen Saturation
Minutes of Life	**SpO$_2$ Range**
1	60%–65%
2	65%–70%
3	70%–75%
4	75%–80%
5	80%–85%
10	85%–95%

Data from Weiner GM, Zaichkin JG. *Textbook of Neonatal Resuscitation*. 8th ed. Elk Grove Village, IL: American Academy of Pediatrics; 2021.

and observation of chest excursion and HR. The infant should respond to effective ventilation with an improvement in HR, oxygen saturations, and spontaneous respiratory effort.[5,13]

Neonates are at high risk for pulmonary air leaks such as a pneumothorax or pneumomediastinum, so ventilating pressures should always be monitored with a manometer. Although pressures up to 30–40 cm H_2O may be initially necessary to open the lungs, the lowest pressures possible to maintain adequate chest rise and oxygenation should be used. Once the infant has established spontaneous respirations and an HR of 100 beats/min, the team should reevaluate the amount of support needed.

If there is no clinical improvement with effective PPV or if PPV is required for more than a few minutes, consider intubation.[5]

An accurate gestational age can help guide the proper depth of endotracheal tube (ETT) insertion and ETT size selection (Table 17.3). For ETT depth, the nasal–tragus length method is validated: the ETT marking at the baby's lip should correspond to the calculated depth of (distance from the baby's nasal septum to the ear tragus) +1.[5] Another easy calculation for the depth of the ETT in patients greater than 750 g is 6 + weight in kilograms = ETT depth. In patients less than 750 g, this calculation could cause the ETT to be secured too deeply.[14]

Careful and immediate evaluation for right or left mainstem or esophageal intubation should be done and effectiveness of ventilation should be assessed. Clinical signs of increasing HR, symmetric chest rise, and equal, bilateral breath sounds suggest successful intubation. End-tidal carbon dioxide detection should also be done with either a colorimetric or waveform device.[5,15,16]

The laryngeal mask airway (LMA) may be a beneficial airway adjunct in patients when PPV with a face mask is unable to achieve effective ventilation or when intubation is unsuccessful or not possible.[9] This may occur when the neonate presents with facial congenital anomalies such as Pierre Robin syndrome. Placement does not require instruments, and the LMA is blindly passed using the clinician's finger to guide it into place. Limitations of the LMA include size constraints, inability to deliver high ventilation pressures, and insufficient evidence that it can be used for intratracheal medications or prolonged assisted ventilation in neonates.[5] The smallest LMA for use in neonates is for those greater than 2 kg.

TABLE 17.3	Endotracheal Tube Size and Depth for Neonatal Patients		
Gestational Age (Weeks)	Weight (g)	ETT Size	Maximum ETT Depth
<28	<750	2.5	6.75
<28	750–1000	2.5	7
28–34	1000–2000	3	8
34–38	2000–3000	3.5	9
>38	>3000	3.5–4.0	10

ETT, Endotracheal tube.
Data from Karlsen K. Learner Manual. The S.T.A.B.L.E. Program. Post-Resuscitation /Pre-Transport Stabilization Care of Sick Infants: Guidelines for Neonatal Healthcare Providers. 6th ed. Park City, UT: S.T.A.B.L.E; 2013.

Chest Compressions

Chest compressions should be initiated if the HR is less than 60 beats/min after 30 seconds of effective PPV.[5] Resuscitation for neonates should be performed at a rate of 120 "events" (compressions or breaths) per minute. Ninety compressions plus 30 breaths on 100% oxygen should occur at a ratio of 3:1. The status of the infant should be reassessed after 60 seconds of resuscitation. If the infant's HR is greater than 60 beats/min, compressions can be stopped. If the HR remains below 60 beats/min, epinephrine should be given.

The recommended technique for chest compressions in neonates is the thumb-encircling-hands technique, preferred over the previously recommended two-finger technique because of the ability to have more control over the depth of compression and delivery of a more consistent pressure.[17] This method appears to provide better peak systolic and coronary artery perfusion pressure. The baby should be placed on a firm surface for delivery of effective compressions, with the caregiver encircling the infant's chest with both thumbs used to depress the infant's sternum. The infant's chest should be depressed to a depth of approximately one-third of the anteroposterior diameter of the chest, and the chest should be allowed to recoil completely by releasing pressure so that the heart can refill.[5]

Drug Support

Less than 1% of neonates will require drug intervention when effective ventilation has been established. If the HR continues below 60 beats/min with effective ventilation and chest compressions for a minimum of 30 seconds or in the absence of an HR, epinephrine should be given. The recommended IV dose is 0.2 mL/kg or 0.02 mg/kg of 0.1 mg/mL epinephrine solution followed by 3 mL flush of normal saline.[5] ETT administration may be more readily accessible, but studies have shown larger doses are required and absorption is unreliable and not as effective as IV administration.[18] If the ETT route is used, administer 1 mL/kg or 0.1 mg/kg of 0.1 mg/mL epinephrine.[5] Administration of ETT epinephrine should be followed by PPV to facilitate absorption by distribution throughout the lungs. If the first dose is given via the ETT and does not elicit an effective response, subsequent doses should be given by IV as soon as vascular access is established.[9] If the HR remains below 60 beats/min, subsequent doses of epinephrine may be given every 3–5 minutes.

Consider hypovolemia in patients with a history of bleeding or if the infant has poor response to resuscitation, pallor, decreased capillary refill, and/or weak pulses that persist even with adequate ventilation, chest compressions, and administration of epinephrine. If hypovolemia is suspected, normal saline should be given in 10 mL/kg aliquots over 5–10 minutes. In very low birth weight (VLBW) infants, this should not exceed 1 mL/min. Uncross-matched type O Rh-negative blood should be considered at 10 mL/kg when severe fetal anemia is documented.

If peripheral vascular access cannot be rapidly achieved, current NRP guidelines for resuscitation in the delivery room recommend emergent line placement into the umbilical vein as the most accessible parenteral route (Fig. 17.2). IO is another vascular access route for those trained in the technique. This approach is a reasonable alternative, especially in the outpatient setting when cannulation of the umbilical vessel may not be possible. All medications and fluids that can be given in an umbilical vein catheter can be given via IO in term and preterm neonates.[5]

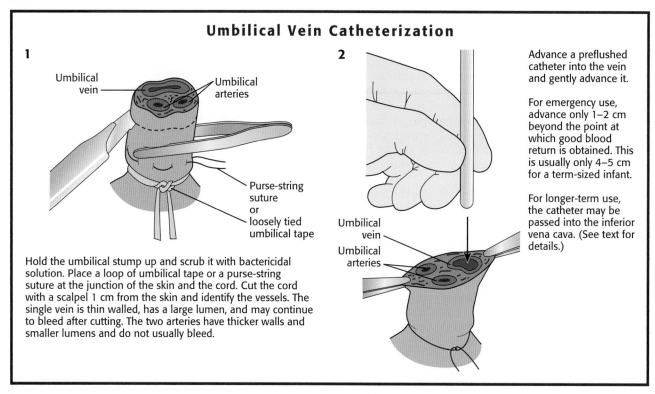

Umbilical Vein Catheterization

1

Umbilical vein — Umbilical arteries

Purse-string suture or loosely tied umbilical tape

Hold the umbilical stump up and scrub it with bactericidal solution. Place a loop of umbilical tape or a purse-string suture at the junction of the skin and the cord. Cut the cord with a scalpel 1 cm from the skin and identify the vessels. The single vein is thin walled, has a large lumen, and may continue to bleed after cutting. The two arteries have thicker walls and smaller lumens and do not usually bleed.

2

Advance a preflushed catheter into the vein and gently advance it.

For emergency use, advance only 1–2 cm beyond the point at which good blood return is obtained. This is usually only 4–5 cm for a term-sized infant.

For longer-term use, the catheter may be passed into the inferior vena cava. (See text for details.)

Umbilical vein

Umbilical arteries

• **Fig. 17.2** Umbilical vein catheterization. (From Zaoutis L, Chiang V. *Comprehensive Pediatric Hospital Medicine*. Philadelphia, PA: Elsevier; 2007.)

Special consideration should be given to product manufacturer recommendations. Many IO products are not approved for usage with patients less than 3 kg and/or 6 lb.

Apgar Scoring

The AAP and American Congress of Obstetricians and Gynecologists encourage the use of an expanded Apgar score for up to 20 minutes for infants who are depressed (score less than 7) at 5 minutes of life (see Table 17.1). The Apgar score is not an accurate indicator of neonatal asphyxia and should not be used to predict mortality or neurologic outcomes.[19–21] Low scores at 5 and 10 minutes can be associated with acute peripartum or intrapartum events.[22] An infant with an Apgar score of 0 at 20 minutes of age can have resuscitative efforts discontinued because of the high probability of poor neurologic outcome if there is confirmation that there has not been a detectable HR (decision individualized on patient and contextual factors).[5,21]

Special Considerations for Preterm/LBW Babies

Preterm and LBW infants are at great risk for cold stress because of their thin skin, large surface area relative to body mass, and decreased fat stores that allow for increased heat loss. In the transport setting, thermal mattresses and plastic wrap can be used to maintain body heat. Monitor temperatures frequently to avoid overheating or underheating and to maintain a goal temperature of 36.5°C.[5]

Preterm infants are at increased risk of neurologic injury because of the delicate capillaries in the germinal matrix. Transport has been associated with an increased risk for IVH in VLBW infants.[23] Evidence supports the practice of neutral head positioning to decrease the risk of IVH.[24] If possible in the transport environment, keep the head in a midline position for the first 72 hours of life along with the head of the bed elevated at 30 degrees.[25] IVH is discussed in further detail later in this chapter.

In the stress of the transport environment, attention should be given to careful handling of the infant. This includes avoiding a head-down position; avoiding overinflation of the lungs, which could result in a pneumothorax; assuring gradual changes in oxygenation and ventilation; and avoiding rapid volume infusions. As mentioned previously, fluid administration should not exceed 1 mL/min in this patient population to avoid the increased risk of intraventricular hemorrhage.

Evaluation of Prolonged Resuscitation

If the neonate has not responded to the initial priorities of delivery room management, the transport team must reevaluate the clinical assessment and management of the infant. Common reasons for an inadequate response to resuscitation include the following:

- Pulmonary sources
  - Dislodged ETT
  - Obstructed airway
    - Obstructed ETT
    - Congenital malformation
  - Pneumothorax
  - Failure of oxygen supply or ventilation device
  - Pulmonary hypoplasia
  - Congenital diaphragmatic hernia (CDH)
- Cardiac sources
- Shock

- Inborn error of metabolism
- Hypothermia
- Hypoglycemia

Noninitiation and Discontinuation of Resuscitation

According to the NRP, when circumstances at birth predict "almost certain early death and when unacceptably high morbidity is likely among survivors, resuscitation is not indicated although exceptions may be appropriate." Situations that may call for noninitiation of resuscitation include:

- Birth weight less than 400 g
- Confirmed trisomy 13
- Anencephaly
- Gestational age less than or equal to 22 weeks
- No response after 10 minutes of ongoing adequate resuscitative efforts
- Severe fetal growth retardation[5,18,26]

Postdelivery Management

History and Assessment

Assessment of the newborn should include history, clinical examination, and laboratory data. The maternal history is a key part of the neonatal history. Obstetric information obtained should include the estimated day of confinement (EDC) or due date based on the mother's last menstrual period and clinical data; maternal age; gravity; parity; abortions; fetal demise; neonatal deaths; number of living children; time since rupture of membranes; and complications of the pregnancy, labor, or delivery. Description of amniotic fluid, such as color, odor, or amount. The presence of maternal fever, instrument-assisted delivery, and any details regarding fetal heart rate monitoring. Maternal medications (both during pregnancy and during the perinatal period) should be assessed, specifically CNS depressants (i.e., SSRIs and magnesium sulfate), along with group B streptococcus (GBS) status and associated treatment, and other maternal infections such as herpes simplex virus, chlamydia, gonorrhea, hepatitis B, syphilis, or human immunodeficiency virus (HIV). Any maternal illicit drug or alcohol use should also be obtained.

Neonatal history should include gestational age, postdelivery age, the delivery type and course, time or membrane rupture and nature of fluids, Apgar scores, resuscitation efforts, initial physical examination, and subsequent clinical course. Laboratory data and radiographic studies should also be reviewed.

A considerable amount of baseline information can be obtained strictly through simple observation before disturbing the infant. This observation should include:

- Neurologic assessment
- Cough, gag, and suck, Moro reflex, palmar grasp, pupils, gaze, fontanelles, tone
- Heart
  - Rate, rhythm, heart sounds, murmurs, extra sounds
- Chest
  - Symmetry and adequacy of air entry, rales, rhonchi, wheezes
- Abdomen
  - Bowel sounds, organomegaly, masses, 2- or 3-vessel umbilical cord
- Pulses
  - Quality

- Comparison between upper and lower and right versus left extremities
- Signs and symptoms of distress
  - Color, respiratory effort, posture, tone
- Obvious morphology.

Once the baseline examination has been established, the rest of the examination should proceed with an organized, systematic approach. For example, the transport team might examine the infant beginning from the head and working downward. The essential components of a detailed examination are outlined in Table 17.4. The potential value of each part of the examination must be weighed against any stress it may cause to an already compromised infant and current physiologic stability.

Glucose and Maintenance Fluids

Before birth, the fetus stores glucose in the form of glycogen to use after birth.[27] The ability of the neonate to maintain glucose stability after birth can be adversely impacted by three factors: glycogen levels, hyperinsulinemia, and glucose utilization. Glycogen storage generally occurs in the latter portion of the third trimester, which puts the preterm infant at risk for hypoglycemia. Small-for-gestational-age (SGA) infants (those in the lowest 10% of the growth curve) stressed in utero use the glucose transferred from the mother via the placenta for growth and survival. This restricts the infant's ability to make or store glycogen.

TABLE 17.4	Key Components of Neonatal Physical Exam
	Assess
Head	Symmetry, shape, caput succedaneum, cephalhematoma
Fontanelles/sutures	Fontanelle number, fullness, depression, size, suture mobility
Symmetry of face	Development, shape, movement
Ears	Shape, position of face, presence of skin tags
Eyes	Shape, position, size, pupils, hemorrhages
Mouth	Cleft palate, teeth, abnormalities, presence of micrognathia
Neck	Webbing, length
Nose	Symmetry, septum, patency
Clavicles	Masses, intactness
Chest	Size, symmetry, shape
Umbilical cord	Number of vessels
Genitals	Development, testes, urethral and vaginal openings
Anus	Patency, meconium
Spine	Masses, symmetry, dimples
Extremities	Symmetry, development, movement, pulses
Hips	Range of motion
Reflexes	Root, suck, Moro, grasp
Tone	Flaccid, normal, jitteriness, flexion

A second factor is hyperinsulinemia, which occurs in infants of diabetic mothers (IDM) and which should be considered in infants who are large for gestational age (those in the top 10% of the growth curve). Abnormal elevation of maternal glucose concentrations will be seen in the fetus; however, maternal insulin does not cross the placenta. The fetus will increase insulin secretion in response to the increased glucose concentration. At delivery, the maternal glucose stops but the infant's insulin remains elevated and can take several days to regulate. IDM babies are also at increased risk for hypocalcemia and hypomagnesemia.

Finally, increased glucose utilization occurs in infants that are stressed or sick because increased energy needs can rapidly deplete their glycogen stores. Some maternal medications can also increase the risk of neonatal hypoglycemia such as terbutaline, beta-blockers, tricyclic antidepressants, sulfonylureas, and thiazide diuretics.[27]

The healthy term infant normally reaches the nadir of the serum glucose level at approximately 2 hours after birth.[28] Glucose screening is therefore recommended for all healthy term infants between 1 and 2 hours of age. Infants identified as high risk should have screening glucose levels as soon as possible after delivery. A widely used neonatal education program for the stabilization of sick infants called STABLE recommends that a glucose less than 50 mg/dL should be corrected with IV therapy and monitored until the glucose stabilizes between 50 and 110 mg/dL on two consecutive measures 15–30 minutes apart.[27]

Hypoglycemia that is symptomatic in the neonate is associated with increased neurodevelopmental impairment. Symptoms of neonatal hypoglycemia include hypotonia, lethargy, poor feeding, jitteriness/tremors, seizures, apnea, tachypnea, and cyanosis. When hypoglycemia is suspected, a screening test should be done while a plasma glucose is sent to the laboratory. Treatment should be initiated before confirmation from the laboratory is received. Not all infants with hypoglycemia are symptomatic, and there is not currently clear evidence that asymptomatic neonatal hypoglycemia impacts neurodevelopmental outcomes. Nevertheless, infants that are asymptomatically hypoglycemic and are sick should be kept in the normoglycemic range.[27]

In the otherwise healthy infant, oral reestablishment of serum glucose is the preferred method; however, critically ill neonates cannot tolerate oral intake. Symptomatic patients will require an IV established and a glucose infusion rate of 4–6 mg/kg per minute. A usual starting dose is 80 mL/kg per day (5.5 mg/kg/min) followed by a bolus of 2 mL/kg (200 mg/kg) of D10W slowly over 5 minutes.[27] Do not bolus with dextrose concentrations over D10. A recheck of the blood glucose should be repeated within 15–30 minutes after a glucose bolus or IV rate increase. When there is continued hypoglycemia, a decision to bolus or increase fluid rates or dextrose concentration must be made on the basis of the fluid requirements and tolerance of the individual baby.

A peripheral vein may be used to administer solutions that contain glucose concentrations up to 12.5% dextrose. At concentrations over 12.5% dextrose, a central venous line should be considered. Treatment of extremely resistant hypoglycemia may include the use of glucagon, glucocorticoids, and diazoxide. Administration of these drugs, however, is beyond the scope of this chapter.

Hyperglycemia (blood glucose levels greater than 125 mg/dL) can be seen in infants less than 32 weeks' gestation or infants that are SGA because of their immature endocrine system. Generally, hyperglycemia is managed by individual program protocol or medical direction.

Glucose monitoring should be conducted frequently during transport to ensure that glucose homeostasis is maintained. A point-of-care glucose check should be assessed within 15–30 minutes after changing IV fluids containing dextrose or increasing or decreasing infusion rates. All abnormal results should be monitored and reported as per protocol or medical direction.

Inborn Errors of Metabolism

In the setting of continued hypoglycemia, metabolic acidosis, and/or hyperammonemia, consideration of inborn errors of metabolism is warranted. This grouping of metabolic derangements are congenital inability to process sugar complexes in the body. Some examples include lactase deficiency, galactosemia, mitochondrial disorders, and phenylketonuria. Symptoms range in severity from diarrhea and mild hypoglycemia to apnea, severe metabolic acidosis, or death. Many states require the testing for these metabolic disorders prior to discharge from the hospital.

Fluid Management

Maintenance of fluid and electrolyte balance in the newborn requires careful, precise calculations. The transport team should precisely calculate the infant's fluid requirement, including any abnormal losses; too much or too little fluid can be detrimental to the progress of the infant.

Generally, sick infants typically need approximately 80 mL/kg per day on the first day of life. This requirement increases by approximately 10 mL/kg per day on the first subsequent day of life. Premature infants, particularly those weighing less than 1500 g, should be given special consideration of potentially increased fluid needs. Insensible water losses, immature skin surfaces, and prolonged exposure to radiant warmers can increase fluid requirements by as much as 50%.

The main sources of neonatal fluid loss are insensible water loss (skin and respiratory fluid losses) and urinary output (UO). Insensible water loss increases significantly in the extremely premature or ELBW infant. Radiant warmers, elevated environmental temperature, and respiratory distress increase insensible water loss. The use of heat shields and warm, humidified air delivered through the ventilator can significantly minimize these losses. In the sick neonate, UO should be measured as accurately as possible with urine bags, diaper weights, or catheterization. With appropriate fluid intake, UO should be 1–2 mL/kg per hour. During the first week of life, the infant averages a 5% to 7% loss of birth weight.[29] Subsequent changes in the baby's fluid intake are based on evaluation of these criteria.

The need for electrolyte evaluation before transport is determined based on the age of the newborn, the length of the transport, and the presence of risk factors for electrolyte imbalance. The addition of electrolytes to IV fluids is usually not necessary in the first 12 to 24 hours. Serum electrolyte levels should be checked before any additional electrolytes are added.

Thermoregulation

It is well documented that unintended hypothermia in neonatal patients adversely impacts morbidity and mortality.[27,30] The neonate is at high risk for hypothermia because of a large skin surface area to body mass ratio and poor thermal insulation. If not corrected, hypothermia can increase metabolism and cause peripheral vasoconstriction. This decreases peripheral perfusion and can lead to metabolic acidosis. Other adverse effects of cold stress include increased oxygen consumption, pulmonary vasoconstriction, and increased glucose demand. Infants with the greatest risk for hypothermia include those that are preterm, SGA, ELBW, sick, requiring a prolonged resuscitation, or those with defects requiring surgery such as myelomeningocele, gastroschisis, or omphalocele.[27]

Compared with the adult, the neonate has a limited ability to increase oxygen consumption, to produce heat by shivering, or to dissipate excess heat through sweating. The neonate maintains body temperature through basal metabolism, muscular activity, and chemical thermogenesis. The infant's primary mechanism of heat production in response to cold stress is chemical thermogenesis by metabolizing brown fat stores. This process requires increased oxygen consumption and increased glucose utilization. Preterm or hypoxic neonates are at increased risk for cold stress because of decreased stores of brown fat and/or their inability to metabolize it for the generation of heat production.[27]

The optimal temperature ranges for the newborn include the following:
- Skin: 36.2°C to 37.2°C
- Axillary: 36.5°C to 37.3°C
- Rectal: 36.5°C to 37.5°C[31,32]

Temperature must be frequently monitored during transport via skin temperature probes in transport incubators. Rectal temperatures are not recommended because of the high risk of perforation of the rectum.

Heat losses occur through convection, conduction, evaporation, and radiation.
- Radiation: Simple heat transfer from the body to the surrounding atmosphere
- Convection: Heat transfer from the body as air flows past (e.g., air currents, breezes)
- Evaporation: Heat transfer to water as it changes from liquid to gas (e.g., a wet infant)
- Conduction: Heat transfer between the body and objects in contact (e.g., a scale)

The neutral thermal environment is the range of environmental temperatures at which the neonate maintains a normal body temperature with minimal metabolic activity and oxygen consumption. During transport, the baby must be in a double-walled isolette set at a temperature that creates a neutral thermal environment.[33]

When managing a baby in the hospital, the baby should be on a radiant warmer. Chemical mattresses and plastic wrap can also be beneficial in preparing the neonate for transport and should be considered for babies less than 32 weeks' gestation or those at high risk for developing hypothermia.[5] Carefully follow manufacturer guidelines with any commercial heat-generating products to prevent overheating or burns. Clear plastic wrap or commercial products can be applied directly (e.g., wrapping the infant) to minimize further heat loss, but avoid the head and airway to prevent suffocation. When transporting a neonate in severe cold conditions, thermal covers may be used over double-walled transport incubators to further maintain a neutral thermal environment for the neonate.

Rewarming neonates that are unintentionally hypothermic is generally done slowly, at rates under 0.5°C/h, to decrease complications such as apnea, hypotension from vasodilatation, and arrhythmias.[27]

The neonate must also not become hyperthermic, which is associated with perinatal respiratory depression.

Respiratory Management: General Considerations

Many ill neonates have some degree of respiratory compromise. The transport team must perform careful and continuous assessment of respiratory status to provide adequate respiratory support before moving the patient to the transport incubator. This minimizes the likelihood of having to remove the baby from the transport incubator to perform interventions in a less controlled environment with fluctuating temperatures.

A normal neonatal respiratory rate is 30–60 breaths/min. Tachypnea can occur in neonates with pulmonary processes that impair gas exchange or from nonpulmonary processes that result in a metabolic acidosis. In either case, the respiratory center will respond by increasing the minute volume in an attempt to compensate for the developing acidosis. It is important to evaluate the baby's respiratory rate, work of breathing, gas exchange, presence of cyanosis, and oxygen saturations in the context of current oxygen supplementation. It can also be helpful to review chest x-rays and blood gas results because these can help guide ventilator and other treatment strategies.

Gas exchange is best evaluated by looking for regular, symmetric chest rise and fall and by listening to lung fields bilaterally for air flow.

Increased work of breathing is evidenced by nasal flaring, grunting, and retractions. Nasal flaring decreases airway resistance to improve air flow. Grunting represents an attempt to increase end-expiratory pulmonary pressures and improve the driving pressure of oxygen across the alveolar–capillary interface. Retractions occur when a neonate with poor lung compliance attempts to increase tidal volumes by using accessory respiratory muscles. This effort increases inspiratory force and draws the chest inward during inspiration, but retractions can also decrease the usable lung capacity and ventilation.

Hemoglobin desaturation can be evaluated by looking at the tongue and mucous membranes and through pulse oximetry. On examination, acrocyanosis is a self-limiting condition in which the neonate's hands and feet remain cyanotic for up to 48 hours after birth. It is generally not a pathologic finding. Central cyanosis (cyanosis in the tongue and mucous membranes) is a more significant finding. Pulse oximetry monitoring greatly enhances the ability to titrate oxygen delivery based on patient response and need. The oxygen saturation probe should be placed on the right hand or wrist to assess preductal oxygenation. This site evaluates oxygenation to the brain and heart, as it evaluates blood that is before the ductus arteriosus, so it is not affected by a ductal-level shunt, if one exists.[5,34] It may take up to 10 minutes for a baby to achieve an oxygen saturation of 95% after birth (see Table 17.2). Immediate care after delivery should be targeted to an age-appropriate saturation. After the first 10 minutes, preductal target oxygen saturations should be maintained between 91% and 95% unless there are conditions present that require adjustment, such as cardiac disease or pulmonary hypertension.[27,35]

Fetal hemoglobin and, accordingly, the fetal oxyhemoglobin dissociation curve, are different than those of adult patients. Fetal hemoglobin (hemoglobin-N) has a higher affinity for oxygen than adult hemoglobin, meaning that it binds oxygen at a lower oxygen tension but is reluctant to release the oxygen molecules. This is beneficial in utero to facilitate placental oxygen uptake. For the neonate, this means that the PaO_2 can be high with little change in oxygen saturation. This relationship is represented by a leftward shift of the oxyhemoglobin dissociation curve.[27,36] Remember that other factors causing a leftward shift are alkalosis and hypothermia, whereas acidosis and hyperthermia shift the curve to the right. With a right shift, it is more difficult to saturate the hemoglobin molecule, but it is easier to release the oxygen to the tissues (Fig. 17.3).

Blood gases supplement pulse oximetry in determining oxygenation along with assessing ventilation and pH. Newly born infants tend to have a mild metabolic acidosis, but usually have more normal blood gases within 48 hours. It is important to know the site from which the sample was drawn because normal values vary among arterial, venous, and capillary blood gas samples. Normal values are included in Table 17.5. It is also important to understand that the blood gas could be an umbilical cord sample, meaning that it typically only assesses pH and base excess. It is only to assess the metabolic condition of the neonate at the time of delivery. The blood gas sample should also be interpreted in the context of the respiratory support being provided at the time the sample was obtained.

Respiratory Support

The first component of respiratory management is ensuring correct opening, positioning, and clearing of the airway. Following that, supplemental oxygen is often administered. Oxygen is a drug with associated risks and side effects, particularly lung injury and retinopathy of prematurity.[35] It is administered by a number of methods.

Blow-by or free-flow oxygen near the baby's face can be used on a short-term basis but has two main drawbacks. First, accurate measurement of the exact amount of supplementation is impossible. Second, the flow of cold oxygen into the neonate's face may result in increased inappropriate heat-generating responses and vagal stimulation.

A low-flow nasal cannula delivers flow rates of 1 L/min or less.[37] Although commonly used, it is difficult to ascertain the inspired oxygen concentration because the baby entrains room air through the mouth and nose in addition to the supplied oxygen.

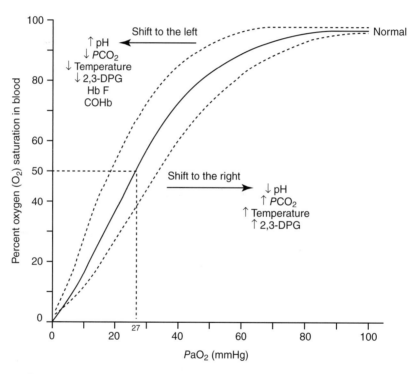

• **Fig. 17.3** Oxyhemoglobin dissociation curves: normal and shifted. (From Schick L, Windle P. *PeriAnesthesia Nursing Core Curriculum: Preprocedure, Phase I and Phase II PACU Nursing.* 3rd ed. St. Louis, MO: Elsevier; 2016.)

TABLE 17.5	Normal Neontal Blood Gas Values			
Site	pH	PCO_2	PO_2	HCO_3^-
Arterial	7.35–7.45	35–45 mmHg	50–90 mmHg (term) 50–80 mmHg (preterm)	22–26 mEq/L (term) 20–24 mEq/L (preterm)
Capillary	0.02–0.05 lower than arterial	8–14 mmHg higher than arterial	30–41 mmHg lower than arterial	2–3 mEq/L higher than arterial
Venous	0.01–0.03 lower than arterial	3–7 mmHg higher than arterial	23–32 mmHg lower than arterial	0.5–1.5 mEq/L higher than arterial

Data from Yapicioglu H, Ozlu F, Ozcan K, et al. Comparison of arterial, venous and capillary blood gas measurements in premature babies in newborn intensive care unit. *Cukurova Med J.* 2014; 39(1):117–124.

In ELBW neonates, low-flow nasal cannula is believed to provide some mild positive pressure to the lungs.

Nasal continuous positive airway pressure (nCPAP) is beneficial for infants with adequate respiratory effort but who exhibit increased work of breathing and/or increased oxygen requirements. It can be delivered via mask or nasal prongs, and mask CPAP can be given while the nCPAP is being set up. The delivery will vary among facilities. Resource-limited programs may use bubble CPAP which utilizes a water source to establish pressure. The early use of CPAP can reduce the need for intubation, mechanical ventilation, and surfactant administration in newborns.[11,38,39] An AAP policy statement described it as the preferred initial approach to prevent neonatal respiratory distress syndrome (RDS). Neonates with an oxygen requirement that exceeds 60%–70% should be evaluated for intubation.

High-flow nasal cannula (HFNC), with flow rates typically between 2 and 8 L/min, is increasingly being used instead of nCPAP devices.[38–41] The nasal prongs are smaller than prongs used with nCPAP and HFNC does not require a seal, which may cause less nasal trauma. It may also be easier to apply, and some believe that it improves carbon dioxide elimination.[37] The role of HFNC is still being evaluated; it appears to be at least not inferior to nCPAP.[42] A small device that heats and humidifies HFNC air is available for transport.

Noninvasive mechanical ventilation is used when the clinician is attempting to avoid endotracheal intubation. Nasal intermittent positive-pressure ventilation augments nCPAP by delivering intermittent positive-pressure breaths via nasal prongs. It is mainly used for infants requiring early support because of apnea or for postextubation. Although there are no current data to support the use of nasal intermittent positive pressure ventilation over nCPAP, early studies suggest nasal intermittent positive-pressure ventilation reduces the frequency and severity of apnea and is better at reducing extubation failures in neonates.[43,44]

Invasive ventilation requires the placement of an ETT, with inherent risks for complications. Mechanical ventilation decreases work of breathing, improves overall gas exchange, and can recruit lung units. ETT and mechanical ventilation should be considered in infants with warning signs of respiratory failure, such as grunting with retractions, inability to maintain O_2 saturations, or respiratory insufficiency, that are not responsive to a trial of CPAP. Patients with inadequate respiratory effort require early intubation, as do babies with pathology that precludes positive pressure by other means, such as a CDH.

There are significant differences amongst providers on the usage of pharmacology for induction during intubation of the neonate. Many providers chose to intubate without induction agents such as sedation or neuromuscular blockade. This process involves swaddling the neonatal and/or physically restraining while making intubation attempt(s). It typically requires more than one attempt to successfully secure the airway due to the continued movement of the neonate. The concern is that deep sedation and neuromuscular blockade are detrimental to neurodevelopment. However, there is not sufficient evidence to support this. Alternatively, the support for usage of induction agents to increase first pass success is gaining traction. Ozawa et al. found in a multifacility, retrospective study of 2260 neonatal intubations that use of sedation with neuromuscular blockade was associated with favorable tracheal intubation outcomes.[45] Further, intubation should be completed by the most trained and proficient provider, which may not be the physician in some cases. The usage of video laryngoscopy has become more favorable to direct laryngoscopy to also increase first pass intubation attempts.

Securing of the endotracheal tube in place is important and should be verified by two providers prior to transport. Commercial devices or tape should be used. Best practices vary between institutions, however significant awareness should be paid to endotracheal tube security with all moves. Given the nature of small airways, one-half centimeter migration could dislodge the tube from the trachea. Confirmation with continuous end-tidal CO_2 is the gold standard during transport. However, this may be difficult with VLBW and ELBW neonates given the additional weight on the endotracheal tube. Coordinated positioning by all team members prior to, during, and at handoff is essential in this process. Confirmation is also completed with the presence of bilateral lung sounds, chest x-ray, and visual inspection with video laryngoscopy.

Traditionally, neonatal transport ventilators have provided time-cycled, pressure-limited ventilation. With this method of conventional mechanical ventilation, tidal volumes can have considerable fluctuation caused by lung compliance changes, ETT leaks, and the baby's spontaneous breathing.[46] Ventilation can also be delivered in a volume-targeted mode, which may be associated with decreased risk for barotrauma and associated chronic lung disease, less risk for pneumothorax, and decreased days of ventilation.[46–48] The goal with either mode is a returned tidal volume between 4 and 7 mL/kg. After ventilation is begun with empiric settings, subsequent adjustments are based on physical examination, chest x-rays, blood gases, and response to treatment.

High-frequency ventilation (HFV) delivers fast rates and small tidal volumes, via high-frequency oscillation ventilation (HFOV), high-frequency jet ventilation (HFJV), and high-frequency flow interruption (HFFI). The use of HFOV and HFJV in transport has historically been limited because of size, weight, battery life, and electromagnetic interference with aircraft avionics. Small, lightweight, pneumatically driven HFV devices are available for the transport environment.

There are differences in the mechanism of how gas exchange occurs with each device, and there are also similarities. For all devices, oxygenation is achieved by titrating FiO$_2$ and adjusting mean airway pressure. HFOV has active exhalation, whereas HFJVs and HFFIs have passive exhalation. Amplitude, which creates chest movement, is adjusted similarly on the HFO and HFFI, whereas HFJV requires conventional breaths to help recruit the lung.

With HFV, mean airway pressure is used to recruit the lung and improve oxygenation. Small changes in tidal volume (amplitude) have a big effect on carbon dioxide removal because alveolar ventilation during HFV is equal to tidal volume squared times frequency. Frequency is set to achieve optimal gas exchange based on the pathophysiology of the lung. Studies suggest that HFV with inhaled nitric oxide (iNO) is more successful in treating patients with severe lung disease and meconium aspiration syndrome than conventional mechanical ventilation, and suggest a benefit to using HFV for infants with CDH.[49–51]

Any infant treated with positive pressure is at increased risk for complications. Abdominal distention can also interfere with adequate ventilation, so patients with invasive or noninvasive ventilation should have a gastric tube in place venting air. Any sudden deterioration in an infant receiving PPV should prompt immediate evaluation, including patients receiving noninvasive PPV. The DOPE mnemonic[52] is a reminder of potential causes of deterioration in an intubated child's condition:

- Displacement of the tube
- Obstruction of the tube
- Pneumothorax
- Equipment failure

Blood Pressure and Perfusion

Assessment of circulatory status should begin with an evaluation of the maternal history along with any delivery room complications. A history suggestive of hypovolemia as a basis for poor perfusion may include compression of the cord or a history of blood loss during the pregnancy, labor, or delivery. A history of maternal fever or infection may result in an infant with distributive or septic shock. Infants with a history of asphyxia may have myocardial dysfunction.

The physical assessment should include the evaluation of serial blood pressures (BPs) and pulses in upper and lower extremities, central capillary refill time (in the context of body temperature, i.e. if the neonate of hypothermic, capillary refill may be prolonged), and preductal and postductal oxygen saturations. For a normal BP, many clinicians use the criterion that the mean arterial BP in millimeters should be maintained at or greater than the baby's gestational age in weeks. Interestingly, this has not been empirically evaluated.[53,54] It is also important to pay attention to the pulse pressure, determined by subtracting the diastolic pressure from the systolic pressure. Normal pulse pressure for a term infant is 25–30 and for a preterm infant it is 15–25. A narrow pulse pressure can suggest heart failure, peripheral vasoconstriction, compression on the heart, or severe aortic valve stenosis. A wide pulse pressure can be suggestive of a patent ductus arteriosus (PDA), other cardiac abnormalities, and/or sepsis from warm shock.[27]

Shock is a major cause of neonatal morbidity and mortality, and sepsis is the most common source of shock in neonates.[55] Shock is characterized by inadequate tissue and organ perfusion that results in cellular dysfunction and, if not corrected, cellular damage can cause end organ failure and potential death. Adequate tissue perfusion is dependent on cardiac output, vascular integrity, and the ability of the blood to deliver oxygen and metabolic substrates and remove wastes.[56] It is important to differentiate simple hypotension from hypotension associated with uncompensated shock. Hypotension and poor perfusion in the absence of other shock symptoms are common problems in the neonate, especially in infants less than 1500 g.[27]

Shock can be classified in three categories: hypovolemic, cardiogenic, and distributive. These etiologies are not necessarily exclusive. In compensated shock, perfusion to vital organs (i.e., brain, heart, liver, kidneys) is maintained with absent or minimal changes noted in vital signs caused by compensatory mechanisms that maintain BP and blood flow. The transport team may observe an increase in capillary refill time; decreased pulse quality; tachycardia; pallor and/or cool peripheral skin; or neurologic changes such as hypotonia, lethargy, and irritability.[57] If the shock is not reversed, the neonate will be unable to maintain compensatory mechanisms, resulting in hypotension. Treatment of shock should begin before the development of hypotension and further cellular dysfunction.[53,57]

Treatment is aimed at restoring adequate perfusion. An initial bolus of 10 mL/kg of normal saline solution infused over 15–30 minutes is a reasonable initial step in babies without evidence of pulmonary edema. If there is acute blood loss, packed red blood cells, including uncross-matched type O negative cells, can be given. Packed red blood cells are typically dosed at 10 mL/kg. Each volume bolus should be followed by an assessment of pulmonary status before continuing to additional volume restoration. If cardiogenic shock is suspected initially or on subsequent examination, an inotropic agent is indicated. Patients with refractory hypotension may benefit from the addition of vasopressors such as dopamine, epinephrine, or norepinephrine. The administration of hydrocortisone can increase BP and reduce catecholamine requirement without serious adverse reactions.[54,58] The management of infection and septic shock is discussed in greater detail elsewhere in this chapter.

Pathologic Conditions of the Neonate

Respiratory Disorders

Surfactant Deficiency

The most common cause of respiratory distress in the preterm infant is RDS, formerly known as hyaline membrane disease (HMD). RDS is primarily caused by a deficiency of surfactant, but can also occur in the presence of extreme stress such as severe hypoxia.

The primary function of lung surfactant is to lower surface tension at the air–water interface of the alveoli, preventing atelectasis and improving compliance. Surfactant decreases surface tension in the alveolus during expiration, which allows the alveolus to maintain a functional residual capacity. The absence of surfactant results in poor lung compliance and atelectasis. Infants with surfactant deficiency have progressive respiratory distress symptoms such as increased work of breathing, accessory muscle use, retractions, nasal flaring and grunting, and increased oxygen support as a result of poor lung compliance. Characteristic radiographic findings include reticular granular pattern in the lungs and hypoexpansion. Infants may require minimal respiratory support to maximal mechanical ventilation. As discussed earlier, early use of nCPAP is recommended for babies with RDS.

Exogenous surfactant was approved for use by the Food and Drug Administration in 1990. Ten years of extensive clinical studies showed that exogenous surfactant treatment substantially reduces mortality, incidence of air leak, pulmonary interstitial emphysema, and other complications such as bronchopulmonary dysplasia.[59,60] Both natural surfactant extracts and synthetic preparations are available. Administration of exogenous surfactant may result in rapid improvement in lung volumes and compliance with subsequent overventilation and air leaks. The team should monitor the baby and the measured ventilator values carefully in the half-hour after surfactant delivery. During this period, suctioning should be limited to allow the surfactant to work. Known complications associated with surfactant administration include pneumothorax and pulmonary hemorrhage. There is not a clear, proven best method to deliver surfactant.[61] Repeated doses at specific intervals may be indicated.[61]

Pneumonia

Pneumonia is typically of bacterial origin and can have early or late onset. Early-onset pneumonia is generally acquired from the mother and is seen within the first 3 days of life. It is often associated with rupture of membranes for more than 12 hours before delivery. However, a respiratory infection can occur in the fetus even in the presence of intact membranes. Symptoms of amnionitis and fetal infection include maternal fever or elevated white count, purulent or foul-smelling amniotic fluid, fetal tachycardia, loss of beat-to-beat variability, and premature labor. Late-onset pneumonia is associated with mechanical ventilation and prolonged hospitalization. See also the discussion of sepsis and septic shock elsewhere in this chapter.

Aspiration Pneumonia

Although aspiration of meconium is the most severe form of aspiration pneumonia, the neonate may also aspirate amniotic fluid or blood at the time of delivery. Typically, meconium aspiration occurs in term or post-term infants when meconium is passed and aspirated causing pulmonary disease, which leads to hypoxemia and acidosis. It is a leading cause of morbidity and mortality in term infants.[62] The presence of meconium in the amniotic fluid should alert the medical team to the possibility of acute or chronic in utero asphyxia, as well as the risk for meconium aspiration pneumonia.

Common symptoms of neonates with meconium or other substance aspiration include respiratory distress soon after birth, the appearance of a barrel chest caused by overinflation, and tachypnea. Radiographic findings may reveal patchy bilateral densities. The presence of meconium in the bronchial tree causes obstruction to air flow and pneumonitis. Complications of meconium aspiration syndrome include pulmonary air leaks and persistent pulmonary hypertension (PPHN).

The transport goals for managing the neonate with aspiration pneumonia are maintaining oxygenation and ventilation and, if mechanically ventilated, minimizing barotrauma. To achieve optimal gas exchange, deep sedation and the use of neuromuscular blockade may be necessary. Agitation can contribute to an increased PVR, right-to-left shunting, and hypoxemia. Careful attention must be paid to maintaining adequate perfusion and BP, and to avoid acidosis. Antibiotic therapy is frequently started in these infants until sepsis has been ruled out as the cause of in utero meconium release.

Pulmonary Air Leaks

Air leaks occur most commonly in neonates with underlying lung disease and are frequently seen with the use of positive airway pressure treatments.[63,64] The most common air leaks are pneumothorax and pneumomediastinum. Uncommonly, pneumoperitoneum and pneumopericardium could also occur. The infant with an air leak may appear nearly asymptomatic, with only muffled heart tones or absent/diminished breath sounds, or the infant's condition may deteriorate rapidly, necessitating immediate intervention. Assessment includes evaluation of breath sounds, shift in the location of point of maximum impulse (PMI), transillumination of the chest, and radiographic confirmation. To transilluminate the chest, place a cold light source on the chest. A normal chest will have a small and symmetric halo around the light source. A large and asymmetric light distribution suggests a pneumothorax. It can be very helpful to compare the light distribution bilaterally.

Neonates with a pneumothorax and minimal symptoms may only need a one-time needle thoracentesis and oxygen, or no treatment other than close monitoring. Infants with severe distress or with clinical indication of a tension pneumothorax need emergent needle decompression without delay for radiographic diagnosis (Figs. 17.4 and 17.5). For babies with an air leak of any type who are mechanically ventilated, minimizing the mean airway pressure will help to prevent the accumulation of air. In the transport setting, medical personnel must consider the impacts of altitude changes on an air leak or air collection. Boyle's law describes that entrapped gas volume expands by about 3% for every 1000-foot increase in elevation. Thoughtful consideration should be given, and the placement of a chest tube may be required, if risk for tension physiology is persistent or suspected during aeromedical transport.

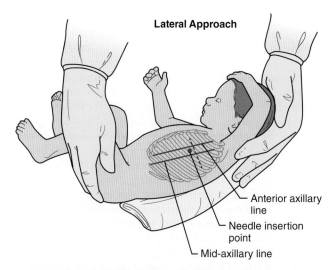

• **Fig. 17.4** Needle insertion point. (Modified from Bleak T, Frakes MA. Care and transport of the newborn. In: ASTNA; Semonin Holleran R, Wolfe AC, Frakes MA, eds. *Patient Transport: Principles and Practice.* 5th ed. St. Louis, MO: Mosby Elsevier; 2017.)

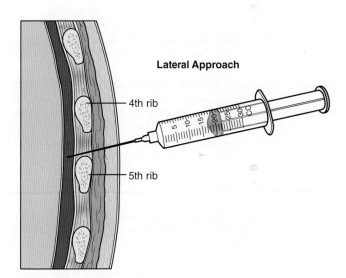

• **Fig. 17.5** Needle insertion. (Modified from Bleak T, Frakes MA. Care and transport of the newborn. In: ASTNA; Semonin Holleran R, Wolfe AC, Frakes MA, eds. *Patient Transport: Principles and Practice.* 5th ed. St. Louis, MO: Mosby Elsevier; 2017.)

Persistent Pulmonary Hypertension in the Newborn

PPHN of the newborn is a syndrome characterized by persistent elevated PVR that results in right-to-left (pulmonary-to-systemic) shunting at the ductus arteriosus or the foramen ovale and leads to hypoxemia in the presence of a structurally normal heart. This disease process is commonly seen in near-term infants with severe asphyxia, meconium aspiration syndrome, CDH, or sepsis. PPHN can also rise from idiopathic vascular abnormalities or arrested vascular development from CDH or other space-occupying chest lesions.

The clinical differentiation between cyanotic heart disease and PPHN can be difficult to make. A preductal and postductal oxygen saturation differential of over 10 mmHg in the presence of profound hypoxemia suggests, but is not exclusive for, PPHN. The shunt can also occur centrally, across the foramen ovale. The hyperoxia test will also help distinguish PPHN from parenchymal disease. In this test, the patient is placed on 100% FiO_2 by hood or ETT for 10 minutes, and then a preductal arterial blood gas is drawn from the right radial artery. A significant increase in the PaO_2 to over 100 mmHg during the test suggests parenchymal disease, whereas the absence of an increase favors PPHN or cardiac disease (i.e., PaO_2 less than 50 mmHg). Patients with PPHN may also demonstrate an improvement with hyperventilation to the high end of the normal respiratory rate range while on 100% oxygen, and those with heart disease will not.[65]

Treatment for PPHN is aimed at maintaining adequate oxygenation until the PVR begins to drop, which normally occurs in the first several days. Oxygen is a potent pulmonary vasodilator that is as effective as iNO when either is administered alone, so patients should receive 100% oxygen initially.[66-68] Maintaining a systemic BP higher than pulmonary pressure discourages right-to-left shunting. Typically, these infants are managed at the upper limits of normal through ensuring adequate circulating volume and cardiac output. Accepted parameters include a mean arterial pressure of 45–55 mmHg or systolic BP of 50–70 mmHg.

Infants unable to maintain adequate oxygenation with 100% oxygen and BP support may be considered for iNO therapy. Nitric oxide is a selective pulmonary vasodilator that targets the vascular smooth muscle cells surrounding the resistance arteries and creates an additive decrease in pulmonary vascular pressures beyond that of oxygen alone.[68] The iNO reduces the need for extracorporeal membrane oxygenation (ECMO) in term and late preterm infants with severe PPHN, but does not reduce non-ECMO mortality, length of stay, or adverse neurodevelopmental development. Up to 40% of babies with PPHN will not respond to, or sustain a response to, iNO.[69]

Once it diffuses into the bloodstream, nitric oxide binds to hemoglobin and is inactivated. This allows for pulmonary bed relaxation with minimal systemic side effects. The ultrashort half-life, under a second, does mean that interruptions of delivery to an NO-dependent patient must be avoided. A usual starting dose of iNO is 20–40 parts per million. If there is not a response within about 20 minutes of initiation, improvement is not usually seen with higher doses.[69-71] There is a trend toward increased off-label use of iNO in preterm infants (less than 34 weeks) that is not supported by evidence.[72]

Patients transported on iNO may benefit from deep sedation with neuromuscular blockade paralytics to minimize oxygen consumption and increases in PVR because of endogenous catecholamine release. Surfactant therapy decreases the need for ECMO in patients with PPHN that is secondary to mild parenchymal lung disease, but not for babies without concomitant parenchymal lung disease. Use varies among centers.[73,74]

Infants with severe PPHN who remain hypoxic even with maximum respiratory support and initiation of iNO may be considered for cardiopulmonary support from ECMO. ECMO is also used to treat neonates with RDS, PPHN, meconium aspiration syndrome, sepsis, and CDH. Indicators of severity of illness are standardized and require the use of calculations of the oxygen index (OI), as shown in the following oxygenation index formula[75]:

Oxygenation Index = $(FiO_2 * Mean Airway Pressure * 100) / PaO_2$

Extracorporeal Life Support Organization severity indications include:
- OI greater than 40 for greater than 4 hours
- OI greater than 20 with lack of improvement despite prolonged (over 24 hours) maximal medical therapy or persistent episodes of decompensation
- Severe hypoxic respiratory failure with acute decompensation (PaO_2 greater than 40) unresponsive to intervention
- Progressive respiratory failure and/or pulmonary hypertension with evidence of right ventricular dysfunction or continued high inotropic requirement.[76]

When the severity of illness criteria has been met, specific criteria are also used for patient selection. Variability exists among ECMO centers on this specific selection criteria; however, examples include the following:
- Birth weight greater than 2000 g
- Gestational age over 34 weeks
- No uncontrolled bleeding
- No major intracranial hemorrhage
- Mechanical ventilation longer than 10–14 days
- No uncorrectable CHD
- No lethal congenital anomalies
- No irreversible brain damage[75-77]

The goal of ECMO is to support the lungs and heart until there is a reversal of the pulmonary and cardiac dysfunction. ECMO cannulation can be venous–venous (VV) or venous–arterial (VA). With VV ECMO, blood is removed from and then returned to the venous circulation. VV ECMO provides only pulmonary support by improving oxygenation and carbon dioxide removal. With VA ECMO, blood is removed from the venous circulation and returned to the arterial circulation. VA ECMO provides support for both the heart and lungs by decreasing cardiac work and oxygen consumption, improving cardiac output, and providing oxygenation and carbon dioxide removal.

Risks associated with ECMO include bleeding, blood clot formation, infection, and transfusion problems along with mechanical failure of the pump. The most common clinical complication is bleeding caused by the anticoagulation therapy required for the implementation of ECMO.[77] Potential hemorrhage sites include but are not limited to insertion sites of cannulas; chest tubes; peripheral IV lines; and intracranial, intrathoracic, and abdominal areas.[77] Intracranial hemorrhages are the most serious complication associated with poor neurologic prognosis.[76,78]

Congenital Diaphragmatic Hernia

CDH occurs within the first few weeks of gestation. The cause has not been well defined; however, it is believed that CDH occurs because of failure of the pleuroperitoneal folds to close normally. Abdominal contents migrate into the thoracic cavity, compressing the developing lungs and blood vessels causing pulmonary hypoplasia and pulmonary hypertension. Generally, CDH is an isolated event, although it can be associated with additional abnormalities. Left-sided defects account for 80%–85% of all CDH and occur more often in males. Right-sided defects are associated with higher morbidity and mortality.[79]

Early detection of this defect is essential to quickly initiate appropriate therapy and surgical intervention, because bowel distention further compromises respiratory function beyond the structural defect. For babies with a prenatal diagnosis of CDH, a large-bore (10-Fr) orogastric tube should be inserted right away with the initiation of low intermittent suction. It is important to manage the airway early because these infants are at high risk for hypoxemia and acidosis, which will increase the risk of pulmonary hypertension. Avoid PPV with a facemask. When ventilation is necessary, immediate endotracheal intubation should be performed. Ventilatory management is aimed at maximizing ventilation while minimizing barotrauma, if possible, with lower inspiratory pressures and, as needed, higher respiratory rates. Preserving spontaneous respiration in these patients, if possible in the transport setting, can be beneficial.

Up to one-third of CDHs are diagnosed in the postnatal period, even in countries with robust ultrasound programs.[80] The typical presentation with postpartum diagnosis of CDH includes the early onset of respiratory distress, unequal or absent breath sounds, a shift in the PMI, and potentially scaphoid abdomen. Although scaphoid abdomen is listed as a classic sign, it is frequently not evident in the delivery room. Bowel sounds may be auscultated in the chest, and abdominal structures will be visible in the chest on a radiograph. The placement of a gastric tube before imaging will help illuminate gastrointestinal (GI) structures.

CDH used to be considered a surgical emergency. Recent studies have supported delayed surgery to permit physiologic stabilization. PPHN and shock frequently complicate the management of these infants. For babies with CDH and PPHN, evidenced by a wide preductal–postductal saturation difference, preserving ductal patency, supporting the right ventricle, and pulmonary vasodilatation can be helpful. Published protocols recommend the use of iNO to treat pulmonary hypertension in newborns with CDH and may provide short-term oxygenation improvement before ECMO cannulation. The safety and efficacy of prolonged INO therapy in these patients has not been well established.[69,81–83]

Neonatal Heart Disease

Congenital heart disease (CHD) is the most common birth defect, and is estimated to occur once in every 110 births in the United States. Maternal factors that would suggest a high risk for cardiac disease are a family history of CHD, congenital infection, prepregnancy diabetes, and exposure to alcohol and drugs.[84,85]

The early signs of congestive heart failure are tachypnea and tachycardia, which makes distinguishing pulmonary inefficiencies from cardiac disease difficult. A detailed history of the onset of symptoms can be helpful. The immediate onset of respiratory symptoms at birth is more likely to indicate the presence of pulmonary disease, because few babies are born in active heart failure. Babies with cardiac disease are often "quietly tachypneic" initially, without other indications of respiratory distress. This may be seen as a respiratory rate of 80–100 without grunting or retractions. A chest x-ray should be obtained and evaluated in concert with clinical findings. An abnormal heart size with increased or decreased vascular markings may be suggestive of a heart defect.[85]

On assessment, tachypnea with low $PaCO_2$ is more indicative of non-pulmonary causes of respiratory distress such as cardiac anomalies or metabolic or neurologic disorders, whereas tachypnea accompanied by increased PCO_2 suggests pulmonary conditions. Cardiovascular findings suggestive of cardiac disease include pathologic murmurs (e.g., diastolic murmurs, systolic regurgitant murmurs, continuous murmurs associated with an abnormal examination), other abnormal heart sounds, hyperactive precordium, discrepant BPs or pulses between upper and lower extremities, and hepatomegaly. A baby with no murmur may still have significant heart disease.[85]

Preductal and postductal oxygen saturation monitoring can be used as a supportive diagnostic tool. Preductal oxygen saturation is measured on the right hand, and postductal oxygen saturation is measured on either foot. Preductal oxygen saturations more than 10 mmHg higher than lower extremity saturations indicate right-to-left shunting from the pulmonary artery across the ductus arteriosus to the aorta. Preductal oxygen saturations less than lower extremity saturations may indicate transposition of great vessels. Remember that intracardiac shunting at the atrial or ventricular level will produce a decreased systemic oxygen saturation but not differential saturation between preductal and postductal sites.

Once the determination has been made that cyanosis in the newborn is caused by a fixed right-to-left shunt, the transport team should attempt to differentiate between shunting caused by PPHN and anatomic heart disease. Typically, infants with CHD present with a low $PaCO_2$ and a compensated or partially compensated metabolic acidosis. As described earlier, the infant who is hypoxic in room air but has a PaO_2 greater than 150 with 100% supplemental oxygen is more likely to have pulmonary disease than cyanotic heart disease or PPHN with a fixed right-to-left shunt. Patients with PPHN may also demonstrate an improvement with hyperventilation to the high end of the normal respiratory rate range while on 100% oxygen, whereas those with heart disease will not.[65]

If other causes of cyanosis have been ruled out and oxygen saturations do not increase greater than 75% even with 100% FiO_2, adequate ventilation, and fluids, a presumptive diagnosis of heart disease should be considered and the patient managed accordingly.

Neonatal cardiology and congenital heart defects represent a complex spectrum of conditions. Understanding normal neonatal anatomy, then considering the circulation effects of the defect and the effects of shunting across the duct (if present), can help conceptualize the patient's presentation and management (see Fig. 17.1). A simplified rubric, which may help make the defects and management more understandable, groups defects into four categories:
- Left outflow tract defects, ductal dependent for systemic blood flow
- Cyanotic defects, not ductal dependent
- Cyanotic defects, ductal dependent for pulmonary blood flow
- All other defects[85]

Approximately 20% of congenital heart defects are those with an anatomic obstruction to systemic blood flow, caused by coarctation or interruption of the aorta, critical aortic valve stenosis, or a hypoplastic left heart. In these patients, closure of the ductus arteriosus dramatically reduces systemic blood flow, causing pulmonary edema and shock. On examination, patients with aortic arch interruption or aortic coarctation classically have a BP gradient between higher upper extremity pressures and lower pressures in the legs. Patients with an obstruction to systemic blood flow benefit from preserved ductal patency by continuous prostaglandin infusion.

Prostaglandin E1 is a continuous infusion medication that dilates the smooth muscle in the ductus arteriosus. It is indicated in patients who are known to have CHD that is ductal dependent for either systemic or pulmonary flow, and is also a reasonable intervention in patients who are persistently cyanotic and in whom the diagnosis of CHD cannot be clearly ruled in or out. This is often the case in the initial stabilization and transport settings.[86] Common side effects include apnea, fever, and hypotension. In consideration of the short half-life and critical nature of the drug, it is best to infuse prostaglandins through a separate IV site and to ensure that a second working IV is always available. Clinicians should consider the possibility of hypotension and apnea when starting prostaglandins on a neonatal patient, particularly at higher doses. There is some evidence that lower doses of the agent may be as effective as currently recommended doses, particularly in patients requiring ductal patency for pulmonary rather than systemic flow, and that lower doses reduce the incidence of side effects.[87,88]

In the patient with a left ventricular outflow tract that is ductal dependent for systemic flow, BP and cardiac output can be managed with volume resuscitation and inotropic medications. Hyperoxia and hypocarbia decrease PVR, increase left-to-right shunting across the ductus, and can worsen systemic perfusion and pulmonary edema. Accordingly, these patients are best managed with target preductal oxygen saturations between 75% and 85% and ventilation to a PCO_2 that is normal or in the higher end of the normal range. Continuous, simultaneous monitoring of the preductal and postductal oxygen saturations can demonstrate changes in the magnitude of the shunt across the ductus.

A number of heart lesions will create cyanosis as a result of the mixing of oxygenated and deoxygenated blood at the atrial or ventricular level but have preserved blood flow through the pulmonary artery and are generally not ductal dependent for pulmonary flow. These cases represent about 15% of CHD patients and include the tetralogy of Fallot, truncus arteriosus, total anomalous pulmonary venous return, and Ebstein's anomaly. Oxygen will improve pulmonary blood flow in these patients. The central mixing and need to balance systemic and pulmonary blood flow make the target preductal oxygen saturation 75%–85% in these patients. Prostaglandin infusions are generally not required, unless there is severe disease represented by a persistent preductal saturation under 75% on supplemental oxygen.

A smaller number, about 9% of patients with CHD, have a defect creating cyanosis from reduced pulmonary blood flow. These patients, therefore, are dependent on an open ductus arteriosus for pulmonary blood flow. These defects include transposition of the great arteries, tricuspid atresia, pulmonary atresia, and the severe forms of tetralogy of Fallot and Ebstein's anomaly. In patients with an obstruction to pulmonary blood flow, higher inspired oxygen concentrations will reduce PVR and improve blood flow, so preserving ductal patency with a prostaglandin infusion is required to preserve pulmonary circulation. As with other patients who have cyanotic CHD, the target preductal oxygen saturation is between 75% and 85%. High levels of oxygen are also a stimulus for the PDA to close, which could worsen ductal-dependent lesions. Preductal and postductal saturations should be monitored continuously to evaluate both vital organ perfusion and a change in shunt magnitude.

Gastrointestinal Disorders

The transport team deals primarily with GI disorders related to obstruction, either functional or anatomic; infection; or externalized abdominal contents. Obstructions of the GI tract can occur anywhere from the esophagus through the anus. The management of all of these disorders primarily centers on decompression of the bowel, fluid management, antibiotic therapy, and respiratory support.

Esophageal Atresia/Tracheoesophageal Fistula

Esophageal atresia (EA) is a congenital defect that results in an interruption of the esophagus causing a loss of connection to the lower esophagus and stomach. The upper esophagus can end in a blind pouch or be associated with an abnormal connection to the trachea called a tracheoesophageal fistula (TEF). The incidence of EA/TEF is about 1 in every 4000 live births in the United States. Of these, 84% have an associated TEF. Interestingly, an "H-type" TEF without EA occurs approximately 4% of the time.[89,90]

These conditions may be difficult to diagnose. An obstetric history of polyhydramnios should increase the suspicion of upper GI obstruction. The accumulation of amniotic fluid occurs because it is not passing through the fetus' GI/renal system. Patient findings suggesting EA include the inability to pass a gastric tube to the stomach, excessive oral secretions, and choking or coughing during feedings. Diagnosis can be confirmed with radiographs, particularly those showing a radiopaque catheter curled in the upper esophageal pouch or supplemented with contrast medium. Careful evaluation of the rest of the GI tract, the cardiovascular system, and the genitourinary system should be completed because of frequently associated anomalies.[89,90]

It is estimated that up to 60% of infants with EA/TEF have additional anomalies, including the VACTERL association. VACTERL is not specific to a genetic diagnosis but includes vertebral, anal, cardiac, TEF, renal, and limb defects.[89,91]

The majority of fistulas occur between the lower esophageal pouch and the trachea.[89] These fistulas allow air to pass from the respiratory tree into the stomach and gastric acid to reflux into the bronchial tree. These infants are at high risk for aspiration either from the oropharynx refluxing from the upper esophageal pouch or aspiration of gastric contents from the lower TEF. PPV should be avoided if possible, because it distends the stomach via the fistula and may interfere with ventilation or result in gastric perforation. A transport team caring for an infant with EA should place the patient in a semi-prone position to minimize aspiration.[92] A gastric tube should be placed in the upper esophageal pouch and placed to suction. If a TEF is suspected, elevate the bed 30 degrees to reduce the risk of gastroesophageal reflux and aspiration.

Intestinal Obstructions

Common initial symptoms of intestinal obstruction include bilious vomiting, abdominal distention, feeding intolerance, large quantities of gastric contents at delivery, absence of an anal opening, and lack of stooling in the first 24 hours. An obstetric history of polyhydramnios suggests a GI obstruction. Although the presence of bilious vomiting in a newborn may be related to other causes, intestinal obstruction should be presumed until ruled out. Abdominal distention may be present depending on the level of the obstruction. The presence of tenderness, metabolic acidosis, or decreasing platelets may indicate a bowel necrosis or peritonitis and should be treated as an urgent problem.

Urgent cases include malrotations with volvulus and those with associated peritonitis, perforation, or suspected bowel necrosis.

Management includes decompression of the bowel with intermittent large-bore gastric suction, IV fluids, antibiotic therapy as indicated, and respiratory support. These infants may have large fluid requirements because of large interstitial fluid losses. Often, one and a half times maintenance fluids will be a required minimum for this patient population during transport. Severe abdominal distention may compromise respiratory status. Evaluation of these neonates should include assessment of oxygen needs and ventilatory capacity with appropriate measures taken to correct deficits. In severe cases of peritonitis, sepsis and shock may also be present and should be treated appropriately.

Necrotizing Enterocolitis

Necrotizing enterocolitis (NEC) is an acquired disease characterized by intestinal damage ranging from mucosal injury to necrosis and perforation. It occurs in up to 10% of VLBW babies, with a mortality rate of up to 50%, but may also affect older, larger, and even term babies. For preterm infants, presentation is usually in the second or third week of life, with earlier onset as birth gestational age declines. For term infants, onset is usually in the first few days after birth, but NEC can present as late as 1 month. The genesis of NEC is poorly understood, with contributing factors believed to include hypoxia, feeding, sepsis, abnormal colonization of the bowel, GI ischemic–reperfusion injury, and the release of inflammatory mediators.[93] There is not a specific microorganism responsible for NEC.

Early recognition of risk factors and symptoms allows for early treatment. Systemic nonspecific signs include apnea, lethargy, poor feeding, and temperature instability. Abdominal symptoms include feeding intolerance with increased gastric aspirates, bile-stained gastric aspirates, increasing abdominal girth, and guaiac-positive stools. Progression of the disease results in increasing abdominal distention to the point of tautness, grossly bloody stools, abdominal wall erythema, and abdominal tenderness. Radiographic findings include dilated bowel loops, thickening of the bowel wall, and the classic sign of air in the bowel wall (pneumatosis intestinalis). Portal gas is a poor prognostic sign, and pneumatosis intestinalis is pathognomonic. The absence of radiographic findings does not rule out the diagnosis of NEC.[93]

The initial course of treatment includes cessation of enteral feedings and gastric decompression. Patients will require IV fluids and parenteral nutrition. They are usually started on broad-spectrum antibiotics such as ampicillin, gentamicin, and clindamycin or metronidazole. Surgery is always a consideration. It is mandatory for perforation or for necrotic intestine, both of which are suggested by pneumoperitoneum.[93]

Omphalocele/Gastroschisis

Although omphalocele and gastroschisis are two separate entities, their treatment during transport is essentially the same. An omphalocele occurs when the abdominal contents that protrude into the extra embryonic coelom at the base of the umbilical cord during embryonic development fail to return to the abdominal cavity in the 12th week. The defect is covered by an amniotic–peritoneal membrane in which the umbilical cord inserts. The membrane may be broken during delivery. The size of the defect may vary from a small hernia to inclusion of a large percentage of the abdominal contents. An omphalocele is often associated with other abnormalities and syndromes.[94] Gastroschisis, on the other hand, is a defect that occurs because of a disruption of the abdominal wall formation in the embryonic period. The defect is usually to the right of the umbilical cord and allows for evisceration of abdominal contents. Because the defect is normally very close to the umbilicus, it is frequently mistaken for an omphalocele. This defect, however, is not covered by a membrane. The defect occurs early in gestation, so the intestines may appear edematous with adhesions because they have been floating in the amniotic fluid for some time. Generally, gastroschisis is categorized as simple, meaning it is not associated with other GI or chromosomal abnormalities.[95]

Both groups of infants are at risk for infection, hypothermia, large fluid losses, hypoglycemia, and impaired bowel perfusion. Treatment includes immediate wrapping of the defect with moist saline gauze and plastic wrap or, alternatively, placement of the neonate in a bowel bag to prevent fluid losses. The infant must have nothing by mouth and gastric suction applied to maintain bowel decompression. If the abdominal opening is extremely small, the patient may be at a high risk for bowel ischemia as a result of the constriction of blood flow. Caring for the infant on its side may help reduce tension on the bowel and improve circulation. Careful monitoring and maintenance of temperature in normal range are essential in the management of these infants with a skin defect. This increased need for thermogenesis also places them at continuous risk for hypoglycemia and hypovolemia.

Neonatal Infections

Neonates are at risk for infections because of their immature immune system. Infections are acquired in utero, in the birth canal, or from external sources after birth. The most common neonatal infections are viral and bacterial pneumonia; sepsis; and infrequently, meningitis. Pneumonia has been addressed in the subsections on respiratory illnesses. Other neonatal infections include congenital cytomegalovirus, rubella syphilis, toxoplasmosis, neonatal hepatitis B, and herpes simplex virus.

Sepsis is categorized as either early-onset (EOS) or late-onset (LOS), differentiated by the appearance before or after 72 hours of life.[96,97] Infants with EOS often present during their hospitalization, whereas infants with LOS are often seen initially in outpatient settings such as emergency departments. Risk factors for EOS include maternal chorioamnionitis, rupture of membranes greater than 18 hours before delivery, premature labor, maternal illness, infection or fever, and maternal GBS colonization. LOS is thought to be caused by environmental organisms.

The infant with sepsis may have mild and subtle onset of symptoms or a fulminating course that results in rapid progression to shock. Common signs and symptoms include temperature instability particularly hypothermia, "does not look well," respiratory distress, tachycardia, apnea and bradycardia, lethargy, irritability, poor tone, and poor feeding. Poor perfusion and hypotension are considered late findings. An infant with any of these symptoms must be evaluated for potential sepsis. If the infant has meningitis, seizures must be added to the list of common presenting signs.

Evaluation of these infants includes a complete blood cell count with differential. A low absolute neutrophil count and an elevated ratio of immature-to-total neutrophils (I/T ratio), although not required for a diagnosis of sepsis, increases the level of suspicion for bacterial sepsis. The ANC is calculated with the equation (white blood cell count) × (segmented neutrophil percentage + band neutrophil percentage + metamyelocyte percentage). Normal ranges vary by postnatal age, and the Schmutz or Manroe chart describes normal values. The I/T ratio is a more rapidly calculated and interpreted guide. The ratio is calculated with the equation (percentage of band neutrophils + percent of metamyelocytes)/(percentage of segmented neutrophils + percentage of band neutrophils + percentage of metamyelocytes). An I/T ratio over 0.2 suggests infection, and an I/T ratio over 0.8 is associated with a higher risk of death from sepsis.[27]

Although the definitive diagnosis of septicemia requires positive blood culture results, infants with highly suspicious signs should be started on an appropriate empiric antibiotic regimen until culture results are available. Classic empiric antibiotic approaches include ampicillin, gentamicin, third-generation or fourth-generation cephalosporins, and antiviral agents. In the case of meningitis with seizures, examination of the cerebrospinal fluid (CSF) via lumbar puncture is indicated but should not delay antibiotic therapy and should probably also not delay transport. For these patients empiric ceftriaxone is usually added to the sepsis regimen.

Patients with severe sepsis or shock will require hemodynamic support with isotonic IV fluids and, as indicated, vasopressors and hydrocortisone.

Neurologic Disorders

Hypoxic-Ischemic Encephalopathy

Brain injuries that are caused by hypoxic ischemia can cause neonatal encephalopathy, which carries risks for significant mortality and long-term morbidity. The mechanism of hypoxic injury can be maternal impaired oxygenation, insufficient placental perfusion, or intrapartum events that impair fetal oxygenation such as cord prolapse, uterine rupture, difficult extraction, or nuchal cord.

Targeted temperature management (TTM) with induced hypothermia is an effective therapy that improves neurologic outcomes in late preterm and term babies (≥36 weeks) with moderate to severe hypoxic-ischemic encephalopathy (HIE). The TTM involves lowering the infant's body temperature to slow biological processes, decreasing disease progression. A meta-analysis of six large published clinical trials showed a number needed to treat (NNT) is six babies with moderate HIE to prevent one death or disability, and seven babies with severe HIE to prevent one death or disability.[98–100] In comparison, the NNT for the benefit of aspirin for patients with ST-elevation myocardial infarction is 42 patients.[101]

Current inclusion criteria require a highly specific age, an indicator of birth hypoxia, and an indicator of neurologic effect:
1. Chronologic
   - Gestational age of 36 weeks or more
   AND
   - 6 or fewer hours of life
2. Perinatal depression
   - Indicator of birth hypoxia: Apgar score of less than 5 at 10 minutes of age
   OR
   - pH less than 7.0, or base deficit greater than or equal to 16 mmol/L in an umbilical cord blood sample or any blood sample within the first hour of birth
   OR
- Need for PPV at 10 minutes of life
3. Abnormal neurologic examination
   - Seizures
   OR
   - Abnormality in three of these categories
     - Spontaneous activity
     - Posture
     - Autonomic nervous system
     - Tone
     - Primitive reflexes
     - Level of consciousness
   OR
   - Moderate (Sarnat stage II) to severe (Sarnat stage III) encephalopathy[98,99]

The Thompson HIE score is a tool used to categorize symptoms into mild, moderate, or severe. The score ranges from 0 to 22. 0 being no symptoms and 22 being most severe. There are nine symptom categories: tone (normal, hyper, hypo, or flaccid), level of consciousness (normal, hyper alert, or lethargic), fits (normal, infrequent, or frequent), posture (normal, fisting/cycling, strong

distal flexion, or decerebrate), Moro reflex (normal, partial, or absent), grasp (normal, poor, or absent), sucking reflex (normal, poor, or absent), respiration (normal, hyperventilation, brief apnea, or apneic), fontanelle (normal, not full tense, or tense). Scores 0–10 are considered mild HIE, scores 11–14 are moderate HIE, and greater than or equal to 15 are considered severe HIE.[102]

The majority of large clinical trials have administered cooling by two methods: whole-body cooling and selective head cooling. There is limited research comparing the two methods, and no clarity demonstrating that either is safer or more effective.[103,104] Similarly, the optimal target temperature for cooling has not been determined. Most study protocols have maintained a temperature between 33.0°C and 35.0°C for 3 days.[99] It is clear that longer and deeper cooling do not improve outcomes.[105]

In the transport setting, both active and passive cooling can be used effectively. Active cooling in transport may increase the risk that babies will arrive with nontherapeutic hypothermia. Servo-controlled devices improve the effectiveness and safety of active cooling in transport.[106–109] Care must also be taken to prevent hyperthermia, which is associated with an increased risk of death and disability.[110] Monitor BP, HR, and capillary refill, and provide appropriate support of vital signs. As the metabolic rate decreases, so does the HR, so hypothermia does often cause a relative bradycardia that is well tolerated. Monitor electrolytes, especially blood glucose, and coagulation labs during active cooling.

Head Ultrasound

A minimally invasive and nonradiographic option for inspection of neonatal neurologic disorders is the head ultrasound (US). With open fontanelles, multiple views of the brain are possible and can lead to diagnosis of hemorrhage, edema, and identification of masses. Many neonatal intensive care institutions require a head ultrasound prior to discharge of VLBW and ELBW infants due to the high risk for germinal matrix injury in the underdeveloped brain.

Obviously in symptomatic neonates (e.g., dropping hematocrit, seizures) or in neonates with abnormal fetal examinations, a head ultrasound should be performed as soon as possible. Magnetic resonance imaging is the imaging modality of choice for hypoxic ischemic encephalopathy in the acute phase, but US even with its lower sensitivity for the detection of early ischemic changes is an important triaging tool.[111]

Intraventricular Hemorrhage

IVH can be graded four ways. Grade I is the least significant, where bleeding is only present in the lining of the ventricles. Grade II includes bleeding in the ventricles with no enlargement or swellings. Grade III is bleeding that has filled the ventricles with enlargement. Grade IV is bleeding that has filled the ventricles and has overflowed into surrounding brain tissue. As mentioned previously in this chapter, ELBW infants are at considerable risk for IVH with transport alone.[25.] Precautions should be taken to limit IV infusion rates, hypoglycemia, hypothermia, maintain neutral head positioning, and practice due diligence to minimize stimulation of the ELBW infant to avoid IVH.

Neural Tube Defects

Neural tube defects (NTDs) are birth defects of the brain, spine, or spinal cord and are the most common congenital central nervous system (CNS) structural anomaly.[112] Failure of development of the neural tube early in gestation may result in a number of defects including anencephaly, encephalocele, meningocele, and myelomeningocele.

Open defects are more common and have exposed neural tissue with associated leakage of CSF. Myelomeningocele is the most common NTD. Patients with myelomeningoceles are at high risk for the subsequent development of a latex allergy, so all medical supplies used in caring for these patients should be latex free.[113] Assess the location, size and whether the defect is leaking CSF. An initial evaluation of spontaneous activity, muscle weakness or paralysis, and anal wink should be noted. The infant should be positioned off the defect during transport. If feasible, prone positioning may be necessary. Infection is a significant concern, so the defect should be covered by a sterile saline-soaked dressing and then covered with plastic wrap to prevent heat loss. Consider antibiotic prophylaxis.

Closed defects are usually on the spine, and neural tissue is not exposed. It is not uncommon to be able to see the abnormality along the spine, which can present as a fluid-filled mass, a tuft of hair at the base of the spinal cord, an area of skin discoloration, or a lesion covered by skin without visible neural tissue. As noted with open lesions, an evaluation of spontaneous activity, muscle weakness, paralysis, and anal wink should be noted on assessment before transport.

Seizures

Seizures commonly occur in ill newborns and are often the first sign of a CNS disorder. There are many etiologies of neonatal seizures. The most frequently occurring are neonatal encephalopathy, intracranial hemorrhage, infection, metabolic disturbances, congenital abnormalities of the brain, and drug withdrawal.[114] Because of the immature nervous system of the newborn, infants rarely exhibit the generalized tonic–clonic seizures seen in adults and older children. Seizures in the newborn can be divided into four categories:

1. *Subtle*: These are frequently overlooked by caretakers. This type may consist of repetitive mouth or tongue movement, bicycling movements, eye deviation, repetitive blinking, staring, or apnea.
2. *Clonic (multifocal or focal)*: These are typically characterized by slow, repetitive, rhythmic contractions of the limbs, face or trunk.
3. *Tonic (generalized or focal)*: These may resemble posturing seen in older infants and children and may be accompanied by disturbed respiratory patterns. This type may also include tonic extension of limbs or tonic flexion of upper limbs and extension of lower limbs.
4. *Myoclonic*: These are characterized by multiple jerking motions of the upper (common) or lower (rare) extremities.

Seizure activity is frequently confused with jitteriness in the newborn. Jitteriness may be distinguished from seizures in the following ways:

- Sensitive to stimulus, whereas seizures are not.
- Characterized by tremors rather than the slow and fast phases of seizure activity.
- Can normally be stopped with flexing of the limb, as opposed to seizures, which do not respond to this maneuver.

In treatment of neonatal seizures, identification of the cause is important because it may prevent further injury. The obstetric and neonatal history may reveal risk factors for seizure disorders. Physical examination should be performed, along with laboratory studies including glucose, calcium, magnesium, sodium, blood gas, and in suspected infection, blood cultures. There is no consensus regarding an optimal treatment strategy, and there is limited helpful literature. Phenobarbital is the most commonly used initial antiepileptic agent in neonates, followed by either repeat doses of phenobarbital or second-line agents such as phenytoin, fosphenytoin, levetiracetam, or a benzodiazepine.[115,116]

There is debate regarding the safety of benzodiazepines in preterm neonates due to potential for continued and/or increased seizures. Benzodiazepines should be avoided for gestational age less than 35 weeks. If considering administration in less than 35 weeks' gestation, a multidisciplinary team consult is suggested. Serious side effects of these drugs may include respiratory or cardiovascular depression.

Head Trauma

There are three distinct extracranial hemorrhages involved with the birthing process. These are typically present after a vacuum-assisted birth. Caput succedaneum and cephalohematoma are mostly benign and will require only observation. However, subgaleal hemorrhage is bleed in the galea aponeurotica of the scalp that can be fatal if left unrecognized. Assessment and treatment include monitoring head circumference, serial lab data, and blood product transfusion.

Developmental Care

It is important to incorporate developmental care interventions while transporting these small patients to decrease the risk of neurodevelopmental complications. Transport teams can consider the use of a gel-filled mattress to decrease the effects of vibration on infants and nesting the infant with rolls or gel donuts serves to reduce stress by providing containment, positioning, and comfort.[25,117] Infants are exposed to excessive noise in the transport environment, which can create negative physiologic responses such as increased heart and respiratory rates and decreased oxygen saturation. Transport teams should consider interventions that decrease the noise levels. The use of earmuffs is associated with a reduction in noise level and adverse neonatal outcomes.[118,119] Eye protection/coverings are indicated in ELBW/VLBW infants or infants receiving phototherapy during transport.

Equipment

The transport of the neonate requires a skilled team and proper equipment. Medical equipment used in air medical operations should be electromagnetic interference–approved for flight.[120,121] If a team engages in multiple simultaneous transports, a full set of functioning equipment and appropriate caregiver skill mix is necessary for each neonate that is transported. The transport team should use safety and best industry practice for securing neonatal patients and also for securing themselves and their equipment.

Credentialling for Advanced Procedures

Neonatal transport professionals should be trained, proficient, and credentialed in advanced procedures to minimize mortality during transport. These procedures vary between institutions; however, some examples include:

- Endotracheal intubation
- Needle chest decompression
- Tube thoracostomy
- Surfactant administration
- Inhaled nitric oxide
- IV/IO insertion
- UVC/UAC insertion
- PICC insertion
- Blood product transfusion
- Servo-controlled active cooling

Summary

Medical transport providers caring for neonates in any out-of-hospital environment must have training in the stabilization and care of the types of infants they may transport.[122] Attention to appropriate team composition and the availability of specialized equipment and medications is necessary to ensure safe transport of these patients. Competency in neonatal care, protocols, and procedures is essential to neonatal transport care.

References

1. Kugelman A, Colin AA. Late preterm infants: near term but still in a critical developmental time period. *Pediatrics.* 2013;132(4):741–751.
2. Orr RA, Felmet KA, Han Y, et al. Pediatric specialized transport teams are associated with improved outcomes. *Pediatrics.* 2009; 124(1):40–48.
3. Commission on Accreditation of Medical Transport Systems. *10th Edition Accreditation Standards.* Sandy Spring, SC: CAMTS; 2015.
4. American Academy of Pediatrics. *Guidelines for Air and Ground Transport of Neonatal and Pediatric Patients.* 4th ed. Elk Grove Village, IL: American Academy of Pediatrics; 2015.
5. Weiner GM, Zaichkin JG. *Textbook of Neonatal Resuscitation.* 8th ed. Elk Grove Village, IL: American Academy of Pediatrics; 2021: xiii, 313.
6. Apgar V, Holaday DA, James LS, et al. Evaluation of the newborn infant; second report. *J Am Med Assoc.* 1958;168(15):1985–1988.
7. Apgar V. A proposal for a new method of evaluation of the newborn infant. *Curr Res Anest Anal.* 1953;32(4):260–267.
8. Mullany LC. Neonatal hypothermia in low-resource settings. *Semin Perinatol.* 2010;34(6):426-433.
9. Wyckoff MH, Aziz K, Escobedo MB, et al. Part 13: Neonatal Resuscitation: 2015 American Heart Association guidelines update for cardiopulmonary resuscitation and emergency cardiovascular care. *Circulation.* 2015;132(18 suppl 2):S543–S560.
10. Al Takroni AM, Parvathi CK, Mendis KB, Hassan S, Reddy I, Kudair HA. Selective tracheal suctioning to prevent meconium aspiration syndrome. *Int J Gynaecol Obstet.* 1998;63(3):259–263.
11. Morley CJ, Davis PG, Doyle LW, et al. Nasal CPAP or intubation at birth for very preterm infants. *N Engl J Med.* 2008;358(7):700–708.
12. SUPPORT Study Group of the Eunice Kennedy Shriver NICHD Neonatal Research Network, et al. Early CPAP versus surfactant in extremely preterm infants. *N Engl J Med.* 2010;362(21):1970–1979.
13. Dawes GS. *Foetal and Neonatal Physiology; A Comparative Study of the Changes at Birth.* Chicago, IL: Year Book Medical Publishers; 1968.
14. Peterson J, Johnson N, Deakins K, Wilson-Costello D, Jelovsek JE, Chatburn R. Accuracy of the 7-8-9 Rule for endotracheal tube placement in the neonate. *J Perinatol.* 2006;26(6):333–336.
15. Garey DM, Ward R, Ric W, Heldt G, Leone T, Finer NN. Tidal volume threshold for colorimetric carbon dioxide detectors available for use in neonates. *Pediatrics.* 2008;121(6):e1524–e1527.
16. Finn D, Boylan GB, Ryan CA, Dempsey EM. Enhanced monitoring of the preterm infant during stabilization in the delivery room. *Front Pediatr.* 2016;4:73.
17. Whitelaw CC, Slywka B, Goldsmith LJ. Comparison of a two-finger versus two-thumb method for chest compressions by healthcare providers in an infant mechanical model. *Resuscitation.* 2000;43(3):213–216.
18. Wyllie J, Perlman JM, Kattwonkel J, et al. Part 11: Neonatal resuscitation: 2010 International Consensus on Cardiopulmonary Resuscitation and Emergency Cardiovascular Care Science with Treatment Recommendations. *Resuscitation.* 2011;81(1):e260–e287.
19. Iliodromiti S, Mackay DF, Smith GC, Pell JP, Nelson SM. Apgar score and the risk of cause-specific infant mortality: a population-based cohort study. *Lancet.* 2014;384(9956):1749–1755.
20. Freeman JM, Nelson KB. Intrapartum asphyxia and cerebral palsy. *Pediatrics.* 1988;82(2):240–249.
21. Watterberg KL, Aucott S, Benitz WE, et al. The Apgar score. *Pediatrics.* 2015;136(4):819–822.
22. Executive summary: Neonatal encephalopathy and neurologic outcome, second edition. Report of the American College of Obstetricians and Gynecologists' Task Force on Neonatal Encephalopathy. *Obstet Gynecol.* 2014;123(4):896–901.
23. Mohamed MA, Aly H. Transport of premature infants is associated with increased risk for intraventricular haemorrhage. *Arch Dis Child Fetal Neonatal Ed.* 2010;95(6):F403–F407.
24. Schmid MB, Reister F, Mayer B, et al. Prospective risk factor monitoring reduces intracranial hemorrhage rates in preterm infants. *Dtsch Arztebl Int.* 2013;110(29–30):489–496.
25. Malusky S, Donze A. Neutral head positioning in premature infants for intraventricular hemorrhage prevention: an evidence-based review. *Neonatal Netw.* 2011;30(6):381–396.
26. Rysavy MA, Li L, Bell EF, et al. Between-hospital variation in treatment and outcomes in extremely preterm infants. *N Engl J Med.* 2015;372(19):1801–1811.
27. Karlsen K. *Learner Manual. The S.T.A.B.L.E. Program. Post-Resuscitation/Pre-Transport Stabilization Care of Sick Infants: Guidelines for Neonatal Healthcare Providers.* 6th ed. Park City, UT: S.T.A.B.L.E; 2013.
28. Committee on Fetus and Newborn, Adamkin DH. Postnatal glucose homeostasis in late-preterm and term infants. *Pediatrics.* 2011;127(3):575–579.
29. Brownell E, Howard CR, Lawrence RA, Dozier AM. Delayed onset lactogenesis II predicts the cessation of any or exclusive breastfeeding. *J Pediatr.* 2012;161(4):608–614.
30. Mathur NB, Krishnamurthy S, Mishra TK. Evaluation of WHO classification of hypothermia in sick extramural neonates as predictor of fatality. *J Trop Pediatr.* 2005;51(6):341–345.
31. Rutter N. Temperature control and its disorders. In: Rennie JM, ed. *Robertsons Textbook of Neonatology* (pp. 267–279). London: Churchill Livingstone; 2005.
32. Knobel RB. Thermal stability of the premature infant in neonatal intensive care. *Newborn Infant Nurs Rev.* 2014;14(2):72–76.
33. Gardner SL, Carter BS, Enzman-Hines MI, Niermeyer S. *Merenstein & Gardner's Handbook of Neonatal Intensive Care.* Philadelphia, PA: Elsevier Health Sciences; 2015.
34. Mariani G, Dik PB, Ezquer A, et al. Pre-ductal and post-ductal O_2 saturation in healthy term neonates after birth. *J Pediatr.* 2007; 150(4):418–421.
35. Manja V, Lakshminrusimha S, Cook DJ. Oxygen saturation target range for extremely preterm infants: a systematic review and meta-analysis. *JAMA Pediatr.* 2015;169(4):332–340.
36. Castillo A, Sola A, Baquero H, et al. Pulse oxygen saturation levels and arterial oxygen tension values in newborns receiving oxygen therapy in the neonatal intensive care unit: is 85% to 93% an acceptable range? *Pediatrics.* 2008;121(5):882–889.
37. Wilkinson D, Andersen C, O'Donnell CP, De Paoli AG, Manley BJ. High flow nasal cannula for respiratory support in preterm infants. *Cochrane Database Syst Rev.* 2016;2:CD006405.
38. Papile L-A, Ambalavanan N, Carlo WA, et al. Respiratory support in preterm infants at birth. *Pediatrics.* 2014;133(1):171–174.
39. Dunn MS, Kaempf J, de Klerk A, et al. Randomized trial comparing 3 approaches to the initial respiratory management of preterm neonates. *Pediatrics.* 2011;128(5):e1069--e1076.
40. Shoemaker MT, Pierce MR, Yoder BA, DiGeronimo RJ. High flow nasal cannula versus nasal CPAP for neonatal respiratory disease: a retrospective study. *J Perinatol.* 2007;27(2):85–91.

41. Sakonidou S, Dhaliwal J. The management of neonatal respiratory distress syndrome in preterm infants (European Consensus Guidelines–2013 update). *Arch Dis Child Educ Pract Ed.* 2015;100(5):257–259.

42. Lavizzari A, Colnaghi M, Ciuffini F, et al. Heated, humidified high-flow nasal cannula vs nasal continuous positive airway pressure for respiratory distress syndrome of prematurity: a randomized clinical noninferiority trial. *JAMA Pediatr.* 2016, Aug 8. doi: 0.1001/jamapediatrics.2016.1243.

43. Lemyre B, Davis PG, De Paoli AG, Kirpalani H. Nasal intermittent positive pressure ventilation (NIPPV) versus nasal continuous positive airway pressure (NCPAP) for preterm neonates after extubation. *Cochrane Database Syst Rev.* 2014;(9):CD003212.

44. Cummings JJ, Polin RA. Noninvasive respiratory support. *Pediatrics.* 2016;137(1):e20153758.

45. Ozawa Y, Ades A, Foglia EE, et al. Premedication with neuromuscular blockade and sedation during neonatal intubation is associated with fewer adverse events. *J Perinatol.* 2019;39:848–856.

46. Klingenberg C, Wheeler KI, Davis PG, Morley CJ. A practical guide to neonatal volume guarantee ventilation. *J Perinatol.* 2011;31(9):575–585.

47. Al Ethawi Y. Volume-targeted versus pressure-limited ventilation for preterm infants: a systematic review and meta-analysis. *J Clin Neonatol.* 2012;1(1):18–20.

48. Wheeler K, Klingenberg C, McCallion N, Morley CJ, Davis PG. Volume-targeted versus pressure-limited ventilation in the neonate. *Cochrane Database Syst Rev.* 2010;11:CD003666.

49. Kinsella JP, Truog WE, Walsh WF, et al. Randomized, multicenter trial of inhaled nitric oxide and high-frequency oscillatory ventilation in severe, persistent pulmonary hypertension of the newborn. *J Pediatr.* 1997;131(1 Pt 1):55–62.

50. Datin-Dorriere V, Walter-Nicolet E, Rousseau V, et al. Experience in the management of eighty-two newborns with congenital diaphragmatic hernia treated with high-frequency oscillatory ventilation and delayed surgery without the use of extracorporeal membrane oxygenation. *J Intensive Care Med.* 2008;23(2):128–135.

51. Honey G, Bleak T, Karp T, MacRitchie A, Null Jr D. Use of the Duotron transporter high frequency ventilator during neonatal transport. *Neonatal Netw.* 2007;26(3):167–174.

52. Kleinman ME, Chameides L, Schexnayder SM, et al. Part 14: pediatric advanced life support: 2010 American Heart Association Guidelines for Cardiopulmonary Resuscitation and Emergency Cardiovascular Care. *Circulation.* 2010;122(18 Suppl 3):S876–S908.

53. Dempsey EM, Barrington KJ. Evaluation and treatment of hypotension in the preterm infant. *Clin Perinatol.* 2009;36(1):75–85.

54. Ng PC, Lee CH, Bnur FL, et al. A double-blind, randomized, controlled study of a "stress dose" of hydrocortisone for rescue treatment of refractory hypotension in preterm infants. *Pediatrics.* 2006;117(2):367–375.

55. Caresta E, Papoff P, Valentini SB, et al. What's new in the treatment of neonatal shock. *J Matern Fetal Neonatal Med.* 2011;(24 suppl 1):17–19.

56. Schmaltz C. Hypotension and shock in the preterm neonate. *Adv Neonatal Care.* 2009;9(4):156–162.

57. Seri I, Markovitz B. Cardiovascular compromise in the newborn infant. In: Gleason CA, Devaskar SU, eds. *Avery's Diseases of the Newborn.* Philadelphia: Elsevier Saunders; 2012:714–731.

58. Ruoss JL, McPherson C, DiNardo J. Inotrope and vasopressor support in neonates. *NeoReviews.* 2015;16(6):e351–e361.

59. Bahadue FL, Soll R. Early versus delayed selective surfactant treatment for neonatal respiratory distress syndrome. *Cochrane Database Syst Rev.* 2012;11:CD001456.

60. Engle WA, American Academy of Pediatrics Committee on Fetus and Newborn. Surfactant-replacement therapy for respiratory distress in the preterm and term neonate. *Pediatrics.* 2008;121(2):419–432.

61. Committee on Fetus and Newborn, American Academy of Pediatrics. Respiratory support in preterm infants at birth. *Pediatrics.* 2014;133(1):171–174.

62. Lee J, Romero R, Lee KA, et al. Meconium aspiration syndrome: a role for fetal systemic inflammation. *Am J Obstet Gynecol.* 2016; 214(3):366.e1–e9.

63. Jeng M-J, Lee Y-S, Tsao P-C, et al. Neonatal air leak syndrome and the role of high-frequency ventilation in its prevention. *J Chin Med Assoc.* 2012;75(11):551–559.

64. Ho JJ, Subramaniam P, Davis PG. Continuous distending pressure for respiratory distress in preterm infants. *Cochrane Database Syst Rev.* 2015;7:CD002271.

65. Warren JB, Anderson JM. Newborn respiratory disorders. *Pediatr Rev.* 2010;31(12):487–496.

66. Steinhorn RH. Neonatal pulmonary hypertension. *Pediatr Crit Care Med.* 2010;11(Suppl 2):S79–S84.

67. Stark AR, Eichenwald ED. Persistent pulmonary hypertension of the newborn. Waltham, MA: UpToDate; 2016.

68. Atz AM, Adatia I, Lock JE, Wessel DL. Combined effects of nitric oxide and oxygen during acute pulmonary vasodilator testing. *J Am Coll Cardiol.* 1999;33(3):813–819.

69. Finer NN, Barrington KJ. Nitric oxide for respiratory failure in infants born at or near term. *Cochrane Database Syst Rev.* 2006;4: CD000399.

70. Ichinose F, Roberts Jr JD, Zapol WM. Inhaled nitric oxide: a selective pulmonary vasodilator: current uses and therapeutic potential. *Circulation.* 2004;109(25):3106–3111.

71. Peliowski A, Canadian Paediatric Society, Fetus and Newborn Committee. Inhaled nitric oxide use in newborns. *Paediatr Child Health.* 2012;17(2):95–100.

72. Kumar P; Committee on Fetus and Newborn; American Academy of Pediatrics. Use of inhaled nitric oxide in preterm infants. *Pediatrics.* 2014;133(1):164–170.

73. Nair J, Lakshminrusimha S. Update on PPHN: mechanisms and treatment. *Semin Perinatol.* 2014;38(2):78–91.

74. Lotze A, Mitchell BR, Bulas DI, et al. Multicenter study of surfactant (beractant) use in the treatment of term infants with severe respiratory failure. Survanta in Term Infants Study Group. *J Pediatr.* 1998;132(1):40–47.

75. Chapman RL, Peterec SM, Bizzarro MJ, Mercurio MR. Patient selection for neonatal extracorporeal membrane oxygenation: beyond severity of illness. *J Perinatol.* 2009;29(9):606–611.

76. Extracorporeal Life Support Organization. *Guidelines for Neonatal Respiratory Failure: Supplement to the ELSO General Guidelines.* *Extracorporeal Life Support Organization.* Ann Arbor, MI: Extracorporeal Life Support Organization; 2013.

77. Carriedo H, Deming D. Therapeutic techniques: neonatal ECMO. *NeoReviews.* 2003;4(8):e212–e214.

78. Stocker CF, Horton SB. Anticoagulation strategies and difficulties in neonatal and paediatric extracorporeal membrane oxygenation (ECMO). *Perfusion.* 2016;31(2):95–102.

79. DeKoninck P, Gomez O, Sandaite I, et al. Right-sided congenital diaphragmatic hernia in a decade of fetal surgery. *BJOG.* 2015; 122(7):940–946.

80. Doné E, Guccisrdo L, Van Miegham T, et al. Prenatal diagnosis, prediction of outcome and in utero therapy of isolated congenital diaphragmatic hernia. *Prenat Diagn.* 2008;28(7):581–591.

81. Campbell BT, Herbst KW, Briden KE, Neff S, Ruscher KA, Hagadorn JI. Inhaled nitric oxide use in neonates with congenital diaphragmatic hernia. *Pediatrics.* 2014;134(2):e420–e426.

82. Puligandla PS, Grabowski J, Austin M, et al. Management of congenital diaphragmatic hernia: a systematic review from the APSA outcomes and evidence based practice committee. *J Pediatr Surg.* 2015;50(11):1958–1970.

83. Mohseni-Bod H, Bohn D. Pulmonary hypertension in congenital diaphragmatic hernia. *Semin Pediatr Surg.* 2007;16(2):126–133.

84. Mai CT, Riehle-Colarusso T, O'Halloran A, et al. Selected birth defects data from population-based birth defects surveillance programs in the United States, 2005–2009: featuring critical congenital heart defects targeted for pulse oximetry screening. *Birth Defects Res A Clin Mol Teratol.* 2012;94(12):970–983.

85. Karlsen KA, Tani LY. S.T.A.B.L.E Cardiac Module: Recognition and stabilization of neonates with severe CHD. Salt Lake City, UT: S.T.A.B.L.E; 2003.

86. Donofrio MT, Moon_Grady AJ, Hornberger LK, et al. Diagnosis and treatment of fetal cardiac disease: a scientific statement from the American Heart Association. *Circulation.* 2014;129(21):2183–2242.

87. Huang F-K, Lin C-C, Huang T-C, et al. Reappraisal of the prostaglandin E1 dose for early newborns with patent ductus arteriosus-dependent pulmonary circulation. *Pediatr Neonatol.* 2012;54(2):102–106.

88. Yucel IK, Cevik A, Bulut MO, et al. Efficacy of very low-dose prostaglandin E1 in duct-dependent congenital heart disease. *Cardiol Young.* 2015;25(1):56–62.

89. Scott DA, et al. Esophageal atresia/tracheoesophageal fistula overview. In: Pagon RA, eds. *GeneReviews.* Seattle, WA: University of Washington, Seattle; 2014.

90. Achildi O, Grewal H. Congenital anomalies of the esophagus. *Otolaryngol Clin North Am.* 2007;40(1):219–244.

91. Shaw-Smith C. Oesophageal atresia, tracheo-oesophageal fistula, and the VACTERL association: review of genetics and epidemiology. *J Med Genet.* 2006;43(7):545–554.

92. Pinheiro PF, Simoes e Silva AC, Pereira RM. Current knowledge on esophageal atresia. *World J Gastroenterol.* 2012;18(28):3662–3672.

93. Gephart SM, McGrath JM, Effken Jam Halpern M. Necrotizing enterocolitis risk: state of the science. *Adv Neonatal Care.* 2012;12(2):77–89.

94. Henrich K, Huemmer HP, Reingruber B, Weber PG. Gastroschisis and omphalocele: treatments and long-term outcomes. *Pediatr Surg Int.* 2008;24(2):167–173.

95. Arnold MA, Chang DC, Nabaweesi R, et al. Risk stratification of 4344 patients with gastroschisis into simple and complex categories. *J Pediatr Surg.* 2007;42(9):1520–1525.

96. Sass L. Group B streptococcal infections. *Pediatr Rev.* 2012;33(5):219–225.

97. Cohen-Wolkowiez M, Moran C, Benjamin DK, et al. Early and late onset sepsis in late preterm infants. *Pediatr Infect Dis J.* 2009;28(12):1052–1056.

98. Committee on Fetus and Newborn, Papile LA, Baley JE, et al. Hypothermia and neonatal encephalopathy. *Pediatrics.* 2014;133(6):1146–1150.

99. Tagin MA, et al. Hypothermia for neonatal hypoxic ischemic encephalopathy: an updated systematic review and meta-analysis. *Arch Pediatr Adolesc Med.* 2012;166(6):558–566.

100. Jacobs S, Hunt R, Tarnow-Mordi W, Inder T, Davis P. Cooling for newborns with hypoxic ischaemic encephalopathy. *Cochrane Database Syst Rev.* 2013;1:CD003311.

101. Randomised trial of intravenous streptokinase, oral aspirin, both, or neither among 17,187 cases of suspected acute myocardial infarction: ISIS-2. ISIS-2 (Second International Study of Infarct Survival) Collaborative Group. *Lancet.* 1988;2(8607):349–360.

102. Thompson CM, Puterman AS, Linley LL, et al. The value of a scoring system for hypoxic ischaemic encephalopathy in predicting neurodevelopmental outcome. *Acta Paediatr.* 1997;86(7):757–761.

103. Allen KA. Moderate hypothermia: is selective head cooling or whole body cooling better? *Adv Neonatal Care.* 2014;14(2):113–118.

104. Atici A, Celik Y, Gulasi S, et al. Comparison of selective head cooling therapy and whole body cooling therapy in newborns with hypoxic ischemic encephalopathy: short term results. *Turk Arch Pediatr.* 2015;50(1):27–36.

105. Shankaran S, Laptook AR, Pappas A, et al. Effect of depth and duration of cooling on deaths in the NICU among neonates with hypoxic ischemic encephalopathy: a randomized clinical trial. *JAMA.* 2014;312(24):2629–2639.

106. Fairchild K, Sokora D, Scott J, Zanelli S, et al. Therapeutic hypothermia on neonatal transport: 4-year experience in a single NICU. *J Perinatol.* 2010;30(5):324–329.

107. Sharma A. Provision of therapeutic hypothermia in neonatal transport: a longitudinal study and review of literature. *Cureus.* 2015;7(5):e270.

108. Chaudhary R, Farrer K, Broster S, McRitchie L, Austin T. Active versus passive cooling during neonatal transport. *Pediatrics.* 2013;132(5):841–846.

109. Akula VP, Joe P, Thusu K, et al. A randomized clinical trial of therapeutic hypothermia mode during transport for neonatal encephalopathy. *J Pediatr.* 2015;166(4):856–861.e1–e2.

110. Laptook A, Tyson J, Shankaran S, et al. Elevated temperature after hypoxic-ischemic encephalopathy: risk factor for adverse outcomes. *Pediatrics.* 2008;122(3):491–499.

111. Maller VV, Cohen HL. Neonatal head ultrasound: a review and update—Part 1: Techniques and evaluation of the premature neonate. *Ultrasound Quarterly.* 2019;35(3):202–211.

112. Parker SE, Mai CT, Canfield MA, et al. Updated National Birth Prevalence estimates for selected birth defects in the United States, 2004–2006. *Birth Defects Res A Clin Mol Teratol.* 2010;88(12):1008–1016.

113. Rendeli C, Nucera E, Ausili E, et al. Latex sensitisation and allergy in children with myelomeningocele. *Childs Nerv Syst.* 2006;22(1):28–32.

114. Silverstein FS, Jensen FE. Neonatal seizures. *Ann Neurol.* 2007;62(2):112–120.

115. Slaughter LA, Patel AD, Slaughter JL. Pharmacological treatment of neonatal seizures: a systematic review. *J Child Neurol.* 2013;28(3):351–364.

116. Hellstrom-Westas L, Boylan G, Agren J. Systematic review of neonatal seizure management strategies provides guidance on antiepileptic treatment. *Acta Paediatr.* 2015;104(2):123–129.

117. Prehn J, McEwen I, Jeffries L, et al. Decreasing sound and vibration during ground transport of infants with very low birth weight. *J Perinatol.* 2015;35(2):110–114.

118. Zahr LK, de Traversay J. Premature infant responses to noise reduction by earmuffs: effects on behavioral and physiologic measures. *J Perinatol.* 1995;15(6):448-455.

119. Duran R, Ciftdemir NA, Ozbek UV, et al. The effects of noise reduction by earmuffs on the physiologic and behavioral responses in very low birth weight preterm infants. *Int J Pediatr Otorhinolaryngol.* 2012;76(10):1490–1493.

120. Bruckart JE, Licina JR, Quattlebaum M. Laboratory and flight tests of medical equipment for use in U.S. Army Medevac helicopters. *Air Med J.* 1993;1(3):51–56.

121. Nish WA, Walsh WF, Land P, Swedenburg M. Effect of electromagnetic interference by neonatal transport equipment on aircraft operation. *Aviat Space Environ Med.* 1989;60(6):599–600.

122. Cross B, Wilson D. High-fidelity simulation for transport team training and competency evaluation. *Newborn Infant Nurs Rev.* 2009;9(4):200–206.

18

Care and Transport of the Pediatric Patient

SHELLIE A. BRANDT

COMPETENCIES

1. List common pediatric medical conditions and unique challenges associated with air medical transport for pediatric patients.
2. Apply age-appropriate assessment techniques and interventions for pediatric patients involved in air medical transport.
3. Create a comprehensive plan of care for a critically ill or injured pediatric patient requiring air medical transport.

Introduction

Pediatric patients have unique considerations and challenges in air medical transport. As healthcare professionals entrusted with the welfare of children during critical moments, it is paramount that we possess a specialized understanding of their distinct physiologic and psychologic needs. In this chapter, we embark on a journey to explore the intricacies of pediatric medical transport, equipping you with the knowledge and skills necessary to provide optimal care and support to this vulnerable population. From neonates to adolescents, we will navigate the nuances of assessment, treatment, and communication, ensuring that each young patient receives the highest standard of care during their journey on ambulances or aircraft. Caring for pediatric patients in transport situations can provoke anxiety. It can be stressful for the patient and family, but also for the transport crew. Intra-hospital transport teams have the advantage of knowing the approximate age and weight of their patients prior to patient contact. This allows for quick preparation of medication with the use of pediatric medication apps and reference guides created by children's hospitals in the United States.[1,2]

A Developmental Approach to Pediatric Assessment

Approaching pediatric assessment from the perspective of nurses and paramedics who care for patients in the air or ambulances underscores the critical importance of adaptability and specialized knowledge in pediatric transport. When working in these high-stress, time-sensitive environments, healthcare providers must be equipped with a keen understanding of pediatric development.

For nurses and paramedics involved in air or ambulance transport, a developmental approach to pediatric assessment serves as the foundation for safe and effective care. It allows them to recognize that infants, toddlers, school-age children, and adolescents have distinct physiologic and psychologic needs, which can significantly impact their responses to illness or injury. When assessing a pediatric patient during transport, professionals must consider age-appropriate vital signs, communication techniques, and comfort measures. For example, ensuring proper restraint systems for transport vehicles or pediatric-sized equipment is crucial for safe transportation. Moreover, recognizing that children may experience anxiety or fear during transport, healthcare providers can employ age-appropriate distraction techniques or offer emotional support to ease the child's distress. This approach not only enhances the quality of care provided but also contributes to the overall well-being of the pediatric patient during a critical and potentially frightening experience.

Pediatric Resuscitation

Resuscitation of the pediatric patient requires that the transport crew is aware of several differences between pediatric and adult patients. The pediatric patient can compensate until approximately 30% of their total blood volume has been lost. Pediatric patients compensate well but once they develop uncompensated shock as evidenced by hypotension, the mortality rate drastically increases.[3] Uncompensated shock in a pediatric patient is a critical medical emergency where the body's compensatory mechanisms have failed to maintain adequate blood flow and tissue perfusion. Recognizing the signs of uncompensated shock in pediatric patients is crucial for prompt intervention. According to Leeper, McKenna, and Gaines, 46% of pediatric patients who develop hypotension will not survive.[4] It is vital that those providing care for pediatric patients are vigilant for other signs and symptoms that indicate that they are critically injured, for instance, tachycardia and tachypnea, which may indicate that the patient is compensating to perfuse their vital organs.[4] Consideration when transfusing a pediatric patient involves the balance of the risks related to lung injury and circulatory overload that may occur as a result.[5] These factors are not typically associated with adult patients because their more developed physiologic systems can better tolerate blood transfusions and substantial intravenous fluid volumes. Experts in the pediatric field came together as part of the Pediatric Critical Care Transfusion and Anemia Expertise Initiative (TAXI) and formulated recommendations to help guide the transfusion process in critically ill pediatric patients.[5] As a result of this collaboration, it became clear that the decision to transfuse should not be taken lightly and not based solely upon the patient's hemoglobin level: evaluation of other signs and symptoms, risks, and benefits or an alternative to transfusion must be considered as well. While there is relatively less research on the use of tranexamic acid in the pediatric population, it could serve as a potential option to mitigate blood loss. However, experts concur that further research is necessary to fully understand its efficacy and safety in pediatric patients.[6]

Resuscitation of the pediatric patient requires that transport team members have the knowledge and skills to care for this population. There are many transport programs located throughout the United States that use specialized pediatric transport teams to support an infant or child during transport. As of 2015, when the last survey was completed, there were 145 specialized neonatal and pediatric teams in the United States, according to the American Academy of Pediatrics.[7] Nonspecialized teams that transport pediatric patients require crew members to acquire additional training and education to support pediatric patients. Once that initial training is completed, there must continue to be ongoing education and use of those skills to remain competent. According to the Commission on Accreditation of Medical Transport Systems (CAMTS), specialty care pediatric transport has a specialized team with the ability to support an infant or child with a life-threatening illness or injury. Specialized pediatric critical care transport teams are experienced, trained, and equipped to deliver definitive care away from the tertiary care center. These specialized teams provide an age-appropriate assessment and stabilization of the critically ill pediatric patient.

When a specialized pediatric transport team is available, they should be considered for the transport of critically ill or complex pediatric patients. Recent publications have shown improved care and better outcomes for neonatal and pediatric patients when the transport was provided by a specialized team.[8–11]

Pediatric Airway Anatomy

The anatomy of the pediatric airway is different from adult airway. These differences, which may affect advanced airway management, include the following[8,12–16]:

- Children possess larger and more vascular tonsils and adenoids in comparison to adults. Manipulating the airway during procedures may result in bleeding and partial airway obstruction, accompanied by altered levels of consciousness.
- In infants and children, the larynx is positioned more anteriorly and cephalad compared to adults. In infants and children, the larynx is situated opposite the C3 to C4 vertebrae, possibly reaching as high as C2 to C3 in some infants. As they grow into late adolescence and adulthood, the larynx descends to around C4 to C5 or even C6. This natural growth pattern in children affects the process of endotracheal intubation, making it more challenging for some providers.

- Children below the age of 3 have a large and flexible epiglottis, while older children have a long, narrow, and flexible epiglottis. In all cases, the epiglottis is angled away from the trachea. Using a straight blade, like the Miller blade, is often necessary and effective in lifting the epiglottis out of the visual field for direct laryngoscopy.
- Some children, particularly those with laryngomalacia, may have an omega-shaped epiglottis, which can result in positional inspiratory stridor.
- The trachea is notably shorter in neonates, measuring only 5 cm, and it elongates to 12 cm in adults. Additionally, the trachea is narrower in younger children compared to adults. The shorter trachea increases the likelihood of right mainstem intubations and self-extubations.
- In children under 10 years old, the narrowest part of the trachea is typically the cricoid process or ring. However, more recent studies suggest that in anesthetized children, the greatest narrowing occurs at the vocal cords. In spontaneously breathing children, the subglottic region remains the functionally narrowest portion. Both cuffed and uncuffed pediatric endotracheal tubes (ETTs) are available. Pediatric Advanced Life Support (PALS) recommends using cuffed ETTs for patients suspected of having elevated airway pressures, such as those with asthma or acute respiratory distress syndrome. Some referring providers may be hesitant to use cuffed ETTs, potentially making it challenging to provide adequate ventilation in cases of significant air leaks, necessitating ETT replacement.
- Pediatric tracheas can experience flexibility or collapse during episodes of agitation or partial airway obstruction, such as those seen in children with croup. In such cases, positive-pressure ventilation (PPV) with a bag-valve-mask (BVM) may be required to stent open a partially obstructed upper airway, serving as an initial rescue measure for these children. If the patient is alert, maintaining a position of comfort is advised. However, if the patient is only semi-conscious, attempting PPV with a BVM may be considered as a rescue measure before securing the airway.
- The narrow tracheal lumen, the space between the tracheal rings, and the small size of the cricothyroid membrane present challenges when attempting needle or surgical cricothyroidotomy in infants or children. For children under 10 years of age, surgical cricothyroidotomy is not recommended as a rescue method. Instead, a needle cricothyroidotomy should be attempted. Based on animal studies, this approach provides oxygenation for an estimated 30 minutes while a definitive airway control method is secured.

The clinical implications affected by the pediatric airway compared with the adult airway include the following[8,12–16]:
- Infants are considered obligatory nose breathers, with the nasal passages accounting for nearly half of their total airway resistance. Any presence of secretions, swelling, or obstruction in these passages can significantly increase the effort required for breathing, potentially leading to respiratory distress in these young children.
- Due to the small diameter of their nasal passages, even a slight amount of swelling or obstruction can substantially impair air exchange, as commonly observed in children with conditions like croup or respiratory syncytial virus (RSV).
- The posterior displacement of the tongue can result in airway obstruction, a condition that becomes more pronounced in the supine position or when a child's level of consciousness is altered.

- Managing the positioning of the tongue and epiglottis with a laryngoscope blade may be challenging.
- The angle between the base of the tongue and the glottic opening is more acute in children, making straight blades more effective for visualizing the glottis in this population.
- Due to the shape of the epiglottis, the Miller or straight blade is preferred over the curved Macintosh blade. The straight blade is positioned beneath the epiglottis to lift it for a clearer view of the vocal cords, while the curved blade is inserted into the vallecula and indirectly elevates the epiglottis away from the glottic opening.
- Blind endotracheal tube (ETT) placement can become snagged at the anterior commissure of the vocal cords, potentially causing trauma and swelling, and further narrowing the airway.
- Appropriately sized ETTs minimize air leakage during ventilation. Cuffed ETTs are acceptable and recommended, especially for children expected to have higher airway pressure requirements, as per Pediatric Advanced Life Support (PALS) guidelines.
- Infants and young children tend to have a higher metabolic rate and consume oxygen at twice the rate of adults. Additionally, they possess a lower functional residual capacity, resulting in reduced intrapulmonary oxygen reserves during periods of apnea or hypoventilation.
- The combination of their higher metabolic rate and lower functional residual capacity means that infants and young children can experience rapid and abrupt desaturation even with adequate preoxygenation before airway interventions, unlike adults.

- Infants and young children have smaller tidal volumes (5–8 mL/kg), and delivering higher volumes or employing more aggressive PPV increases the risk of causing iatrogenic barotrauma in these young patients.
- The parasympathetic nervous system has a more significant impact on the nervous system of infants due to the immaturity of the sympathetic nervous system. This increases the potential for bradycardia in response to hypoxia and further reduces oxygen delivery.
- Infants and young children exhibit a heightened vagal response to airway suctioning or the use of laryngoscope blades.
- In cases of airway difficulty, children deteriorate more rapidly than adults if left without intervention.

A list of airway adjuncts for managing respiratory distress can be found in Table 18.1.[8,17–20]

Pediatric respiratory distress can be managed with noninvasive ventilation, and the most frequently employed modalities are detailed in Table 18.2.[12,14–18,21,22]

Pediatric Airway Management/Respiratory Distress

Roughly 200,000 neonates and children are annually transported to advanced care facilities in the United States. According to Schmidt et al., nearly half of all pediatric transports are attributed to respiratory distress, emphasizing the importance of proactive measures by transport teams to address the respiratory status of

TABLE 18.1 Airway Adjuncts for Respiratory Distress in the Pediatric Patient

Nasal cannula (NC)	• Low-flow use only • 4%–44% FiO_2 with flows 1–6 L/min • Should try to use humidity for all pediatric patients; best used with a bubble humidifier • During transport may not be humidified
Simple oxygen mask	• 35%–60% FiO_2 with flows 6–10 L/min • Higher concentrations of oxygen compared with an NC • May be used for transport
High-flow nasal cannula or Vapotherm	• Provides relative humidity of nearly 100% FiO_2 when warmed to 34°C–37°C • Reduces work of breathing by washing out carbon dioxide from the upper airway, humidification helps clear mucus from airways • Flow rates >2 L/min up to 30 L/min • Recent studies showing increased use in ED and during prehospital or interfacility transports
Nonrebreather mask with reservoir	• FiO_2 95% with flows 10–15 L/min • Reliably supplies the highest concentration of oxygen to a spontaneously breathing patient • Tight mask fit required to deliver higher concentrations of oxygen • If the bag deflates patient may breathe in large amounts of exhaled carbon dioxide
Face tent	• A clear, plastic shell surrounds the child's head and upper body • 40%–50% FiO_2 using high-flow oxygen up to 15 L/min • Not sufficient if oxygen requirement >30% because of mixing of room air when the tent is opened
Oxygen hood	• Oxygen hoods are clear, plastic cylinders that encompass the infant's head • 80%–90% FiO_2 with flow rates of >10–15 L/min • Usually not large enough for children over 1 year of age
Oropharyngeal airway (sizes 00 mm for neonates up to 110 mm for the extra-large adult patient)	• A plastic flange that displaces the tongue from the posterior pharynx and provides an oral opening for ventilation and suction • Placed with a tongue depressor and direct visualization in the unconscious child in those whose airway maneuvers (jaw thrust and chin lift) were unsuccessful at opening the airway • Contact with tongue and supraglottic structures may stimulate vomiting • Size determined with external measurement, with the flange at the level of the mouth, the tip should reach the angle of the jaw

TABLE 18.1	Airway Adjuncts for Respiratory Distress in the Pediatric Patient—cont'd
Nasopharyngeal airway	• A flexible rubber tube that provides a conduit for air or oxygen from the nares to the posterior pharynx and provides ability to suction from the posterior pharynx • Tolerated in responsive or awake patients • Sizes determined with external measurement, with the airway approximated to equal the length from the tip of the nose to the tragus of the ear • Used in children with soft-tissue upper airway obstruction • Lubricate well and gently insert into nares to avoid bleeding or injury
Self-inflating ventilation bag	• FiO_2 95%–100% with reservoir • Used to provide assisted ventilation and oxygen • Unable to provide blow-by oxygen • Does not require an oxygen source to function
Flow-inflating ventilation bag	• FiO_2 100% • Used to provide assisted ventilation and oxygenation • Able to provide blow-by oxygen • Must have an oxygen source to function • May require experience with use to be reliable

Pediatric respiratory distress can be managed with noninvasive ventilation, and the most frequently employed modalities are detailed in Table 18.2.
Data from references 8,17–20

TABLE 18.2	Noninvasive Ventilation Used in Pediatric Patients in Respiratory Distress
NIV	• The delivery of assisted ventilation without the use of an advanced airway • NIV improves alveolar ventilation, oxygenation, and work of breathing • NIV avoids risks associated with advanced airways such as laryngeal injury and ventilator-induced lung injury
CPAP	• CPAP provides constant flow to maintain a set pressure to the lower airways • CPAP starts at 4–5 cmH_2O; adjust pressures to effect based on physiologic response up to 8–10 cmH_2O • CPAP increases functional residual capacity, which increases oxygenation, reduces airway resistance, and decreases work of breathing • Several positive-pressure methods available to deliver CPAP such as nasal prongs, face masks, nasal mask
BiPAP	• BiPAP provides two levels of positive airway pressure • Higher IPAP ranging from 2 to 25 cmH_2O • Lower EPAP ranging from 2 to 20 cmH_2O • Initial settings of IPAP of 8–10 cmH_2O and EPAP of 4–5 cmH_2O
HFNC	• Heated, humidified oxygen delivered by nasal cannula at high flow rates to decrease entrainment of room air • Comfortable and tolerated better than face masks or nasal masks • Improves oxygenation and ventilation, decreases work of breathing, reduces the need for intubation, and allows earlier extubation • Mechanism of action of this mode is washout of nasopharyngeal dead space, which improves alveolar ventilation, decreases airway resistance, and improves pulmonary compliance, leading to lung recruitment • Positive-pressure varies depending on flow rate and leakage around nares • Initial flow of 1–2 L/kg. Max flow is generally 25–30 L • Recent studies demonstrating increased use in emergency departments and during prehospital or interfacility transports

BiPAP, Bilevel positive airway pressure; *CPAP*, continuous positive airway pressure; *EPAP*, end-expiratory positive airway pressure; *IPAP*, inspiratory positive airway pressure; *NIV*, noninvasive ventilation; *HFNC*, heated high-flow nasal cannula.
Data from references 12,14–18,21,22

these patients. Rapid decompensation leading to respiratory failure can occur.[11]

Numerous factors can contribute to respiratory complications, including:
• Upper airway issues such as obstruction due to foreign bodies or anatomic abnormalities.
• Lower airway problems, including conditions like asthma and bronchiolitis.
• Lung tissue diseases, encompassing infectious processes and pulmonary hypertension.

• Central nervous system (CNS) factors, such as ingestion and head injuries.

A review of prehospital crews across the United States revealed that 34 states have protocols in place to manage respiratory distress in the pediatric population. Some states go a step further by specifying distinct diagnoses within respiratory distress, such as asthma, croup, epiglottitis, and anaphylaxis. These protocols vary in detail, covering specific medications, dosages, age groups affected, and the type of monitoring required. The authors underscored the evidence-based practice of administering steroids to asthmatic patients and its positive impact on reducing hospital stays.[23]

Regular protocol reviews are essential to ensure compliance with the latest recommendations. Additionally, chart and peer reviews are crucial to confirm that crews adhere to established protocols, guaranteeing the delivery of the highest-quality patient care.

Acute respiratory failure or arrest is the main cause of morbidity and mortality in critically injured or ill children. Airway management is one of the first steps initiated in stabilizing a pediatric patient for transport. It is essential for the transport provider to be able to anticipate, rapidly recognize, and initiate appropriate interventions and treatment to prevent respiratory failure, cardiopulmonary arrest, or death. Without clearing or establishing an airway, resuscitation efforts, regardless of the quality of chest compressions, may prove ineffective. Respiratory failure is a result of the inability to provide oxygen to the tissues and remove carbon dioxide to meet the metabolic demands of the child.[24–30]

Respiratory distress in children can be categorized into three levels: mild, moderate, or severe.

- Mild respiratory distress is characterized by no noticeable changes in color, mild or absent retractions, mildly reduced air entry, and normal level of consciousness (LOC). In some cases, the child may display restlessness when stimulated.
- Moderate respiratory distress presents as no significant changes in color, moderate retractions, moderately reduced air entry, and increasing anxiety or restlessness with stimulation.
- Severe respiratory distress is marked by the child appearing pale, dusky, or cyanotic. Retractions become severe, involving the use of accessory muscles. Air entry is significantly diminished, and the child's LOC is deteriorating, with possible lethargy. Severe respiratory distress is a critical condition that, without prompt intervention and treatment, can progress to failure or arrest in infants and children.

Trained transport providers should be able to recognize the severity of dyspnea, increasing tachypnea, decreased or inadequate air entry, tachycardia, cyanosis, signs of impending fatigue, changes in LOC, and alterations in respiratory status. Preparation for immediate intubation is highly suggested. Refer to Table 18.3 for the most common causes of respiratory failure in children.[24–31] There are features of the pediatric airway and its development that predispose pediatric patients to respiratory distress and failure at higher rates when compared with adults. Refer to Table 18.4 for anatomic and physiologic causes for increased risk of respiratory failure in infants and children.[12,13,16,25]

The objective of airway management is to establish a secure airway and ensure sufficient tissue oxygenation and ventilation. Achieving effective airway management in the prehospital environment can be challenging due to diverse injury patterns or conditions, including facial trauma, pharyngeal injuries, or restricted access to the patient's airway. Additionally, the presence of congenital airway anomalies can complicate airway management in pediatric patients. Pierre Robin sequence is a congenital anomaly with possible airway obstruction requiring airway management. Pierre Robin sequence is a triad of symptoms of micrognathia, glossoptosis, and laryngomalacia or tracheomalacia. Prone positioning may be effective in less severe presentations and if necessary a nasal airway may suffice for transport.[24–31]

Acquired upper airway obstructions the transport provider might encounter may be infectious or noninfectious. These include severe tonsillitis with adenoid enlargements such as with infectious mononucleosis, retropharyngeal and peritonsillar abscess, epiglottitis, croup, bacterial tracheitis, foreign body aspiration (FBA),

TABLE 18.3	Common Causes of Respiratory Distress or Failure in Children
Upper airway obstruction	• Croup • Epiglottitis • Foreign body aspiration
Lower airway obstruction	• Bronchiolitis • Status asthmaticus • Bronchopulmonary dysplasia
Lung disease	• Pneumonia • Acute respiratory distress syndrome • Pulmonary edema • Near-drowning
Causes affecting ventilation	• Neuromuscular disorders or myopathies • Infant botulism • Guillain–Barré syndrome • Chest wall trauma or malformations • Severe congenital scoliosis • Pleural effusion or pneumothorax
CNS issues affecting ventilation	• Status epilepticus • CNS infection • Trauma • Apnea of prematurity
Inability to meet oxygen demands of the body	• Hypovolemia • Septic shock • Cardiac insufficiency • Metabolic disorders

CNS, Central nervous system.
Modified from Hammer J. Acute respiratory failure in children. *Pediatr Respir Rev.* 2013;14(3):2–13.

anaphylaxis and angioedema, thermal injury from burns, caustic ingestion, or damage from referral endotracheal intubation or tracheostomy.[24] Certain topics will receive a more comprehensive discussion later in this chapter. Furthermore, it is worth noting that referral facilities may lack expertise or have apprehensions regarding pediatric intubation. Unsuccessful or protracted intubation efforts can carry adverse outcomes in pediatric cases. While various airway devices are accessible for neonatal and pediatric patients (see Table 18.2), it is crucial to emphasize that endotracheal intubation (ETI) remains the preferred and sole definitive method for safeguarding the child's airway, ensuring proper oxygenation and ventilation, and averting aspiration.

Pediatric endotracheal intubation demands a high level of skill, experience, and recurrent training for providers to maintain proficiency, as highlighted in numerous studies.[24–30] While intubation is a preferred approach for some providers, it carries inherent risks. After intubation, it is imperative to employ proper bagging or ventilator management techniques to avoid potential harm. Transport providers must exercise caution to prevent ventilator-induced lung injury (VILI), as discussed earlier.

In the case of ventilated pediatric patients, it may be more appropriate to entrust their care to specialized pediatric transport teams, given the frequency with which they manage such cases. Research has indicated that the utilization of specialized pediatric teams results in fewer adverse events.[32] A study by Stansell and Cherry demonstrated that even nonspecialized teams can benefit from the use of a checklist specifically designed for appropriate

TABLE 18.4	Anatomic or Physiologic Causes for Increased Risk of Respiratory Failure in Infants and Children Compared with Adults	
Anatomic/Physiologic Cause	**Impact**
• High metabolic rate • Rapid desaturation	• Increased oxygen consumption to more than double that of adults • Lower functional residual capacity
• Increased risk of apnea • Increased risk of bradycardia	• Prematurity resulting in immature control of breathing • Incomplete maturation of sympathetic nervous system
• Increased resistance to breathing • Increased upper airway resistance	• Obligate nose breathers (usually up to 6 months of age) • Large tongues relative to the size of oral cavity • Epiglottis is large, floppy (impacts visualization of airway structures during direct laryngoscopy) • Smaller airway size, narrower at subglottic level (cricoid ring) • Airway softer, more pliable increasing chance of compression, collapse, or obstruction (e.g., agitation, illness, or pressure applied) • Larynx, trachea, and bronchi more compliant
• Increased resistance to breathing • Increased lower airway resistance	• Smaller airway size • Airway softer, more pliable, increasing chance of compression, collapse, or obstruction (e.g., agitation or illness) • Increased airway chest compliance • Decreased elastic recoil
• Smaller lung volumes • Reduced surface area for gas exchange	• Significantly smaller number of alveoli (incomplete development) • Limited collateral pathways of ventilation (given that obstructed airways prevent alveoli to be ventilated by these alternative means predisposes those <3 years of age to atelectasis, hypoxia, and hypercapnia)
• Decreased efficiency of respiratory muscles	• Decreased efficiency of diaphragm (poorly prepared to sustain increased workload of breathing) • Highly compliant ribs (horizontal ribs) • Poorly developed intercostal muscles
• Decreased endurance of respiratory muscles • Proportionately larger head, particularly the occiput in infants and children	• Increased respiratory rate • Increases anatomic airway obstruction in supine position without a roll under shoulders for neck flexion • Inadequate positioning obstructs visualization of glottic opening during direct laryngoscopy

Data from references [16,23,24,27]

ventilation strategies in pediatric patients.[32] For teams that do not regularly transport ventilated pediatric patients, having general guidelines with established parameters can be invaluable in guiding ventilator management.

This research includes the checklist, which provides a step-by-step process for making ventilator adjustments based on the patient's response to changes.[32] Prior to implementing the checklist, the authors found that 41.3% of intubated pediatric patients were outside the established guidelines. However, after the checklist was introduced, there was a significant improvement within a relatively short period (7 months), with the number of pediatric patients falling outside established parameters decreasing to just 10.0%.[32]

Initial Management of Respiratory Distress/Arrest in the Pediatric Patient

Conduct a swift assessment of the child, as respiratory distress in children can rapidly progress to cardiac arrest without timely intervention. Here are the steps to follow:

1. Open the airway using either a jaw thrust or chin lift maneuver.
2. Perform suctioning as needed and appropriately position the patient.
3. Administer oxygen and assist with breathing using bag–mask ventilation or any of the airway adjuncts listed in Tables 18.1 and 18.2.
4. Be prepared for the potential need for intubation.

Advanced Management of Respiratory Distress in the Pediatric Patient

Based on the initial quick assessment of the patient, transport providers may opt for the use of noninvasive ventilation (NIV) and conduct frequent reassessments to gauge the patient's tolerance. NIV serves as a valuable adjunct and carries a lower risk compared to invasive ventilation, as it mitigates the potential for ventilator-induced lung injury.[33] Until recently, NIV had limited adoption in transport settings and was predominantly employed by specialized pediatric transport teams. NIV encompasses techniques like continuous positive airway pressure (CPAP) and high flow nasal cannula (HFNC).[33]

A systematic literature review conducted by Cheema et al. examined the incidence of patient decompensation during transport while on NIV, the need for escalated care within 24 hours of admission, and instances of intubation during hospitalization.[33] The review revealed that among patients transported with NIV, 0.4% required escalated care during transport, including intubation, and 10% needed intubation within the first 24 hours of admission.[33] When considering intubation at any point during hospitalization, the collective data from seven reviewed studies indicated that 13% of patients required intubation, with individual study figures ranging from as low as 10% to as high as 35%.[33]

Patients who present with respiratory distress or progress to respiratory failure will need more aggressive support than opening the airway and providing oxygen via an airway adjunct.

• BOX 18.1 Bag-Valve-Mask Ventilation

- Successful BVM ventilation requires selecting the correct mask size, sustaining an open airway with a tight seal between the mask and the patient's face, and assessing effectiveness.
- BVM ventilation is performed by a two-handed technique or if at all possible a two-person technique, with one hand or person securing the mask to the child's face, and the other providing bag ventilation.
- BVM is best performed with proper head positioning. The child should be managed with a head tilt chin lift maneuver, and hand positioning needs to ensure that the submental area is not depressed and occluding the patient's airway.
- If a cervical spine injury is suspected in a child, BVM should be performed while maintaining the cervical spine in a neutral position. This may require manual control of the cervical spine if the immobilization device is not in place or removed.
- Optimal positioning for airway patency and effective ventilation is in a neutral sniffing position for infants and with a roll or towel placed under the head and neck of toddlers. A variety of head and neck positions may be attempted to find the optimal position for effective ventilation in the absence of cervical injury.
- Provide 100% oxygen for all ventilation BVMs. This is best performed with a self-inflating bag-valve device with an attached reservoir. Anesthesia bags may also be used, but may require practice and experience to be successful. Remember, if congenital heart disease is suspected, 100% oxygen may be detrimental to those dependent on a patent ductus arteriosus.
- An oropharyngeal or nasopharyngeal airway (depending on the patient's level of consciousness) is helpful in providing more effective oxygenation/ventilation.
- Gastric distention is a complication of BVM positive-pressure ventilation leading to vomiting and possible aspiration. Gastric distention affects ventilation by restricting movement of the diaphragm. Insertion of a gastric tube decreases gastric distention during BVM ventilation and is an important consideration in the pediatric patient.
- Cricoid pressure (Sellick's maneuver) in the unconscious or sedated patient is often used in rapid sequence intubation in pediatrics to prevent gastric distention or passive regurgitation of gastric contents during BVM ventilation.
- Most self-inflating bags have a built-in pressure-limiting pop-off valve to prevent high airway pressures during BVM ventilation. When providing BVM ventilations during CPR, the bag should not have a pop-off valve or it needs to have a valve that may be occluded to inactivate it in the event airway resistance is high or there is poor lung compliance and requires more pressure to ventilate the patient.

BVM, Bag-valve-mask; *CPR,* cardiopulmonary resuscitation.
Data from references 12–17,25–27,30–33

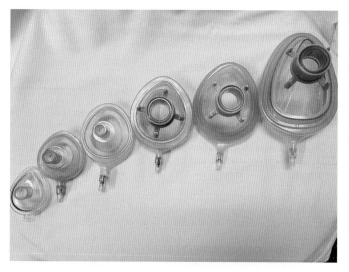

• Fig. 18.1 Different sizes of resuscitation masks.

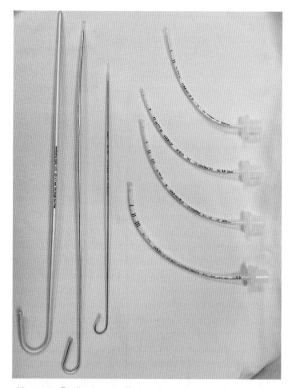

• Fig. 18.2 Pediatric uncuffed endotracheal tubes and stylets.

These patients may need support from BVM ventilation (see Box 18.1[12–17,25–27,30–33]) with or without endotracheal intubation. The transport provider should remember the best airway in a child is one with which you can oxygenate and ventilate the patient. Research has demonstrated there is not a clear neurologic or survivable advantage between endotracheal intubation and BVM in pediatric patients 12 years of age or younger in the prehospital setting. According to the 2015 American Heart Association (AHA) guidelines, BVM ventilation may be effective and safer than endotracheal intubation for short transport times or short out-of-hospital resuscitation. Endotracheal intubation for longer transport times is recommended given that it is difficult to maintain effective BVM ventilations for long periods and even harder in a moving vehicle.[8,14,15,17,24–27]

Refer to Fig. 18.1 for various sizes of resuscitation masks. See Fig. 18.2 for various-sized uncuffed pediatric ETT with stylets.

Endotracheal Intubation

Endotracheal intubation is considered one of the most effective and reliable methods of airway management in pediatric patients for an array of reasons, which include the following:[8,12–14,24–31]

- Pediatric airway can be isolated with an improved probability of adequate oxygenation and ventilation.
- Aspiration risk is decreased when there is a loss of protective airway reflexes in the unresponsive patient or those at risk for aspiration of blood or vomit.
- Ventilations with chest compressions can be more efficient and coordinated.
- Improved control of inspiratory times and pressures.
- Positive end-expiratory pressure (PEEP) can be delivered.

- Endotracheal medications may be given during resuscitation measures when IV access cannot be obtained.
- Pulmonary toilet can be performed.

Indications for ETT in pediatric patients include[8,12–14,24–31]:
- Anatomic or functional airway obstruction.
- Inadequate oxygenation from pneumonia or congestive heart failure.
- Inadequate ventilation based upon lab values, i.e., pH and $PaCO_2$.
- Respiratory distress leading to respiratory insufficiency, respiratory failure, or respiratory arrest.
- The need for mechanical ventilatory support.
- If patient transport is anticipated and the patient is experiencing any of the previously mentioned issues.
- Intubation to protect the pediatric patient's airway during long transport times.

Airway management is an initial step in stabilizing the pediatric patient. The reason for achieving airway control is to adequately oxygenate and ventilate the pediatric patient while decreasing the potential for aspiration. Pediatric patients are at risk for rapid deterioration during intubation with an increasing risk of bradycardia with desaturation from prolonged attempts. In addition, airway management in pediatric patients requires specialized equipment because of the differences in anatomy based on the patient's size and age.[2,8,24–30]

Endotracheal intubation in the pediatric patient requires initial training, unique skill sets, clinical judgment, ongoing training, and experience to reliably perform in an effective, timely, and safe method. Endotracheal intubation requires specialized training to attain and maintain competency for a wide range of pediatric patients regarding age and size. Research has demonstrated that specialized critical care transport teams achieve higher success rates when performing intubations in pediatric patients. Clinical experiences are becoming more limited because of the increased use of noninvasive ventilation devices available. Simulation offers the transport provider opportunities to develop, practice, and improve endotracheal intubation skills without injury to a child using a number of different types of simulations from low fidelity to high fidelity. The high-fidelity–enhanced simulation is effective for the individual provider, team training, and system optimization and is a suitable tool for the assessment of the competency of the provider and team interaction during intubation of the pediatric patient.[2,8,17,24–30]

Pediatric healthcare providers must possess the skills to assess, anticipate, and intervene promptly in cases of respiratory distress among children. It is critical for these providers to identify which patients require aggressive airway management. The narrowest segment of the pediatric airway, particularly in children under 8–10 years of age, is at the subglottic level, specifically at the cricoid ring. Traditionally, this anatomic feature led to the use of uncuffed endotracheal tubes (ETTs) for intubation in these pediatric patients. However, recent literature challenges the previously held notion that the pediatric airway is extremely narrow.[6–11,23,24] The 2015 American Heart Association's Pediatric Advanced Life Support (PALS) guidelines recommend the use of either cuffed or uncuffed ETTs for emergency intubations in children. Research has established that cuffed ETTs are just as safe as uncuffed ones. PALS guidelines advise using cuffed ETTs for children when there is an anticipated or suspected need for high airway pressures, such as in cases of asthma or acute respiratory distress.

Cuffed ETTs have been proven to reduce the necessity for multiple intubations due to air leakage around an uncuffed ETT,

without increasing adverse outcomes like damage to the airway mucosa or subglottic area across all age groups. Pediatric cuffed ETTs are designed for safe use, allowing cuff pressure management either through a cuff manometer or by monitoring the air leak around the tube. This approach minimizes the risk of harm to the subglottic area.

When selecting a cuffed ETT, if the transport provider opts for one, it should be approximately one-half size smaller than the uncuffed ETT estimated based on standard calculations. The healthcare team must be proficient in determining the appropriate tube size, tube positioning, and cuff inflation pressure, which should be maintained below 20 cm H_2O of water pressure.[2,8,12–15,24–31]

There are several methods the provider may use to select the correct ETT size in pediatric patients including:
- Matching the outside diameter of the ETT to the child's little finger or nares
- Use of length-based resuscitation tapes, such as Broselow tape or Handtevy
- For children older than 2 years, the formulas are:
  Endotracheal tube size = 16 + (age in years/4)
  Or
  Uncuffed endotracheal tube size (mm ID) = (age in years/4) + 4
  Or
  Cuffed endotracheal tube size (mm ID) = (age in years/4) + 3

The depth of the ETT placement can be approximated by multiplying the internal diameter by 3 (e.g., 3.5 mm ETT × 3 is inserted to 10.5 cm). Often, pediatric patients experience respiratory distress before it becomes apparent to parents and referral staff. By this point, their abdominal area may have become notably distended. Furthermore, if the patient has undergone bag-mask ventilation, it can lead to stomach overdistention, which, in turn, can impede the full expansion of the lungs. Gastric decompression is necessary in pediatric patients and selecting the correct size nasogastric or orogastric tube can be estimated by multiplying 2 by the size of the ETT.[8,12–15,21,30,31]

Preparing for endotracheal intubation is a critical step that must not be overlooked. The pediatric provider who is prepared for complications that may occur can often prevent life-threatening events during this procedure. The necessary equipment is listed in Box 18.2.[7–10,23,24,27,28,33–36]

See Fig. 18.3 for examples of laryngoscopes both fiberoptic and video. See Fig. 18.4 for CO_2 detectors (choose the correct one for patient weight).

The pediatric provider should have a backup plan in place in the event the provider is unable to ventilate or oxygenate the pediatric patient. Consider using oral or nasal airway adjuncts and attempt intubation. If unable to intubate the pediatric patient, consider using supraglottic rescue devices. If these devices are unsuccessful, consider needle or surgical airway procedures.[17–22,24,33,34,37]

Rapid sequence intubation (RSI) is considered to be the universal method used for obtaining definitive airway management in the emergency setting. It is the combined efforts of pre-oxygenation, sedation, and a neuromuscular blockade used in rapid succession to optimize endotracheal intubation in critically ill or injured patients. RSI is the appropriate method used in pediatric patients to facilitate intubation. The provider must be adequately prepared for RSI in pediatric patients, which includes the readiness for unexpected situations or complications.[38,39]

Rapid sequence intubation sedatives commonly used in pediatric patients are listed in Table 18.5.[39] Common neuromuscular blockade medications used for pediatric RSI are listed in Table 18.6.[39]

• BOX 18.2 Equipment Necessary for Intubation

- Oxygen delivery system (e.g., blow-by, nasal cannula, simple mask, nonrebreather, self-inflating bag, or flow-inflating bag)
- Bag-valve-resuscitation bag without pop-off valve
- Resuscitation masks of all pediatric sizes
- Oral and nasopharyngeal airways of all pediatric sizes
- Suction devices with pediatric-sized catheters
- Pulse oximeter with pediatric probes
- Cardiac monitor
- If sedation and paralytics are used, rescue/reversal medications (e.g., naloxone) should be available
- Pediatric endotracheal tubes, sizes to include both uncuffed and cuffed 2.5, 3.0, 3.5, 4.0, 4.5, 5.0, 5.5 mm and 6.0, 6.5, 7.0, and 8.0 mm cuffed (see Fig. 18.2)
- Pediatric laryngoscope blade sizes 00 to 4 straight (e.g., Miller) and 1 to 4 curved (e.g., MacIntosh).
- Pediatric stylets for endotracheal tubes sizes 2.5–8.0 mm
- Magill forceps both pediatric and adult
- End-tidal CO_2 detectors (disposable or in line) both pediatric and adult
- Rescue airway devices such as supraglottic airways
- Securing tape or device

Data from references 7–10,23,24,27,28,33–36

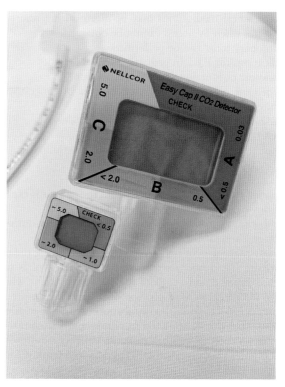

• **Fig. 18.4** Colorimetric CO_2 detectors.

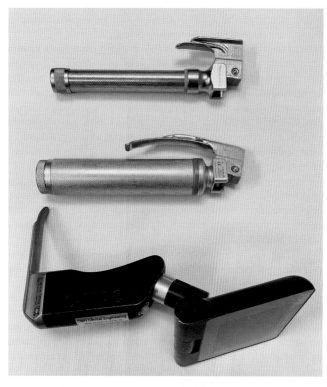

• **Fig. 18.3** Laryngoscopes both fiberoptic and video.

Atropine sulfate may be used to block the vagal responses in infants and pediatric patients during emergent endotracheal intubation.[40–42] According to the 2015 PALS update, pretreatment with atropine is not routinely recommended prior to intubation. It remains a recommendation in specific cases where the patient may be more prone to bradycardia, such as when certain medications are utilized for intubation such as succinylcholine. A single-center study also found that the use of atropine did not affect the incidence of bradycardia significantly.[40–42]

TABLE 18.5	Sedatives Commonly Used in Pediatric Rapid Sequence Intubation (RSI)	
Sedative	**Advantages**	**Disadvantages**
Etomidate	• Hypotension rare • Effects observed quickly • Efficient	• Possible adrenal suppression seen with septic shock • Long-acting NMB affects efficacy
Ketamine	• Potential for hypertension in patients exhibiting shock • Potentially may prevent post-RSI hypotension • Efficient	• Slower rate of administration compared to NMB • Increased systemic vascular resistance may cause harm to patients with cardiogenic shock
Fentanyl	• Hypotension is rare • Efficient	• Possible rigid chest with rapid administration
Propofol	• Effects observed quickly • Efficient	• Potential hypotensive issues
Versed	• Rapid onset of action • Amnesia	• Potential hypotensive issues

NMB, Neuromuscular blockade; *RSI*, rapid sequence intubation.
Data from Mittiga MR, Rinderknecht AS, Kerrey BT. A modern and practical review of rapid-sequence intubation in pediatric emergencies. *Clin Pediatr Emerg Med.* 2015;16(3):172–185.

TABLE 18.6	Neuromuscular Blockade Commonly Used in Pediatric Rapid Sequence Intubation (RSI)	
Neuromuscular Blockade	Benefits	Risks
Succinylcholine	• Effects observed quickly • Short-acting • Efficient	• Short-acting and may need additional dosing • Hyperkalemia may occur • Additional dosing may cause bradycardia
Rocuronium	• Safe to use with renal clearance (hyperkalemia) • Effects observed quickly (more efficient than vecuronium)	• Long-acting, which may cause an issue if unable to intubate the patient • Shorter duration compared with vecuronium
Vecuronium	• Safe to use with renal clearance (hyperkalemia)	• Long acting (longer compared with rocuronium)

Data from Mittiga MR, Rinderknecht AS, Kerrey BT. A modern and practical review of rapid-sequence intubation in pediatric emergencies. *Clin Pediatr Emerg Med.* 2015;16(3):172–185.

Proper ETT placement is verified immediately after intubation by several methods:
- Positive end-tidal CO_2 ($ETCO_2$) indicator via colorimetric detector or capnography is considered the most definitive by the American Academy of Pediatrics.[43]
- Auscultation of bilateral breath sounds begins high in the axillae with equal chest rise.
- Direct visualization of the ETT through the cords.
- Absence of breath sounds or gurgling sounds in the stomach.
- Chest radiograph results should verify proper tube depth.

Evidence and controversy in pediatric prehospital airway management exist and options include BMV, endotracheal intubation, and supraglottic devices. Supraglottic airways have increased in popularity and use in the prehospital and emergency room settings because these devices are so easy to use, training is relatively simple, and they are dependable and quick to insert. Supraglottic devices do not offer a definitive airway in the prehospital setting. However, newer, more advanced devices are offering greater seal pressures and the capacity to decompress gastric secretions to decrease potential aspiration. Supraglottic devices are usually used as rescue devices. Supraglottic airways have revealed a decrease in hands-on time during resuscitation, yet it is ambiguous as to whether any advanced airway offers a neurologic survival advantage compared with simple BVM in the prehospital setting. Supraglottic airways are considered to be first- or second-generation devices. The first-generation supraglottic airways are simple airways attached to a mask resting over the glottic opening. The second-generation supraglottic airways have a gastric access channel for the placement of gastric tubes or venting of gastric contents. Second-generation supraglottic devices offer several advantages compared with the first-generation devices such as an improved airway seal with the ability to reduce the risk of gastric insufflations, which ultimately allows for improved PPV and some protection against aspiration.[34,37,38,41]

Children who are designated as having a difficult airway or are unable to be intubated by direct laryngoscopy may benefit from using supraglottic airways because they are potential conduits for endotracheal intubation. The pros of using a supraglottic airway as an adjunct for intubation include the ability to be able to provide oxygen during intubation and relief of any upper airway obstruction in children designated with a difficult airway. Supraglottic airways are available in pediatric sizes and include the laryngeal mask airway (LMA), LMA Unique, LMA Supreme, and LMA ProSeal. The King LT-D and King LTS-D are available in pediatric >12 kg to adult sizes. The I-gel is available in neonatal 2 kg to adult >90 kg sizes. Air-Q and Air-Q SP are available in

pediatric <7 kg to adult and pediatric <4 kg to adult sizes. Research comparing specific supraglottic airway devices, BVM, and ETT and associated neurologic outcomes has not been performed. Esophageal obturator airways such as the Combitube and oxygen-powered breathing devices are both not recommended in the pediatric population because of limited patient-appropriate sizes.[34,37,38,41]

No matter which advanced airway modality is used, the transport provider must confirm proper placement, provide adequate ventilation and oxygenation, and promptly recognize displacement of the airway to improve pediatric advanced airway management during the prehospital or interfacility transports. Pulse oximetry, which is a noninvasive measurement of arterial blood oxygenation, has become a standard method of monitoring respiratory status for pediatric patients in prehospital or interfacility transports. Pulse oximetry is affected by movement, hypothermia, vasoconstriction, and poor perfusion, which are all common in the pediatric patient requiring transport.[6,15,44]

$ETCO_2$ measurement is used to confirm the correct placement of the airway and effectiveness of assisted ventilations. Research has shown capnography improves time to detection of a dislodged ETT and the corrective actions necessary in pediatric patients. Freeman et al. demonstrated that continuous capnograph waveforms may be useful for the assessment of pediatric ventilation regardless of airway (ETT, BVM, or supraglottic).[45] Current literature and the 2015 AHA guidelines support BVM over endotracheal intubation in the prehospital setting and using continuous capnograph may be an essential tool to ensure adequate ventilation in pediatric patients. Providing an adequate mask seal, with effective chest rise and breath sounds, is difficult to maintain and assess as providers are confronted with multiple tasks, environmental factors, limited space, and continuous movement from the mode of transport in the prehospital or interfacility setting. A useful tool for assessing adequate ventilation via ETT, BVM, or supraglottic device appears to be continuous capnography.[6,15,45]

Intubated pediatric patients are at high risk of extubation when the child is being loaded and unloaded in an aircraft or ground ambulance. If a change in the child's status occurs, consider the mnemonic DOPE to help identify the problem[6,45]:

D: Displacement of the ETT
O: Obstruction of the ETT
P: Pneumothorax
E: Equipment failure

Needle Cricothyroidotomy

Surgical airway in a child is rarely performed, but when it is, it is potentially a lifesaving intervention. The pediatric provider must be able to recognize and manage the difficult airway in a child. Failing to recognize and respond in an appropriate manner can cause significant morbidity and mortality in that child. The inability to secure and control the child's airway via BVM, ETT, a supraglottic device, or because of facial injuries or airway obstruction is an emergent situation requiring the pediatric provider to consider a surgical airway. An invasive airway in a pediatric patient is rare. A needle cricothyroidotomy is used for children 10 years of age or less. The Seldinger cricothyroidotomy may be used on children older than 5 years of age. A surgical airway can be placed through the cricothyroid membrane in children older than 10 years of age if the structures can be palpated.[20,21,33] This procedure affects oxygenation. Passive exhalation occurs when using the needle cricothyroidotomy method. The size of this airway is small and limited because of the lumen size, and it is more effective in oxygenation than ventilation. The child can only be oxygenated for about 30–45 minutes using this technique. Needle cricothyroidotomy is a temporary method to control a child's airway until ETT can be placed or the airway obstruction is removed.[35,38,40,45]

Indications for needle cricothyroidotomy include the following:
- Complete airway obstruction
- Severe orofacial injuries
- Laryngeal tear or transection
- Inability to secure the airway with the less invasive methods

The procedure for a needle cricothyroidotomy is shown in Box 18.3.

• BOX 18.3 Cricothyroidotomy

1. Place the patient in a supine position.
2. Attach a 14-gauge, 8.5-cm over-the-needle catheter to a 10-mL syringe.
3. Surgically prepare the neck with antiseptic swabs.
4. Palpate the cricothyroid membrane between the thyroid and cricoid cartilage.
5. Stabilize the trachea with the thumb and forefinger to prevent lateral movement.
6. Puncture the skin in the midline over the cricothyroid membrane with the 14-gauge needle attached to the syringe. A small incision with a #11 blade may facilitate passage of the needle.
7. Direct the needle at a 45-degree angle caudally.
8. Carefully insert the needle into the lower half of the cricothyroid membrane, aspirating as the needle is advanced.
9. Aspiration of air signifies entry into the tracheal lumen. Saline in the syringe may also be used. When aspiration occurs bubbles will be seen.
10. Remove the syringe and stylet while gently advancing the catheter downward into position, taking care not to perforate the posterior trachea.
11. Oxygen can then be delivered in a variety of ways. Commercial jet insufflators are available for this purpose. Oxygen can also be supplied by attaching the adapter from a #3.0 endotracheal tube to the catheter and ventilate with a resuscitation bag. Oxygen tubing can be cut with a hole toward the end of the tubing, which is then attached to the catheter hub. Once attached to an oxygen source of 50 psi or greater, oxygen can be delivered by occluding the hole with the thumb. Regardless of the oxygen delivery source, inspiration should be provided for 1 second while passive exhalation is provided for 4 seconds. Another alternative is to use the barrel of a 3-mL syringe attached to a 7.5 ETT adapter. The BVM easily fits onto the adapter for oxygenation.

From Holleran RS, ed. ASTNA Patient Transport: Principles and Practice. 4th ed. St. Louis, MO: Mosby Elsevier; 2010.

Complications of a needle cricothyroidotomy include the following:
- Inadequate ventilation that leads to hypoxia and death
- Aspiration of blood
- Esophageal laceration
- Hematoma
- Posterior tracheal wall perforation
- Subcutaneous or mediastinal emphysema
- Thyroid perforation

Selected Diagnoses and Their Effect on the Pediatric Population

Asthma

Asthma prevalence in children is progressively increasing annually, with an estimate of 6.8 million children currently diagnosed with asthma, or 9.3% of all children under the age of 18 years in the United States.[46,47] Asthma is not curable, nor can it be prevented, but it can be controlled. Asthma has a higher prevalence in children compared with adults. In children less than 18 years of age, males have a higher prevalence compared with females. Racial and socioeconomic differences exist, with higher prevalence in Hispanic and African American children. In addition, children living below the federal poverty level also have a higher prevalence of asthma.[46,47]

Asthma is one of the most common chronic childhood diseases and is characterized by chronic airway inflammation, airway hyper-responsiveness, and intermittent and reversible bronchial constriction or obstruction. Pediatric asthma exacerbation is an acute episode that does not respond to standard therapy, leading to a medical emergency. Recent reports show that there are over 750,000 emergency room visits and 200,000 hospitalizations due to asthma every year.[48] Asthma is also the leading cause of missed school days and work absences.[36,46,47]

Obesity is a risk factor for developing asthma. Some obese pediatric patients have not only increased airway microphages but some of those airway microphages are less responsive to treatment.[49] The macrophages also contribute to inflammation. Other factors impacting asthma development or exacerbation include environmental factors, allergens, and respiratory viruses.[36,46,50–53] Approximately 80% of asthma exacerbations are caused by viral respiratory infections: (a) rhinovirus, (b) respiratory syncytial virus (RSV), (c) coronaviruses, (d) influenza A and B, (e) parainfluenza viruses, (f) adenovirus, (g) human metapneumovirus, (h) human bocavirus, and (i) enteroviruses are all related to exacerbations. Rhinovirus is the most common pathogen causing exacerbations in older children, and RSV is the most common in younger children.[53]

Clinical Presentation

A hallmark finding in patients experiencing an exacerbation is expiratory wheezing. Asthma is the most common cause of chronic cough in children. Acute exacerbation signs and symptoms include coughing, dyspnea, chest tightness, and wheezing. Younger children reveal shortness of breath as decreased activity or verbalization. In children 5 years of age and younger, wheezing is the most common symptom associated with asthma. The child may present with nonspecific signs of respiratory distress including retractions, nasal flaring, cyanosis, accessory muscle use, and altered mental status. Coughing triggered by asthma may be recurrent or persistent and is usually associated with wheezing. Recurrent shortness of breath or during exercise increases the chance of an asthma diagnosis. A child who presents with hypoxia or saturations less than 92% may require aggressive treatment. Severe exacerbations in children may cause tachypnea, tachycardia, and occasionally pulsus paradoxus. Accessory muscle use may indicate a severe asthma exacerbation. In severe exacerbation, poor air exchange and movement without wheezing, known as a silent chest, is a sign of impending respiratory failure. Agitation or decreased mental status are also signs of impending respiratory failure in children.[36,46–48,50–55] A helpful easy assessment tool is to ask the child simple questions or have them recite their ABCs to assess how many words they can speak.[56] Generally, the fewer words or sounds, the more severe the asthma exacerbation is.

A detailed medical history is an important tool for the transport provider in the assessment of a child with wheezing. It is essential in determining causes other than asthma in a first-time wheezing patient. Questions to ask include the age of the patient, onset of symptoms, associated symptoms, history of asthma, history of ED visits, intensive care unit admission including if the child was on a ventilator within the past year, use of a short-acting beta-agonist (SABA), compliance with controller medications, number and frequency of home treatments, and history of greater than or equal to 3 days of oral steroids in the last 3 months. A significant indicator of asthma exacerbation in a child is a recent ED visit for asthma.[36,48,50–55,57–59]

There are three reliable asthma scoring tools available for the provider to use to assist with the severity of the asthma exacerbation (Table 18.7).[36]

Treatment

The primary goal of asthma treatment is the reversal of hypoxemia and the control of contributing inflammatory responses. First-line therapy consists of supplementation of oxygen, the repeated administration of inhaled short-acting bronchodilators (SABA) and anticholinergics, and early administration of corticosteroids either orally or intravenously. The most common bronchodilators and anticholinergics are albuterol and ipratropium bromide nebulized aerosols. A distinguishing characteristic of asthma is the response to bronchodilator or corticosteroids when symptomatic. In children, asthma is a clinical diagnosis.[36,48,50–55,57–59] In the review of the prehospital protocols in 34 states, all of them recommended the use of albuterol. Seventeen of the states required wheezing prior to administration while 12 of them allowed for its use based upon the suspicion of bronchoconstriction. The danger is that when patients have a severe exacerbation, they may not be moving enough air to cause wheezing.[21,56]

SABAs are the most effective treatment to relieve bronchospasm and reverse airway obstruction. SABAs use their sympathomimetic effects to exert bronchodilating effects by relaxing airway smooth muscle to relieve bronchospasm. They also have secondary effects that enhance water output from bronchial mucous glands and improve mucociliary clearance. Albuterol and levalbuterol are the two available SABAs used in children. Airway inflammation occurs with an asthma exacerbation, and corticosteroids are the most common treatment by suppressing cytokine production, granulocyte–macrophage colony-stimulating factor, and nitric oxide synthase activation and decreasing airway mucous production.[36,48,50–55,57–59] Seven of the states surveyed in the study referred to above allow for administration of IM epinephrine in their prehospital guidelines.[21]

Most guidelines suggest the use of steroids in an exacerbation when the child does not respond to one inhaled SABA treatment. Prednisone, prednisolone, or dexamethasone are the most common corticosteroids administered for asthma exacerbation in children.[59] However, in the study of the protocols of 34 states, there were only two states that included steroid use, including IV or oral.[21] It is difficult when pediatric patients are struggling to breathe to give oral medication effectively. Often, they will vomit because of gastric distention that is already present as they are struggling to breathe. Studies show that the earlier that steroids are administered, it reduces the symptoms and may even help prevent the need for hospital admission.[21]

Ipratropium bromide (Atrovent) is an anticholinergic medication used in children to promote bronchodilation without inhibiting mucociliary clearance. This medication has demonstrated its effectiveness in decreasing hospitalization rates and shortening the duration of a child's hospital stay.[21] Children presenting with severe exacerbation are often dehydrated because of poor oral intake and increased insensible losses from increased minute ventilation. The transport provider needs to consider a 20-mL/kg fluid bolus during transport and reassess. IV or subcutaneous terbutaline is a selective beta-2 agonist and may be used in the management of acute severe asthma exacerbation in children. It is important that the bolus is started or, even better, finished prior to administering magnesium sulfate as it can cause a decrease in blood pressure. Magnesium sulfate is a bronchodilator used in the treatment of severe asthma by blocking calcium channels in respiratory smooth muscle. Magnesium also depresses muscle fiber excitability by inhibiting acetylcholine release and promoting bronchodilatation. Magnesium can also have an anti-inflammatory effect.[54] According to Aniapravan et al., patients treated with magnesium sulfate have 66% less chance of requiring admission. Of the states that have prehospital protocols concerning the administration of

TABLE 18.7	Pediatric Asthma Scores: Tools Used to Assist the Provider in Classifying the Severity of Exacerbation		
	Preschool Respiratory Assessment Measure (PRAM)	**Pediatric Asthma Severity Score (PASS)**	**Pediatric Asthma Score (PAS)**
	• A reliable, valid, and responsive tool to measure severity of airway obstruction in children 2–17 years of age	• A valid, reliable tool that determines pediatric asthma severity based on the physical exam findings in children 1–18 years of age	• A measurement tool with excellent face validity and good inter-observer agreement for children >2 years of age
	• Measures suprasternal retractions, air entry, wheezing, respiratory rate, and oxygen saturation	• Is limited because it only measures three clinical measures: wheezing, prolonged expiration, and work of breathing	• Measures respiratory rate, oxygen saturation, auscultatory findings, retractions, and dyspnea

From Kline-Krammes S, Robinson S. Childhood asthma: a guide for pediatric emergency medicine providers. *Emerg Med Clin North Am.* 2013;31(3):705–732.

magnesium sulfate, the dose ranges from 25 mg/kg up to 50 mg/kg IV generally with a maximum dose of 2 g.[54] An additional treatment that may be used in children is leukotriene receptor antagonists, such as montelukast (Singulair), which block the production of natural mediators involved in bronchoconstriction. Singulair is a daily medication that is used in maintenance therapy. Heliox is a gas blend of 20% oxygen and 80% helium that may be used for asthma exacerbation in children. Heliox can reduce turbulent flow and increase laminar gas flow, which ultimately improves airflow resistance in small airways. Heliox improves particle dispersion of aerosol treatments in the distal lungs, which helps remove carbon dioxide and decrease the work of breathing in the child. If hypoxemia is present this therapy is not recommended, which severely limits its use as many of these patients are also hypoxic. An additional method used in severe exacerbation is noninvasive PPV (NiPPV) as an option to avoid intubation in children and improve their outcomes. ETI is indicated for children who are apneic or unresponsive and should be considered for those presenting with intractable hypoxemia, unresponsive respiratory acidosis, unresponsive to first-line asthma therapy medications, or worsening LOC.[36,48,50–55,57–59]

COVID-19

A new virus swept the world in 2019–20 and came to be known as SARS-CoV-2, or COVID-19. It was first identified in Wuhan, China in December 2019. Initially, it seemed to cause only mild,

if any, symptoms in the pediatric population.[60] Much like the disease itself, the first known reported pediatric cases originated in Shanghai, China in March 2020. Of the 2135 children affected, there were varying degrees of illness, with the majority (51%) having mild symptoms, 38% with moderate symptoms, and only 6% exhibiting severe symptoms such as hypoxia and respiratory failure.[61] Of the children affected by COVID-19, over 30% of them had other illnesses or comorbid conditions that perhaps predisposed them to be more susceptible to the infection.[61] There are various symptoms associated with COVID; most frequently, the child has some sort of respiratory symptoms (16%) followed by gastrointestinal symptoms (13.9%), rash (8.1%), and finally, neurologic symptoms (4.8%) (Table 18.8).[61] Of the children affected worst by COVID-19, two categories emerged. These cases were first identified in April of 2020.[60] The first was termed *severe acute COVID-19 illness* that, by definition, affected one or more organ systems, and then a small group emerged with what came to be known as a *multisystem inflammatory syndrome in children* (MIS-C).[60–64] According to the CDC, to meet the criteria for MIS-C, the patient must exhibit a fever, elevated inflammatory markers, multiple systems must be involved and recent SARS-CoV-2 infection (Table 18.8). Minority populations seemed more likely to be diagnosed with both severe acute COVID and MIS-C.[61]

Caring for a COVID-positive patient necessitates careful crew considerations, particularly regarding the use of appropriate personal protective equipment (PPE). The type of transport can pose

---

TABLE 18.8   Differentiation Between Severe Acute COVID and MIS-C

	Severe Acute COVID	MIS-C
Symptoms	• Younger age: 0–5 years old or 13–20 years old • Obesity or other risk factors such as chronic pulmonary, neurologic, and cardiovascular disease. Medically complex, sickle cell disease or immunosuppression • Hypoxia on admission • Increased WBCs, positive COVID test (RT-PCR), elevated CRP, procalcitonin, BNP and platelet count, LDH • Bilateral infiltrates on x-ray. CT is gold standard: 1st phase halo sign (nodules/masses) surrounded by ground glass; 2nd phase widespread ground glass; 3rd phase consolidative opacities	• Less than 21 years old (median age 8–11 years old) • Majority are previously healthy • Fever • Severe abdominal pain and vomiting • Elevated inflammatory markers (CRP), liver enzymes, D-dimer, ferritin, elevated BNP and troponin. Low levels of platelets and absolute lymphocyte count • Multisystem (>2) organs involved. GI most prevalent. Ventricular dysfunction • No alternative diagnoses • Positive for current or recent SARS-CoV-2 infection (within past 2–6 weeks) • Hypotension and shock • Black and Hispanic patients are more likely to have MIS-C than severe COVID
Treatment	• Baseline ECG should be obtained/chest x-ray, possibly CT • Manage acute respiratory failure-supplemental O$_2$, NIV, or intubation with mechanical ventilation • Adequate mean arterial BP without fluid overload • Inotropic support as needed • Intubation: RSI – phenylephrine/epinephrine in case of hemodynamic instability • Ventilator settings: lung protective strategies – tidal volume 5–7 mL/kg; PEEP – initial 8–10 cmH$_2$O. Titrate PEEP/FiO$_2$ for goal O$_2$ saturation 0.88–0.92 in severe ARDS • Goal: driving pressure <=15, peak pressure <28–32	• Resuscitation: cautious with fluids due to cardiac involvement • Broad-spectrum antibiotics • Vasopressor support (epinephrine or norepinephrine). The need for BP support is much more common in MIS-C as compared to severe COVID • Intubation: supportive, not usually pulmonary-related • IVIG • Corticosteroids • Anticoagulation • Low-dose aspirin • Biologic agents (anakinra) • Daily CBCs, BMP, D-dimer, troponin every 6 hr and BMP every 48 hr • ECG every 48 hr, ECHO every 1–2 weeks

ARDS, Acute respiratory distress syndrome; BMP, basic metabolic panel; BNP, brain natriuretic peptide; BP, blood pressure; CBC, complete blood count; CRP, C-reactive protein; CT, computed tomography; ECG, electrocardiogram; ECHO, echocardiogram; GI, gastrointestinal; IVIG, intravenous immunoglobulin; LDH, lactate dehydrogenase; MIS-C, multisystem inflammatory syndrome in children; NIV, non-invasive ventilation; PEEP, positive end-expiratory pressure; RSI, rapid sequence intubation; RT-PCR, reverse transcription polymerase chain reaction; WBC, white blood cells.

Modified from: Kalyanaraman M, Anderson MR. COVID-19 in children. *Pediatr Clin North Am.* 2022;69:547–571.

challenges in maintaining proper PPE. It is imperative to apply bacterial/viral filters to the expiratory circuit when a patient is intubated. Employing a closed ventilator circuit with inline suctioning is crucial for safeguarding crew members from potential exposure.

Given the potential requirement for higher pressures, it is expedient to intubate using a cuffed endotracheal tube (ETT). Studies have indicated that administering paralytics during the initial 24–48 hours is beneficial.[62] This approach helps prevent patient–ventilator dyssynchrony, facilitates proning, and reduces the risk of elevated peak plateau pressures.

Escalation of care may include the use of inhaled nitric oxide (iNO), high-frequency oscillatory ventilation (HFOV), and even extracorporeal membrane oxygenation (ECMO).[63] From the literature reviews, the resiliency of pediatric patients shows that the mortality is low (2%), with the majority of children going on to recover.[60]

Croup

Croup is a common childhood upper airway viral infection called laryngotracheitis. It is the second most common cause of respiratory distress in younger children.[65] It usually occurs in children ages 6 months to 3 years of age and in the fall and winter months. Sporadic cases may occur any time of year in older children.[8,20,66]

Clinical Presentation

Croup symptoms mimic other respiratory diseases, requiring the pediatric provider to make the appropriate differential diagnosis to ensure proper and effective interventions. Croup resulting from a viral infection is most frequently caused by human parainfluenza type 1 and occasionally type 3. Diagnosis is usually determined from the history and physical examination. In most cases of viral croup, the symptoms are self-limiting and resolve on their own. Patients generally present with an upper respiratory tract infection, low-grade fever, and coryza. As the symptoms progress, inspiratory stridor may be present characterized by a barking cough with mild to moderate respiratory distress including nasal flaring, respiratory retractions, and stridor. The most reliable symptoms to establish the severity of the disease are stridor and severity of retractions, indicating narrowing of the subglottic area. A chest x-ray (CXR) will exhibit the "steeple" sign. If the inflammation extends to the bronchi, rhonchi and wheezing will be present. The provider must rule out epiglottitis and retropharyngeal abscesses because croup presentation is so similar. When assessing a child with suspected croup, it is essential to keep the child calm by allowing the parent to continue to hold the patient to prevent exacerbation of respiratory distress symptoms and excessive narrowing of the child's airway.[8,20,66] A small subset of these children may go on to be diagnosed with recurrent croup. This is unique in that it is not associated with a virus but is more of an anatomic issue of narrowing and these children tend to be older. These children are typically well and then suddenly develop stridor, usually at night.[67] These children typically have a rapid onset, unlike those with viral croup who typically have 2 days of minor illness leading up to their stridor. They also resolve quickly and it can tend to recur. These children may be evaluated by subspecialists who can fully investigate the symptoms and with further testing, include laryngoscopy, bronchoscopy, and esophagoscopy, and can develop a specialized plan of care.[67]

Treatment

The recommended treatment of choice for croup is a single dose of systemic corticosteroid. Steroids have been shown to reduce symptoms, reduce the number of hospital admissions, reduce the length of admission, and reduce the number of ICU admissions.[65] The current evidence supports using dexamethasone as the preferred steroid based on its longer half-life. Current evidence recommends nebulized epinephrine for children with moderate to severe croup. The provider must remember nebulized epinephrine has a 10- to 30-minute onset of action and a 2-hour or less duration and the child may rebound.[65] Of those states with prehospital respiratory distress protocols, 79% of them recommend racemic epinephrine administration. Twenty-six percent recommend the use of dexamethasone.[21] The time that dexamethasone takes to start reducing swelling is anywhere from 30 minutes to 6 hours, so keeping that in mind, it is not too unusual that a second or even more doses of racemic epinephrine may be required. Different facilities have varying protocols but studies have shown that the patient is more likely to be admitted if they receive more than one dose of racemic epinephrine. The study by Bagwell et al. found that those pediatric patients who did receive more than one breathing treatment were less likely to return to the emergency department within 7 days from their first visit.[65] On rare occasions, severe croup may exhibit upper airway edema or obstruction requiring endotracheal intubation for oxygenation and ventilation of the child.[8,31,66]

E-Cigarette or Vaping Product Use-Associated Lung Injury

E-cigarette or vaping product use-associated lung injury, also known as EVALI, is an illness that first became apparent in the middle of 2019.[68] E-cigarettes have been around in the United States since 2007 and were first marketed as a way to help those addicted to cigarettes be able to stop smoking. The marketing for these products could be argued to be directed toward youth because of the fruity flavors that appeal to them.[69] According to Kaslow et al., between 2019 and 2020, there has been an astonishing 1000% increase in the number of those in high school that have started using vapes and a 400% increase in middle schoolers.[70]

In the summer of 2019, health departments across the country started investigating what would become known as EVALI.[68–70] According to the Centers for Disease Control,[71] as of February 2020, there have been a total of 2807 people that have been diagnosed with EVALI and 68 deaths due to it.[71] It is unclear what causes the symptoms of EVALI. Some sources postulate that it is due to substances contained in the e-cigarette, whether it is THC variations or even heavy metals like chromium, nickel, or lead.[70] Regardless of the exact cause, the changes seen in the lungs show varying degrees of alveolar damage, pneumonitis, bronchiolitis, and organizing pneumonia.[69]

Clinical Presentation

These patients usually present with some form of respiratory complaint, whether it be cough, shortness of breath, or chest pain. The respiratory complaint is accompanied by an array of other symptoms such as fever, nausea, vomiting, or headache. Generally, these patients may be afraid to admit to vaping and it may be revealed when other diagnoses continue to be ruled out. When COVID became widespread, it was even more difficult to diagnose, as both COVID and EVALI can have similar signs and symptoms. To be diagnosed as EVALI, there must be some evidence, either on an x-ray or CT, of infiltrates or ground-glass opacities.[68] There have been reports of patients with seemingly normal chest x-rays but then abnormalities show up on CT. These patients also have abnormal pulmonary function tests and of those that had bronchoscopies, the majority of them had inflammatory cells as well as lipid-laden macrophages.[72] Their blood work may show signs of inflammation with elevated LDH, CRP as well as leukocytosis.[72] Some of these patients also present with elevated bleeding times (PT, PTT, INR) as well as procalcitonin, D-dimer, and ferritin. COVID-19 should be ruled out by confirming a negative PCR as well as other respiratory viruses by completing a respiratory viral panel.[73] There must be a history of e-cigarette use within the past 90 days prior to the onset of symptoms as well as no other potential diagnoses based on the patient's medical history, in order to be diagnosed with EVALI, according to the CDC.[71]

Treatment

On transport, supporting their respiratory system will be key, whether they just require a nasal cannula to HFNC or even intubation. It is difficult to state what the typical treatment is as there need to be further widespread studies concerning EVALI and how best to treat it. High-dose steroids are used to help blunt the body's inflammatory response. While not all sources agree on the use of steroids or for how long, they are commonly used. Tapering of the steroids is important as not adhering to this has been shown to necessitate readmission.[70] It is important to educate the patient on the importance of avoiding vaping in the future. Patients should follow up shortly after discharge, within 24–48 hours, as a small percentage of them may require readmission, especially if there is not compliance with discharge instructions.[70]

Epiglottitis

Epiglottitis is a rare bacterial infection of the supraglottic larynx, which is the area of the larynx superior to the vocal folds. If not recognized and treated properly, it becomes a potentially life-threatening condition. Epiglottitis primarily affects children 2–6 years of age before the introduction of the conjugated *Haemophilus influenzae* type B (Hib) vaccine. Epiglottis may be seen in older children and adults presenting with atypical symptoms. Epiglottitis risk factors include lack of immunity for Hib and immunodeficiency.[8,31]

Clinical Presentation

A child presenting with epiglottitis has a toxic appearance with a history of rapid onset of symptoms of high fever, noisy breathing, sore throat, and inability to tolerate secretions. Epiglottitis is second only to croup as a cause for infectious stridor and muffled voice. Presenting symptoms include fever, drooling, or spitting up of secretions caused by supraglottic edema and suprasternal and subcostal retractions. The child presents anxious and in the classic tripod positioning by leaning forward with arms extended for support and jaw thrust forward or in the sniffing position with head up, neck forward with mouth open to maintain the airway. These positions help increase air entry. Altered mental status, mottled skin and cyanosis are impending signs of airway obstruction and circulatory collapse. The provider must be able to recognize these signs because of the potential for life-threatening airway obstruction.[8,31]

Treatment

Assessing a patient with suspected epiglottitis is rapid, with the patient remaining in a position of comfort, usually in the parent's lap, and never forced to change positions or become agitated. Obtain a history from the parents on time of onset of symptoms, any sick contacts, immunization status, medications, and their last meal. The provider must be prepared to secure the airway if necessary. The most qualified personnel available to secure the airway in the event of an acute obstruction should be called to the bedside. Noninvasive monitoring can usually be applied without upsetting the patient. The presence of hypoxia may represent impending airway obstruction. The toxic-appearing patient must have their airway secured by an anesthesiologist or the ear, nose, and throat physician before any other intervention should be completed such as laboratory work or obtaining IV access. A lateral neck x-ray may help rule out other causes of stridor and respiratory distress. An edematous epiglottis will have a "thumb print" appearance on a lateral neck x-ray if epiglottitis is present. The aryepiglottic folds may also appear enlarged. Airway management, if possible, should be performed in the operating room. Because of the high risk of this procedure, the plan for securing the airway is discussed with the most experienced physician providers available and they are the only ones allowed to intervene. Securing the airway is a critical procedure requiring equipment for endotracheal intubation, cricothyroidotomy and tracheostomy and it must be ready and in the patient's room. If the airway cannot be secured by intubation and the patient begins to deteriorate, the provider must be prepared to do a tracheostomy. Once the airway is secured, obtain cultures and begin third-generation cephalosporins; ceftriaxone and cefotaxime are the treatment of choice because they are able to eliminate Hib infection.[8,31]

Foreign Body Aspiration

Foreign body aspiration (FBA) is a common pediatric emergency and a significant cause of morbidity and mortality in children. FBA is the sixth most common cause of accidental deaths in children. FBA occurs when a foreign object is accidentally lodged anywhere within a child's respiratory tract. Seventy percent of FBA occurs in children 3 years of age and younger, with the peak incidence at 2 years of age. Factors increasing the risk for aspiration include immature dentition, poor chewing ability and swallowing coordination, the epiglottis positioned higher, the ease with which toddlers and infants are distracted, talking or crying while eating, and oral exploration. Organic foreign bodies such as nuts and grapes are the most common types of items aspirated by children. Other organic items include food, food-related items, fruits, and bones. The most common inorganic foreign objects aspirated are coins, pins, beads, small toy parts, small batteries, and pen caps. Organic foreign objects produce an inflammatory response and may make the obstruction worse and shorten the asymptomatic period. The inorganic foreign objects may remain asymptomatic for longer periods.[74-79]

Button batteries are smooth, shiny, and appealing to young children, and the incidence of battery foreign body ingestion has increased 80% over the last 10 years in young children. An ingested battery can pass the esophagus and remain uneventful through the gastrointestinal (GI) system. However, the complications can be devastating if the battery becomes lodged in the esophagus or nasal cavity. Once the battery is impacted in either the esophagus or nasal cavity it releases a toxic alkaline solution causing significant liquefactive necrosis in the surrounding tissues. Full thickness injury can occur in as little as 15 minutes.[80] Button battery aspiration or ingestions should be considered a medical emergency.[74–83]

Clinical Presentation

Foreign objects are aspirated into the right mainstem bronchus most often followed by the left mainstem bronchus; the trachea; the larynx; and finally, both bronchi. Upper airway aspiration or ingestion may cause a mechanical obstruction of the airway with asphyxiation if it becomes lodged in the larynx. There is a 45% mortality rate if the larynx is completely obstructed. Balloons are the most common cause of mortality in children. The transport providers must consider FBA or ingestion as a differential diagnosis when a child presents without any symptoms or presents with acute onset of respiratory symptoms regardless of the initial lack of evidence to support it when the physical examination and CXR are normal. The most sensitive predictor of a true FBA in a child is a positive history or witnessed event from the parents. Choking or coughing has a high sensitivity associated with a proven FBA or ingestion. Physical examination of a child with suspected FBA is not as sensitive as a positive history. Only 40% of children will present with the classic triad of symptoms such as choking, coughing, and unilateral wheezing or decreased air entry, which indicates that the foreign object is in the bronchial tree.[74–83]

Most children who present with FBA or ingestion are often not witnessed. The clinical presentation of children suspected of FBA will depend on the location of the foreign object. Tracheal FBA may present with various levels of respiratory distress, stridor, or an acute life-threatening obstruction. The most common symptom is paroxysmal cough, which is a natural defense response to remove the foreign body from the airway. Other clinical symptoms include stridor, cyanosis, unilateral decreased air entry, fever, wheezing, and dyspnea.[74–83]

Children may present with *upper airway obstruction* from an FBA with stridor, hoarseness, drooling, and some degree of respiratory distress depending on the location of the aspirated foreign object. *Lower airway obstruction* in children may present with wheezing and unilateral decreased breath sounds on the affected side in children with FBA. Persistent coughing can present in both upper and lower airway obstructions as well.[74–83]

FBA or ingestion necessitates prompt diagnosis and management. Delaying the diagnosis for more than 24 hours is associated with a 2.5 times increased risk of serious acute complications. The delayed diagnosis of a foreign body may result in an unrelenting cough, recurrent pneumonia, atelectasis, emphysema, laryngeal edema, laryngeal trauma, and hypoxic encephalopathy. Additional complications include pneumothorax, hydropneumothorax, pneumomediastinum, subcutaneous emphysema, pleural thickening, bronchiectasis, bronchial stenosis, or pulmonary abscess.[74–83]

The most common signs and symptoms of button battery aspiration or ingestion include vomiting, difficulty feeding, mild abdominal pain, cough, and bloody nasal discharge. Button battery ingestion and impaction is misdiagnosed as an upper respiratory tract infection in the absence of a history of battery ingestion. The damage caused by button batteries is a result of the alkalinity of the object. Some studies have shown that administering honey or sucralfate is helpful in that they are mild acids and can help neutralize, thereby protecting the esophagus until the object can be emergently removed.[80] A magnet is another object increasingly being ingested by young children. Most magnets are smooth and will pass through the GI tract without complications; however, multiple magnets attract each other and will attract through different loops of the bowel causing the movement to stop and potentially cause mural pressure necrosis leading to bowel perforation, fistula formation, volvulus, obstruction, abdominal sepsis, and ultimately, death.[74–83]

Treatment

If a child presents with complete obstruction, emergent airway procedures must be initiated. This may include the Heimlich maneuver, jaw thrust chin lift maneuver, and opening nasal or oral airways. If these procedures do not improve the child's respiratory distress, direct laryngoscopy may be required to either remove the foreign body with Magill forceps or to place an ETT past the obstruction. If unable to remove the object, the provider may need to push the object past the point of obstruction where it can be retrieved by bronchoscopy. If all of these interventions are unsuccessful, an emergent cricothyroidotomy or tracheostomy is essential to prevent morbidity or mortality in the child. Partial airway obstructions in a child with FBA are more common than the complete obstruction of the child's airway. These children should be treated as if they are heading for an emergency. Allow these children to remain with their parents and in a position of comfort while preparing for an emergent intervention should the airway become completely obstructed. Preparation includes preparing intubation equipment for airway management such as the bag and mask, ETTs, stylet, and Magill forceps for foreign body removal, and set up for an emergent needle or surgical cricothyroidotomy.[74–83]

The emergent treatment of FBA is based on the child's presentation with or without symptoms. It is imperative to obtain a history of possible FBA in a child, physical examination, and CXR. If there is a lack of clinical symptoms, additional diagnostic testing is required to confirm FBA in children. If an object is radiopaque it will be easily seen on CXR, but not all foreign objects are radiotransparent. The indirect findings on CXR, if the object is not radiopaque, will be overinflation, atelectasis, lung infiltrates, or consolidation. Normal CXRs have been found in 30% of children presenting with FBA. A multidetector computed tomography (MDCT) with virtual bronchoscopy is a noninvasive diagnostic tool that may be used. The disadvantage is the radiation exposure the child will endure from the CT. The rigid bronchoscopy was the procedure of choice in the past for retrieval of foreign objects in children and was considered the gold standard treatment for children. The disadvantage of this modality is that the child requires general anesthesia and the inability to reach the peripheral airways. The most popular modality currently used is the flexible bronchoscopy to remove foreign objects in children and as a diagnostic indicator. This treatment is relatively easy and safer than a rigid bronchoscopy and only requires local anesthesia. The flexible bronchoscopy is able to reach the distal airways to remove the foreign object, remove mucous or blood plugs, and allow bronchoalveolar lavage and vacuum aspiration if necessary. The only limitation of the flexible bronchoscopy is if the foreign object is too large to pass through the scope or the forceps are unable to grasp the object.[74–83]

Bronchiolitis

Bronchiolitis is the most common lower respiratory tract infection affecting infants and toddlers. It is the leading cause of pediatric admissions related to respiratory diseases for children under the age of one.[84] It is an acute infection with an inflammatory component resulting in obstruction of the small airways. Bronchiolitis typically occurs in children between the ages of 0 and 24 months of age with peak incidence occurring at 3–6 months of age. It is diagnosed clinically with the primary symptoms of difficulty breathing, coryza, poor feeding, coughing, rhinorrhea, and wheezing on auscultation. It is important to note that neonates may present as having had a brief resolved unexplained event, or BRUE, with apnea and cyanosis.[85] Bronchiolitis is associated with viral infections with the most common being RSV, which aligns seasonally beginning in the winter through to the spring typically. The seasonal aspect of bronchiolitis has changed since the COVID-19 pandemic. Children's hospitals are now seeing it year-round, including the summer.[85] The typical patterns of infection, including RSV and flu, have been altered since 2020. Additional viruses associated with bronchiolitis include rhinovirus, parainfluenza, adenovirus, metapneumovirus, and *Mycoplasma*. Bronchiolitis caused by rhinovirus infects the lower respiratory tract and can trigger asthma exacerbation in children. This viral pathogen is associated with a higher morbidity.[84–86]

Clinical Presentation

The incubation period for bronchiolitis caused by RSV is between 2 and 8 days; children will shed this virus for 3–8 days and infants have been found to shed RSV for up to 4 weeks. Bronchiolitis presents with a 1- to 3-day history with signs and symptoms of upper respiratory tract infection including nasal congestion or discharge, cough, and low-grade fever; after the third day of wheezing, signs of respiratory distress with increased work of breathing and retractions are seen. Bronchiolitis patients have a higher fever with the causative agent adenovirus compared with RSV in children. Presenting signs and symptoms typically include tachypnea, mild intercostal and subcostal retractions, expiratory wheezing, prolonged expiratory phase with coarse or fine crackles on auscultation, and hypoxemia, which is present with oxygen saturations less than 93%. The child's clinical course may be mild in severity or severe with signs of apnea and deteriorating respiratory status requiring hospitalization. The severity of bronchiolitis is determined after an assessment of the child's fluid status, tachypnea, nasal flaring, retractions, grunting, cyanosis, change in LOC, and apnea.[86–88]

Treatment

Bronchiolitis diagnosis is determined based on patient history and physical findings. Treatment of bronchiolitis is based on the infant or toddler's signs and symptoms and is supportive. The goal of therapy is to maintain adequate oxygenation and hydration. Infants having difficulty eating will need to have IV fluids for hydration or a nasogastric tube for feeds. An infection of the airway in infants and young children increases the risk of respiratory failure because infants are obligate nasal breathers. Infants exhibiting respiratory distress may require supplemental oxygen to maintain oxygen saturations higher than 90%. Evidence supports nasal suctioning of children with bronchiolitis but not deep suctioning of the pharynx or larynx, to provide temporary relief. Bronchodilator use with bronchiolitis is controversial, and the evidence demonstrates inconsistent improvement when using bronchodilator therapy. Steroids may be given to potentially assist with reducing airway inflammation and edema. Additional treatments for bronchiolitis include nebulized 3% saline but the most recent evidence has not shown conclusive improvement when treated with hypertonic saline.[84,85] There has been increased usage of high-flow nasal cannula (HFNC) with the delivery of heated and humidified oxygen from 8 to 40 L/min. Typically, flow rates for HFNC should not exceed 2 L/kg. If a higher flow is needed, the child will likely need admission to a pediatric intensive care unit where they can be closely monitored for further deterioration. The goal for oxygen saturation in these patients is also variable, depending on which recommendation is followed. In general, the low is 90% with a median of 92% recommended.[84] The clinical course is usually self-limiting, usually lasting 7–10 days in healthy children, and requires longer (up to 28 days) recovery time for those children with preexisting conditions or premature infants. An increased risk for severe bronchiolitis occurs in premature infants, those less than 36 weeks' gestation, infants less than 12 weeks of age, and children with preexisting illnesses such as congenital heart disease (CHD) or chronic lung disease. Children in severe distress who are unresponsive to treatment may need endotracheal intubation and mechanical ventilation.[86–88]

Pneumonia

Community-acquired pneumonia (CAP) is a major cause of mortality and the leading cause of hospitalization in children 5 years of age or younger. The majority of pathogens detected are viral and include RSV, rhinovirus, adenovirus, parainfluenza, and coronaviruses (not COVID-19). RSV is the most common cause of pneumonia in children 2 years of age or younger. Rhinovirus is the next most common cause of pneumonia in children. Adenovirus, parainfluenza, and coronavirus are the next most common. Bacterial pathogens are also a source of pneumonia in children. The most common bacterial pathogens causing pneumonia in children less than 2 years of age include *Streptococcus pneumoniae*, group B streptococci, Gram-negative bacilli, *Staphylococcus aureus*, and *Chlamydia trachomatis*. The bacterial pathogens causing pneumonia in children 2–5 years of age include *S. pneumoniae* and *S. aureus*. The most common bacterial pathogens causing pneumonia in children older than 5 years of age include *S. pneumoniae* and *Mycoplasma pneumoniae*. The best prevention of pneumonia in children is vaccination.[89–91]

Clinical Presentation

The World Health Organization (WHO) considers a diagnosis of CAP when a previously healthy child presents with signs of lung disease caused by an infection acquired outside of the hospital. Clinical signs of pediatric pneumonia are nonspecific in mild to moderate pneumonia in young children, making it difficult to diagnose, which leads to unnecessary antibiotic therapy. Refer to Table 18.9 for risk factors and signs and symptoms of community-acquired pneumonia.[92]

CXRs are not effective in differentiating viral and bacterial CAP or mild to moderate infection. Pneumonia, bronchiolitis, and reactive airway disease in children have similarities in clinical presentation and CXRs in children less than 5 years of age.[89–92]

Treatment

There has been a significant diversity in the use of diagnostic tests and antibiotic selection and use for CAP in children. The Pediatric Infectious Diseases Society and the Infectious Diseases Society of America developed guidelines in 2011 for the clinical management of CAP in the pediatric population, and these have been accepted by the American Academy of Pediatrics (AAP) and the American College of Emergency Physicians (ACEP). These guidelines were established to promote appropriate diagnostic testing

TABLE 18.9	Community-Acquired Pneumonia (CAP) in Children
Factors associated with incidence and severity	• Prematurity • Congenital heart disease • Gastroesophageal reflux disease • Reactive airway disease • Smoke exposure • Neuromuscular disease • Immunosuppressed • Malnutrition • Underweight • Low socioeconomic status • Childcare attendance

Common physical findings	• Initial physical findings (key in clinical diagnosis of CAP)
	  • Fever
	  • Tachypnea (most significant clinical sign in children)
	  • Increased work of breathing
	  • Breath sounds: crackles, rhonchi, wheezing
	  • Coughing
	• Indicators for hospitalization
	  • Oxygen sats <92%
	  • Delayed capillary refill
	  • Lethargy
	  • Decrease LOC

Diagnostic testing	• Chest x-ray (CXR)
	  • Often used to diagnose CAP
	  • CXR or ultrasound rule out effusions
	  • Pleural effusions are most significant predictor of bacterial pneumonia
	  • Alveolar infiltrate suggests bacterial over viral
	  • Interstitial infiltrates may be viral or bacterial
	• Lab work
	  • CRP, CBC/D, procalcitonin, ESR (limited use in bacterial diagnosis of CAP)
	  • Nasopharyngeal swab: PCR assay (tests for eight respiratory viruses)
	  • Tracheal aspirate (limited use in diagnosis)
	  • Blood cultures (studies indicate cultures do not change management)

Antibiotic treatment	• Amoxicillin
	  • First choice for children 60 days of age to 5 years of age
	• Azithromycin (Zithromax)
	  • For patients allergic to penicillin or beta-lactam antibiotics
	  • Children 5–16 years
	• Clarithromycin (Biaxin)
	• Erythromycin

Supportive care	• Acetaminophen (Tylenol) or ibuprofen (Motrin) used to treat additional symptoms accompanying CAP in children
	  • Fever
	  • Localized and referred pain in the chest and/or abdomen
	  • Headache
	  • Arthralgia

CBC/D, complete blood count with differential; *CRP*, C-reactive protein; *ESR*, erythrocyte sedimentation rate; *LOC*, level of consciousness; *PCR*, polymerase chain reaction.
From Koppolu, R., Simone S. *Medical and surgical management of pediatric pneumonia.* https://www.napnap.org/sites/default/files/userfiles/education/2015SpeakerHO/213-%20 Koppolu%20%26%20Simone.pdf; 2016.

and a reduction in excessive use of broad-spectrum antibiotics in pediatric patients with CAP. The pediatric CAP guidelines recommend not obtaining diagnostic laboratory work or radiographic imaging as well as reducing or preventing excessive use of broad-spectrum antibiotics in children presenting with mild to moderate CAP in the ambulatory care setting. This includes not routinely obtaining blood cultures in children who are fully immunized and are nontoxic. A strong recommendation is that CXRs are not necessary for suspected CAP unless presenting with respiratory distress with hypoxemia, or for children who failed to improve after initial antibiotic treatment. These guidelines do recommend diagnostic testing, including complete blood count; C-reactive protein (CRP); procalcitonin; influenza and viral polymerase chain reaction (PCR) testing, which screens for influenza A and B; parainfluenza 1, 2, and 3; adenovirus; RSV; and human metapneumovirus. Also recommended are a blood culture as well as a CXR along with the initiation of narrow-spectrum antibiotics for children presenting with moderate to severe CAP.[89–96] The goal is to use the narrowest spectrum antibiotic for the shortest effective time.[97]

The treatment approach for pediatric pneumonia primarily revolves around providing supportive care. When a child exhibits mild respiratory distress with oxygen saturations below 92%, the initial step is to commence oxygen therapy using a nasal cannula. However, if there is a moderate increase in the effort required for breathing, nasal cannula alone may not suffice. These patients might display signs of atelectasis, and restrictive or obstructive lung issues, with oxygen saturations at 90% or lower while breathing room air or through a nasal cannula. In such cases, additional support, such as high-flow nasal cannula (HFNC) or Vapotherm, may be necessary, particularly in a hospital setting.

Certain pediatric specialty teams can transport patients while providing heated HFNC. It is crucial to choose the appropriate cannula size, and the initial flow rate typically starts at 2 L/min/ kg, with a maximum flow rate of around 15 L. Commencing with a higher flow rate may facilitate a quicker weaning process, both in terms of flow and FiO_2. Starting HFNC therapy earlier in the treatment process may help circumvent the need for escalated support measures such as noninvasive ventilation or intubation.

If the patient deteriorates and advances to severe respiratory distress or failure with tachypnea, apnea, hypoxia, or fatigue, they may require noninvasive ventilation or advanced airway management with an ETT and mechanical ventilation.

Children with CAP may need fluid resuscitation or hydration and need IV access because of their inability to take fluids by mouth caused by their respiratory status or insensible fluid losses. It is necessary to obtain blood cultures if initiating antibiotics in these patients. Patients who present with moderate to severe respiratory distress, worsening respiratory status, toxic appearance, have changes in LOC, fail to respond to antibiotics, dehydration, and are less than 6 months of age should be admitted to the hospital.[89–96,98]

Pertussis

Pertussis or whooping cough is an endemic, vaccine-preventable, highly contagious disease. It is caused by *Bordetella pertussis*, which is a Gram-negative coccobacillus that is a highly contagious acute infection of the human respiratory tract responsible for a significant increase in morbidity and mortality, especially in infants younger than 6 months of age. According to the CDC, children are considered fully vaccinated once they have received five doses of DTaP (2, 4, 6 months, between 15 and 18 months, and then between 4 and 6 years of age) or four doses if the fourth dose was administered on or after the fourth birthday.[99] Pertussis usually spreads to susceptible individuals through respiratory droplets aerosolized through paroxysms of coughing or sneezing by those infected who are in close contact. Most infants are infected by their parents or siblings. If pertussis is suspected, an important question for the transport team to ask would be if the parent's immunizations are up to date. Pertussis is commonly referred to as whooping cough or the 100-day cough. The incidence of pertussis is highest among infants, children 7–10 years of age, and adolescents in the United States. Despite widespread vaccination, the incidence of pertussis has increased dramatically over the past 25 years with identified contributing factors being parental refusal of immunizations and potential waning immunity after acellular pertussis vaccinations.[100–102]

Clinical Presentation

The most common clinical signs of pertussis infections are prolonged and paroxysmal coughing and inspiratory stridor, which makes the classic whooping cough sound. A pertussis diagnosis is difficult in young children and may go unrecognized when coinfections are present, such as RSV and adenovirus. The classic presentation of pertussis includes paroxysms of coughing, an inspiratory whoop, and post-tussive emesis. These classic symptoms occur as a primary infection in unvaccinated children younger than 10 years of age. It may also occur in vaccinated children and adults, but the symptoms are usually not as severe.

Pertussis, the cough of 100 days, is divided into three stages. The catarrhal stage presents with symptoms similar to an upper viral respiratory infection with a cough and coryza, and fever is uncommon or low grade. The cough in this stage gradually increases in severity instead of improving, and the coryza remains the same. This stage usually lasts 1 to 2 weeks. The risk of transmission is greatest during the catarrhal stage. In the second, or paroxysmal stage, the coughing spells increase in severity. The paroxysmal cough is distinctive with a long series of coughs with little or no inspiratory effort. The child may gag, become cyanotic, or appear to be struggling to breathe. The whoop noise is forced inspiratory effort following a coughing spell and is not always present. Post-tussive emesis is common, especially in children younger than 1 year of age. Infants develop severe complications including failure to thrive (FTT), apnea, respiratory failure, seizure, and death. The paroxysmal stage usually lasts 2–8 weeks with the coughing episodes increasing in frequency during the first couple of weeks. It remains the same for 2–3 weeks, and then the coughing will gradually decrease. The convalescent stage is when the cough subsides and lasts over several weeks to months.[100–104]

Treatment

When a case of pertussis is identified, all exposed individuals should be notified and offered preventative treatment if necessary. This preventative treatment should include the team that transported the patient. Supportive care is the primary management for pertussis. Antibiotic therapy is imperative, or the child will remain contagious throughout the majority of the illness. Treatment with antibiotics is important for infants younger than 6 months of age because they have an increased risk for severe complications. Pertussis is identified by either a pertussis culture or positive PCR within 6 weeks of cough onset in children less than 1 year, or 3 weeks of cough onset in children older than 1 year. The initiation of antibiotic therapy should be started based on

clinical suspicion and not waiting on laboratory confirmation since it may take up to a week for the result. The most common antibiotic used to treat pertussis is azithromycin. Consider admitting children less than 6 months of age to the hospital because they have an increased risk of severe or fatal pertussis.[100–104]

Anaphylaxis

Anaphylaxis is a serious and potentially life-threatening systemic reaction in children occurring after contact with an allergy-triggering substance. The systems affected include cutaneous, mucosal (80%–90%), respiratory (70%), cardiovascular (45%), GI (45%), and central nervous systems ([CNS] 15%). The incidence of allergic or anaphylactic reactions in the pediatric population is increasing annually. It is imperative for prehospital providers to rapidly assess, diagnose, and treat anaphylaxis appropriately to decrease mortality and morbidity in the pediatric population.[105,106]

Clinical Presentation

Anaphylaxis is a clinical diagnosis. A complete blood count and a comprehensive metabolic panel have been long established as unreliable and not practical in identifying anaphylaxis in children. The three most common allergens causing anaphylaxis in children are food (e.g., tree nuts, peanuts, fish, shellfish, eggs, fruits, dairy products), medications (e.g., penicillin), and insect stings and bites (e.g., honeybees, bumblebees, yellow jackets, hornets, wasps). Refer to Table 18.10 for signs and symptoms of pediatric anaphylaxis.[105–107]

Treatment

Initial treatment of the pediatric patient experiencing anaphylaxis begins with a quick, thorough assessment of the child's airway, breathing, and circulation and rapid administration of intramuscular (IM) epinephrine, which is the treatment for controlling symptoms and decreasing morbidities and mortalities. Epinephrine is the drug of choice for treating pediatric anaphylaxis and should be given as soon as a diagnosis is suspected. If administered prior to arrival at the hospital, it is less likely that the patient will require hospital admission and require less time of observation in the ER.[108] The initial recommended dose of epinephrine is 0.01 mg/kg of a 1:1000 solution IM, such as in the child's thigh. The max for children is 0.3 mg and for adolescents it is 0.5 mg. This dose may be repeated every 5–15 minutes. Even though most patients experiencing anaphylaxis respond to one or two doses of epinephrine, the prehospital provider must be prepared for advanced airway management in a child experiencing an anaphylactic reaction because deterioration in respiratory status may occur quickly. If the child does not respond to epinephrine and upper airway edema occurs, rapid sequence intubation medications are not recommended, and if unable to place an ETT, the child may require a needle cricothyroidotomy. Capnography use during transport assists in detecting early ventilatory changes in children with anaphylaxis, because hypoxemia may be a late sign of impending airway compromise in children.[105–107,109] Some additional treatments for anaphylaxis, once epinephrine has been administered, are antihistamines and both H_1 and H_2 blockers. In addition, steroids, bronchodilators, and fluids may also be given to help blunt the effects of the reaction.[110]

Metabolic Acidosis

Metabolic acidosis is a common finding in pediatric patients. The anion gap (AG) is used to classify pediatric causes of metabolic

TABLE 18.10	Signs and Symptoms of Pediatric Anaphylaxis

Signs and Symptoms

Cutaneous/mucosa	• Urticaria (hives)
	• Angioedema
	• Flushing
	• Pruritus
	   • Periorbital
	   • Lips, tongue, palate
	   • Throat, uvula

Upper respiratory	• Stridor • Dysphonia • Hoarseness • Swollen lips, tongue, or palate • Sneezing • Rhinorrhea • Bronchospasm • Upper airway obstruction
Cardiovascular	• Chest pain • Tachycardia • Bradycardia • Hypotension • Dysrhythmias • Cardiac arrest
Gastrointestinal	• Abdominal pain • Nausea, vomiting • Diarrhea
Central nervous system	• Sense of impending doom • Fussy, irritable • Drowsy, decreased LOC • Dizziness • Confusion • Headache • Anxiety

Treatment Options

1st-line therapy	• Epinephrine IM (anterolateral thigh)
2nd-line therapy	• Antihistamines • Corticosteroids • Aggressive fluid resuscitation

IM, Intramuscular; *LOC*, level of consciousness.
Data from Tiyyagura GK, Arnold L, Cone DC, Langhan M. Pediatric anaphylaxis management in the prehospital setting. *Prehosp Emerg Care*. 2014;18(1):46–51; and Zilberstein J, McCurdy MT, Winters ME. Anaphylaxis. *J Emerg Med*. 2014;47(2):182–187.

TABLE 18.11	Pediatric Causes of Metabolic Acidosis

Large Anion Gap	Normal Anion Gap	Small Anion Gap

MUDPILES
M = methanol
U = uremia or chronic
   renal failure
D = diabetic ketoacidosis
P = propylene glycol
I = infection, inborn
   errors or metabolism
L = lactic acidosis
E = ethanol
S = salicylates
	Renal tubular
	   acidosis
	Vomiting
	Diarrhea
	Addison's disease
	Acetazolamide
	Enteric fistulas
		Hypoalbuminemia
		Nephrotic
		   syndrome

Data from Kher K, Sharron M. Approach to the child with metabolic acidosis. In: UpToDate, July 2016. Kim MS (ed.), UpToDate, Waltham, MA. https://www.uptodate.com/contents/approach-to-the-child-with-metabolic-acidosis#H628739007; 2016.

obvious clinical finding in acute metabolic acidosis caused by respiratory compensation is tachypnea. In metabolic acidosis, respiratory compensation results in a lower PCO_2 and will raise the pH in the direction of normal. Inadequate compensatory response may be an indication of unrecognized respiratory insufficiency, disease, or impending failure. Metabolic acidosis is diagnosed by obtaining a blood gas with a pH less than 7.35, a decrease in blood HCO_3 levels, and a decrease in PCO_2 with respiratory compensation. A 1-mmHg decrease in PCO_2 usually results in a 1 mmol/L decrease in HCO_3 levels. Identifying the cause of metabolic acidosis is essential in guiding treatment options. Initial evaluation includes a detailed history, physical examination, and basic laboratory testing, and with the initial diagnostic tests, an AG is needed. Identification and management of the underlying cause of metabolic acidosis is essential and needs to occur quickly. Pediatric causes of metabolic acidosis are listed in Table 18.11.[8,111]

Endocrine and Metabolic Emergencies

Children presenting with a suspected endocrine or metabolic disorder are a challenge for providers if there is no underlying condition because the signs and symptoms of these disorders are nonspecific and similar to those seen in children experiencing other emergencies. These nonspecific symptoms may lead to a delayed or missed diagnosis resulting in serious morbidities and mortalities such as cerebral dysfunction leading to coma or death, which may be seen in diabetic ketoacidosis (DKA), hypoglycemia, or adrenal insufficiency. Refer to Table 18.12 for signs and symptoms common to these emergencies.[112,113]

Hypoglycemia

Hypoglycemia is when the blood glucose concentration is 60 mg/dL or lower, with alterations in LOC occurring with 50 mg/dL in plasma and 44 mg/dL in whole blood. If hypoglycemia continues beyond 48 hours, it requires an evaluation of the underlying cause. The causes of hypoglycemia are age-dependent. Hypoglycemia in children from birth to 6 months of age is the result of an increase in glucose utilization as seen with hyperinsulinism, small-for-gestation age infants, asphyxiated neonates, infants born to diabetic

acidosis. The AG is usually calculated as the difference between sodium (Na^+), a major cation, and the major measured anions chloride (CL^-) and bicarbonate (HCO_3^-) using the following formula: AG (mEq/L) = (Na^+) – (Cl^- + HCO_3^-). An elevated AG is caused by an increase in unmeasured anions such as lactate or beta-hydroxybutyrate in the blood. AG can also be elevated with hypokalemia, hypocalcemia, or hypomagnesium. In newborns, an elevated AG is greater than 16 mEq/L, and in children, it is greater than 14 mEq/L.[8,111]

There are no clinical features of pediatric metabolic acidosis; instead, infants and children present with symptoms of their underlying condition. An example of this is lactic acidosis, which presents with signs and symptoms of sepsis or shock with poor tissue perfusion, cool extremities, and hypotension. The most

TABLE 18.12	Signs and Symptoms of Pediatric Endocrine and Metabolic Emergencies		
CNS Impairment	**Cardiovascular**	**Metabolic Acidosis**
• Lethargy • Irritability • Tremors • Seizures • Altered LOC • Coma • Hypotonia • Cheyne–Stokes respirations	• Tachycardia • Hypotension • Shock	• Kussmaul's respirations • Nausea • Vomiting • Poor feeding • Weight loss • Failure to thrive

LOC, Level of consciousness.
Data from Adramerina A, et al. How parents' lack of awareness could be associated with foreign body aspiration in children. *Pediatr Emerg Care.* 2016;32(2):98–100.

mothers, Beckwith–Wiedemann syndrome, defects in ketone production, carnitine deficiency, inadequate fat stores, infection, or fever. Causes of decreased hepatic glucose are enzyme deficiencies, inadequate glycogen stores, or liver failure. Children 6 months to adolescence experience hypoglycemia either from increased glucose utilization or decreased hepatic glucose production.[112,113]

Treatment

Initial labs are bedside glucose, serum glucose, liver function tests, electrolytes, and urinalysis including ketones. Hypoglycemia treatment is initially nonspecific until the underlying cause is identified. The goal is to restore normal glucose concentrations to support the CNS and renal metabolic needs of the child. Emergent treatment is usually 2–3 mL/kg of dextrose 10% and ongoing dextrose infusion 5%–20% to maintain euglycemia. It is important to note that the maximum dextrose concentration that should be given peripherally is 12.5%. Reassess glucose levels after interventions. More intensive laboratory work is required to diagnose the underlying cause if it continues beyond the first 48 hours of life.[112,113]

Adrenal Insufficiency

Adrenal insufficiency causes are either central, which are abnormalities in the hypothalamus or pituitary gland, or primary to the adrenal glands. If a child is receiving steroids to treat asthma, leukemia, organ transplantation, an autoimmune disorder, or replacement steroids for central or primary hypoadrenalism, they are at risk of an adrenal insufficiency crisis during an acute, febrile illness. Adrenal insufficiency from any cause results in the inability of the child to maintain electrolyte balance, plasma volume, blood pressure, and glucose levels when experiencing stress, and may have a fatal outcome without glucocorticoid replacement.[112,113]

Treatment

Children with adrenal insufficiency may exhibit weakness, anorexia, vomiting, weight loss, salt cravings, and hyperpigmentation. The child with adrenal insufficiency will present with tachycardia, hypotension, and signs of shock including pale color, poor perfusion, cool clammy skin, alterations in LOC, or coma. The comprehensive metabolic panel will demonstrate

adrenal insufficiency with hyponatremia, decreased bicarbonate, increased chloride level, a normal AG, metabolic acidosis, and a low glucose level. The initial treatment for children with adrenal insufficiency crisis is to restore tissue perfusion with a 20-mL/kg bolus of normal saline to treat hypotension or dehydration. Hypoglycemia is treated with a glucose bolus of 2–3 mL/kg of 10% dextrose and a stress dose of a glucocorticoid such as hydrocortisone 2–3 mg/kg.[112,113]

Hyponatremia

Hyponatremia is noted when serum Na^+ is less than 135 mEq/L. Causes of hyponatremia are considered to be disorders of sodium homeostasis when the movement of free water into the extracellular space surpasses its loss. Fundamental causes of hyponatremia include hypovolemia from renal losses caused by diuretics, mineralocorticoid deficiency, renal tubular dysfunction, cerebral salt wasting, vomiting, diarrhea, and burns. Other causes include nephrotic syndrome, acute or chronic renal failure, or water intoxication.[112,113]

Treatment

Initial signs and symptoms of hyponatremia are CNS changes from cerebral edema with anorexia, lethargy, or apathy, which may progress to the child being disoriented and agitated and experiencing seizures, Cheyne–Stokes respirations, hyporeflexia, and coma. Neuromuscular weakness and vomiting may be present. The comprehensive metabolic panel is the initial laboratory test. Hyponatremia treatment is usually initiated when the sodium level is below 125 with a hypertonic 3% saline solution of 1 mL/kg per hour IV infusion, which will correct the sodium level by 1 mEq/L per hour and monitor serum sodium levels during infusion.[112,113]

Hypernatremia

Hypernatremia is a disorder of water metabolism. The loss of free water from the kidneys or GI tract exceeding the loss of sodium will lead to hypernatremia. Osmotic diuresis, diabetes insipidus, gastroenteritis or excessive sodium intake either by mouth or intravenously will lead to hypernatremia. Patients with a normal thirst mechanism rarely experience hypernatremia.[112,113]

Treatment

The signs and symptoms of hypernatremia result from intracellular CNS dehydration. Rapid correction of hypernatremia may result in cerebral edema. It is recommended to correct the serum sodium level slowly by less than 0.5 mEq/L per hour to decrease any unwanted side effects. In hypovolemic children, isotonic 0.9% saline is used initially to correct fluid deficits over a 36- to 48-hour period of time and then transition over to 0.45% saline solution for maintenance. If the child is experiencing diabetes insipidus, then the drug of choice is desmopressin. If the child is in a hypervolemic state, such as those with Cushing's syndrome, then they will require diuretic therapy using hydrochlorothiazide.[112,113]

Diabetic Ketoacidosis

Diabetes mellitus is one of the most common pediatric and adolescent diseases worldwide. A major complication of diabetes is DKA, which is the leading cause of overall morbidity and mortality in children and adolescents with type 1 diabetes. Cerebral edema is the cause of morbidity and mortality in children with DKA. It is estimated that cerebral edema results in less than 1% of all DKA presentations, and 50%–60% of those children will not survive. DKA is characterized by the metabolic triad of hyperglycemia, AG metabolic acidosis, and ketonemia resulting from an absolute or relative insulin deficiency and an excess of counterregulatory hormone. DKA presents with hyperglycemia leading to osmotic urinary diuresis with subsequent dehydration. The body responds to dehydration by stimulating a stress response with counterregulatory hormone production, leading to greater insulin resistance, which results in a vicious cycle of hyperglycemia and continued fluid losses. Ultimately DKA causes severe dehydration and electrolyte abnormalities in these children.[114–117]

Clinical Presentation

DKA typically presents with the classic triad of symptoms of polyuria, polydipsia, and weight loss with or without polyphagia. Abdominal pain nausea and vomiting are also common presenting symptoms. Late signs and symptoms result in changes in mental status, Kussmaul respirations, and fruity, sweet-smelling breath. DKA is diagnosed if a child presents with hyperglycemia with a blood glucose level greater than 200 mg/dL, venous pH less than 7.3 or bicarbonate (HCO_3) concentration less than 15 mmol/L, ketonuria, and ketonemia. DKA severity has three different presenting categories: mild DKA presents with a venous pH less than 7.3 and HCO_3 less than 15 mmol/L, moderate DKA presents with venous pH less than 7.2 and HCO_3 less than 10 mmol/L, and severe DKA presentation is a venous pH less than 7.1 and HCO_3 less than 5 mmol/L.[114–117]

The goal of therapy for DKA is a reversal of the ketoacidosis and not the return of glucose levels to normal. Important initial labs are venous blood gas, complete blood count, comprehensive metabolic panel, and beta-hydroxybutyrate or urine ketones. Current practice guidelines recommend pediatric resuscitation if necessary in these patients, obtaining IV access, monitoring hourly vital signs, neurologic checks, monitoring blood glucose, and accurate fluid intake and output. Children with new-onset DKA younger than 5 years of age or with significant acidosis, hypocapnia, or azotemia are at a higher risk of developing cerebral edema. DKA management is fluid resuscitation to rehydrate and improve tissue perfusion and glomerular filtration rate, corrections of ketoacidosis and hyperglycemia through the inhibition of lipolysis and ketogenesis with insulin infusion, restoration of electrolyte balances, and the prevention of complications such as cerebral edema.[114–117]

Treatment

Initial fluid resuscitation in pediatric patients is a 10- to 20-mL/kg fluid bolus over 1–2 hours. This dose can be repeated if the patient is hemodynamically unstable. To prevent the risk of cerebral edema and herniation, fluid resuscitation must not go beyond 40–50 mL/kg in the first 4 hours of treatment. The total replacement fluids include both maintenance and deficit replacement fluids and should not exceed two times the maintenance rate.[114–117]

Initial replacement fluids are normal saline in pediatric DKA patients. Initially, no dextrose is in the replacement fluids, but as the hyperglycemia improves from the insulin infusion, a dextrose infusion is started and titrated to control the drop in the blood glucose levels while maintaining the insulin infusion. If the child's blood glucose is higher than 250 mg/dL, then replacement fluids

are only normal saline. Once the blood glucose level falls below 250 mg/dL, replacement fluids should change to a two-bag system with one being normal saline and the other 5% dextrose to slow the decline of the patient's blood glucose levels. If the patient's blood glucose falls below 150 mg/dL, then the dextrose should be changed to 10% solution.[114–117]

Rehydration alone can slowly drop the blood glucose levels in pediatric DKA patients, but an insulin infusion is essential to suppress the lipolysis and ketogenesis that controls DKA. Insulin infusion treatment is started after volume resuscitation has started and initial labs are obtained to know the patient's potassium level. Low-dose insulin infusion at 0.1 units/kg per hour is started and continues at this rate until the ketoacidosis has resolved. The patient's high glucose levels usually will improve or be close to normal before the acidemia resolves. Because of this, the insulin infusion must continue until the ketoacidosis is resolved with a pH greater than 7.3, HCO_3 greater than 15 mmol/L, beta-hydroxybutyrate less than 1 mmol/L, and closure of the AG. During fluid replacement for DKA patients, the dextrose fluids are titrated to prevent hypoglycemia from occurring while maintaining the insulin infusion. The fluids used for rehydration must also contain electrolytes to help replenish them, for example, potassium phosphate and potassium acetate.[118] It is imperative to monitor frequent blood glucose levels and the neurologic status of these children.[114–117]

Heart Disease

Congenital Heart Disease

Congenital heart disease (CHD) defects are those present at birth. These defects change the blood flow through the heart and may involve the interior walls of the heart, valves in the heart, or the arteries or veins that carry blood to or away from the heart. CHD may present as a simple heart defect without any presenting symptoms to complex heart defects presenting with life-threatening symptoms. CHD is now the most common type of birth defect. It is estimated that there are close to one million adolescents and young adults worldwide living with CHD.[119–122]

A universal screening tool for newborns for critical CHD is endorsed by the AAP, AHA, and the American College of Cardiology. The Centers for Disease Control and Prevention (CDC) reported in 2015 that almost all states have established legislation, regulations, or hospital guidelines supporting newborn screening for CHD. This tool was designed to screen newborns before discharge using pulse oximetry. Screening should be performed after 24 hours of life or as late as possible before discharging the patient home. Screening performed before 24 hours is not as reliable as later screening because the child may still be in transition from intrauterine to extrauterine conditions. A positive screen indicates the patient needs further evaluation to identify the cause and may require the child to be transferred to a designated center capable of treating CHD.[122]

Clinical Presentation

Acyanotic heart defects are defects in which oxygenated blood is shunted from the left (systemic) side of the heart to the right (pulmonary) side. Cyanotic heart defects are defects in which blood from the right (pulmonary) side of the heart mixes with oxygenated blood from the left (systemic) side and enters the systemic circulation. This defect will present itself within minutes of delivery to the first few weeks of life when the patent ductus arteriosus (PDA) closes. The PDA may provide the only means of pulmonary blood flow requiring prostaglandin E_1 (PGE) to be started. These defects may require a shunt in the newborn period. The mixing blood flow heart defects may require emergent surgical palliation or surgery to survive. Patients with mixing blood flow heart defects may present extremely ill with severe acidosis and in a shock state, for example, if the child is born with transposition of the great arteries (TGA) and has a patent septum and no septal defect is present. Total anomalous pulmonary venous return (TAPVR) defects are a surgical emergency if the veins are obstructed below the diaphragm and do not allow blood to return to the heart. The child born with a left ventricular outflow tract resulting in an obstruction to blood flow out of the heart will be critically ill if the ductus arteriosus has closed. Transport providers must remember that any neonate presenting in shock that is not responding to airway control, fluid resuscitation, and vasopressors has left ventricular outflow tract obstruction until proven otherwise, and PGE must be started immediately. Refer to Table 18.13 for signs and symptoms of CHD.[119–122]

Acquired Heart Disease

Acquired heart disease occurs after birth and is a result of damage to the heart from an inflammatory process affecting the endocardium, myocardium, pericardium, conduction system, or coronary arteries from a viral or bacterial infection.[119–121]

Kawasaki Disease

Kawasaki disease (KD) is the leading cause of acquired heart disease in children. There is no definitive test to diagnose KD. The hallmark of KD is a fever of at least 5 days, and the presence of four of these symptoms: conjunctivitis; erythema of the lips and oral mucosa; rash; unilateral cervical adenopathy; and erythema to the palms and soles, with induration and desquamation to the fingers. The goal of initial management is to reduce the inflammation and reduce the risk of coronary artery damage or aneurysms. Treatment in the acute phase includes aspirin and IV immunoglobulin.[119–121]

Myocarditis

Myocarditis is an inflammation of the cardiac muscle and the leading cause of dilated cardiomyopathy in children. Congestive heart failure (CHF) is the hallmark sign of myocarditis, and myocarditis is the most common cause of acute CHF. The child has a viral illness 10–14 days before onset of symptoms. Treatment is inotropes, afterload reducers, diuretics, antibiotics, and support therapy.[119–121]

TABLE 18.13	Congenital Heart Defects, Presenting Signs and Symptoms			
Classification	**Acyanotic Heart Defects**	**Cyanotic Heart Defects**	**Mixed Blood Flow Defects**	**Obstructive Blood Flow Defects**
PBF	Increased PBF	Decreased PBF	Mixed PBF	Left-sided obstructive blood flow
Shunt	Left-to-right shunting	Right-to-left shunting	Shunting direction depends on size and pressure in the lungs	Obstructed blood flow
Early signs	Tachypnea caused by excessive PBF	Cyanosis, may present at birth or in first few weeks of life when PDA closes PDA may be only source of PBF	May be a surgical emergency at birth if TGA does not have an ASD or large patent foramen ovale for mixing of blood It is also a surgical emergency in TAPVR if veins are obstructed	Must start PGE immediately or will quickly develop metabolic acidosis and shock if PDA closes
Congenital heart disease	PDA, ASD, VSD, atrioventricular canal defect (atrioventricular canal)	Tricuspid atresia, pulmonary atresia, tetralogy of Fallot, pulmonary stenosis, Ebstein's anomaly	TGA, TAPVR, truncus arteriosus	Coarctation of the aorta, aortic stenosis, interrupted aortic arch, hypoplastic left heart syndrome
Presenting signs and symptoms	Respiratory distress, diaphoresis with feeds or activity, poor weight gain, FTT, enlarged heart, pulmonary edema, CHF	Murmur, tachypnea, shortness of breath, irritable, diaphoresis, difficulty feeding, poor weight gain, FTT, fatigues easily, may need to start PGE to reopen or maintain PDA, CHF, cardiomegaly, arrhythmias	Cyanosis, CHF, murmur may or may not be present, tachypnea, emergent atrial septostomy may be needed to stabilize TGA, may require PGE infusion to open or maintain PDA TGA on chest x-ray may appear as an egg on a string TAPVR may appear as a snowman on chest x-ray	Tachycardia, tachypnea, decreased perfusion, pallor, cyanosis, murmur may or may not be present, CHF, decreased pulses, cardiomegaly on chest x-ray Without PGE to open PDA will quickly deteriorate to metabolic acidosis and shock

ASD, Atrial septal defect; *CHF*, cardiac heart failure; *FTT*, failure to thrive; *PBF*, pulmonary blood flow; *PDA*, patent ductus arteriosus; *PGE*, prostaglandin; *TAPVR*, total anomalous pulmonary venous return; *TGA*, transposition of the great arteries; *VSD*, ventricular septal defect.
Data from references 121,122

Pericarditis

The hallmark of pericarditis is inflammation of the pericardium. The most common cause in infancy is a virus such as coxsackie, AV, or influenza. Acute pericarditis may be secondary to *S. pneumoniae* or *S. aureus*. Postpericardiotomy syndrome occurs following cardiac surgery. Symptoms of acute pericarditis include precordial chest pain made worse by breathing, coughing, or movement; pericardial friction rub; and fever. Treatment requires blood cultures and nonsteroidal antiinflammatory medications to treat discomfort. If an infectious cause is suspected, pericardiocentesis may be required.[120,121]

Endocarditis

Endocarditis is inflammation of the endocardium affecting a valve. Infective endocarditis (IE) is an uncommon but life-threatening infection in children. CHD is a significant risk factor for IE. A fever and murmur are always present. The child usually presents with fulminant disease with a septic appearance. If the patient presents with sepsis, then severe valvular dysfunction, conduction disturbances, or embolic events may occur and empirical antibiotic treatment must be initiated until the specific organism is able to be isolated for appropriate antibiotic treatment.[119–121]

Cardiomyopathy

Cardiomyopathy is a disease of the myocardium. The heart muscle becomes abnormally thick, stiff, or enlarged, affecting the heart's ability to pump and maintain its rhythm. Dilated cardiomyopathy is the most common type. The heart becomes enlarged and weakened and has many causes that may be familial. Hypertrophic cardiomyopathy occurs when one or more of the ventricles become thickened, and usually affects adolescents. It is associated with abnormal heart rhythms and can lead to sudden death. Hypertrophic cardiomyopathy runs in families. Restrictive cardiomyopathy is the rarest form affecting children. The chambers of the heart become stiff, are unable to fill adequately with blood, and have associated abnormal heart rhythms. Symptoms in infants include difficulty breathing, diaphoresis, poor weight gain, and irritability, and older children may have a heart murmur, fatigue, heart palpitations, dizziness, fainting, and difficulty exercising. Treatments include diuretics, fluid restriction, inotropes, antiarrhythmic medications, pacemakers, or a heart transplant.[121–123]

Arrhythmias

Cardiac arrhythmias in children are often caused by an underlying CHD, especially following open heart surgery. Certain CHDs are associated with a higher incidence of cardiac arrhythmias including tetralogy of Fallot, corrected TGA, TAPVR, large atrial and ventricular septal defects, atrioventricular canals, aortic and subaortic stenosis, congenital mitral stenosis. The most common postoperative arrhythmias include supraventricular tachycardia, ventricular tachycardia, sick sinus syndrome, and complete heart block. Other causes of arrhythmias in children include congenital complete heart block, Wolff–Parkinson–White syndrome, and long QT syndrome. Acquired heart diseases associated with arrhythmias include viral myocarditis, KD, and cardiomyopathies.[121–123]

Congestive Heart Failure

Congestive heart failure (CHF) occurs when the cardiovascular system is unable to deliver oxygen and nutrients to the tissues at a rate that meets the metabolic demands, or the supply is inadequate for demand. CHF affects preload, afterload, contractility, and heart rate. CHD is the most common cause of CHF in children. Symptoms of CHF include poor feeding, which is a red flag to the provider; the patient is diaphoretic and tachypneic with feeds; slow weight gain or FTT; and small for age. Symptoms include tachypnea, retractions, nasal flaring, cardiomegaly, hepatomegaly, tachycardia with weak pulses, diaphoresis, cool extremities, a gallop, pulmonary effusions, and decreased urine output. Treatment of CHF includes decreasing oxygen consumption with bed rest, sedations, nutrition, antipyretics, and if necessary mechanical ventilation to improve oxygen delivery to the body. Medical management includes medications to increase contractility of the heart such as digoxin, decreasing workload, diuretics, and milrinone. If these are ineffective, surgical intervention may be required.[119–121]

Advanced Trauma Life Support: ABCDEs of Trauma Care

The American College of Surgeons (ACS) established the systematic approach for the rapid assessment of traumatic injuries and implementation of lifesaving interventions of the patient's identified injuries, vital signs, and mechanism of injury (MOI). The systematic approach involves a rapid primary survey to identify life-threatening injuries, resuscitation, a secondary survey, and the initiation of definitive care. This process is considered to be the ABCDEs of trauma care, and it helps the provider to identify life-threatening injuries by using the following sequence:

A: Airway maintenance with cervical spine protection
B: Breathing and ventilation
C: Circulation with hemorrhage control
D: Disability–neurologic status
E: Exposure/environmental control

This process was initially developed for the adult trauma patient, but the principles of the ABCDEs of initial assessment are the same for children.[8,123]

Pediatric Trauma

Pediatric trauma is the leading cause of morbidity and mortality in children over 1 year of age. Head injuries are the most common injury reported. Motor vehicle collisions (MVCs) are the leading cause of severe pediatric trauma and deaths. Research, education, and injury prevention programs designed to decrease pediatric-related trauma injuries including MVCs and related injuries are a priority for trauma centers, regulatory governmental agencies, trauma support groups and societies, and the automotive industry.[124–126]

Physiologic and Psychologic Considerations

Almost all medical transport providers have heard about how children are not smaller versions of adults but rather unique and continually evolving. A child's anatomic, physiologic, and psychological differences separate them considerably from the adult. The unique anatomic and physiologic differences in children as well as the severity of injuries support the need for children to be transported to facilities that are experienced; that have pediatric-appropriate equipment; and that are capable of recognizing, diagnosing, and treating pediatric traumatic injuries, and that embrace family presence. Research studies have demonstrated an increase in survival rates and a decrease in mortality and morbidities when pediatric patients are treated at pediatric trauma centers (PTCs) or adult trauma centers with pediatric capabilities.[124–126]

Size and Body Surface Area

A significant physical characteristic of children is their smaller size, which exposes their vulnerability. The intense energy transferred from falls, car bumpers, or any form of blunt force trauma results in a greater force applied per unit of body area in children. This is because children have smaller total body mass, lesser amounts of elastic connective tissue, a pliable skeleton, and a compact location of internal organs. These features have been shown to increase the incidence of multiple organ injuries in children. Children have thinner skin, less subcutaneous tissue, and a higher body surface area to mass ratio compared with adults. These factors result in an increased thermal energy loss and reduce the child's ability to autoregulate their temperature or maintain normothermia. Brief exposure can quickly lead to hypothermia, which can prolong coagulation, alter CNS function, and increase the risk of mortality in pediatric trauma.[124–127]

Skeletal Structure

Children have pliable incomplete calcification of their skeletons and many active growth plates. The pliability of the pediatric patient's skeletal structures may result in their internal organs being injured without damage to the overlying bony structures. An example would be the pediatric patient presenting with a pulmonary contusion from blunt force trauma in the absence of any rib fractures. Pediatric patients have many active growth centers or plates, which if injured, require a pediatric orthopedic surgeon consult to prevent any long-term morbidities. A child should be suspected of having significant trauma to underlying organs and structures if skeletal thoracic fractures are identified because it takes a massive amount of energy to cause these fractures.[123–125]

Psychologic Status

Interacting with pediatric patients requires the provider to understand age-appropriate developmental levels and key milestones. Transport providers must interact with injured children according to their developmental level. An ill or injured child may regress to an earlier developmental stage. Interactions with children should be based on the developmental level depicted. Medical transport providers should become familiar with normal developmental milestones in children so they will know when the child is age-appropriate or regressing developmentally from the stressful event (see Tables 18.14 and 18.15).[8,127,128]

TABLE 18.14 Developmental Stages and Approach Strategies for Pediatric Patients

Stage of Development	Major Fears	Characteristics of Thinking	Approach Strategies
Infants	Separation and strangers	–	• Provide consistent caretakers • Reduce parent anxiety because it is transmitted to the infant • Minimize separation from parents
Toddlers	Separation and loss of control	• Primitive • Unable to recognize views of others • Little concept of body integrity	• Keep explanations simple • Choose words carefully • Let toddler play with equipment (stethoscope) • Minimize separation from parents
Preschoolers	• Bodily injury and mutilation • Loss of control • The unknown and the dark • Being left alone	• Highly literal interpretation of words • Unable to abstract • Primitive ideas about the body (e.g., fear that all blood will "leak out" if a bandage is removed)	• Keep explanations simple and concise • Choose words carefully • Emphasize that a procedure helps the child be healthier • Be honest
School-age children	• Loss of control • Bodily injury and mutilation • Failure to live up to expectations of others • Death	• Vague or false ideas about physical illness and body structure and function • Able to listen attentively without always comprehending • Reluctant to ask questions about something they think they are expected to know • Increased awareness of significant illness, possible hazards of treatments, lifelong consequences of injury, and the meaning of death	• Ask the child to explain what they understand • Provide as many choices as possible to increase the child's sense of control • Reassure the child that they have done nothing wrong and that necessary procedures are not punishment • Anticipate and answer questions about long-term consequences (e.g., what the scar will look like, how long activities may be curtailed)
Adolescents	• Loss of control • Altered body image • Separation from peer group	• Able to think abstractly • Tendency toward hyperresponsiveness to pain (reactions not always in proportion to event) • Little understanding of the structure and workings of the body	• When appropriate, allow adolescents to be a part of decision-making about their case • Give information sensitively • Express how important their compliance and cooperation are to their treatment • Be honest about consequences • Use or teach coping mechanisms such as relaxation, deep breathing, and self-comforting

From Sanders MJ. *Mosby's Paramedic Textbook*. 2nd ed. St. Louis, MO: Mosby; 2000.

TABLE 18.15 Age-Specific Development and Injury Patterns

Age	Development	At-Risk Injuries
Infant 0–4 months	Feeding, holding, bonding, and dependence on caregivers	Aspiration, sudden infant death syndrome, bathing injuries (burns, near-drowning), environmental exposures (heat and cold), abuse, neglect, homicide, sexual assault, MVCs without proper restraint
Infant 4–8 months	Introduction of solid foods, teething, rolling side to side, sitting up, crawling	Falls, electrocution from cords and outlets, foreign body aspiration, toxic ingestions, MVC without proper restraint, burns, near-drowning, abuse, neglect, homicide, sexual assault, lacerations, fractures, head and spine injuries
Infant 8–12 months	Crawling, walking, increased motor coordination (opening doors, latches, etc.)	Falls, aspiration, foreign body ingestion, toxic ingestion, pedestrian versus vehicle injuries, near-drowning, electrocution, motor vehicle collision without proper restraint, burns, suffocation, abuse, neglect, homicide, lacerations, fractures, head and spine injuries
Child 15 months to 3 years	Walking well and running, increased climbing skills, increased use of riding toys, use of utensils and cup, advanced motor skills (latches, doorways, match/lighter use) Emotionally, have increased desire for autonomy but have stranger anxiety Beginning to speak simple sentences	Falls, strike by vehicle as pedestrian or bike rider, burns, suffocation, near-drowning, toxic ingestions, foreign body aspiration, electrocution, MVC without proper restraint, abuse, neglect, homicide, lacerations, fractures, head and spine injuries
Child 4–9 years	Bike riding; swimming skills; entry into school systems; use of tools, firearms, and weapons Increased exposures to nonfamily members, involvement in team sports Use of seatbelts Emotionally continue to increase autonomy with heightened body awareness and sensitivity to invasive examinations/procedures Rapidly increasing verbal skills	Toxic ingestions, foreign body aspiration, electrocution, MVC without proper restraint, abuse, neglect, homicide, sexual assault, lacerations, fractures, head and spine injuries
Child 10–12 years	Rapid physical growth; learning complex social skills; beginning of alcohol, tobacco, and drug experimentation; increased sexual experimentation; and involvement in largely physical team sports Use of motorized vehicles Emotionally, have heightened awareness in gender differences, intense need for privacy, sense of responsibility, and need to be involved in decision-making May experience clinical depression	Falls, strikes by vehicle as pedestrian or vehicle rider, burns, near-drowning, toxic ingestions, drug or alcohol overdose, foreign body aspiration, electrocution, MVC without proper restraint, abuse, neglect, homicide, sexual assault, suicide, complications of pregnancy or contraception, lacerations, fractures, head and spine injuries
Child 12–16 years	Increased incidence of risk-taking behaviors; increased autonomy in decisions of daily living; begin driving car; begin part-time jobs; increased sexual behavior; increased drug, alcohol, and tobacco use Emotionally, have increased body image disturbances, increased need for independence/decision-making May suffer from clinical depression	MVC, falls, occupational injuries, strikes by vehicle as pedestrian or bike rider, burns, near-drowning, toxic ingestions, drug or alcohol overdose, foreign body aspiration, electrocution, abuse, neglect, homicide, suicide, sexual assault, complications of pregnancy or contraception, lacerations, fractures, head and spine injuries

MVC, Motor vehicle crash.

Evidence has demonstrated that family presence during resuscitation and invasive procedures is beneficial to patients and their families. Family presence at a child's bedside meets the psychologic needs of the patient in a time of crisis and helps the parents understand the severity of their child's condition and witness all the efforts by the medical team to help their child. Family presence has been shown to improve medical decision-making, patient care, communication with the healthcare team, and patient and family satisfaction.[129,130]

Approximately 200,000 specialty neonatal and pediatric critical care transports occur each year, making family-centered care a relevant issue. A majority of pediatric critical care transport teams support parents going along with their child on ground transports, but because of aircraft performance issues with weight and balance, configuration, or individual program policy constraints, a smaller number of transport programs allow parents on air medical transports. Parental accompaniment has now become a measure of quality in pediatric critical care transports.[129,130]

Long-Term Effects of Traumatic Injury

Long-term quality of life in children following traumatic injuries, and the subsequent effects on their growth and development, is a significant concern. Pediatric patients have to recuperate from a traumatic injury as well as continue the process of normal growth and development. The physiologic and psychologic effects of traumatic injuries may impact the child's long-term quality of life, especially if the injury affects physical characteristics by altering functionality and growth, leaving physical scars, or causing traumatic brain injury type changes cognitively and behaviorally. Evidence has shown children may have alterations in cognition and behavioral changes up to a year following an injury. Social, affective, and learning disabilities are present in a large number of seriously injured children. Data have shown that up to 25% of children in an MVC experience post-traumatic stress disorder. Most children and their parents will experience resolution of mild trauma symptoms without the need for psychologic or psychiatric treatment. However, traumatic experiences can impact children and their families long after the actual event. Some children and their families may benefit from psychosocial support or interventions. Pediatric injuries and hospitalizations also create a considerable burden on parents and siblings including financial burdens, time away from work, and separation from their other children. All medical facilities should have a multidisciplinary team of social workers, child life specialists, psychiatrists, psychologists, and chaplains to help patients and their families deal with the long-term results of traumatic experiences.[8,123,126,131,132]

The Primary Survey

The goal of the primary survey is to rapidly survey the injured child to identify underlying injuries and reverse potential life-threatening conditions. During the primary survey, the assessment and management were the same for adults and children. The differences include the amount of blood, fluids, and medications; size of the child; degree and swiftness of heat loss; and injury patterns. The ABCDE algorithm identifies life-threatening injuries by following the sequence in order of airway maintenance with cervical spine protection, breathing and ventilation, circulation with hemorrhage control, disability and neurologic status, and exposure/environmental control including complete removal of clothes to expose the patient and prevent hypothermia. The primary survey includes frequent reassessments following interventions to confirm or exclude injuries requiring immediate intervention. Remember to consider the pediatric patient's unique physiologic and anatomic differences because they are essential for proper assessment and treatment.[8,123,126]

Airway and Cervical Spine Protection

Airway patency is critical to prevent severe morbidities and mortalities in pediatric patients. Airway management is an initial step in stabilizing the pediatric trauma patient. Achieving adequate airway control is necessary to adequately oxygenate and ventilate the pediatric patient while decreasing the potential for aspiration. Failure to provide early and aggressive airway management in children leads to hypoxia, respiratory failure, and arrest.[8,14,123,126,133]

An open airway is the number one priority in the initial assessment. The pediatric airway is anatomically different from the adult airway. The child's larger tongue and the position of the larynx being anterior and more cephalic in the neck increase the level of difficulty during laryngoscopy compared with adults. Children have a disproportion between the size of the head and midface. The child's large occiput forces passive flexion of the cervical spine while the child is lying supine, and the airway is more likely to be compromised and obstructed. In the absence of trauma, the pediatric

patient's airway is best protected by placing the child in the "sniffing" position, which is a slightly superior and anterior position of the midface. In the presence of trauma, the "neutral" position best protects both the cervical spine and ensures adequate airway opening. Placing a towel or blanket of approximately 2- to 3-cm thickness under the shoulders and posterior thorax will help the child achieve a more anatomically neutral position. In the pediatric trauma patient, the neck should be kept immobilized to prevent hyperextension at C1–C2 and prevent hyperflexion at C5–C6. With traumatic injuries, manual stabilization of the cervical spine should be maintained during airway management and until the child is immobilized. (Immobilization of the cervical spine is addressed later in the chapter.)[8,25,123,126,133]

The airway in the unresponsive child should be opened using the jaw thrust without a head tilt maneuver to open the airway while a team member maintains manual stabilization to protect the cervical spine. If the child is unconscious, an oropharyngeal airway will give support to keep the tongue out of the hypopharynx but may cause vomiting if the child has an intact gag reflex. An oral airway should be placed with direct visualization with a tongue blade to prevent oral trauma and bleeding.[8,25,44,123,126,133]

Once the airway is opened and suctioned for debris or secretions, supplemental oxygen should be provided. Patients with inadequate respiratory rates, impaired ventilation, or an inability to protect the airway from secretions or emesis should have the airway protected with ETI. BVM ventilation with 100% oxygen is the best method to use initially to provide assist ventilations in the unresponsive child while preparing for ETI. The transport provider should remember the best airway in a child is one you can oxygenate and ventilate. Research has demonstrated there is no clear neurologic or survivable advantage between ETI and BVM in pediatric patients 12 years of age or younger in the prehospital setting. According to the 2015 AHA guidelines, BVM ventilation may be effective and safer than ETI for short transport times or short out-of-hospital resuscitation.[8,14,17,24–27,39,41,45,123]

Nonelective nasal intubations should not be performed on children younger than 12 years of age because of the acute angle to the glottis. This makes this procedure extremely difficult for maintaining a neutral cervical spine position. Needle (<10 years of age) or surgical (>10 years of age) cricothyroidotomy may be necessary to control the child's airway if intubation is unsuccessful or facial trauma prevents ETI.[8,35,39,41]

Rapid sequence induction standardized medication protocols exist for the majority of transport programs to simplify rapid sequence intubation and allow efficient airway management of the critically injured child. Pediatric patients are at risk of rapid deterioration during intubation with an increased risk of bradycardia with desaturation for prolonged attempts. These standardized protocols outline the use of IV medications to facilitate ETI while avoiding potential complications associated with induction, such as bradycardia and desaturations.[8,39,41,123,133]

Currently, the National Association of EMS Physicians (NAEMSP), ACEP, and ACS Committee on Trauma (COT) support the use of drug-assisted intubation in the prehospital environment. Differences continue to exist between transport programs concerning which RSI medications are the best or preferred for children who have suffered traumatic injuries.[8,38,39,41,123,132,133]

It is necessary to have an accurate patient weight to provide proper medication dosages during the RSI procedure. Infants and children have a pronounced vagal response to ETI, and many RSI protocols use atropine sulfate as the initial medication to block the vagal response to laryngoscopy, depending on the age of the child.[8,38,39,41,123,132,133]

Hypoxia is a major cause of bradycardia in pediatric patients, which is another reason preoxygenation is performed in children. Bradycardia should be treated rapidly during any airway procedure using the BVM for assisted ventilation with supplemental oxygen and atropine if not already administered. Atropine is followed by a short-acting sedative and a short-acting neuromuscular blocking agent. Several rapid-sequence intubation medications fulfill these requirements and can be safely used in children. The medications used in RSI and management of the pediatric airway were discussed in more detail earlier in this chapter.[8,38,39,41,123,132,133]

Rescue airways such as the esophageal obturator or the Combitube are not usually recommended in the pediatric population because of limited patient-appropriate sizes. Supraglottic airways have increased in popularity and use in the prehospital setting because of ease of use, relatively simple training, dependability, and quick insert. Supraglottic devices do not offer a definitive airway in the prehospital setting; however, newer more advanced second-generation devices are offering greater seal pressures and the capacity to decompress gastric secretions, which decreases potential aspiration. Supraglottic devices are usually not used as rescue devices in the prehospital setting. Supraglottic devices were discussed in more detail earlier in the chapter.[8,37–39,44,123]

ETI is the most reliable method of establishing a secure airway and oxygenating and ventilating a pediatric trauma patient. ETI indications, procedure, and AHA and PALS recommendations for cuffed or uncuffed ETT use with pediatric trauma patients was discussed in detail earlier in this chapter.[15,27]

Breathing

After control of the airway and cervical spine immobilization has been achieved, attention is then turned to oxygenation and ventilation of the pediatric trauma patient. All trauma patients need supplemental oxygen. Evaluation of the child's respiratory status and the ability to recognize early signs of distress are essential in the management of pediatric trauma patients because subtle findings of respiratory distress are often missed. The patient's respiratory rate is the first assessment step when evaluating respiratory status. Children have varying normal rates of respiration that decrease with age. It is important to know what the normal respiratory rates are for the different pediatric ages. For example, a healthy infant breathes 40–60 times per minute, whereas an older child will have normal respiratory rates of 20 breaths/min. Tachypnea is an early but nonspecific sign of respiratory distress. Bradypnea is a late sign of distress and often signifies impending cardiopulmonary arrest. Hypoxia is the most common cause of respiratory arrest in children. When viewed with other physical findings, the assessment of a child's respiratory rate provides a much more accurate assessment of the overall respiratory status.[8,123,126]

A child's work of breathing increases with respiratory distress. Increased work of breathing in children may present with any of the following clinical signs and symptoms:

- Nasal flaring
- Retractions: intercostals, subcostal, substernal, clavicular, supraclavicular
- Head bobbing
- Grunting
- Tripod positioning
- Stridor

- Snoring
- Altered respiratory rate: tachypnea, bradypnea, or apnea
- Adventitious breath sounds: wheezing, rales, or rhonchi
- Paradoxical respirations: seesaw respirations
- Pallor
- Decreased gag reflex
- Decreased or absent breath sounds
- Cyanosis, which is a late sign of distress

Any of these changes call for supplemental oxygen support and, depending on the severity of the child's respiratory distress, may necessitate BVM ventilations or advanced airway control with ETT.[8,123,126]

Selected Traumatic Injuries Contributing to Respiratory Distress

Chest trauma accounts for approximately 10% of all trauma affecting children. However, it is quite significant because of the considerable mortality associated with it. Chest trauma is either nonpenetrating or blunt trauma (does not involve opening the chest) and usually involves a high-energy impact to multiple areas of the body, or penetrating trauma (causes an open wound). More than 80% of pediatric thoracic trauma results from blunt injury.[8,123,134] Injuries as a result of blunt force chest trauma can be classified into four types:

1. Chest wall injuries causing rib fractures, sternal fractures, or a flail chest
2. Pulmonary injuries causing pulmonary contusion, pneumothorax, hemothorax, tracheobronchial disruption, or diaphragmatic injury
3. Cardiovascular injuries resulting in myocardial contusion, cardiac tamponade or rupture, aortic disruption, or pulmonary vascular injury
4. Esophageal injuries, including an esophageal rupture

Chest trauma is second only to head injuries as a cause of accidental death in children. The physiologic differences in pediatric patients change the patterns of injury. Chest or thoracic trauma is a common cause of respiratory distress in children. The compliant nature of the pediatric thoracic cage allows for significant blunt force trauma that compresses the ribs and sternum without any fractures, which allows the transfer of high-energy trauma to a child's internal structures and organs. The most common pattern of pediatric chest trauma is a high-energy blow that may involve other regions of the body. Over half of children with chest trauma also have head, abdominal, and limb injuries. The elastic consistency of the ribs protects children from sustaining rib fractures or mediastinal injury or it may prevent rib fractures from occurring; thus, rib and mediastinal fractures are uncommon in children. The provider should be concerned about the underlying organs if rib fractures are present. The thinness of the chest wall may cause the respiratory assessment to be more difficult because breath sounds may be referred from one area of the chest to another, making diagnosis more difficult. The mobility of the mediastinal structures increases the susceptibility of pediatric patients to develop a tension pneumothorax. Pneumomediastinum is rare and relatively benign in the majority of pediatric cases.[8,123,134]

Tension Pneumothorax

A tension pneumothorax occurs when air enters into the pleural space on inspiration and is unable to escape on expiration. The air leaks into the thorax and pressures rise rapidly affecting ventilation on that side, which relocates the mediastinum toward the contralateral side and the pressure then interferes with venous return. Tension pneumothorax presents with distention of the hemithorax, dyspnea, hypotension, absence of breath sounds, and hyperresonance together on the affected side, with increased jugular venous pressure, cyanosis, and tracheal deviation (which is a late sign). Subcutaneous emphysema may be noted with tactile examination of the chest. Intubation with mechanical ventilation may increase the risk of a tension pneumothorax because PPV increases intrathoracic pressure. Tension pneumothoraces are diagnosed clinically indicating emergent intervention without the delay of CXR confirmation.[8,123,134,135]

Treatment for Tension Pneumothorax

Adequate treatment can be a needle decompression followed by a chest tube or insertion of the chest tube. The most common initial treatment is a needle decompression with a large-bore IV catheter placed into the intrapleural space at the second intercostal space midclavicular line of the affected side of the chest. The placement of an age-appropriate size chest tube at the fifth intercostal space at the anterior midaxillary line on the affected side is the definitive treatment. Chest tubes should have a one-way flutter valve attached or be placed to water seal drainage to prevent reaccumulation of air. Tension pneumothoraces should always be treated before transport.[8,123,134,135]

Simple Pneumothorax

A simple pneumothorax may be caused by either blunt or penetrating trauma. In pediatric patients, a simple pneumothorax occurs in the absence of rib fractures from blunt trauma occurring during inspiration when the glottis is closed causing an abrupt increase in the intrathoracic alveolar pressure and subsequent alveolar rupture. The lung will collapse when air enters the potential space between the visceral and parietal pleura. As the lung tissue collapses, ventilation and perfusion are affected because blood perfusing the collapsed area is no longer oxygenated. Signs and symptoms of a simple pneumothorax are dyspnea, decreased or absent breath sounds on the affected side, hyperresonance on the affected side, and chest pain that radiates to the shoulder area. Respiratory distress may be present or develop over time or with ascent in a fixed-wing aircraft. Subcutaneous emphysema may be present with tactile examination of the chest.[8,134,135]

Treatment for Simple Pneumothorax

Treatment of a simple pneumothorax consists of the placement of an age- and size-appropriate chest tube in the fifth intercostal space at the anterior midaxillary line on the affected side. Chest tubes should be attached to one-way flutter valves or water seal drainage to prevent reaccumulation of air. A suspected simple pneumothorax without signs of severe respiratory or cardiovascular compromise should be evaluated by CXR secondary to other conditions (e.g., traumatic diaphragmatic hernia) and may have similar clinical findings. All pneumothoraces greater than 20% or any pneumothoraces present in patients who are intubated and on mechanical ventilation or will need PPV should be treated with a chest tube before transport or ascending in an air medical transport vehicle.[8,134,135]

Open Pneumothorax

An open pneumothorax occurs when a penetrating injury allows free movement of air in and out of the pleural space causing collapse of the lung with impaired ventilation. Open pneumothorax is characterized by the presence of a penetrating chest wound, dyspnea, chest pain, hyperresonance, and decreased breath sounds over the affected side of the chest. An audible "sucking" sound may be heard during inspiration and expiration.[8,134,135]

Treatment for Open Pneumothorax

Treatment for an open pneumothorax requires treatment for both the lung collapse and the penetrating chest wound. A sterile occlusive dressing, taped on three sides, should be immediately placed over the wound. The dressing is taped on three sides to allow for venting of the pleural space by lifting the dressing should reaccumulation of air in the pleural air occur. If untreated, reaccumulation of pleural air can lead to a tension pneumothorax. After the wound is treated, a chest tube should be inserted as discussed previously to treat lung collapse and prevent a tension pneumothorax during transport. A chest tube should be placed remotely from the penetrating wound to decrease the risk of intrathoracic infection and initiate antimicrobial treatment.[8,134,135]

Hemothorax

Hemothorax occurs when blood collects in the pleural space from either blunt or penetrating trauma. The most common causes are lung lacerations or lacerations of an intercostal vessel producing a potentially severe or massive hemothorax, which would require immediate drainage and a possible blood transfusion in pediatric patients. Massive hemothorax of this type is rare in children. Hemorrhage exceeding 20%–25% of the child's blood volume not only will cause hypovolemic shock but also restrict the intrathoracic space, necessitating an intervention. Blood losses of 4% per hour require surgical intervention, but this rarely occurs in pediatric patients. Signs and symptoms of a hemothorax present with dyspnea, chest pain, decreased or absent breath sounds over the affected side, and dullness to percussion on the affected side of the chest. Tachycardia, tachypnea, cool, pale, diaphoretic skin, and hypotension (signs of shock) may also be present.[8,123,134,135]

Treatment for Hemothorax

Management of hemothorax should begin with resuscitative efforts with oxygenation, ventilation, control of external bleeding, and fluid resuscitation if needed. Aggressive fluid resuscitation can dilute the remaining blood and clotting factors, which interferes with the body's ability to form clots, control bleeding, and hemostasis. Once a hemothorax exceeds 20%–25% of the child's blood volume mark, signs of hypovolemic shock will be present. Initial treatment may be intubation and mechanical ventilation, and the placement of age- and size-appropriate chest tube in the fifth intercostal space of the anterior midaxillary line. The chest tube then needs to be placed to water seal drainage with suction. These interventions will allow time for transport to a surgical center or for the decision for an emergent thoracotomy. This rarely occurs in pediatric patients. A venous hemorrhage may stop with an increase in intrathoracic pressures, which will allow the patient to stabilize without surgical intervention. Remember that clamping the chest tube is a temporary measure until an emergent open thoracotomy can be performed. Fluid resuscitation for blood loss may be needed.[8,123,134,135]

Flail Chest

The elasticity of children's ribs protects against fractures, even in the presence of significant energy transfer or blunt force trauma. A significant blunt force causing multiple adjacent rib fractures in several places along the chest wall allowing a segment of the chest to move and separate from one another is a rare incident in pediatric trauma but may be the most common severe pediatric injury providers treat. Multiple and extensive rib fractures damage the rigidity of the rib cage and produce a flail chest. A flail chest leads to a paradoxical respiratory effort in which the thoracic wall collapses during inspiration and compromises gas exchange. It may be rare in pediatric patients but usually has underlying lung involvement or damage when it does occur. A flail chest may occur more often in older adolescents. In addition to the paradoxical chest wall movement on the affected segment during inspiration and expiration, chest pain, dyspnea, hypoxia, and cyanosis are present.[8,134–137]

Treatment for Flail Chest

A flail chest in pediatric patients is often diagnosed by CXR. CT of the chest may be indicated to assess the extent of underlying injuries. Most rib fractures do not require specific interventions except for pain control and supportive interventions. However, when the rib cage is unstable in children presenting with multiple fractures in multiple places, it may be helpful to use adhesive bandages or other methods in an attempt to make the chest wall more rigid and prevent paradoxical movements. If this method is ineffective, and a flail chest cannot be stabilized, the child will require intubation and mechanical ventilation, which is the only intervention to preserve adequate gas exchange. Management focuses on supportive measures to control pain and prevent atelectasis and pneumonia. The underlying pulmonary contusion associated with a flail chest is a major concern in pediatric patients. These injuries can be difficult to manage because the contusion to the lungs is sensitive to being over- and under-resuscitated.[8,134–137]

Pulmonary Contusion

Pulmonary contusion and lacerations are the most common pediatric thoracic injuries. Pulmonary contusion can occur in the absence of overlying rib fractures and is an injury resulting from direct compression of the parenchyma by a significant blunt force high-energy trauma or the violent displacement of the lung, which can lead to more severe life-threatening injuries. A pulmonary contusion can occur even in the absence of rib fractures. Pulmonary contusion occurs when kinetic energy from some form of blunt force is transferred to a child's chest wall damaging the lung parenchyma. This results in damage to the alveolar spaces, hemorrhage, and edema, and the contusion may interfere with gas exchange affecting the respiratory status of the child. Damage to the child's lung includes alveolar collapse from extravasation of fluid into the interstitium and inactivation of surfactant as well as ventilation–perfusion mismatch, which causes hypoxia. If left untreated, respiratory arrest may occur. Presenting symptoms of a pulmonary contusion in children include dyspnea, tachypnea, bloody sputum, and possibly obvious chest wall injuries. Clinical appreciation of pulmonary contusions on examination may be difficult; however, the provider should maintain a high index of suspicion for pediatric patients with thoracic injuries or those involved in rapid deceleration injuries. Radiographic changes may not appear until 24 hours after injury. Pulmonary contusions can be reabsorbed and the lung repaired after several days, but this can cause substantial damage, which may increase the risk of an infection. If the child also has a lung laceration with the contusion, it is usually associated with air leaks, pneumothorax, and eventually a hemothorax.[8,134–137]

Treatment for Pulmonary Contusion

Pulmonary contusion treatment management in children centers around oxygenation, ventilation, cardiovascular support, and the immediate management of life-threatening injuries. Initially, pulmonary contusions in children may be associated with significant MOIs and multiorgan involvement, and the initial assessment may require life-threatening complications to be addressed. Pulmonary contusions may not be symptomatic and present with a normal CXR that is not indicative of a contusion. When the child presents asymptomatic, this phase deteriorates within 24–72 hours from the initial traumatic event, and diagnosis is made by CXR and the child exhibiting signs of respiratory distress.[8,134–137]

Complications associated with pulmonary contusion are pneumonia or acute respiratory distress syndrome. Diagnosis may be made if the provider is highly suspicious of a significant MOI to the chest, or the child is complaining of chest pain and tenderness, or if external contusions are noted. These symptoms and injuries are associated with additional internal injuries such as pneumothorax or hemothorax. Most pulmonary contusions are scarcely symptomatic by themselves. In these rare situations, the affected area is large and will limit gas exchange surface area resulting in hypoxia, hypercarbia, and acidosis.[8,134–137]

Definitive treatment of pulmonary contusion in children is supportive with rigorous monitoring for respiratory deterioration, supplemental oxygen, assisted ventilation, and other supportive interventions such as pain control, inhaled nitric oxide, and positioning. There is limited evidence demonstrating any benefits of broad-spectrum antibiotic administration to prevent an infection from damaged lung tissue, but it is widely accepted and ordered. Extracorporeal membrane oxygenation (ECMO) is regarded as a supportive therapy for pulmonary contusions in pediatric patients unable to oxygenate and ventilate to prevent further lung damage from barotraumas.[8,134–138]

Diaphragmatic Rupture

Traumatic diaphragmatic rupture (TDR) usually results from blunt or penetrating injuries to the upper abdomen or lower thorax resulting in rupture or herniation of the diaphragm. It is a relatively uncommon injury in pediatric patients but should be considered in cases of thoracoabdominal injury. TDR commonly affects the left side more frequently because the internal structures on the left side are weaker and the liver offers extra protection and support to the right hemidiaphragm. On rare occasions, a penetrating instrument may tear the diaphragm directly, but more often TDR is a result of high-energy blunt force trauma to thoracoabdominal structures. Blunt force trauma severe enough to tear the diaphragm usually has spleen or liver involvement. Diagnosis of TDR is often difficult because the signs may not stand out on CXRs, the presenting symptoms may resemble other conditions or injuries, or the severity of the other injuries distracts the provider from detecting diaphragmatic injuries. Rapid diagnosis and identification of TDR injuries and any other associated injuries are essential to prevent life-threatening herniation from the abdominal organs being pushed into the thorax causing lung compression, shifting of mediastinal structures, obstruction, ischemia, sepsis, and death. TDR is characterized by dyspnea, dysphagia, chest pain, sharp shoulder pain, auscultation of bowel sounds over the lower thorax, and decreased breath sounds over the affected side of the chest.[8,134,136,137,139]

Treatment for Diaphragmatic Rupture

Pediatric traumatic rupture of the diaphragm is a rare event that occurs more often on the left side and always requires surgical treatment. CXR and multidetector CT (MDCT) are the most commonly used modalities used to diagnose TDR. The definitive treatment for diaphragmatic rupture is surgical repair. Clinical support with intubation, mechanical ventilation, and gastric decompression are necessary before transport or surgical intervention. Adequate gastric decompression must be provided to these patients during air medical transports. The definitive treatment for TDR is surgical repair.[8,134,136–139]

Tracheobronchial Injuries

Tracheobronchial ruptures (TBRs) caused by blunt chest trauma are rare but potentially fatal in pediatric patients. TBRs are life-threatening ruptures of the trachea or bronchi usually located between the cricoid cartilage and the carina or division of the bronchi. The majority of these injuries are a result of blunt force trauma, usually from MVCs. The elasticity of the thoracic cage of young children protects them from sustaining injuries to the external chest wall. However, in the presence of severe blunt force trauma, the child's intrathoracic structures may be compressed without any external evidence of injury. High-energy blunt force trauma or crush syndrome can cause a rapid increase in tracheobronchial pressure and may account for the blowout perforation of the trachea without the presence of rib or sternal fractures. The majority of tracheal injuries occur close to the carina with the right mainstem bronchus affected more frequently than the left. Major tracheobronchial injuries are life-threatening, resulting in severe respiratory distress and hemodynamic instability requiring rapid interventions. Any damage to the tracheobronchial wall permits air leaks, which potentially can present as a tension pneumothorax, pneumomediastinum, and subcutaneous emphysema. Presenting signs and symptoms of tracheobronchial injury may include dyspnea; hemoptysis; coughing; palpable subcutaneous emphysema of the neck, face, and thoracic areas; respiratory distress; absent breath sounds on the affected side of the chest; persistent air leak from a pneumothorax that reaccumulates after insertion of the chest tube. Hamman's sign, a crunching or rasping sound auscultated over the precordium synchronized with the patient's heartbeat, may also be appreciated with mediastinal emphysema. The transport provider should suspect tracheobronchial injury in a child if, after successful chest tube placement, a pneumothorax reaccumulates after chest tube insertion while continuing to water seal drainage and suction.[8,134–138,140]

Treatment for Tracheobronchial Injuries

Pediatric patients with major tracheobronchial trauma usually die from associated injuries before reaching the hospital. This injury's initial clinical presentation may be inconsistent and vague, making management extremely difficult or the child presents in severe cardiopulmonary distress. Prompt recognition, diagnosis, and surgical treatment are essential prognostic indicators for survival in these rare injuries with high mortality rates. Manage the patient's airway with intubation and mechanical ventilation, and begin resuscitation for hemodynamic instabilities. Perform needle decompression for tension pneumothoraces, and chest tube placement for drainage is indicated. A persistent, large-volume air leak despite adequate chest drainage is a significant indicator of a large tracheobronchial tear or injury. A large tracheobronchial tear could develop a massive pneumothorax and become a life-threatening event. In these cases, air under tension accumulates not only in the pleural space but also in the mediastinum and neck and even in the subcutaneous tissue. A CXR is the most informative diagnostic tool for this injury. Any disturbance of the tracheobronchial air column, massive atelectasis, deep cervical emphysema, and pneumomediastinum,

in association with the pneumothorax, are highly suggestive of a severe TBR. The fallen lung sign is pathognomonic of a total rupture of one of the main pulmonary bronchi. A critical diagnostic tool for diagnosing TBR is bronchoscopy. It should be performed by experienced thoracic surgeons or pulmonologists and remains the gold standard for establishing this diagnosis. All of these patients must be closely monitored for reaccumulation of air that may result in a tension pneumothorax during transport. If chest tube and ventilation management fail to reestablish patient stability, ECMO heart and lung supportive therapy may be used for ventilatory support in the absence of severe bleeding or intracranial hemorrhage. Surgical intervention for repair of TBR injuries is necessary.[8,134–138,140]

Sternal Fractures and Rib Fractures

The elasticity and flexibility of the thoracic cage protects children from being subjected to chest wall injuries such as rib fractures, flail chest, or sternal fractures. Rib and sternal fractures are rather rare in children but are seen in adolescent patients. Infants presenting with rib fractures should raise a red flag for the provider to consider child abuse. Infants presenting with rib fractures from suspected child abuse are a result of an anteroposterior compression of the chest seen in the shaken and squeezed child. A single or isolated rib fracture is not a common occurrence in children and should be investigated further by the provider for associated or underlying injuries because of the significant blunt energy transfer needed to accomplish this injury.[8,134,136,137,141,142]

Blunt force trauma or compression of the chest causes rib fractures in children. Rib fractures in children are associated with an increased risk of severe injuries, and the transport provider should be prepared to manage the potential for severe internal injuries. Rib fractures from blunt force trauma may puncture the pleural cavity, resulting in a pneumothorax, or lacerate the intercostal artery, an internal mammary gland, or the lung parenchyma, which may result in a hemothorax. Rib fractures from blunt trauma cause more internal injuries in children compared with compression injuries. Chest wall compression resulting in rib fractures presents with lateral segments of the ribs fracturing outward. Fractures of the sternum are rarely seen or occur in children. It takes a substantial blunt force to the chest of a child for this injury to occur. The transport provider should be cognizant of damage to the underlying internal structures of children presenting with rib and or sternal injuries or fractures. Cardiac contusions, pulmonary contusions, and aortic injuries may be detected with sternal and/or rib fractures. Rib fractures in children are a common source of pain and discomfort, affecting the depth and quality of the child's respiratory effort, and splinting of respirations, dyspnea, ecchymosis, and possibly crepitus may be seen. Sooner or later, untreated rib fractures will damage underlying structures.[8,134,136,137,141,142]

Treatment of Sternal Fractures and Rib Fractures

It is essential to control the pain of children presenting with rib or sternal fractures. These children may require ventilatory support and will need a physical examination and diagnostic testing to evaluate underlying structure damage. A CXR is usually an adequate diagnostic tool to identify rib fractures. The oblique views may help identify nonaccidental injury and should be considered if child abuse is suspected. CT of the chest should be considered to rule out intrathoracic injuries if the child has first rib fractures, sternal fractures, and posterior sternoclavicular fracture dislocations.[8,134,136,137,141,142]

Laryngotracheal Injuries

Pediatric laryngotracheal injuries result from blunt neck trauma and are extremely rare in children. Presenting symptoms in children may be nonspecific and without the provider suspecting this diagnosis early it is easily overlooked, especially in those presenting with multisystem injury involvement. Laryngotracheal injuries are potentially fatal in children if the provider fails to recognize them early and initiate appropriate interventions. The incidence of pediatric neck trauma with motor vehicle accidents is increasing in the pediatric population from rapid deceleration. Other MOIs for pediatric laryngotracheal trauma include clothesline injuries to the neck while riding motorcycles, all-terrain vehicles, and snowmobiles when the child strikes a stationary object. Also, high-impact sports and martial arts can cause a clothesline injury. Other MOIs include direct trauma to the neck from fists, feet, or blunt weapons, strangulation from hanging, ligature suffocation, manual choking, and falls.[143,144]

Treatment of Laryngotracheal Injuries

The signs and symptoms of laryngotracheal injuries include hoarseness, dysphonia, aphonia, odynophagia, dysphagia, cervical tenderness, cervical crepitus, hemoptysis, stridor, and respiratory distress. It is important to determine when managing a suspected laryngotracheal trauma whether the child is stable or unstable. An injury classification exists for laryngotracheal injuries from group one, which includes minor hematoma without fracture, to group five, which includes a complete laryngotracheal separation. Children who are unstable with laryngotracheal trauma or suspected trauma may be in respiratory distress and require interventions. The provider should use supplemental oxygen, a jaw thrust or a chin lift to open the child's airway and begin gentle mask ventilation. It is important to avoid aggressive BVM to prevent or decrease the worsening of cervical emphysema, which will affect adequate ventilation. Intubation is a high risk with laryngotracheal trauma because of the potential to lose the airway. If the child is unstable, a tracheostomy is considered the standard method for securing the airway for a suspected laryngotracheal injury in the field. Laryngotracheal injuries are associated with additional injuries to the cervical spine, esophagus, and vascular structures of the neck. Chest and neck x-rays are required to evaluate cervical spine fractures, subcutaneous emphysema, pneumothorax, or pneumomediastinum. A CT scan will provide information about the child's airway anatomy, cartilage fractures, cervical spine fractures, or vascular injuries. Airway management is controversial because of the extremely high risk of losing the airway with this injury.[143,144]

Diagnostic Adjuncts for Thoracic Trauma

Thoracic trauma is second only to accidents and unintentional injuries as the leading causes of morbidity and mortality in pediatric patients. In children, more than 80% of all thoracic injuries are the result of blunt trauma. Pediatric trauma patients frequently present first to an outside hospital (OH) before being transported to a Level I PTC for specialized and definitive care. Frequently, the OHs have already performed a CT scan before transfer. This imaging is often unnecessary, according to ATLS recommendations, which stress that CT scans should not be performed at the OH when transferring the child out for treatment, or if they are not clinically indicated. OHs obtaining CT scans on pediatric trauma patients before transfer to PTC results in a delay of care, exposes the child to excessive radiation, and increases health care costs. CT imaging has dramatically increased over the last few years, and

with this escalation comes considerable risk to the pediatric patient. Children are still experiencing growth and development and concern is growing that exposure to ionizing radiation may predispose children to radiation-induced malignancies. Taking into account the risks of radiation-induced cancer from CT scans, PTCs have adopted a variety of dose-reduction techniques and reconstructive models that substantially decrease radiation exposure without decreasing the diagnostic quality of the images produced.

ATLS guidelines recommend using CXRs as the initial diagnostic tool for the assessment of thoracic injuries after physical examination. CXRs are quick, portable, and can promptly diagnose common thoracic complications such as pneumothorax, hemothorax, and mediastinal irregularities. There are no established guidelines for using chest CTs instead of CXRs for pediatric blunt trauma patients. The lack of regulation or guidelines contributes to the remarkable increase in the use of chest CT and the resultant decrease in CXRs for initial diagnostic imaging for pediatric blunt chest traumas. Many studies evaluated the MOI, rib fractures, contusions, and pneumothorax in pediatric blunt thoracic injuries and demonstrated that CTs were not necessary in the majority of trauma cases because the added information obtained frequently did not change the plan of care for these patients. This information suggests the importance of developing a strict imaging guideline for pediatric blunt trauma patients to limit excessive exposure to CT radiation while not compromising the quality of useful diagnostic information. Chest CT offers enhanced imaging of intrathoracic structures and increases the diagnosis of pediatric intrathoracic injuries; however, this added information does not frequently change the overall care of the pediatric trauma patient. CXR is a valuable screening tool for pediatric blunt trauma patients, and the provider should manage this patient without a routine chest CT being performed. After obtaining the initial CXR on these trauma patients, those presenting with an abnormal mediastinal silhouette on CXR should proceed with a chest CT to evaluate the child for vascular injuries. Also, a chest CT should be done on pediatric patients with suspected thoracic spine injuries and fractures because the thoracic spine is the most commonly injured section of the pediatric patient.[8,145,146]

Circulation

In the initial trauma assessment, circulation is the third step of the primary survey to determine the circulatory status of the patient. In trauma, the assessment of circulatory status focuses on the estimation and treatment of fluid and blood loss associated with traumatic injuries. The physiologic differences in pediatric patients make this assessment more difficult than in adults, especially if the provider is not aware of these differences. The provider should also know the pediatric patient's normal vital sign parameters. Together with the knowledge of the physiologic differences in pediatric patients, this will help the provider establish an accurate diagnosis. In pediatric trauma patients, the evaluation and management of the circulation status includes recognition of circulatory compromise, an accurate estimation of the pediatric patient's weight and circulatory volume, fluid resuscitation, blood replacement, venous access, assessments of the adequacy of resuscitation with urine output, and thermoregulation status.[8,123,126,132]

Physical Examination

Pediatric patients with traumatic injuries resulting in fluid and blood loss may present with the following clinical signs and symptoms[8,123,126]:

- An altered LOC. Preverbal children may be unable to recognize parents or caregivers.
- A decreased response to stimuli or the environment. This is often recognized when the child exhibits a decreased response to painful procedures such as IV starts or a reduction of fractures.
- Restlessness or anxiety.
- Confusion or irritability.
- Dry mucous membranes or absence of tears.
- Tachypnea.
- Tachycardia. In the early stages of shock, tachycardia may be the only indicator of blood loss or shock.
- A change in the child's skin color. Pediatric patients may appear ashen, pale, mottled, or cyanotic.
- Capillary refill greater than 3 seconds, which may be a sensitive indicator of circulatory status in children. It is important to monitor the child's thermoregulation because hypothermia will also increase the capillary refill time.
- Peripheral pulses change and become weak and thready with severe shock in children.
- Skin is cool mostly in the extremities and diaphoretic.
- Difficulty in obtaining blood pressure in pediatric patients is caused by vasoconstriction from catecholamine release and decreased cardiac output (CO).
- Children have unique compensatory mechanisms in moderate to severe shock states to maintain normotensive blood pressure because of sustained catecholamine response.
- Blood pressure is a late indicator of circulatory status in children. Other clinical indicators as listed earlier are often more sensitive indicators. Hypotension and bradycardia after traumatic injuries in children are ominous late clinical findings and need to be treated aggressively.
- Decreased or absent breath sounds.
- Decreased urine output.
- Placing a urinary catheter early in the care of traumatically injured children is essential for assessment of circulatory status and effectiveness of resuscitation.
- End-organ perfusion (i.e., kidneys) decreases with fluid or blood loss and is reflected with oliguria or anuria.
- Maintenance of 1–2 mL/kg per hour of urine output is the goal of circulatory support in the pediatric patient.
- Circulatory compromise in children can often be subtle and must be found with a careful physical examination. Waiting for major changes in vital signs or laboratory studies increases patient morbidity and often makes resuscitation more difficult.
- Monitoring of the patient is necessary during the assessment and resuscitation of children with traumatic injuries. Cardiac monitoring and pulse oximetry monitoring can aid in the initial assessment and monitoring of ongoing patient status.
- A normal pulse oximetry reading does not accurately reflect tissue oxygenation, which is an indicator that trauma patients should receive supplemental oxygenation.

Laboratory studies helpful in the assessment of the pediatric trauma patient's circulatory status include the following:

- A complete blood cell count, especially hematocrit levels.
- Serum, finger, or heel stick glucose measurement.
- Electrolytes.
- Arterial and venous blood gases. A decrease in the pH indicates acidosis is developing from oxygen debt and anaerobic metabolism. Elevated $PaCO_2$ indicates respiratory acidosis and impaired ventilation. A decreased PaO_2 is indicative of hypoxia in the child. A decreased HCO_3 is indicative of the buffering of acidosis. Blood gases are helpful in the initial assessment of ventilation and fluid status in the injured child.
- Lactate level.
- Urinalysis for measurement of specific gravity.

Diagnostic studies that may be helpful in the assessment of the circulatory status of trauma patients include:

- Chest radiography for evaluation for hemothorax, aortic injury, or pulmonary contusion.
- Head and cervical spine CT scan for evaluation of intracranial bleeding and spinal cord injury (SCI).
- Abdominal and pelvic CT scan.
- Pelvis radiography for evaluation of pelvic fractures.
- Long-bone radiography, especially of the femurs, which can account for considerable blood loss in children.

Once the circulatory status is revealed, concentrated efforts are aimed at the prevention of further fluid loss by controlling external bleeding and the replacement of fluid or blood loss. Fluid resuscitation is discussed at length later in this chapter.[8,123,126]

Selected Traumatic Injuries that can Lead to Fluid or Blood Loss or Circulatory Compromise

Any injury causing bleeding or fluid loss potentiates hemodynamic instability without treatment. The following injuries are high risk for major blood or fluid loss in the pediatric trauma patient.[8,123]

Head Injuries and Scalp Lacerations

The head is the most frequently injured area in a child and the most common cause of traumatic brain injury (TBI) in the pediatric population. Causes of TBI in children vary by age. Falls are the most common cause of TBI in younger children. Motor vehicle accidents, other accidents, and sports injuries are the most common in older children and teenagers. MVCs are reported to be the major cause of TBI-related deaths in children. Nonaccidental trauma (NAT) is a significant cause of TBI in infants and any child with an unexplainable head injury.[8,123,126]

Pediatric patients have an estimated circulating volume of 80 mL/kg. Infants have a proportionately larger head-to-body ratio, and an associated larger blood volume in their head leads to hypovolemia in the presence of intracranial hemorrhage. Infants with open fontanelles and open cranial sutures may have increased bleeding and intracranial pressure (ICP). Epidural, subdural, subarachnoid, and intraventricular hemorrhages are four types of internal bleeding on the brain in a child; they can cause significant to lethal amounts of blood loss in pediatric patients. Scalp and head lacerations are vascular, and bleeding may be profuse with the potential for substantial blood loss to occur in children and may require aggressive fluid resuscitation and direct pressure. Support of the child's circulatory status with fluid resuscitation may take precedence over the treatment of increased ICP with TBI. (Head injuries are discussed in depth later in the chapter.)[8,114,123,126]

Facial and Mandibular Injuries

Facial fractures are relatively uncommon in pediatric patients, with mandibular fractures being the most common of all facial fractures of childhood. MVCs, fall from a height, bicycle injury, sports-related injury, violence or assault, and NAT are the most common MOIs. Concomitant injuries with pediatric maxillofacial injuries include concussion, intracranial hemorrhage, cervical spine injury (CSI), and skull fractures. Concomitant intracranial, chest, abdominal, and extremity injuries emphasize the high-energy impact required to induce mandibular fractures in children. The bony structures of the skull are incredibly vascular, and like facial injuries, they bleed copiously when injured. Patients with LeFort fractures or open mandibular fractures may need aggressive resuscitation. The majority of profuse bleeding associated with pediatric facial trauma may be from lacerations and soft-tissue injuries. The vascularity of the face makes clinical findings often obvious with frank external bleeding noted. After airway control is achieved, some patients may need oral and retropharyngeal packing to control bleeding. Marked facial swelling and ecchymosis may also be present with these injuries. Monitor for cerebrospinal fluid leakage in children with maxillofacial injuries.[8,132,147–149]

Treatment of Facial and Mandibular Injuries

Evaluating pediatric facial injuries involves following the principles of trauma management with the initial or primary survey of the child's airway to clear and secure the airway, breathing, and bleeding control while maintaining immobilization of the cervical spine because of concomitant injuries. Be cautious with the application of cervical immobilization devices with these types of fractures. The device may depress the soft tissue and occlude the airway. Hypovolemic shock may result in children from excessive blood loss from injuries to the extremely vascular face. Bleeding may require resuscitation because of the amount of blood loss, especially with open LeFort fractures. Consider that the patient may have a TBI and maintain adequate systolic blood pressure to ensure adequate cerebral perfusion pressure (CPP) when resuscitation measures are needed. Depending on the child's response to crystalloid support during resuscitation, blood products may be needed until bleeding is under control. After the child is stabilized, move on to the secondary survey for a more detailed examination of the child's head, face, and neck to identify any additional injuries.[8,132,147–149]

Cardiac Injuries

Blunt cardiac injury (BCI) is uncommon in children. It is usually associated with high-energy mechanisms such as MVCs. Diagnosis of BCI is difficult in children because presenting signs and symptoms and external signs are limited or absent. The child presenting with any of the following symptoms—ecchymosis, abrasions, or deformity to the chest wall; focal rib tenderness; muffled heart tones; new-onset murmur; abnormal upper and lower extremity pulses; rib fractures; and pulmonary contusion in the presence of blunt force trauma—should be considered at risk for BCI.[8,141,150,151]

The chest wall of a child is more susceptible to underlying injuries such as BCI because of the elastic, compliant rib cage, which transmits more kinetic energy to a child's intrathoracic internal structures without fractures in blunt force trauma. Most BCIs may not be diagnosed and will resolve without interventions, and those who are diagnosed usually have additional presenting symptoms on CXR, abnormal electrocardiogram (ECG), or physical examination.[8,141,150,151]

Treatment for Cardiac Injuries

BCI occurs most often from MVCs, falls, and crush injuries. Direct impact to the precordium from a projectile is less common but increasing in frequency. Rapid deceleration is the most common MOI resulting in BCI. BCI in children is associated with pulmonary contusion and rib fractures. Prehospital management of BCI is difficult in the field. Follow the principles of ATLS with rapid transport to the closest trauma center. Children with blunt chest trauma may present with respiratory or cardiac compromise or immediate life-threatening injuries, and an initial rapid assessment is necessary to initiate control of the airway, breathing, and circulation. Immediate interventions are implemented to treat life-threatening injuries such as cardiac tamponade, commotio cordis, or injury to the great vessels.[8,134,141,150–153]

Commotio Cordis

Commotio cordis is a type of BCI that occurs in athletes and is increasing in frequency because of sports-related injuries. Commotio cordis results from a projectile, such as a baseball, striking the child's chest during a susceptible time in the cardiac cycle resulting in ventricular fibrillation and sudden cardiac death in the child.[8,141,150–153]

Treatment for Commotio Cordis. Perform the primary survey, which is the initial rapid assessment and stabilization of the child; identify life-threatening injuries; and initiate immediate treatment for any BCI in children. If commotio cordis is suspected or witnessed, immediately begin cardiopulmonary resuscitation (CPR). Survival for this BCI requires immediate CPR and early automated external defibrillator use for survival; without these two interventions, survival is poor in children.[8,141,150–153]

Cardiac Tamponade

Cardiac ventricular rupture is rare in children but is the most common cause of death from blunt trauma. The right ventricle is the chamber most frequently injured because the location is anterior to the chest and under the sternum. Because of the increased pliability of the pediatric rib cage, rib fractures may be absent in a child with a cardiac injury. Pericardial tamponade most frequently occurs with injury to the heart or great vessels. It can be caused by either blunt or penetrating trauma to the chest. Children with blunt thoracic injuries commonly have few signs and symptoms to suggest a cardiac injury is present. The classic triad of jugular venous distension, muffled heart sounds, and hypotension (referred to as Beck's triad) is difficult to detect in pediatric patients. Another classic sign of cardiac tamponade is pulsus paradoxus, which is when the child's blood pressure falls more than 10 mmHg during inspiration. Data indicate this occurs in less than 50% of pediatric patients with pericardial tamponade, so it is not reliable for the diagnosis of pericardial tamponade. Jugular venous distention, and an elevated central venous pressure, can be missed in smaller children because of smaller necks and increased subcutaneous tissue and cannot be a reliable sign. Remember that other clinical conditions may occur, such as hypovolemia, or environmental concerns, such as noise, can make this diagnosis difficult. It only takes a small amount of blood to interfere with cardiac activity because of the child's small pericardial sac. Fortunately, the removal of this small amount of blood will drastically improve cardiac function.[8,141,150–153]

Cardiac tamponade should be considered in all patients with blunt or penetrating thoracic injuries. Pulseless electrical activity in the absence of tension pneumothorax and hypovolemia is highly suggestive of cardiac tamponade. Another sign of cardiac tamponade is pulsus paradoxus, which is described earlier and is not reliable for the diagnosis of pericardial tamponade. Kussmaul's sign, which is a rise in venous pressure with inspiration when breathing spontaneously, is a true paradoxical venous pressure abnormally associated with cardiac tamponade. Both of these are extremely difficult to assess in the transport setting but can be indicative of cardiac tamponade.[8,141,150–153]

Treatment of Cardiac Tamponade. The treatment of cardiac tamponade includes immediate supportive treatment with IV crystalloid to transiently increase filling pressure and improve CO, but definitive treatment includes pericardiocentesis to evacuate fluid. The most optimal method would be under ultrasound guidance, but this is not part of the transport provider's normal arsenal of equipment.

Pericardiocentesis. Treatment for cardiac tamponade is rapid pericardiocentesis to decompress the pericardium. A subxiphoid approach with a spinal needle or an over-the-needle catheter attached to a 30-mL syringe with a three-way stopcock is the preferred method of aspiration of blood from the pericardial sac. The needle is directed to the pericardium at a 45-degree angle during aspiration. Cardiac monitoring to assess for ventricular arrhythmias or irritability is essential. Aspiration of a small amount of pericardial nonclotting blood may be all that is needed to temporarily relieve symptoms and see an improvement in hemodynamic status caused by the injured myocardium's ability to self-seal. Pericardiocentesis may not be diagnostic or therapeutic when the blood in the pericardial sac has clotted. Transport to an appropriate facility for definitive cardiac care is always necessary.[8,123,141,150–153]

Myocardial Contusion

Myocardial contusion occurs when blunt force is delivered to the myocardium causing injury. Cardiac contusion is the most common cardiac injury after blunt trauma. With relatively smaller amounts of subcutaneous fat and cartilaginous ribs, children are at great risk for this injury. Only mild symptoms, such as palpitations or precordial or chest pain, may be present following injury. Additional symptoms such as arrhythmias and decreased CO may occur but are not common in the immediate post-injury period. The absence of obvious chest wall trauma does not rule out the diagnosis of cardiac injury. Pediatric patients with blunt thoracic trauma serious enough to cause pulmonary contusion or rib fractures are at high risk for myocardial contusion. Because of the potential for complications and the difficulty in making a definitive diagnosis, a high index of suspicion for myocardial contusion should be held in patients with blunt chest trauma. Monitor the patient for complications of myocardial contusion, which include hypotension, conduction abnormalities, or wall motion abnormalities on echocardiography. Common arrhythmias include premature ventricular contractions, unexplained sinus tachycardia, atrial fibrillation, and bundle branch blocks (primarily on the right); ECG may show ST-segment abnormalities indicating myocardial infarction.[8,123,141,150–153]

Treatment of Myocardial Contusion. Treatment of myocardial contusion is supportive. Patients need at least 24 hours of cardiac monitoring. The risk for sudden arrhythmia decreases greatly after 24 hours. Significant arrhythmias should be treated with advanced cardiac life support (ACLS) and PALS protocols, and cardiology consultation may be indicated.[8,123–125]

Traumatic Aortic Disruption

Traumatic aortic disruption or blunt aortic injury (BAI) resulting from blunt chest trauma is a rare injury in children and most die at the scene of the traumatic injury. The chance of survival is increased with rapid detection and surgical intervention. Rapid deceleration is the most common MOI resulting in BAI from MVCs or falls from great heights. Children who survive may present with hypotension, unequal upper and lower pulses or decreased blood pressures in the lower extremities compared with upper extremities, and paraplegia.

Occasionally, children may present with minimal or no evidence of chest wall trauma. If the child has rib fractures or suspected pulmonary contusion, suspect BAI. If CXRs are available, a widened superior mediastinum, an abnormal contour of the aortic knob, and a left hemothorax or pleural effusion may be seen. Patients with aortic rupture who have a chance of survival are those with a partial laceration at the level of the ligamentum arteriosum and survive because of a contained hematoma at the site. Unexplained persistent hypotension is usually not related to this injury, and other bleeding sources should be sought. A transected aorta that bleeds freely into the left chest can cause profound hypotension but is quickly fatal (in minutes) without operative intervention. Clinical signs and symptoms of this injury are often absent, and a high index of suspicion must be maintained for patients with MOIs that involve rapid deceleration. CXR findings that may be indicative of major vessel injury are listed in Box 18.4. False-positive and negative x-ray findings are possible, so any patient with suspected aortic injury should receive more testing. Angiography continues to be the gold standard for diagnosis, but a CT scan of the chest and transesophageal echocardiography may also show aortic injury.[8,123,150–153]

Treatment of Traumatic Aortic Disruption. Transport the patient to a center capable of caring for a child with a cardiothoracic injury. Treatment of this injury is operative repair either with resection and grafting or primary repair. Hemothoraces should be treated as described previously, and fluid resuscitation should be provided based on the patient's hemodynamic status.[8,123,152,153]

Penetrating Cardiac Trauma

Research is limited regarding pediatric penetrating cardiac trauma. Penetrating cardiac trauma may be associated with a hemopericardium and tamponade. Penetrating trauma resulting from gunshot wounds tends to cause larger injuries to the chest and presents with blood loss and hypovolemia. Small penetrating injuries to the pericardium can heal spontaneously over time. The right ventricle is injured more often in penetrating trauma because of its anterior location. Penetrating injury to multiple chambers of the heart has a significant mortality attached. Rapid resuscitation and early transfer to the operating room at a definitive facility will significantly decrease mortality.[8,123,152,153]

Abdominal Injuries

Abdominal trauma is the most common cause of unrecognized fatal injury in children. Blunt abdominal trauma is the third most common cause of trauma-related deaths in children. Approximately 90% of abdominal trauma is blunt force and 10% is penetrating. Intra-abdominal injuries are more common in patients with seatbelt signs than those children without. The presence of the seatbelt abrasion sign should trigger the provider to suspect significant intra-abdominal injuries that may require acute interventions. The anatomic differences in children predispose them to abdominal injuries. Children have larger solid organs in relation to their size, less subcutaneous fat, and less developed musculature of the abdomen resulting in less protection from injury. They also have a protruding abdomen placing vital organs closer to impacting forces and a small thorax with elastic compliant ribs that decrease protection, especially to the liver and spleen. The spleen and liver are the most frequently injured organs, followed by the kidneys, small bowel, and pancreas.[8,123,126,154–157]

The most common MOIs for blunt abdominal trauma in children are MVCs, auto versus pedestrian injury, bike versus car, and falls. Bicycle handlebar injuries, sports, incidents involving all-terrain vehicles, and NAT are additional MOIs causing internal abdominal injuries in children. The mortality rate in children after blunt abdominal trauma is rare but increases as more abdominal structures are identified as injured. It is difficult to perform examinations of abdominal injuries of pediatric patients because of their fear of being examined or the pain from other injuries that distract the child and interfere with the assessment. Preverbal children are unable to describe or relate pain. Abdominal findings can be subtle and are often missed on initial examination. The transport provider should maintain a high index of suspicion or awareness for potentially serious underlying injuries in children presenting with multiple traumatic injuries.[8,123,126,154–158]

Treatment of Abdominal Injuries

The initial management of children with suspected intra-abdominal injury (IAI) should follow the ATLS or program guidelines for diagnosis and treatment of immediately life-threatening injuries. During stabilization, children with signs of IAI and hemodynamic instability that do not respond to fluid resuscitation and blood transfusion call for an emergent laparotomy. Following the primary survey, the provider should begin the secondary survey of hemodynamically stable children who are suspected of blunt IAI to identify any missed injuries. The secondary survey helps identify other indicators for observation or laboratory evaluation. Imaging with a focused assessment with sonography for trauma (FAST) is a useful tool in the initial and secondary evaluation, or an emergent laparotomy may be needed in unstable patients.[8,123,126,154–158]

Penetrating abdominal trauma in children from gunshot or stab wounds accounts for approximately 10% of all abdominal injuries. Bullets may cause extensive damage from the high kinetic energy of the projectile, and the blast effect can change the route of the bullet after it enters the body, increasing damage along the bullet's path. The small intestine is injured more often than the large bowel, which is injured more than the liver in penetrating abdominal trauma. Penetrating trauma is usually easily identified in the primary survey through inspection.

The risk of complications may be expected by the presentation of clinical shock, number of organs injured, amount of blood transfusions the child required, and other associated thoracic injuries. Exploratory laparotomy is currently the gold standard for managing penetrating abdominal injuries in children.[8,123,126,154–158]

New data are emerging indicating that selective nonoperative management may be a safe treatment option for children who are hemodynamically stable after clinical examination and radiographic evaluations are performed. Minimally invasive laparoscopic surgery may be used for those patients who are hemodynamically stable. The Pediatric Emergency Care Applied Research Network (PECARN) conducted a study and established a prediction rule encompassing seven patient history and physical examination variables, without labs or ultrasonographic information, that were able to identify children with blunt torso trauma at very low risk for IAI, which successfully limited CT scans and invasive treatment methods.[8,123,126,154–159]

Blunt abdominal trauma must be suspected and discovered from historical information, MOI, and physical examination. During the secondary survey, the provider monitors closely for subtle signs of hemorrhagic shock such as compensation for hypovolemia with tachycardia that progresses to a narrowed pulse pressure (20 mmHg or less); delayed capillary refill time; pallor; mottling; cool, clammy skin; decreased urine output; or altered mental status in children. Although not definitive, these findings may indicate ongoing intra-abdominal hemorrhage. Remember, children can lose up to 30% of their blood volume before systolic blood pressure begins to trend down, which allows a significant intra-abdominal hemorrhage to occur. Physical signs indicating increased suspicion for IAI in children include ecchymosis, especially in the umbilical or flank areas; abrasions; tire track marks; seatbelt sign in restrained passengers; abdominal tenderness; abdominal distention; peritoneal irritation indicated with abdominal wall rigidity; or pain in the left shoulder induced by palpation of the left upper quadrant (Kehr's sign); or absent bowel sounds indicating a prolonged ileus. Signs of abdominal injury are variable and may evolve over time, which necessitates serial examinations. The stomach and bladder (unless contraindicated because of injury) need to be decompressed and the child examined for abrasions and contusions. If the child remains awake and alert, gentle palpation may demonstrate significant pain and tenderness, but the accuracy of the provider's assessment may be affected if distracting injuries are present.[8,123,127,154–159]

Seatbelt Sign (Syndrome) and Injuries

Seatbelt use in an MVC is the single most effective process to decrease morbidity and mortality in children. The use of lap and shoulder seatbelt restraints reduces the risk of fatal injuries to children 5 years of age and older. It is important to ensure the child is using the seatbelts correctly and has the lap belt positioned correctly low across the thighs and not across the abdomen, which will reduce intra-abdominal injuries in children. Seatbelt sign or syndrome presents with erythema, ecchymosis, or abrasions across the abdominal wall, intra-abdominal injuries to both hollow (more common) and solid (less common) organs, and spinal fractures of the lumbar spine (Chance fracture, which is most often from L2 to L4 in children). Additional signs and symptoms may include abdominal pain or tenderness indicating an increased risk of internal injuries.[8,123,127,160–162]

The MOI related to the seatbelt sign is a rapid deceleration resulting in compression of the lower abdomen and sudden hyperflexion of the upper torso around the seatbelt, leading to crushing of the abdominal content against the spine. The MOI related to the seatbelt sign is a significant force being transmitted to the abdomen and spine necessitating a thorough examination by the provider. Children who present with seatbelt signs are considerably more likely to sustain intra-abdominal injuries involving the mesentery, bowel, and pancreas, compared with those without seatbelt signs. There is not a reported association of solid organ (liver or spleen) injuries involved with this presenting sign. Intra-abdominal injuries are more common in patients presenting with the seatbelt sign than without. The transport provider should be cognizant and prepared to provide rapid interventions for the child with a seatbelt sign. In addition, an SCI presents in half of the children with a seatbelt sign.[8,123,127,155,160–162]

Treatment for Seatbelt Sign. The initial management of children with suspected IAI resulting from the seatbelt sign or syndrome is to follow the ATLS guidelines for diagnosis and treatment of immediately life-threatening injuries. The provider needs to maintain a high level of suspicion for internal injuries in these patients and perform serial clinical examinations and appropriate diagnostic tests in patients not proceeding immediately to laparotomy. Treatment may include observation, IV fluids, blood transfusion, labs, emergent laparotomy (unstable), and potential CT (stable).[8,123,127,155,160–162]

Diagnostic Adjuncts for Abdominal Trauma

The FAST is a quick noninvasive method for evaluating for free intraperitoneal fluid suggestive of abdominal injuries, but CT remains the gold standard for diagnosing abdominal injuries. Treatment is trending toward serial monitoring of hematocrit, bed rest, and additional imaging studies, and less toward surgery. CTs are associated with significant radiation exposure, and now there are data suggesting children exposed to CT will develop cancer (such as thyroid cancer), later in life. The diagnostic peritoneal lavage (DPL) can be used to quickly diagnose or exclude the presence of internal bleeding. The DPL is a diagnostic tool used less often because of the increased use of CTs and FAST modalities. DPL is used more often in unstable children or those presenting with inconsistent examinations.[8,123,127,154–156]

Nonaccidental Abdominal Trauma

Abdominal injury in NAT is a documented reason why children are hospitalized. Abdominal injuries in children from NAT are frequently significant with an escalating need for surgical interventions. If a child presents with an abdominal injury and NAT is known or suspected, CT of the abdomen and pelvis with contrast should be performed for both diagnostic testing and forensic evidence. NAT injuries of the bowel have a high rate of occurrence, but the liver, spleen, and pancreas are injured more often in children. The abdominal injuries present in a child suspected of NAT are frequently quite severe and may require surgery. Abdominal trauma is the second most common cause of fatal child abuse after head injuries. Children with abdominal injuries from NAT will usually also present with coexisting injuries including head injuries, thoracic trauma including rib and clavicle fractures, and pulmonary contusions. Identifying NAT in the setting of known abdominal trauma is important to protect the child from future abuse and also guide diagnostic investigation. Recognition of abdominal injuries in the presence of NAT or suspected abuse is challenging as a result of unclear clinical histories, delayed presentations, and vague or nonspecific patient complaints. Delays in diagnosing abdominal injuries from NAT may contribute to poor outcomes in these children. A large number of children with abdominal injuries from NAT may not have any physical signs such as bruising or their x-ray does not demonstrate changes indicative of NAT. Physical signs may include hypoactive bowel sounds or abdominal bruising. Labs are not always clear-cut and helpful in diagnosing NAT. Findings of anemia and leukocytosis are not reliable indicators of abdominal trauma and may occur without significant injuries. Patients with aspartate aminotransferase

(AST) or alanine aminotransferase (ALT) greater than 80 IU/L should trigger the transport provider to suspect abdominal trauma. Additional labs to consider are lipase, amylase, and urinalysis. The transport provider should maintain a high level of suspicion for NAT in children who have both hollow viscous injuries and solid organ injuries.[8,123,127,154–156,163]

Spleen and Liver Injuries

The liver and spleen are the most common, potentially life-threatening organs injured in children. The majority of injuries to the liver and spleen are from blunt force trauma in children. The prognosis for both types of injury depends mainly on the presence or absence of associated injuries, especially TBI and chest trauma. Solid organ injuries are common in pediatric patients who suffer major or multisystem trauma. With isolated or single-system trauma, the spleen is the most commonly injured abdominal organ. The ribs of children only partially protect the liver and spleen, and the remainder of these organs extend below the rib cage. The pliability of a child's rib cage, the large segments of the spleen and liver extending below the ribs, less subcutaneous fat, and weak musculature of the abdomen all increase the risk of internal injuries to the liver and spleen when the MOI is from a blunt force.[8,123,154–158]

The MOI may be a direct force on the epigastric area, tearing away the blood supply as a result of rapid deceleration, penetrating injury from a fractured rib, or crushing injury against the spinal column. The liver and spleen are incredibly vascular, and disruption of the vascular supply to these organs can result in massive hemorrhage. Clinical signs may be subtle but may include point and rebound tenderness, radiation of pain to the left shoulder from injuries to the spleen, ecchymosis or abrasion to the upper abdominal quadrants, lower rib fractures, and abdominal distension. Signs of shock may be present when there is significant injury to these organs.[8,123,154–158]

Treatment of Spleen and Liver Injuries

Initial assessment of an injured child should follow the ATLS guidelines to identify life-threatening injuries that have a negative effect on the airway, breathing, and circulation. Identification of abdominal injuries occurs with the secondary survey after the pediatric patient is stabilized through interventions performed in the primary survey.[123]

Clinical signs of injury to the spleen or liver will include signs and symptoms of hypovolemia shock with tachycardia, delayed capillary refill, pallor, altered mental status, decreased urine output, hypotension, abdominal contusions with signs of ecchymosis, abrasions as a result of seatbelt or bicycle handlebars injuries, or abdominal distention. Other clinical signs are tenderness over the abdominal areas, right upper quadrant tenderness that may indicate an injury to the liver, or left upper quadrant tenderness that may indicate an injury to the spleen. Orogastric tube insertion facilitates the abdominal examination by reducing aspiration of gastric contents and decreasing distention from swallowed air. Patients presenting with signs and symptoms of hypovolemia require fluid resuscitation with crystalloid solutions and possibly blood transfusions to reverse the hypovolemic shock until definitive treatment is received to control bleeding of the liver or spleen. Unstable children with blunt trauma to the abdomen who do not improve with fluid resuscitation of 40–60 mL/kg of normal saline or lactated Ringer's solution IV, followed by packed red blood cells of 10 mL/kg IV, require emergent exploratory laparotomy. Transport pediatric trauma patients to a definitive center capable of performing serial observations or damage control surgery to stop the hemorrhage.[8,123,154–158,163]

Nonoperative management of the hemodynamically stable pediatric trauma patient with spleen or liver (solid organ) injuries is a treatment option with low rates of failure; nonoperative failure is when the child requires surgical intervention. Obtaining a CT following blunt abdominal trauma has provided the recognition of active bleeding of the spleen or liver by identifying the IV contrast or blush, which is a reliable indicator of significant organ injury. Nonoperative management of blunt abdominal trauma with suspected liver or spleen injury is the standard of care for the stable pediatric trauma patient. Unstable pediatric patients may require surgical intervention with a splenectomy. Research has shown that pediatric patients presenting with contrast blush on CT were successfully treated with the nonoperative method following serial examinations, labs (especially hematocrit), treatment with blood products, and, if necessary, angiography. This method demonstrated far less blood product requirement for children than the surgical intervention of a splenectomy, which sets up the child for post-splenectomy sepsis.[8,123,154–159,163]

Nonaccidental Solid Organ Injuries

The liver and pancreas are the most frequently injured solid organs from NAT. The left lobe of the liver is the most frequently injured in NAT and most likely from central assault, which is the opposite injury sustained in accidental traumas. In NAT, liver lacerations may be present without signs or symptoms. Liver lacerations can be identified by checking for abnormal levels of transaminase. Transaminase assists in the detection of occult liver injuries and these levels may help determine the age of the hepatic injury. The determination of the age of the hepatic injury may not only help identify the individual responsible for inflicting the blunt force injuries to the child but may help the provider recognize a fabricated history of how the child was injured. In children with NAT liver injury, the ALT may be higher than the AST, indicating that the liver injury is older than 12 hours. Hepatic and splenic injuries from NAT present with MOIs similar to accidental traumas and include lacerations, fractures, hematomas, and rupture and hepatic lacerations, which are the most common. Linear lacerations through the liver, known as bear claw lacerations, are the most common in children and are identified at imaging, and are a result of compression applied to the hepatic parenchyma. The majority of blunt NATs affecting the liver or spleen are treated nonoperatively.[123,154–158,163]

Pancreatic Injuries

The pancreas is the fourth most common solid organ injury in children following injuries to the spleen, liver, and kidneys. The pancreas is not as vascular as the liver and spleen, and major blood loss is very rare. Blunt trauma injury to the pancreas is difficult to diagnose immediately after the injury because of the retroperitoneal location of the trauma, the lack of reliable signs and symptoms, and the limited sensitivity of common imaging modalities. The most common complications are the formation of pancreatic fistulas, pancreatitis, and the development of pancreatic pseudocysts, which usually present weeks after injury. The nonoperative management of minor pancreatic injury is well accepted with grade I and II injuries. Grade III and higher are more serious pancreatic injuries with capsular, ductal, or parenchymal disruption in pediatric patients, and the treatment is controversial. Pancreatic injury is determined by elevated serum amylase, lipase levels, and CRP, CT, ultrasonography, or endoscopic retrograde cholangiopancreatography (ERCP).[8,123,154,155,157,158]

The most common MOIs are pedestrian versus automobile, NAT, injuries received in an MVC, or handlebars of a bicycle. The actual MOI usually involves compression of the pancreas against the rigid spinal column or direct blunt force. Severe pancreatic intra-abdominal injuries may require immediate surgical intervention and other less severe injuries may be treated with nonoperative management. An isolated pancreatic injury may have a delay of hours or days before the onset of abdominal symptoms. The symptoms following injury include abdominal pain, nausea, vomiting, and fever and may be nonspecific but should increase the level of suspicion for pancreatic injury following blunt abdominal trauma. An example would be a bicycle handlebar injury. Serum amylase levels are obtained for all children with blunt abdominal trauma, but they do not correlate to the severity of the injury and should not be used as a diagnostic measure in patients. A CRP level greater than 150 mg/dL at 48 hours helps differentiate between mild or severe pancreatitis. The serum lipase level may be used only to exclude salivary amylase in cases of head and neck injuries.[3,117,149]

CT imaging obtained on admission is a valuable tool when positive for pancreatic injury because it identifies the location of the trauma and grading of injuries is usually accurate. CT should not be used as a study of exclusion. The failure of the CT scan to detect pancreatic injuries on admission does not suggest diagnostic inaccuracy, but rather the evolving nature of pancreatic injuries. Grade III injuries missed on initial CT scans are typically later diagnosed on ERCP. Such injuries are allowed to progress to pseudocysts. Ultrasound scans are used to document and follow-up in children in whom pseudocysts develop during hospitalization. Management of pancreatic injuries is determined by the severity and location of the injury and the presence or absence of associated abdominal injuries. Pancreatic injury is an unusual complication of blunt abdominal trauma, usually minor (grade I or II), with pancreatic ductal disruption occurring in a minority of cases (grade III or higher). Children with pancreatic injuries without ductal disruption do not appear to suffer increased morbidity following conservative management, and children presenting with ductal disruption may require operative intervention.[8,123,154,155,157,158]

Nonaccidental Pancreatic Injuries

The average age of a child with NAT pancreatitis is less than 3 years of age and is younger than children with pancreatitis from other MOIs. The majority of traumatic pancreatitis is secondary to NAT. In the absence of a plausible history, such as an MVC or bicycle handlebar injury, the provider should suspect that the traumatic pancreatitis is from NAT. Imaging to detect pancreatic injury in children may be limited. If the CT is obtained immediately after the trauma it may not detect a majority of injuries to the pancreas. The most common CT finding following a NAT pancreatic injury in children is fluid in the lesser sac. Any finding of any peripancreatic fluid without other abdominal injuries is indicative of pancreatic injury.[163]

Hollow Viscous Injuries

Blunt abdominal trauma is common in pediatric patients but rarely results in significant hollow visceral injuries. For children to have damage to hollow visceral organs requires powerful blunt force mechanisms that cause associated injuries to the solid visceral organs resulting in a delayed diagnosis and treatment of the hollow viscous organs. The most common hollow visceral injury is a jejunal perforation, followed by injury to the duodenum, colon, and finally the stomach. Most of these injuries result from a direct force such as an MVC, seatbelt injury, bicycle handlebar injury, or falls. The MOI is usually rapid acceleration or deceleration of the intestinal structures near a fixed anatomic point, such as the ligament of Treitz, or the trapping of the bowel between the seatbelt and the spine. Definitive management of children evaluated for hollow viscous injury as a result of blunt abdominal trauma is dependent on the child's clinical findings. Most of these injuries will require surgical intervention.[8,123,154,157,164]

Nonaccidental Hollow Viscous Injuries

Hollow viscous injuries account for just over 10% of all intra-abdominal injuries in NAT that require hospitalization. Bowel injury resulting from NAT is significantly higher than accidental bowel injuries. The duodenum and proximal jejunum are the most commonly injured hollow viscous organs in NAT. Other associated NAT injuries are to the gastric area, bladder, and colon. The duodenum and proximal jejunum are high-risk injuries in NAT secondary to their location at the ligament of Treitz and the concentration of force from a punch or kick to the epigastric area. Bowel injuries from NAT can range from localized hematoma to bowel perforation, or an intramural hematoma, which is the most common bowel injury associated with NAT. Bowel injuries may also have mesenteric tears or contusions. A disruption of the mesentery from NAT may cause bowel ischemia. Children presenting with bowel perforation and peritonitis frequently go directly to surgery without any imaging. Free air on CXR is indicative of intraperitoneal free air and that the bowel has perforated. The provider must remember that NAT injuries often involve both the peritoneal and the retroperitoneal duodenum, and a plain x-ray may not be sufficient to identify and diagnose all NAT injuries. Bowel perforation from blunt trauma secondary to NAT may not be identified on a CT scan, making it a difficult diagnosis. Findings of pneumoperitoneum or leakage of oral contrast material are diagnostic of intestinal perforation but are insensitive and are seen most frequently in patients with clinical peritonitis who would proceed to surgery regardless of the CT results. The most common finding in bowel or mesenteric injury is unexplained intraperitoneal fluid. However, this finding is not predictive of injury, and patients with isolated intra-abdominal free fluid at CT can follow a nonoperative approach that includes serial abdominal examinations.[163,164]

Stomach Injuries

Stomach injuries rarely occur as a result of blunt abdominal trauma but may occur as a result of a lap belt, airbag, or handlebar injury. Abdominal pain occurring after blunt abdominal trauma should have the provider suspecting hollow visceral organ injury. Perforation is the most common gastric injury. Pediatric trauma patients develop gastric dilatation from crying or assisted ventilation which may lead to circulatory and respiratory compromise if untreated. All pediatric patients with multisystem injuries or those who need assisted ventilation should have their stomachs decompressed with a gastric tube to prevent these complications. Gastric tubes can be used if the patient does not have known or suspected facial or head injuries. Orogastric tubes are safer than nasal tubes until facial and head trauma are eliminated. Initial management of children with suspected blunt hollow viscous injuries requires adherence to ATLS guidelines related to immediate life-threatening injuries for diagnosis, treatment, and appropriate resuscitation. Peritonitis is more common in patients with perforations of the stomach.[8,123,155-157]

Duodenal Injuries

The most common hollow viscous injury is the jejunal perforation. This injury is suggestive of NAT if there is no other history of abdominal trauma in children. High-energy blunt forces, direct blows to fixed points such as the ligament of Treitz or the ileocecal valve, or sudden deceleration causing a shearing force at the mesenteric attachment may cause injuries to the jejunum. A mesenteric injury may affect the blood supply to the small intestine and may lead to delayed perforation from ischemic necrosis. This injury presents with pain and tenderness to palpation 12–24 hours after the injury. Peritoneal signs are vague because the jejunal contents are not as acidic as those of the stomach. The small intestine contents are less acidic than the stomach contents and have limited or no signs of peritoneal irritation. The bacterial count is low but still has the potential to cause sepsis, abdominal abscess, or infection. Treatment is supportive and requires surgical intervention. MVCs are the most common cause of duodenal injuries in children followed by NAT.[8,123,155,157-159]

Nonaccidental Duodenal Injuries

Duodenal injuries require special consideration given their high association with NAT in young children. In children 3 years of age and younger the majority of duodenal injuries are caused by NAT. A duodenal hematoma may be the first recognizable sign indicating NAT. Clinical presentation in cases of NAT is often delayed, and delay in presentation with duodenal injuries carries a higher rate of complications, with increased rates of abscess formation and sepsis.[163]

Genitourinary Injuries

Traumatic injuries to the genitourinary system are rarely fatal in children, but they may be associated with hemorrhage and hypovolemic shock. In pediatric blunt abdominal trauma, the most injured solid organ is the kidney. Children are at a greater risk of kidney injury because of the pliable elastic rib cage permitting compression during rapid deceleration. The kidneys are anatomically large for the child's abdomen and pelvis size, and the lack of perirenal fat contributes to increased risks of renal injury in children exposed to blunt abdominal trauma. The management goals of pediatric renal trauma are to protect the renal parenchyma and minimize patient morbidity by treating life-threatening injuries. Life-threatening emergencies are rapidly recognized and evaluated by using ATLS rapid primary assessment with the objective to decrease or limit unnecessary surgical interventions. Clinical findings may be subtle, and hematuria is not considered a sensitive indicator of injury.

Treatment of these injuries is supportive and may require surgical evaluation. Most blunt pediatric renal injuries are low, grade I to III, and are seen more in male children usually older than 6 years of age. Management is evolving toward a conservative approach with a high rate of success in grade IV renal injuries in which no life-threatening bleeding is present. The most frequent causes of renal trauma in children include all-terrain vehicles, dirt bikes, falls, MVCs, bicycles, and sporting activities. The majority of pediatric abdominal renal trauma is handled without surgical intervention. The anatomic position of the pediatric bladder offers protection from pelvic fractures. Bladder rupture is more common in children than adults and occurs as a result of the child's shallow pelvis. The genitourinary system in children can be injured by vehicle restraints in deceleration injuries or by falls with direct blunt trauma. As with many abdominal injuries, a high index of suspicion must be maintained for patients with MOIs likely to cause trauma to the genitourinary system.[8,123,154,158–160,163–167]

Nonaccidental Kidney Injuries

Isolated hematuria or renal injury may occur in 25% of cases of IAI secondary to NAT. NAT resulting in renal injuries is common in children hospitalized with intra-abdominal trauma. Reported NAT injuries include hematomas, contusions, and renal vascular injuries. Renal injuries should be graded using the American Association for the Surgery of Trauma Organ Injury Scale. Renal lacerations are graded by the involvement of the renal collecting system. CT imaging requires testing during the excretory phase to detect urinary bleeding. NAT resulting in low-grade lesions, such as ill-defined hypoattenuating parenchymal contusions and small subscapular hematomas, will usually resolve without long-term sequelae. A shattered kidney (multiple lacerations and fragmentation) and complete renal devascularization are the most severe (grade V) renal injuries. Treatment of NAT renal injuries is aimed at renal preservation, with the first choice being nonoperative management.[163]

Pelvic Injuries

Pediatric pelvic fractures are rare injuries and are associated with higher morbidity and mortality than any other orthopedic injuries. Pelvic fractures are rare in children and are caused by a high-energy mechanism. The pediatric pelvis contains more cartilage, is more elastic, and can absorb a greater amount of force without causing fractures to occur. One of the most disturbing complications related to pelvic fractures is extensive bladder and/or urethral injuries (BUIs). Patients with these injuries often require multiple urologic procedures and experience long-term sexual and psychologic dysfunction. Bladder injuries are uncommon regardless of sex, and urethral injuries are seen more often in males. The diagnosis of a pelvic fracture with associated BUI is often difficult to make in the field or the ED, particularly in female children. The reason for this is likely multifactorial, such as BUIs are often sustained after major trauma involving multiple organ systems; the provider may be treating life-threatening injuries during the trauma resuscitation; younger children may not be able to adequately communicate and localize their pain, increasing the risk for an unrecognized injury; and last, the classic signs and symptoms associated with urethral injuries, such as blood at the meatus or perineal hematoma, are often absent. When pediatric pelvic fractures occur they are associated with a higher likelihood of morbidity and mortality. One major cause of this morbidity is BUI. When BUI is missed, the outcome is often poor. Up to 23% of BUIs may be missed on the initial examination on males and up to 40% on females. On average, these missed injuries may not be detected until almost 3 days later. If the diagnosis of BUI is delayed, patients may develop a wide variety of complications including septic shock, pelvic abscess, peritonitis, myonecrosis of the thigh, and bladder entrapment.

The key to a good outcome without complications lies in the early detection of BUI. The majority of children with pelvic fractures, however, are severely injured and do not have BUI.

Children have more pliable bones with thicker periosteum in their pelvic bones. In pediatric patients, avulsion fractures of the pelvis and isolated pelvic ring fractures are more common. Significant force is required for the child to sustain a complete pelvic ring disruption involving the posterior elements. Pelvic fractures are rare in young children but can be common traumatic injuries in late adolescence. MOIs include MVCs and falls with direct blunt trauma. Fatal hemorrhage in the retroperitoneal area is associated with these fractures and requires prompt immobilization and aggressive fluid resuscitation. Clinical findings include obvious visual asymmetry, instability, pain to palpation, pain with adduction of the legs, and ecchymosis. These findings may also present with profound hypotension and shock.[8,123,165–170]

Treatment of Pelvic Injuries. Debate continues on the most appropriate method to use for stabilizing pediatric pelvic fractures for transport. Each transport program should have pediatric protocols related to pelvic support during transport. Stabilization with sheet strapping and external immobilizers are splinting options, dependent on the fracture patterns and orthopedic surgeon availability. Pelvic fractures without hemodynamic instability may only need close observation during transport. Fatal hemorrhage seen in adults is rare in pediatric pelvic fractures. The bleeding that occurs with pediatric pelvic fractures is usually associated with solid organ injuries. Identification and treatment of life-threatening injuries should be the primary focus of the initial acute management in children presenting with pelvic fractures. More aggressive immobilization should be used for pediatric patients with clinical signs of hemorrhage or hypovolemic shock. Fluid resuscitation with crystalloids (normal saline or lactated Ringer's solution) and blood products may be necessary. Plain x-rays have limited sensitivity for detecting pediatric pelvic fractures. CT scan is the gold standard for pelvic fracture diagnosis and assessment in children, but the advantages of CT should be considered against any long-term risks or effects of excessive radiation exposure.[8,123,165–170]

Femur Fractures

Femur fractures in children can cause a significant amount of blood loss. Femur fractures are rare but are the most common cause of hospitalization for pediatric orthopedic injuries. The treatment for femur fractures is based on age and injury with a tendency toward operative stabilization. The femur is the largest bone in the body. In pediatric trauma, a child with a suspected femur fracture may also have associated injuries or life-threatening injuries when linked to high-impact trauma such as an MVC. In infants and toddlers, NAT and falls are the most common causes of femur fractures. In toddlers to older children, falls are the most common cause of femur fractures. Motor vehicle versus pedestrian collisions, MVCs, and sports-related injuries are the most common causes of femur fractures in older children and teenagers. A pediatric injury pattern involving children who are hit by a motor vehicle and sustain a femur fracture, severe head injury, and chest and abdominal injury is commonly called Waddell's triad. Femur fractures are associated with significant trauma in children, and one should suspect multiple injuries in any child who is involved in any trauma with significant blunt force.[8,123,171,172]

Treatment of Femur Fractures

Most femur fractures in children may be diagnosed based on clinical presentation. Common presenting symptoms include localized tenderness, swelling, obvious deformity, shortening, and/or crepitus on palpation. Monitor for indications and associated proximal femur fracture, such as pain in the hip joint and other signs such as an externally rotated leg position. The skin needs to be carefully inspected for signs of an open fracture. Initiate antibiotics as soon as possible with any open fracture. All fractures should include a careful neurovascular examination distal to the fracture site before and after splinting to make sure the fracture has not damaged arteries or nerves. Pediatric femur fractures are considered to be a significant injury with the potential to lose a large amount of blood, which mandates early and urgent interventions. Pediatric patients with femur fractures who have been involved in a high-speed MVC should undergo ATLS standard trauma evaluation to establish an airway and cervical spine immobilization as well as evaluation for breathing and circulation compromise requiring vascular access for fluid resuscitation caused by blood loss in the femur.[8,123,171,172]

After assessment of neurovascular function and administration of appropriate analgesics, fractured femurs should be aligned and immobilized. Traction splints, air splints, or a variety of commercial splints can be used for immobilization. Monitor air splints for pressure increase or decrease with altitude changes. After alignment and immobilization of the child's femur, a neurovascular assessment should always be repeated. Fluid resuscitation with crystalloid and blood products may be necessary. For those children with isolated femur fractures, immobilization and pain management are the goals of treatment.[8,123,171,172]

Vascular and Venous Injuries

Trauma is one of the leading causes of morbidity and mortality in children. Vascular injuries in children are relatively uncommon. In children, vascular trauma creates challenges because of the child's small arteries, vasospasm of these small arteries, decreased intravascular volume, the vessel growth potential, and the significance of long-term durability. Early identification and rapid interventions for vascular injuries are essential to prevent significant morbidity and mortality from massive blood loss in these children. It is challenging in pediatric vascular trauma patients to pinpoint a diagnosis because the signs and symptoms of an internal vascular injury may be cloaked by the child's physiologic ability to compensate hemodynamically for an extended period of time. Providers must maintain a high index of suspicion for associated injuries. Knowledge of the potential patterns of injury and management options is essential to limit long-term disability. Vascular injuries in children resulting from blunt trauma most often occur via the sharp edge of fractured bones. Vascular injury in pediatric trauma may be associated with significant morbidity and mortality from acute or delayed ischemia secondary to acute blood loss, arterial dissection, hematoma, aneurysm, or thrombosis.[173,174]

Treatment of Vascular and Venous Injuries. Clinical imaging techniques such as ultrasound, CT, CT angiography, traditional angiography, and DPL may be used as diagnostic aids, and the use of newer imaging modalities such as MDCT scanning may be the preferred method for assessing pediatric vascular trauma. Nonoperative management of traumatic venous injuries is rarely supported because a delay in definitive management may be detrimental to survival. Consideration for operative intervention is the preferred management of venous injuries, especially if coexisting arterial injury is suspected. Surgical repair of venous injuries in children requires specialist surgical techniques, instruments, and perioperative support. To allow for growth later in life, interrupted sutures may be used for primary repair of venous injuries in children. Synthetic grafts are usually not effective for venous repair in younger children.[173,174]

Poor prognostic indicators of increasing mortality risk in pediatric trauma patients are poor surgical access, blunt MOI with a shearing mechanism, delayed diagnosis, and the presence of additional traumatic injuries such as a head injury. Mortality in pediatric traumatic venous injuries is increased if the inferior vena cava or hepatic veins were injured. Pediatric vascular injuries are primarily caused by blunt force mechanisms and affect the upper and lower extremities. Definitive management for pediatric vascular injuries is operative management. Repair techniques are graft or patch angioplasty, end-to-end anastomosis, and interposition grafts. Pediatric vascular injuries have an increase in morbidity as a result of the small size of the damaged arteries, the need for blood vessel growth along with a child, and long-term patency of the vascular repairs. Children presenting with vascular or venous injuries, or both, should be transferred to a designated PTC for surgical intervention to decrease morbidity and mortality and optimize long-term patient outcomes.[173,174]

Disability

The fourth step in the primary survey is the neurologic assessment of an injured child, which is the disability component of the primary survey. Traumatic head or brain and spinal cord injuries are the most common causes of disability in pediatric trauma patients. Head injuries continue to be the leading cause of death in children injured from traumatic events. Children have anatomic differences that predispose them to head injuries, such as their relatively large head size compared with their body surface area; open fontanelles; cranial sutures, which can allow for a significant increase in intracranial swelling; and poorly developed neck and upper extremity musculature offering less protection to the head and neck.[8,123,126]

The neurologic assessment of the primary survey includes a quick assessment of the child's neurologic function by evaluating pupillary responses and calculating the child's Glasgow Coma Scale (GCS) or the Alert, Verbal, Pain, Unresponsive (AVPU) Pediatric Response Scale. This should be done at the end of the primary survey or before administration of sedatives, narcotics, or paralytics. Assessment of the child's neurologic status should be repeated for any improvement or deterioration. The more extensive neurologic evaluation should be deferred until the secondary survey to evade interruption or slowing down of the primary survey. It is important to establish a baseline GCS in children with a TBI to evaluate an evolving intracranial injury and the associated neurologic status changes. A rapid neurologic assessment evaluates a child's LOC, pupil size and reaction, and motor response, which help assess the level of an SCI. The GCS should be calculated using age-specific criteria. The three main components of the GCS are eye-opening, verbal responses, and motor response; the motor response score is the best predictor of outcome after TBI. Pupillary assessment includes an evaluation of pupil size and response to light and can easily and rapidly be assessed. Causes of a decreased LOC in an injured child include TBI, hypoxemia, poor cerebral perfusion, or hypovolemic shock.[8,123,126,173–178]

Level of Consciousness

The rapid and reliable assessment of LOC is essential to identify the neurologic status of an acutely ill or injured child and to recognize early signs of deterioration. Neurologic status is obtained quickly with the assessment of pupil response to light and use of one of the standard scoring tools used in pediatrics such as the AVPU Pediatric Response and the GCS. The causes of a decreased LOC in children can be numerous and include respiratory distress or failure with hypoxia or hypercarbia, hypoglycemia, seizures, infection, shock, brain injury, or trauma.

Determining LOC is a crucial step in the management of a critically ill or injured child. The GCS is the most commonly used standard scoring tool and provides a reliable, objective assessment of neurologic status by measuring eye opening, verbal response, and extremity movements. This scoring tool is validated in the assessment of children with head injuries and universally accepted for the assessment of LOC in all other neurologic injuries or illnesses. The GCS score is the most commonly used and reliable indicator of the severity of TBI in all patients. The GCS is a validated standard scoring tool but requires skill for the provider to use consistently between patients. The use of the AVPU mnemonic (A is awake and alert, V is only responsive to verbal stimuli, P is only responsive to painful stimuli, and U is completely unresponsive) is a simplified version of the GCS. The AVPU scale is a commonly used assessment tool to rapidly measure the child's LOC and is accepted by the AHA PALS course. The AVPU responsiveness scale appears to provide a rapid, simple method to assess the critically ill child's LOC and is an easier LOC scoring tool for prehospital personnel to use with children. Transport teams that are dedicated to neonatal or pediatric carriers will tend to use the more common GCS for children. The AVPU is far easier to use and remember for the prehospital provider who is not a pediatric specialist.[8,123,126,175,176,179]

Pediatric Traumatic Brain Injury

Pediatric TBI is a leading cause of morbidity and mortality in the United States. For the most part, TBIs in children occur secondary to falls, being struck by an object or struck against a stationary object, MVCs, sports, bicycles, and NAT. The GCS is a clinical classification tool used to quantify the severity of TBI using the patient's best pupil, verbal, and motor responses. A mild TBI is considered to have a GCS range of 13 to 15, a moderate TBI score between 9 and 12, and a score of 8 or less is deemed to be a severe TBI. Long-term quality of life in children who have sustained a TBI can range from mild to severe deficits in academic, neurocognitive, neurobehavioral, and psychosocial skills.[176,179,180]

Etiology of Pediatric TBI

Causes of pediatric TBI can vary by age in children. In young children, falls are the most common cause of TBI. Younger children have large heads compared with body size and while they are developing coordination skills they frequently fall. In older children and adolescents, MVCs, other accidents involving a bicycle or motorcycle, and sports injuries are the most common causes of TBI. The older child age group starts to exhibit risk-taking behaviors, which increases the opportunity for brain injuries to occur. The majority of deaths related to TBI in children older than 1 year of age are the result of MVCs. In infants less than 1 year of age, NAT is the most common cause of TBI and is considered a significant problem. Any child who presents with an unexplainable head injury should be considered NAT until ruled out. A clinical sign used to predict an intracranial injury along with a head injury is the presence of a scalp hematoma. A scalp hematoma in the temporal/parietal or occipital areas of the child's skull increases the risk of an associated linear skull fracture being present. Any time the child presents with a scalp hematoma, the transport provider needs to suspect a linear skull fracture until proven otherwise. The infant who has an open anterior fontanelle may allow a large amount of blood loss into this space before the child will decompensate.[176,180–182]

Table 18.16 lists the low-risk predictors established by the PECARN predictive rule for the identification of a significant brain injury in children without advanced imaging or interventions. A child presenting without any of these symptoms usually does not require CT scans or invasive interventions; instead, observation of these children is performed. Table 18.17 lists the

TABLE 18.16	Pediatric Emergency Care Applied Research Network (PECARN) Rule: A Validated Prediction Tool Used to Identify Children with Low Risk of a Significant TBI
Age in Years	Clinical Criteria[a]
<2	• GCS <15 • Parental reports of child not acting normal • Altered mental status reported • >5 second loss of consciousness • Mechanism of injury severe (e.g., MVC, fall >3 feet) • Temporal, parietal, or occipital scalp hematoma • Palpable skull fracture is detected
≧ 2–18	• GCS <15 • Altered mental status reported • Documented loss of consciousness • Mechanism of injury severe (e.g., MVC, fall >3 feet) • Vomiting • Severe headaches • Signs of a basilar skull fracture detected

[a]Children presenting without any of the following established predictors are considered low risk for a significant TBI and CT is not recommended.
GCS, Glascow Coma Scale; *MVC*, motor vehicle crash; *TBI*, traumatic brain injury.

TABLE 18.17	TABLE Signs/Symptoms Observed in Children Considered a Moderate and High Risk for a TBI	
Moderate Risk		**High Risk**
Treatment Indicates Observation or Probable Neuroimaging by CT Scan or MRI		*Treatment Crucial for Emergent Neuroimaging by Either CT Scan or MRI*
• Vomiting that resolves without intervention • Brief or unknown LOC • Headache • History of lethargy or irritability with infants may be resolved • Parents report infant not acting right • Severe mechanism of injury (e.g., MVC, fall >3 feet) • Scalp hematoma (e.g., temporal, parietal, or occipital) • Skull fracture >24 hours • Unwitnessed traumatic injury • Any traumatic injury in infant <3 months		• Suspicion of NAT in infants or children • Persistent vomiting • New onset seizure activity following injury • Altered mental status • Prolonged LOC • Bulging fontanelles in infants • Focal neurologic findings • Basilar or depressed skull fracture

LOC, Level of consciousness; *MVC*, motor vehicle crash; *NAT*, nonaccidental trauma.
Data from references 146,176–178,180,182,183

moderate and high risks associated with clinically significant TBI signs and symptoms in children and the recommendations for either neurologic observation or the need for neuroimaging with a CT scan or MRI.[146,176,180–183]

Pediatric Primary Brain Injuries

Brain injuries are classified as either primary or secondary. Primary brain injury is the result of a mechanical force or damage incurred by the initial injury to the brain. The most common mechanisms causing a primary brain injury are when an object strikes a child's head, when the brain strikes the inside of the skull, or an acceleration-deceleration type of accident. Primary brain injuries are classified as focal or diffuse and may occur simultaneously. Focal injuries are scalp injuries, skull fractures, soft tissue injuries, or extra-axial hemorrhages such as an epidural, subdural, subarachnoid, or intraventricular hemorrhage. Diffuse injuries are intracranial lesions such as diffuse axonal injuries, cortical contusions, intraparenchymal hemorrhages, or vascular injuries. These injuries are usually a result of acceleration–deceleration forces.[176,180–182]

Pediatric Secondary Brain Injuries

Secondary brain injuries are not mechanically induced; instead, they are the result of events occurring after the initial brain injury and are a result of hypotension, hypoxemia, hypercapnia, hypoglycemia, and intracranial hypertension. Secondary brain injuries may develop rapidly within minutes of the initial insult to the brain and continue to evolve over hours to days. The most common causes of pediatric secondary brain injury are hypotension and hypoxemia which are associated with increased morbidities and mortalities in children. Research shows that correcting hypoxemia in a child with a TBI prior to or during transport is associated with a significant increase in survival and a decrease in morbidities. This makes secondary brain injury prevention a critical intervention and primary goal of prehospital patient transport, EDs, and pediatric intensive care management.[176,180–183]

Standard Trauma Guidelines

Recommendations are for patients with a primary TBI to receive cardiopulmonary and hemodynamic support resuscitation to decrease or reduce secondary brain injuries caused by hypoxia, hypotension, and increased ICP. If the ICP is uncontrollable with positioning and medical management with sedation, then narcotics, paralytics, and osmotic diuretics may be needed. The two most common scoring tools are the AVPU Pediatric Response Scale and the GCS, which were discussed in more detail in a previous section.[176,177,184]

Pupillary Response

The pupils should be assessed for size, equality, and light response. Pupils that are fixed, dilated, unequal, sluggish, poorly reactive, or nonreactive to light and accommodation may be indicative of intracranial hypertension, increased ICP, or brainstem involvement. Direct trauma to the eye may also cause pupillary dysfunction; therefore, ocular findings should be correlated with the rest of the neurologic assessment. The transport provider needs to assess the child's pupils before administration of medications for intubation, seizure control, or paralytics.[8,176,179]

Motor Responses

Children with increased ICP have decreased or abnormal responses to pain. Decorticate and decerebrate posturing may be

present. Flaccidity with severe head injury and paralysis from spinal cord injuries may be found on initial examination. The GCS has three areas assessed: eye-opening, verbal responses, and motor response to stimulation with the motor response score being the best predictor of long-term outcomes in children after TBI. The motor response is regarded as a good indicator of the ability of the child's CNS to function properly to stimulation. The best way to elicit motor responses in a child with altered LOC is to apply pressure to one of the child's fingertips, pinch the trapezius muscle at the base of the child's neck and upper shoulder area, and apply pressure to the supraorbital notch. The child will respond with normal or abnormal flexion motor responses or no response using these three methods. Normal flexion will occur rapidly after stimulation and the arm will move away from the child's body. Abnormal flexion will respond slowly to the applied stimulation, the arm will move toward the body and across the chest with the forearm rotating and thumb clenched, and the child's legs will extend to the stimulation. Factors affecting motor responses in children include spinal cord injuries, peripheral nerve injuries, extremity injuries affecting movement, pain, or the inability to understand the provider or developmental delays.[8,123,126,176,179]

Pediatric TBI: Airway Control, Initial Stabilization, and Cervical Spine Immobilization

For children with TBI, prehospital providers should provide an initial rapid assessment of the patient's airway, breathing, circulatory status, and GCS for any other indicators of disability. The goals of initial stabilization and resuscitation include providing adequate oxygen delivery and ventilation, fluid resuscitation, and prevention of secondary damage to the child's brain. Cervical spine (C-spine) immobilization is recommended for all patients with possible cervical spine or SCI and is included in the initial stabilization of a child with TBI. Children with head injuries may have associated spinal injuries and should be C-spine immobilized and secured on a pediatric-designed immobilization device for transport until an SCI can be ruled out. Cervical spine injuries are closely associated with TBIs in children. The MOI causing the head injury is closely associated and increases the risk of cervical injuries in children. Maintaining manual C-spine immobilization is essential during airway control and stabilization to prevent any cervical damage to these children.

Airway control and stabilization of the child with a TBI begins with the provider securing a stable airway with ETI. In children who are hemodynamically unstable or have low GCS scores, medications to intubate and secure an airway may not be used to potentially prevent hypotension causing a secondary brain injury. Rapid sequence intubation uses analgesia, sedatives, and paralytics to create optimal conditions to perform an emergent intubation. Caution must be observed during the use of RSI medications to prevent hypotension from occurring after administration. RSI sedative medications midazolam and propofol may cause hypotension in these children and subsequent secondary brain injury while controlling the airway. Paralytics such as vecuronium prevent neurologic examination for an extended period and should be avoided. The most commonly used paralytics for RSI include succinylcholine and rocuronium which are the most frequently used in pediatric patients with TBI. Evidence supports the use of etomidate for intubation with a decrease in ICP. Fentanyl is another popular RSI medication for children. There is conflicting research on the usefulness of lidocaine with intubations in children. It is an optional medication that may have the ability to lessen the effects of ICP. Most Emergency Medical Service (EMS) programs and specialty transport teams have established protocols concerning which medications are appropriate for intubating children with TBIs.[8,123,126,176,180,184,185]

Adequate Ventilation

Pediatric patients requiring assisted ventilation via bag and mask or ETI benefit from end-tidal CO_2 ($ETCO_2$) monitoring to ensure hyperventilation and hypoventilation do not occur. Hyperventilation occurs when the PCO_2 is less than 35 mmHg and decreases cerebral blood flow, which may contribute to cerebral ischemia and secondary brain injury. Transient hyperventilation with an $ETCO_2$ goal of 30–35 mmHg can be performed on the pediatric patient with signs of increased ICP and herniation and in the patient with increased ICP refractory to osmotic agents. It is essential to maintain control of the child's airway and maintain adequate ventilation with an $ETCO_2$ of 35–40 mmHg. This will significantly decrease any long-term morbidities in these children. The pediatric TBI guidelines recommend avoiding mild hyperventilation with a $PaCO_2$ less than 35 mmHg and severe hyperventilation with a $PaCO_2$ less than 30 mmHg to decrease the risk of secondary brain injury. Pediatric TBI research has shown that avoiding hypercapnia and hypocapnia for the first 48–72 hours after the initial head injury is associated with the child's survival. Guidelines for prehospital transport of pediatric patients with a TBI recommend that after gaining control of the child's airway it is essential to maintain adequate ventilation management and the use of $ETCO_2$ monitoring. This is the most effective method used to monitor the child's ventilatory efforts during transport.[176,180,184–186]

Circulation

Fluid resuscitation in children begins with isotonic fluid boluses of 20 mL/kg with consideration given to the need for blood products in a pediatric patient who sustained a significant blood loss. Hypotension in pediatric patients with TBI is a predictor of poor outcomes. Evidenced-based TBI guidelines support CPP thresholds, and new research has shown that CPP targets should be age-specific. These thresholds for CPP goals are above 50 mmHg or 60 mmHg in adults, above 50 mmHg in 6- to 17-year-olds, and above 40 mmHg in 0- to 5-year-olds and seem to be appropriate targets for preventing cerebral ischemia and secondary brain injury. Recent studies demonstrated that systemic hypotension had an inconsistent relationship to events of low CPP, but an elevated ICP was significantly related to all low CPP events across all age groups. This data stressed the importance of controlling the child's ICP at all times and treating systolic blood pressure at specific moments. Hypotension after severe TBI increases the risk of secondary brain injury resulting in reduced perfusion to the child's brain. After initial resuscitation, it is important for the transport provider to maintain the child's circulatory status with an effective blood pressure. This is crucial to the child with TBI to ensure that autoregulation of the CPP is not impaired. Children are able to preserve their blood pressure and may initially only exhibit signs of hypovolemia as tachycardia. Tachycardia in a child with suspected TBI requires immediate evaluation. The preservation of a stable mean arterial blood pressure is important to provide adequate cerebral perfusion and oxygenation and decrease secondary brain injury.[176,180,187]

Intracranial Hypertension and Treatment Options

Primary and secondary injuries may lead to increased ICP in children with TBI. When the ICP is high, the direct brain tissue damage impairs the cerebral blood flow and metabolic regulation. In children with a TBI, a GCS of less than or equal to 8 indicates severe TBI with an increased risk of intracranial hypertension. Elevated ICP is one of the causes of secondary brain injury in these children and is associated with poor outcomes. Low GCS scores on the motor response section of the GCS may indicate intracranial hypertension. Increased ICP occurs frequently in children with severe TBI who do not demonstrate spontaneous motor function with the GCS evaluation. When the provider can successfully decrease ICP in children with TBIs, evidence shows a significant improvement in clinical outcomes with decreased morbidities. There are several methods available to help reduce ICP and secondary brain injuries: positioning the patient with the head elevated and midline, the use of sedation, hyperosmolar medications such as mannitol and 3% hypertonic saline, and paralytic medications. Hyperosmolar therapy decreases elevated ICP through an osmotic effect, which is accomplished with either mannitol at 1 g/kg or 3% hypertonic saline at 5–10 mL/kg in children. Both mannitol and 3% sodium have a low penetration across the blood–brain barrier, creating an osmotic gradient effect in the patient's circulating blood, but this osmotic effect requires an intact blood–brain barrier for it to be effective. Recent studies have shown that 3% hypertonic saline given as a bolus was more effective than mannitol in lowering the cumulative and daily ICP spikes after a severe TBI in children. Additional studies have shown these two hyperosmolar medications are equally effective in treating increased ICP in pediatric TBI patients. Successfully controlling the child's ICP improves clinical outcomes in children by preventing secondary brain injuries.[176,180,187–189]

Seizures after TBI or Antiseizure Prophylaxis

Post-traumatic seizures may occur following TBI in children. The percentage of occurrence is directly related to the severity of the brain injury. Seizures are more common in children less than 3 years of age with severe head injuries, depressed skull fractures, cerebral edema, or intraparenchymal hemorrhages. Seizures increase the child's metabolic demands of the brain resulting in increased ICP leading to secondary brain injury. Antiseizure prophylaxis decreases the incidence of post-traumatic seizures in children with TBI. Common medications used for antiseizure prophylaxis are fosphenytoin, phenytoin, and levetiracetam. Common medications for post-traumatic seizures include lorazepam and diazepam, which both can be given rectally, and midazolam, which may be given nasally or rectally. Other medications include fosphenytoin, phenytoin, or phenobarbital. Monitor the patient's vital signs closely with administration of these medications to prevent hypotension and secondary brain injury from a decrease in CPP.[8,176,180]

Positioning

Maintaining the patient's head up at 30 degrees while secured on a pediatric immobilization device while maintaining the patient's head midline with commercial devices or towel rolls unless prohibited by other injuries will assist in decreasing ICP in the child by promoting venous drainage and consequently improving CPP.[8,176,180]

Environmental Issues

Control of noise, especially in the transport setting, is important in controlling acute elevations in ICPs. Unless prohibited by patient injury, earplugs or earmuffs can decrease noise stress on patients. Adequate sedation and pain management can help decrease ICP.[8]

Reevaluation

Continuous monitoring and reevaluation of the patient is performed during primary and secondary surveys, especially with children experiencing a neurologic impairment. It is necessary during transport to assess for deterioration of patient status, increases in ICP, and effectiveness of medical interventions.[176]

Imaging in Mild to Moderate TBI

The goal of caring for children with mild to moderate TBI is to identify significant intracranial injury while limiting unneeded imaging and unnecessary radiation exposure. Most children with mild TBI are at low risk for long-term neurologic complications or deficits. The prevalence of intracranial hemorrhage in children with mild TBI is relatively low and increases if the child has an underlying neurologic disorder such as ventriculoperitoneal shunt, scalp laceration, visible skull fracture, and neurologic findings. PECARN developed the childhood head injury predictive rule, which identifies children at high risk for necessitating neurosurgical intervention and at medium risk for having a brain injury on imaging.[176,183]

Spinal Cord Injuries

Spinal cord injuries (SCIs) in children are rare and increase in prevalence in adolescents. SCIs occurring in children are rarely observed as isolated injuries but are more often combined with additional injury patterns. Because of their anatomic differences, children are predisposed to cervical spinal injuries (CSIs). Pediatric CSIs are rare but devastating, resulting in the child's death or life-changing neurologic damage. Pediatric CSIs are rare because the level of injury is different and they carry a much higher morbidity and mortality compared with adults. It is important to understand pediatric CSI patterns in relation to MOI, treatment, and neurologic outcomes in children. An accurate, rapid diagnosis and management are necessary to avoid potentially devastating injuries to children. The size of the head in a child is proportionally larger compared with their body, resulting in acceleration and deceleration at high-impact speeds, which causes more stress to the upper cervical spine. The fulcrum sits at the C2–C3 level in a child, and as the child ages it

tends to move lower to the C5–C6 level. The incomplete ossification of the vertebral bodies, underdeveloped spinal processes, and ligamentous laxity are the reasons children have a decreased incidence of CSIs. The anatomic and developmental differences, cervical spine stability, and injury patterns in pediatric patients are significantly different from the adult. After 10 years of age, the injury pattern begins to be similar to that of an adult. The most common types of pediatric CSIs are fractures of the vertebral body, followed by subluxation. Table 18.18 lists the CSI MOI and injury classification based on the age of the child.[190–193]

SCI without any radiographic abnormality (SCIWORA) affects older children more often. All three of these types of CSIs are commonly associated with comorbid head injuries. SCIWORA is the diagnosis given to children experiencing neurologic deficits associated with the cervical spinal cord in the absence of abnormalities on radiographs or CTs. Magnetic resonance imaging (MRI) has become a common imaging modality in spinal trauma because of its enhanced ability to identify soft-tissue lesions such as discoligamentous injuries, cord hematomas, cord edema, cord transections, and neurocompressive injuries, which are not seen on radiographs or CT scans. MVCs, falls, and NAT are more common MOIs for children younger than 8 years of age diagnosed with SCIWORA. Sports-related injuries such as gymnastics, diving, horseback riding, football, and wrestling are more common MOIs in older children.[190–193]

Imaging to Detect Traumatic Injuries of the Cervical Spine in Children

CSI may be rare in children but the potential consequences are devastating. The most sensitive and specific methods of clearing cervical spines in children are not known. Over the last decade, cervical spine CT for pediatric patients has increased considerably making it the standard modality used to detect CSIs in children. A cervical spine CT scan is not only costly but the long-term risk of radiation exposure to children is an increasing concern because the use of CT imaging has become more popular in evaluating patients. Cervical radiation exposure increases the risk of developing thyroid cancer in children. Ionizing radiation doses delivered by CT scans are 100 to 500 times higher than conventional x-rays.

TABLE 18.18 **Cervical Spine Injury MOI and Injury Classification Based on the Age of the Child**

Age of Child	Mechanism of Injury for CSI	Injury Classification of CSIs
<2 years of age	• MVC • Falls	• Axial area affected • Most common area is atlanto-occipital dislocation,[a] which affects the occiput through C2 • Uncommon for young children to experience SCIWORA
2–7 years of age	• MVC • Falls • Child versus motor vehicle	• Axial area affected • Atlanto-axial rotator subluxation[b] • Atlanto-occipital dislocation most common (occiput through C2)
8–15 years of age	• Sports injuries • MVC • Falls • Diving accidents	• Subaxial injuries occur with subaxial vertebral body fractures, which affects C3–C7 more frequently (are common and often miss diagnosed) • SCIWORA is more common in this age group

[a]Atlanto-occipital dislocation—highly unstable, potentially devastating ligamentous neurological injury.
[b]Atlanto-axial rotator sublaxation—injury to C1–C2 causing impairment in rotation of the neck.
CSI, Cervical spine injury; *MVC,* motor vehicle crash; *SCIWORA,* spinal cord injury without any radiographic abnormality.
Modified from Leonard JR, Jaffe DM, Kuppermann N, Olsen CS, Leonard JC. Cervical spine injury patterns in children. *Pediatrics.* 2014;133(5):e1179–e1188.

There has been a growing interest in creating guidelines for the clearance of the pediatric cervical spine to reduce significant exposure to CT scan radiation and yet be effective in clearing CSIs. Two commonly validated clinical decision guidelines established to clear the adult cervical spine are the National Emergency X-Radiography Utilization Study (NEXUS) criteria and the Canadian C-Spine Rule (CCR). The NEXUS criteria and the CCR do not specifically address clearance of the pediatric cervical spine. One guideline in the literature was the NEXUS criteria adapted to minimize radiation exposure while clearing the pediatric cervical spine. Protocols have been developed to facilitate safe clearance of pediatric cervical spines clinically or through the use of modalities exposing children to less extreme forms of radiation. Based on concerns about ionizing radiation exposure, the University of Iowa Trauma Service developed a Pediatric Cervical Spine Clearance Protocol for children younger than 10 years of age. The guidelines are moving away from CT scan as the primary modality; initial imaging is plain x-rays and then decide if additional imaging with MRI or CT is warranted.[193–196]

Plain Radiography

Anteroposterior and lateral plain x-rays are commonly used as initial screening x-rays. They can identify the majority of cervical spine fractures but may need to be repeated for a more adequate visualization. The lateral plain radiograph should be the first test to screen for pediatric CSI. The sensitivity of the lateral neck x-ray is relatively high and increases with children older than 8 years. Anteroposterior views usually do not increase sensitivity. In the cooperative child who is over 5 years of age and able to follow commands, the odontoid open mouth x-ray is an additional view that is used to detect burst fractures of C1. An oblique view provides enhanced views of the posterior elements of the neck and subluxation. The odontoid and oblique views are not recommended for initial examination but can be considered when initial views are indeterminate or the clinical scenario suggests a specific bony injury is present. Flexion-extension x-rays are additional views of the cervical spine. These may be considered in the stable trauma patient who has persistent neck pain regardless of normal lateral and anteroposterior x-rays.[195,196]

Magnetic Resonance Imaging

An MRI does not have the ionizing radiation risks associated with CT. Compared with CT, MRI has higher sensitivity for spinal cord and soft-tissue injuries but is less sensitive than CT in detecting bony injuries. The MRI is more difficult to obtain compared with the CT scan in an acutely injured child because of limited availability, and the length of time required to obtain adequate MR images frequently requires sedation in children. The role of MRI in CSI is in the detection of significant CSIs in obtunded patients who cannot be examined clinically. An obtunded patient with a normal MRI finding can have his or her cervical spine safely cleared and can reduce the length of time in a cervical collar. MRI imaging may be cost-efficient if used appropriately. An MRI protocol for obtunded children has saved each patient a significant amount of money likely related to a shorter immobilization time and hospital stay.[195,196]

Computed Tomography

CT scans are superior in sensitivity for detecting acute CSIs compared with plain x-rays. However, current evidence does not support the use of CT scans as a standard screening tool for children with a potential traumatic CSI. In children, most injuries found on cervical spine CT are also noted on plain radiography. CT scans in children are associated with a longer ED length of stay, higher resource use of ED staff, and significant exposure to ionizing radiation to the child. Children are more sensitive to the carcinogenic effects of ionizing radiation. Among the plain x-rays, MRI, and CT imaging technologies, CT scans are of the greatest concern regarding children because of the high levels of ionizing radiation associated with this technology and the estimated increase in the child's lifetime cancer risk associated with the scans. Long-term radiation risks associated with CT scans in children is the rationale for why the industry is adopting other modalities to evaluate CSIs in children. CT scans expose patients to significantly more radiation than plain x-rays. As an example, one head CT scan before the age of 10 years results in one excess brain tumor per 10,000 patients. An approach to reducing radiation exposure for pediatric patients in which a cervical spine CT is indicated is a focused CT. The CT focuses a beam directly to a specific level of concern. A focused CT from occiput to C3 increases sensitivity for diagnosing CSI while limiting radiation exposure.[195,196]

Spinal Protection

A review of the literature was unable to determine whether the effect of full spinal immobilization in pediatric trauma patients was helpful or harmful to the child's mortality, neurologic injury, spinal stability, or adverse effects. There are two goals for spinal protection in children: to limit current damage and prevent a secondary injury. Full spinal immobilization is considered the standard of care for all children meeting the injury criteria for transport to a trauma center with the conviction that maintaining the child's spine in a neutral position and minimizing spine motion during transport will limit neurologic injury. Children who sustain blunt trauma are frequently placed in full spinal immobilization to protect the cervical spine from further injury. However, given the rare association of CSIs in children, the potential harmful effects, if they present themselves, may prevail over any potential benefit of immobilization for most children.[197–202]

The American College of Emergency Physicians (ACEP) states that spinal motion restriction should be the preferred practice because true spinal immobilization is impossible. Without sufficient data, there is only guidance from experts in the field of pediatric trauma, which recommends full spinal immobilization of pediatric trauma patients to protect a child's cervical spine. There is insufficient data in children to support standards of treatment; instead, there are recommendations from the Congress of Neurologic Surgeons, the American College of Surgeons Committee on Trauma (ACS-COT), and the National Association of EMS Physicians (NAEMSP) for spinal immobilization of all patients in the presence of either suspicion of a CSI or an MOI with the potential to cause CSI in a child. The recommendations suggest fully immobilizing the child using a cervical collar and an appropriately sized backboard for transporting children to minimize the risk of CSI after trauma. If at all possible, try to use a pediatric-designed backboard. Adult backboards are unable to immobilize and restrict a child correctly, and they promote neck flexion in a child. Use of either a blanket or padding to elevate the shoulders and upper thoracic area or a backboard with an occipital recess to bring the pediatric spine into better neutral alignment is recommended. The padding or blanket should extend continuously from the shoulders through the thoracic and lumbar spine to the pelvis to maintain a neutral alignment of the child's entire spine. Padding under the shoulders only flexes the thoracic and lumbar spine of a child. Additionally, if you are using an adult backboard or an oversized backboard on a child, consider adding padding between the edges of the board and the child. This will pad the open areas between the sides of the backboard and the child under the straps and fill the open triangle area preventing lateral movement of the child on the backboard.[197–202]

Devices for younger children include the Pedi-Pac, Pedi-Boards, Pedi-Air, MedKids Baby Board, pediatric vacuum mattresses, Papoose board, and Kendrick Extrication Device (KED), which have demonstrated safe and effective immobilization tools for providers. The KED can be used for both extrication and immobilization but still requires a blanket or padding to maintain a neutral position.[197–202]

Application of Proper Spinal Immobilization

The most important intervention in the transport of children with known or suspected SCI is proper spinal protection. Before the application of cervical collars and a backboard, jewelry and necklaces should be removed to prevent interference with radiologic examinations and possible pressure injuries. Care should also be taken to remove sharp debris, such as glass, from the patient to prevent further injury. One provider will maintain manual stabilization of the child's cervical spine while the other places an appropriately sized firm cervical collar. An improperly sized collar can interfere with respirations or cause inappropriate extension of the child's cervical spine. An appropriately fitting cervical collar has the child's chin rest in the chin piece with the collar below the child's ears, and resting on the clavicles. Cervical collars are designed and available to fit newborns up to adults. Infants may be too small for a properly fitted cervical collar or the transport provider may not have the appropriately sized collars available. In these circumstances, a towel roll may be used to immobilize the cervical spine. A towel roll must prevent flexion and extension and align the cervical spine in a neutral position. If a towel roll cannot achieve these goals, manual control may need to be continued until the child is transported to a definitive center.[197–202]

Once a cervical collar has been applied, the child is then logrolled and placed on a backboard. One person should provide manual control of the collared cervical spine, with another person at the child's shoulders and hips and another at the child's hips and legs. Opposite the patient, one person should be in place to position the backboard. The person controlling the cervical spine may then lead the command to turn the patient as a unit onto their side. This is the time for the provider not involved in the logrolling of the patient to inspect and palpate the patient's back and spine, assessing for step-offs, injuries, or pain. Inspection and palpation of the head, neck, and spine should be performed to assess for lacerations, hematoma, cerebrospinal fluid (CSF) bloody drainage from the ears or nose, depressed skull fractures, or step-off in the spinal column. All inspection and palpation should be performed on children while maintaining manual cervical spine control and logrolling with spinal precautions in place.[197–202]

Although evaluation of the spine and back are not technically part of the primary survey, these assessments are best performed with the patient placed on a backboard, which is necessary for transport protection of the cervical spine. Children younger than 8 years of age have disproportionately large heads, so padding under the shoulders on the board is necessary to keep the cervical spine in a neutral position. As mentioned earlier, the entire spine of the child needs to be in a neutral position so the blanket or padding should continue to the child's pelvis. The backboard can be positioned at a 30- to 45-degree angle and the child then rolled onto it. Once the patient is centered on the board, lateral stabilization of the cervical spine with blanket rolls or blocks and securing

the head with straps or tape should be performed. The final step in spinal immobilization is securing the body to the board with straps (securing the chest, hips, and knees). Straps should be secure enough to allow turning the board from side to side without movement of the patient's body. This turning may be necessary for the unintubated patient who has periods of emesis during transport. Suction should be readily available for any patient secured to a backboard. A neurologic examination should precede and follow all spinal immobilization procedures.[197–202]

Even with expert guidance, the diligence of consistent spinal immobilization with appropriately sized equipment for children is highly variable or not done at all. Children younger than 2 years of age are more vulnerable and at a higher risk for severe high-level cervical injuries and are unable to communicate effectively any signs or symptoms of the injury, yet these are the ones who are not fully immobilized with a cervical collar and pediatric-sized backboard. A study found a correlation between eight factors and CSIs in children suggesting the need to provide full spine immobilization. They include altered mental status; focal neurologic findings; neck pain; torticollis; substantial torso injury; and medical conditions predisposing the child to CSI such as Down syndrome, diving injury, or high-risk MVC.[197–202]

Removal of a Child From a Child Safety Seat With Maintenance of Spinal Immobilization

Infants and young children up to about 8 years of age may still require car seats or booster seats when riding in a car. Those secured correctly may never need spinal immobilization. The literature reports controversy over whether to remove a child from their car seat or to transport them in their car seat. Any child with an unstable airway, respiratory, or circulatory status must be removed from their car seat. If the child remains in their car seat, it is impossible for the transport provider to perform a full primary and secondary survey of the child and potential injuries may be missed. Children with an ejected car seat, damage to the car seat, or a car seat with a high back should always be removed from their car seat. Without doing so the transport provider would be unable to provide emergent interventions including intubation, aspiration prevention, or venous access.[8,123,200]

Removing a child from a car seat requires the initiation of manual cervical spine immobilization by one provider. The other provider will remove or cut the shoulder harness and move the safety bar out of the way. Position the child safety seat at the foot of the backboard. Tip the child safety seat back and lay it down on the backboard. One person then slides their hands along each side of the patient's head until they are behind the patient's shoulders. The head and neck are now supported laterally by that person's arms. A second person should then take control of the patient's body. On the instruction of the person holding the head, slide the child out of the safety seat onto the backboard and immobilize as described previously.[8,123,200]

Adverse Effects of Spinal Immobilization

Full spinal immobilization is common in children who are victims of blunt trauma to protect the child's cervical spine from further injury. Because children infrequently suffer cervical injury the potential harmful effects of full spine immobilization may outweigh any potential benefit for the majority of children. Studies have documented that children who are immobilized following a traumatic incident report more pain, experience increased pain on arrival to the ED, and are at a higher risk of undergoing radiographic imaging of the cervical spine and a higher hospital admission rate compared with those children who are not immobilized in the field, regardless of the injury severity reported. Pain caused by spinal immobilization may be confused with the actual traumatic injury, which may lead to unnecessary diagnostic evaluations and exposure to ionizing radiation from a CT scan of the cervical spine. Additional adverse effects include an increased risk of aspiration and skin breakdown if left on a hard backboard for an extended period of time.[8,198,200–202]

Exposure and Environment

The final segment of the primary survey is exposure of the traumatically injured child. The child's clothing is removed to allow a visual inspection of the body for rapid identification and to decrease the chance of missing any obvious injuries and initiate treatment of multiple injuries if warranted. This step requires a team effort to maintain manual cervical spine stabilization and logroll the child. This allows the provider to assess and inspect the child's back and spine for step-offs or other deformities, tenderness, or other external injury. If warranted, a rectal examination may be done at this time. Even though this is not officially part of the primary survey, it falls into place naturally because very little additional time is needed to complete it and the child must be logrolled anyway to be placed on a backboard for transport. Remember to place a pad or blanket under the shoulders down to the pelvis to maintain a neutral spinal alignment, especially for children younger than 8 years of age. Immediately cover the child with warm blankets after exposing the child for examination to minimize heat loss. It is important to be more vigilant with infants and young children because they are more vulnerable to heat loss secondary to their large surface area (head) in relation to their body volume. The patient's temperature should be obtained in this step and reassessed during transport. Additional methods used to help prevent heat loss include increasing the room if in an ED or the ambulance for transport and Bair Hugger or overhead heat lamp if available.[8,123,126,180,203]

Hypothermia

Hypothermia is a decrease in the body's core temperature caused by inadequate body temperature regulation or excessive environmental cold stress. Hypothermia can be accidental, such as an environmental exposure, or intentional, such as with therapeutic hypothermia. Hypothermia can occur rapidly with submersion injuries or gradually as a result of exposure to ambient temperatures. Hypothermia is a core temperature below 35°C (95°F). The stage of hypothermia has a major impact on both recognition and treatment. Hypothermia is considered mild with a core temperature of 32°C to 35°C (90°F–95°F), moderate with a core temperature of 28°C to 32°C (82°F–90°F), or severe with a core temperature below 28°C (82°F). Infants and children are at a higher risk of hypothermia because of their larger ratio of surface area to body mass, limited glycogen stores to support heat production, a young infant's inability to increase heat production through shivering, and a decreased ability to recognize and avoid hypothermic exposure. Heat is lost from the body by radiation, conduction, convection, evaporation, and respiration. The clinical features of hypothermia depend on the stage of hypothermia. See Box 18.5 for the stages and clinical features of hypothermia.[8,123,203]

Management of Hypothermia

Successful management of the hypothermic child depends on the stage of hypothermia and rapid assessment of the patient following

---

• BOX 18.5 Stages and Clinical Signs of Hypothermia

Mild Stage: Core temperature 32°C–35°C or 90°F–95°F
Signs: Conscious, mild tachycardia, shivering, piloerection, cyanosis, pallor, acrocyanosis, vasoconstriction, delayed capillary refill time, increased metabolism, possible hypertension

Moderate Stage: Core temperature 28°C–32°C or 82°F–90°F
Signs: Loss of compensatory shivering, altered mental status, lethargy, clumsiness, confusion or delirium, irrational behaviors such as paradoxical undressing, slurred speech, decreased heat production, circulatory insufficiency and instability, vasodilatation starts, hypovolemia, decreased metabolism, decreasing cerebral blood flow, diuresis, extravasation of fluids, decreasing blood pressure and heart rate, decreasing respiratory depression and ventilation

Severe Stage: Core temperature less than 28°C or 82°F
Signs: Unconscious – suspended cerebral activity, no shivering, loss of thermoregulation, vasodilatation, decreased heart rate and cardiac output, decreased stroke volume, decreased cardiac conduction, increased cardiac irritability, slowed nerve conduction, vital signs may or may not be present, erythema and edema, muscle rigidity, stupor or coma, bradycardia progressing to absent pulses, fixed and dilated pupils, ventricular fibrillation, asystole

Data from Corneli HM. *Hypothermia in Children: Clinical Manifestations and Diagnosis.* In: UpToDate, August 2016. Wiley JF (ed.). Waltham, MA: UpToDate. https://www.uptodate.com/contents/hypothermia-in-children-clinical-manifestations-and-diagnosis (accessed on September 16, 2023); and Corneli JM. *Hypothermia in Children: Management.* In: UpToDate, Dec 2016. Wiley JF (ed.). Waltham, MA: UpToDate. https://www.uptodate.com/contents/hypothermia-in-children-management (accessed September 16, 2023).

---

the ABDCDEs of the primary survey along with the treatment of the injury or other medical conditions including effective rewarming interventions. In the prehospital environment, suspicion of hypothermia is vital and should be considered with not only the children exposed to the environment but also those who may have an altered mental status. Accurate core temperature in children with hypothermia is essential for proper treatment and interventions. Prehospital providers must avoid exertion and excessive handling of the hypothermic patient during rescue or securing on the stretcher. Patients with hypothermia because of these actions may mobilize cold and acidic blood to the heart increasing the potential for cardiac arrhythmias or arrest. Many patients arrive at the hospital colder than at the scene. Patient rescue, transport, and treatment of hypothermic patients involve risks of iatrogenic cooling. During transport the prehospital provider provides passive rewarming strategies by doing everything possible to prevent further heat loss by removing wet clothing, gently covering the patient with blankets, increasing the ambient temperature in the mode of transport, warming IV fluids if possible, and giving heated humidified oxygen. External rewarming of children with moderate to severe hypothermia in transport is usually avoided because it requires active external rewarming, which is difficult in the transport environment.[8,125–127]

Active external rewarming techniques include applying heat externally to the child using a forced air rewarming device, radiant heat, and applying heat packs. Active external rewarming has the potential to promote further cooling, hypotension from rewarming shock, ventricular fibrillation, or asystole in patients. It is important to warm the trunk before the extremities.

Active internal rewarming techniques are invasive ways to rewarm a child. These include continued efforts from the passive and active external rewarming with heated humidified oxygen and warmed IV fluids. Invasive techniques of rewarming used for severe hypothermia include heated saline lavage of the pleura, bladder, stomach, or peritoneum. Another method of active internal rewarming is ECMO which is used for severe hypothermia in children who are unresponsive to the other methods or have absent circulation.[8,125,203,204]

Treatment of Mild Hypothermia

Patients with environmental exposure and mild hypothermia respond well to passive rewarming by removing wet clothing and drying the skin, active external rewarming with a forced air heating blanket and radiant heat lamp, and administering warmed IV normal saline. Continual monitoring of core temperature, and continuous monitoring of cardiac rhythm and circulatory status is essential to demonstrate that the child is responding to the appropriate methods of rewarming.[8,125,203,204]

Determine the underlying cause of the child's mild hypothermia if environmental exposure is not the cause. The most common causes of mild hypothermia in children are sepsis, hypoglycemia, hyponatremia, hypothyroidism, adrenal insufficiency, and burns. Hypothermia is most frequently associated with sepsis in infants and children with Gram-negative sepsis. Drugs affecting the child's CNS or endocrine or metabolic diseases may be the underlying cause of mild hypothermia in children. Diagnostic testing and appropriate treatment should be initiated to correct the hypothermia.[8,125,203,204]

Treatment of Moderate or Severe Hypothermia

Children with moderate to severe hypothermia require intensive support of the airway, breathing, and circulation in addition to rewarming. Hypoventilation may be a physiologic finding in moderate or severe hypothermia. Gentle respiratory support is safe and should be provided as needed by providing warmed humidified 100% oxygen via a nonrebreather mask for all patients. If the status is deteriorating, initiate BVM ventilation and prepare for intubation. ETI is performed if the child continues to deteriorate and respiratory failure occurs along with uncompensated shock or cardiac arrest. ETI should not be delayed in the hypothermic child if the child's status indicates it is needed. Monitor closely for cardiac arrhythmias during intubation. In children with severe hypothermia, intubation may be more difficult because of muscle rigidity. In children with severe hypothermia, the heart rate and respiratory effort may be slow and difficult to detect. Research shows that compressions should be initiated immediately if no signs of life are found in a child with severe hypothermia. Hypothermia induces vasoconstriction making vascular access difficult in children. Vascular access is imperative for the child to improve because the aggressive infusion of warmed IV fluids for volume expansion is one of the primary treatments for moderate to severe hypothermia. It requires the placement of two large-bore peripheral IVs or, if this is not possible, placement of an intraosseous (IO) needle or a central line in the femoral vein and initiation of normal saline 20 mL/kg of volume using high-capacity warmers and tubing and rapid infusion of warm saline. The child may require another 20 mL/kg fluid bolus because aggressive and ongoing volume expansion is usually required while treating hypothermia. Hypoglycemia is a common finding with hypothermia and requires treatment. Rhythms associated with moderate to severe hypothermia include perfusing bradycardic rhythms such as sinus bradycardia, first-degree heart block, and atrial fibrillation. In moderate to severe hypothermia, these rhythms are considered adequate for maintaining sufficient oxygen delivery. Atropine and epinephrine are usually not given because rewarming usually corrects these rhythms to a more normal rhythm. The nonperfusion cardiac rhythms include ventricular fibrillation, ventricular tachycardia without a pulse, and pulseless electrical activity or asystole, and are commonly seen with moderate to severe hypothermia.[8,125,203,204]

Aggressive active internal rewarming or extracorporeal rewarming with ECMO are usually the primary treatments for these children. If a perfusing rhythm does not return with rewarming, immediately begin CPR and continue aggressive rewarming measures. The efficacy of epinephrine is decreased with severe hypothermia. There is limited data to support the administration of epinephrine during rewarming strategies. To promote the return of spontaneous circulation (ROSC), follow the 2015 pediatric cardiac arrest algorithm along with aggressive rewarming techniques, but avoid excessive doses of epinephrine. Attempts at rewarming the child should not delay transport to a critical care facility that can provide all the necessary treatments to reverse the severe hypothermia including extracorporeal capabilities with ECMO.[3,84,125–127]

Heatstroke

Hyperthermia is a life-threatening condition with a core temperature greater than or equal to 40°C (104°F) with CNS dysfunction in patients with environmental exposure to heat. Classic heatstroke occurs from environmental exposure to heat and is common in younger children who are unable to escape from a hot environment, such as those left in a car or those with underlying chronic medical conditions that impair thermoregulation such as cystic fibrosis and CHD. Exertional heatstroke occurs in young healthy children who are engaging in heavy exercise during times of high ambient temperature and humidity, such as teenage athletes. Heat-related illness is the third major cause of death in adolescents behind traumatic and cardiac causes of death. The highest rate of nonfatal heat illnesses is in high school athletes, especially football players.[8,205]

Children receive serious heat-related injuries when the critical thermal maximum (CTM) is exceeded, which is the degree of elevated body temperature and the duration of heat exposure before cell damage occurs. Evaporation is the primary mechanism of heat loss in a hot environment. The diagnostic criteria for children with heatstroke are elevated core temperature greater than or equal to 40°C (104°F) and CNS abnormalities following environmental heat exposure. Temperature elevation increases oxygen consumption and metabolic rate, causing hyperpnea and tachycardia. CNS symptoms may be subtle or cause impaired judgment or inappropriate behavior, seizures, delirium, hallucinations, ataxia, dysarthria, or coma. Additional clinical signs associated with heatstroke include tachycardia, tachypnea, flushed and warm or diaphoretic skin, and vomiting and diarrhea. Patients with heatstroke may present with coagulopathy, with purpura, hemoptysis, hematemesis, melena, or hematochezia. Above 42°C (108°F) patients are at risk for multiorgan failure.[8,205]

Treatment of Heatstroke

Any child with an LOC with exertion in warm weather or found in a heated car should be treated as a child with heatstroke. The diagnosis of heat-related illness is challenging in the prehospital setting. The core temperature may not be obtained and by the time of arrival of EMS some cooling measures have usually already been performed. The prehospital provider's best method of cooling pediatric patients is removal from the source of heat stress, and rapid initiation of cooling treatment. The risk of morbidity and mortality in children with heat-related illness is associated with the duration of hyperthermia exposure. One treatment method is ice water immersion, if the equipment and trained personnel are available, or an evaporative external cooling in the field. Prehospital cooling should start before or at the same time EMS is activated. Evaporative cooling methods in the field or the ambulance are done by spraying the patient with water or saline. Additionally, decrease the ambient temperature in the ambulance with air conditioners at high speed and manually fanning the patient. Apply ice packs to the child's axilla, groin, and neck, along with the administration of room temperature IV fluids.[8,205]

Initial stabilization may include the need for basic or advanced control of the airway and breathing if CNS effects are causing respiratory depression from coma or seizure activity. All patients with heatstroke require venous access either with two large-bore IVs, IOs, or central access. Fluid resuscitation is dependent on the type of heatstroke. The provider can administer IV fluids at room temperature, but monitor closely to prevent fluid overload. Children with classic non-exertional heatstroke are only mildly to moderately hypovolemic, but with exertional heatstroke, they are more moderately to severely hypovolemic and may require 20–40 mL/kg of normal saline or more. Altered mental status may resolve after oxygenation and adequate tissue perfusion, and normothermia is achieved. If seizures develop, treat with benzodiazepines as needed.

All children with heatstroke after stabilization and rapid cooling should be admitted to a pediatric critical care unit because the child remains at high risk for end-organ failure and metabolic and coagulation abnormalities. The child with heatstroke is at risk and should be evaluated for rhabdomyolysis with hyperkalemia, hypocalcemia, hyperphosphatemia, disseminated intravascular coagulation, acute kidney injury, hyponatremic dehydration, cardiogenic shock with low systemic vascular resistance (SVR), cerebral edema, and liver failure.[8,205]

Near-Drowning

Drowning and submersion injuries are the leading causes of accidental death and morbidities in children. Over 500,000 deaths globally each year are attributed to drowning. The CDC reported in 2010 that drowning was the leading cause of accidents and death in children aged 1–4 years, the second leading cause of death in children aged 5–9 years, and the third leading cause of death in children aged 10–14 years. Drownings can be broken down by the type of water (i.e., freshwater or saltwater) and temperature. Warm water drownings occur in temperatures greater than or equal to 20°C (68°F), and cold water drownings occur in temperatures less than or equal to 20°C (68°F). The most common locations of drowning in children occur in freshwater, including lakes, rivers, and other natural bodies of water; followed by swimming pools; then bathtubs or buckets; and then saltwater, which is the smallest percentage. Infant drownings are highest in swimming pools at home.[8,206]

Risk factors identified for children are epilepsy, congenital long QT syndrome, catecholaminergic polymorphic ventricular tachycardia, hyperventilation before swimming, hypoglycemia, and hypothermia. In older children, alcohol and illicit drugs are contributors to drowning. The drowning process usually begins with voluntary breath holding then small amounts of water are aspirated into the airway, triggering a coughing reflex and laryngospasm. The child cannot breathe because of the laryngospasm so the exchange of gas stops, leading to hypoxia, hypercarbia, and acidosis. As arterial oxygen tension decreases, laryngospasm is relieved and additional water is aspirated by the child, leading to cerebral hypoxemia, which causes the child to lose consciousness and become apneic followed quickly by cardiac arrest. The entire drowning process usually takes place within seconds to minutes. Intrapulmonary shunting of blood through poorly ventilated lungs is the primary pathophysiologic process of drowning. Contributing to this process of intrapulmonary shunting include bronchospasm, impaired alveolar–capillary gas exchange from the aspirated fluid within the alveolar space, surfactant inactivation, and washout, decreased surfactant production because of alveolar damage, atelectasis causing pulmonary edema and a ventilation/perfusion mismatch. After 24 hours an infectious or chemical pneumonitis may occur from aspiration of gastric contents or type of water from near nonfatal drowning. Hypoxia, acidosis, and hypothermia contribute to cardiovascular dysfunction or dysrhythmias. Permanent neurologic damage is common in the survivors of near-drowning. The amount of damage is determined by the duration and severity of the initial hypoxic–ischemic injury.[8,206]

Management of Near-Drowning

Pediatric survivors of near-drowning almost universally have two things in common: limited submersion times and excellent initial resuscitative care. The priority in managing a child who has a near-drowning event is to reverse hypoxemia by restoring adequate oxygenation and ventilation. Initial efforts focus on airway, breathing, and circulation. Oxygen, with or without mechanical ventilation support, is the first line of therapy. The child breathing spontaneously and able to maintain oxygen saturation greater than 90% or a partial pressure of oxygen greater than 90 mmHg with a fraction of inspired oxygen of 0.5 may be able to remain on the nonrebreather mask with oxygen therapy alone. Children who are apneic or exhibiting respiratory depression require ETI using a rapid sequence induction technique. Intubation not only secures an airway but also protects against aspiration of gastric contents and allows for suctioning of the airway and effective oxygenation and ventilation if copious pulmonary edema develops. Mechanical ventilation with PEEP should be used. In the event of suspected CSIs, the provider needs to avoid hyperextension of the neck during resuscitation. Immobilization of the cervical spine is based solely on the history of submersion by witnesses. The most frequent complication of children who drown is regurgitation and aspiration of stomach contents, which causes more damage to the lungs and affects oxygenation. All victims of drowning with evidence of shock need IV fluid resuscitation with normal saline, with the initial fluid boluses starting at 20 mL/kg. If IV access cannot be obtained promptly because of ongoing CPR or extreme vasoconstriction, IO access should be performed. Decreased CO with high systemic and pulmonary vascular resistance occurs secondary to hypoxia associated with near-drowning. This injury may persist even after adequate oxygenation, ventilation, and perfusion have been established, requiring the initiation of inotropic agents to improve CO and reestablish adequate tissue perfusion. Reverse the child's hypothermia slowly.[8,206]

The Secondary Survey

The secondary survey begins after the primary survey (ABCDEs) is completed and resuscitative efforts are initiated. A complete head-to-toe evaluation of the trauma patient should be completed to assess for non–life-threatening injuries, including a complete history, physical examination, and reassessment of vital signs and interventions. This evaluation requires each region of the body to be examined completely by inspection, palpation, and, where appropriate, auscultation and percussion. Ideally, this survey should take place during transport rather than at the scene of injury. The potential for missing an injury or for the referral facility to not recognize the impact of an injury is significant, especially in the unresponsive or unstable patient. Assessment for lacerations, fractures, abrasions, ecchymosis, ocular and dental injuries, and areas of swelling or edema are included in the secondary survey. Any part of the body not fully assessed during the primary survey should now be evaluated for injury. A full set of vital signs should also be completed. A complete neurologic examination is performed, including repeating the GCS score. If time permits, dressing of wounds and immobilization of fractures can now take place. Frequent reassessment of the patient's primary survey and the effectiveness of medical interventions should be ongoing during transport. Neurovascular assessments before and after immobilization of fractures are necessary. Obtain the child's weight either by caregiver history or by use of a length-based resuscitation tape. Cardiac monitors and pulse oximeters (if not already in place) should be applied. A radio report to receiving facilities should also be completed at this time and before arrival at the receiving facility.[8,123,126]

Nonaccidental Trauma or Neglect

According to the CDC, abusive head trauma is an injury to the skull or intracranial contents of a baby or child younger than 5 years of age caused by intentional abrupt impact and violent shaking. NAT is a leading cause of childhood traumatic injury and death in the United States. Physical and sexual abuse of children is a frequent, disturbing, and significant problem. When a child is harmed, those who provide emergency care, such as prehospital providers, may be the first to respond to the child's injury or situation. The ability to detect NAT, maltreatment, and neglect is a necessary skill for any person involved in the care of children. Adequate education and training are imperative for prehospital providers. They should know how to assess, suspect, report, and document concerns of NAT. This will not only help the child but also improve the overall quality of pre-hospital care of these children. Careful consideration of patient findings and caregiver history is crucial in the identification of children in need of intervention.[8,125,207]

Abuse may be physical, emotional, or sexual. Acts that deprive children of their basic needs such as food and clothing are more appropriately called neglect. Children born premature or with multiple medical conditions are at a higher risk of experiencing NAT. Shaken baby syndrome is a common form of NAT identified in these children and described by a triad of symptoms, which includes subdural hematoma, retinal hemorrhage, and encephalopathy suggesting MOI with tearing of the bridging veins secondary to shaking the child. All states have statutes that require reporting of suspected maltreatment or neglect. It is important to be aware of the local statutes and community support options available in your area. Physicians, nurses, police officers, social workers, prehospital personnel, and other adults who interact with children should all be aware of historical and physical findings that are indicators of abuse or neglect. These findings are provided in Boxes 18.6 and 18.7. Keep in mind that some of these injuries can occur in the absence of abuse. A careful history

• BOX 18.6 **Historical Indicators of Child Abuse, Neglect, or Maltreatment**

- Caregiver history incongruent with the mechanism of injury and actual injuries
- Caregiver history incongruent with child's developmental abilities
- Delay in seeking medical treatment
- Patterned or unusual marks on the child's body
- Injuries of various age or injuries of multiple types
- A caregiver who denies knowledge of how an injury occurred
- A caregiver whose response to the child's injury is not appropriate
- A caregiver who expresses over- or under-concern for the seriousness of the child's injury
- A recent change in caregivers
- No preexisting medical condition that describes the child's injury
- Inconsistencies or changes in the history provided
- Emphasis of unimportant details or unrelated minor problems by the caregiver
- Previous treatment for suspicious or unexplained injuries
- Caregivers who seek medical attention for the child's injuries in other area hospitals
- Bypassing a closer emergency department to seek care at a department further away
- Tension or hostility between caregivers or tension or hostility directed at the child or staff
- An uncooperative caregiver
- Injuries that could have been prevented with closer supervision

From Holleran RS, ed. *ASTNA Patient Transport: Principles and Practice.* 4th ed. St. Louis, MO: Mosby Elsevier; 2010.

of mechanisms and supervision is critical in children with these clinical findings. Emergency care providers are required to report abuse and to make sure to document the case number in the charting.[3,207,208]

Federal legislation provides the foundation for state laws on child injury by identifying a minimum set of injuries and behaviors that classify abuse and neglect of children. The Federal Child Abuse Prevention and Treatment Act (CAPTA) and the CAPTA Reauthorization Act of 2010 outline the minimum standards of child abuse and neglect for states to follow with their classifications.

Sexual Abuse

Children who suffer sexual abuse may present with vague somatic symptoms or behavioral changes. Sexual abuse should always be considered in patients with equivocal clinical findings. Other children may present for care after revealing abuse to a caregiver. Sexual abuse of children occurs primarily in the preadolescent years. Females are more likely to be sexually abused than males in the preadolescent group, with males less likely to report sexual abuse. Refer to Table 18.19 for signs and symptoms of sexual abuse in children. Care in the transport setting should include treatment of medical issues with psychologic support of the patient.[8,208]

Shock and Shock Management

Shock in pediatric patients is one of the leading causes of morbidity and mortality because of the failure to supply enough oxygen to meet the tissue oxygen demand. This causes tissue hypoxia and increases anaerobic metabolism. Elevated serum lactate levels reflect the anaerobic metabolism related to cellular hypoxia and

• BOX 18.7 Clinical Sign and Symptoms of Child Abuse, Neglect, or Maltreatment

- Behavioral
- Inappropriate reactions to procedures
- Frightened of caregiver
- Goes easily to strangers; uncharacteristic for child's age
- Extreme apprehension with other children's crying
- Bruises: Potentially inflicted bruises include the following:
  - Bruises to the face, neck, chest, abdomen, back, flank, thighs, or genitalia
  - Bruises in various stages of healing
  - Bruises suggestive of being struck by an object
  - Pinch marks; pairs of crescent-shaped bruises
  - Fingerprint or thumb patterns
  - Bruises suggestive of being kicked
  - Bruises to the mouth, gums, or buccal mucosa
  - Multiple or symmetric bruises or marks
- Burns: Characteristics of intentionally inflicted burns include the following:
  - Immersion burn; circumferential and often symmetric "stocking" pattern burns to the feet, "glovelike" pattern
  - Burns to hands, doughnut pattern burn to buttocks
  - Burns with sharply demarcated edges without splash burns
  - Ligature or rope burns to wrists, ankles, torso, or neck
  - Cigarette or cigar burns, especially on typically concealed areas
  - Contact burns: dry uniform print may be in the configuration of an object used to cause the burn (e.g., grill)
  - Symmetric burns
  - Splash patterns in unusual sites (e.g., genitals) or splash patterns with separated areas

- Burn to the dorsum of the hand
- Delays in seeking treatment
- Bites and other marks: Characteristics of potentially inflicted marks include the following:
  - Downturned lesions at the corners of the mouth, caused by being gagged
  - Human bites; crescent-shaped bruises with circular lesions; individual tooth marks may be present; a distance greater than 3 cm between the third tooth and canine on each side indicates a bite caused by an adult or child older than 8 years of age
- Head injuries suggestive of abuse include the following:
  - Skull fractures; multiple complex or bilateral skull fractures in an infant
  - Cerebral edema with retinal hemorrhages (common in shaken baby syndrome)
  - Subdural hematoma or subarachnoid hemorrhage
  - Traction alopecia and scalp swelling from hair pulling
- Skeletal fractures suggestive of abuse include the following:
  - Multiple fractures in different stages of healing or untreated healing fractures
  - Unusual fractures: ribs, scapula, sternum, vertebrae, distal clavicle
  - Metaphyseal injuries that have the appearance of tufts, chips, or "bucket handles" causing arcs of bone
  - Spiral fractures of long bones
  - Transverse fractures
  - Repeated fractures at the same site, multiple bilateral or symmetric fractures

From Holleran RS, ed. *ASTNA Patient Transport: Principles and Practice.* 4th ed. St. Louis, MO: Mosby Elsevier; 2010.

TABLE 18.19 Sign and Symptoms of Sexual Abuse in Children

Physical Signs	Behavioral Signs	Emotional Signs
Sexually transmitted infections	Less communication than usual; secretive behavior	Mood changes (e.g., increase in aggression, anxiety, hyperactivity)
Explained bleeding/bruising/abrasion/laceration in genital area; blood on clothing, sheets	Regressive behaviors (e.g., bed-wetting, thumb-sucking)	Decreased self-confidence
Foreign body in genitourinary cavity	Sexual knowledge and behaviors/activities inappropriate for age and development	Fear or avoidance of being alone with specific people or being away from primary caregiver[a]
Inflammation, irritation, pain/burning in genitourinary tract	Avoidance of nudity (e.g., refusing to bathe, change clothes); change in hygiene	New sleep disturbances (e.g., fear of sleep/dark; night terrors, nightmares)
Frequent urinary tract infection; pain on urination and/or defecation	Overly compliant	Depression; social withdrawal from friends and family
Vaginal or penile discharge	Unusual increase in time spent alone	Excessive fear, phobias[a]
Chronic headache	Change of appetite; loss of appetite/anorexia[b]	
Unexplained gastrointestinal symptoms (e.g., abdominal pain, chronic constipation)	Compulsive masturbation	
Pregnancy in young adolescent	Self-harm, suicidal ideation	

[a]Especially if new behavior.
[b]Often resulting in weight loss.
Data from ASTNA; Holleran RS, Wolfe AC, Frakes MA, eds. *Patient Transport: Principles and Practice.* 5th ed. St. Louis, MO: Mosby Elsevier; 2018; Bechtel K, Bennett BL. Evaluation of sexual abuse in children and adolescents. In: UpToDate, March 2017. Wiley JF (ed.), UpToDate, Waltham, MA.

are considered to be an important indicator of impaired tissue perfusion in patients.[8,209,210]

Shock can develop from an array of conditions resulting in insufficient circulating blood volume (preload), changes in vascular resistance (afterload), heart failure (contractility), and obstruction to flow. Early recognition of shock and prompt treatment is essential for reversing the effects and improving patient outcomes.[8,209,210]

The current American College of Critical Care Medicine recommendations are that the diagnosis of shock include early fluid resuscitation with crystalloids such as normal saline or Ringer's lactate, followed by initiation of vasoactive medications such as dopamine or epinephrine as a first line, epinephrine for cold shock and norepinephrine for warm shock, and hydrocortisone for those with potential risk of adrenal insufficiency.[8,209,210]

There are several etiologies of shock, and the underlying pathology is inadequate tissue oxygenation. The goal of shock management is the support of oxygen delivery and CO.

Etiologies of Shock

There are several etiologies of shock:

- *Hypovolemic shock* is the most common type of shock experienced by children. It develops when intravascular volume is insufficient to maintain tissue perfusion. The decrease in intravascular volume results in a decreased preload, which decreases CO leading to an increase in SVR and increased capillary refill. Sources of volume loss include vomiting; diarrhea; osmotic dieresis; capillary leak from sepsis; and intra-abdominal processes with third space losses such as pancreatitis, intussusception, appendicitis, burn injuries, hemorrhage, inadequate fluid intake, or insensible losses.[8,209–211]
- *Distributive shock*, also called vasodilatory shock, results from a decrease in system vascular resistance, with abnormal distribution of blood flow resulting in inadequate tissue perfusion. Causes of distributive shock include sepsis, anaphylaxis reaction, and acute injury to the spinal cord or brain (neurogenic shock). Sepsis is the most common etiology seen in children. Anaphylaxis is another cause and manifests as an immediate, potentially life-threatening systemic reaction to an external source, which is usually an allergic IgE-mediated immediate hypersensitivity reaction. Neurogenic shock is a relatively rare occurrence following an acute injury to the spinal cord or CNS resulting in a loss of sympathetic venous tone.[8,209–211]
- *Cardiogenic shock* results from pump failure because of intrinsic cardiac disease resulting in the inability of the heart to provide adequate CO. This decreased cardiac contractility is a result of CHD, myocarditis, myocardial contusion, myocardial ischemia, cardiomyopathy, or cardiac arrhythmia. Physiologic signs of cardiogenic shock include tachycardia, increased SVR, and decreased CO.[8,209–211]
- *Obstructive shock* is caused by an acquired obstruction of systemic blood flow from the heart, which causes abrupt impairment of CO resulting in blood flow physically obstructed with an increased vascular resistance. Obstructive shock is caused by cardiac tamponade, tension pneumothorax, massive pulmonary embolism, CHD with ductal-dependent lesions such as hypoplastic left heart syndrome or critical aortic stenosis. It may also present when the ductus arteriosus closes during the first few weeks of life.[8,209–211]

Assessment and Diagnosis

Children can compensate for circulatory dysfunction by increasing heart rate, SVR, and venous tone while maintaining normal blood pressures with poor tissue perfusion present. The challenge for providers is to recognize children in shock before hypotension develops, which is a late sign. The cause of shock is not always known before treatment must be initiated. A systematic approach is needed to assess and diagnose children presenting with poor perfusion. This is done by the provider identifying features of the child's history, physical examination, and ancillary studies that may suggest the underlying condition. The goals of an initial evaluation of shock in children require immediate identification of life-threatening conditions, rapid recognition of circulatory collapse, and early classification of the type and cause of the shock.[8,211,212]

Historical data to help the provider identify the condition causing shock include the following[8,211]:

- A history of fluid loss caused by vomiting, diarrhea from gastroenteritis, DKA, or GI bleeding.
- Hypovolemic shock caused by hemorrhage caused by a solid organ injury from blunt abdominal trauma, obstructive shock with a tension pneumothorax or cardiac tamponade, or neurogenic shock with an SCI.
- Fever or immunocompromise caused by chemotherapy, sickle cell disease, or inherited immunodeficiencies may indicate septic shock.
- A history of exposure to an allergen such as a bee sting or food causing anaphylactic shock.
- Septic shock may develop as a result of exposure to toxins such as beta-blockers, calcium channel blockers, or cardiac glycosides.
- Cardiogenic shock may present in patients with chronic heart disease such as cardiomyopathy or complex CHD.
- Adrenal crisis must be considered in a patient at risk for adrenal insufficiency, such as children receiving chronic steroid therapy, hypopituitarism, or neonates with sepsis.

Signs and Symptoms

The clinical presentation of shock in children is variable with several common signs and symptoms including tachycardia and signs of poor perfusion. Common clinical signs and symptoms of shock include the following[8,213]:

- Tachycardia is a common and important indicator. It is also a nonspecific finding and is seen with other common childhood conditions such as fever, pain, and anxiety, which can cause tachycardia without poor perfusion.
- Skin changes are present in most shock states because of the child's regulatory processes compensating for decreased or poor effective tissue perfusion. Vasoconstrictive mechanisms redistribute blood from the peripheral, splanchnic, and renal vessels to maintain coronary and cerebral perfusion resulting in the child's skin being cool, clammy, pale, mottled, or diaphoretic. Conversely, in early distributive shock, the child has peripheral vasodilation and the skin may be flushed and hyperemic. This is also seen when there is a failure of the child's regulatory mechanisms to maintain peripheral vascular resistance and is a sign of irreversible shock.
- Impaired LOC in children is a sign of impaired cerebral perfusion. The child may initially be listless, restless, anxious, confused, irritable, show decreased levels of responsiveness to the environment, be agitated, or not interact with parents. The

child's mental status will continue to deteriorate and become obtunded, and coma results as shock worsens.

- Tachypnea is present.
- Decreased or absent urine output occurs with a decreased glomerular filtration rate secondary to shunting of renal blood flow to other organs.
- Lactic acidosis develops resulting in progressive tissue hypoperfusion, which is caused by inadequate delivery of oxygen to the tissues and decreased clearance of lactate by the kidneys, liver, and skeletal muscle.
- Decreased or absent bowel sounds.
- Changes in pulse quality may occur with pulses being weak, thready, or absent.
- May have difficulty obtaining blood pressure.
- Hypotension is a late and ominous sign in children. The compensatory vasoconstriction that is very effective early in the shock state with systemic blood pressure maintained in the normal range along with poor perfusion present begins to fail. Bradycardia and hypotension should be recognized as ominous signs and should be aggressively treated in children.
- According to the AHA PALS guidelines, shock can be primarily separated into stages: compensated, decompensated, and irreversible. See Table 18.20 for a description of each stage.[8,210,211]

Many of the preceding clinical signs and symptoms are not specific to shock and need to be considered in relation to history and patient presentation. Measures of end-organ perfusion such as LOC, urinary output, heart rate, and pulse quality may be the most helpful assessment factors in patients with suspected shock.

Diagnostic aids for children in shock include the following[8,211]:

- Cardiopulmonary monitor.
- Pulse oximeter. If the child is exhibiting poor perfusion this may prevent an accurate reading, but a normal reading does not rule out the child's need for supplemental oxygen.
- CXR to rule out cardiomegaly, pulmonary infection, pneumothorax, or hemothorax.
- Laboratory studies to obtain include a complete blood count, glucose, and electrolytes with a lactate level.
- Arterial or capillary blood gases help monitor the child's acidosis caused by oxygen debt and anaerobic metabolism but also monitor the child's oxygenation and ventilation status. Obtaining serial blood gases can be useful to monitor the effectiveness of interventions.
- For suspected septic shock, cultures of blood, body fluids, sputum, CSF, wounds, and indwelling devices may be obtained to determine whether there is a source of potential infection.
- A urinary catheter should be placed for accurate measurement of the child's urine output.
- Urinalysis to assess for the presence of blood, ketones, bacteria, glucose, and specific gravity measurement.

Treatment of Shock

Successful management of children with shock requires the rapid initiation of aggressive treatment. The provider should implement a goal-directed or systematic approach for most patients presenting with shock because the cause is not always known. During initial stabilization, assessment, and observation, indications that help determine the etiology of the shock should be sought. This will provide the most optimal therapy and quickly identify children who may be harmed by the therapy or who are not responding to the initial approach.[8,209,210,212]

- Rapid assessment to quickly determine the presence and suspected type of shock.
- Initial management of hypovolemic, distributive, and cardiogenic shock should focus on fluid resuscitation with an isotonic crystalloid solution appropriate to the type of shock and specific pharmacologic therapies, as indicated, once the etiology of shock is identified.
- Interventions must be administered in a rapid sequence, with the evaluation of physiologic indicators before and after each intervention.
- Physiologic indicators include blood pressure, central and peripheral pulses, mental status, and urine output.
- Several physiologic indicators can be monitored noninvasively during the initial management of shock such as mean arterial pressure. Clinical experience suggests that the quality of central and peripheral pulses, skin perfusion, mental status, and urine output are useful signs for assessing response to therapy interventions.
- Heart rate is an important physiologic indicator of circulatory status. For children with shock, tachycardia is a compensatory response to poor tissue perfusion. A positive response to treatment would be a decrease in the child's heart rate with fluid therapy.
- Continue monitoring and provide supportive treatment for the child after showing signs of improvement in perfusion.
- Achieving normal blood pressure is essential for a patient who has hypotensive shock.

TABLE 18.20   Stages of Shock and Physiologic Response

Compensated	Decompensated	Irreversible
• Homeostatic mechanisms rapidly compensate for diminished perfusion and systolic blood pressure maintained within normal range • Heart rate initially increased • Signs of peripheral vasoconstriction with cool skin, decreased peripheral pulses, and oliguria can be found as perfusion becomes more compromised	• Compensatory mechanism become overwhelmed • Heart rate markedly elevated and hypotension develops • Signs and symptoms of organ dysfunction such as alert mental status result of poor brain perfusion appear • Systolic blood pressure is maintained in normal limits in children until they have lost 30%–35% of their circulating volume • Once hypotension develops, the child deteriorates rapidly to cardiovascular collapse and cardiac arrest	• Progressive end-organ dysfunction leads to irreversible organ damage and death • Tachycardia may be replaced by bradycardia and blood pressure becomes very low • Process is often irreversible regardless of resuscitative efforts

From Waltzman ML. Pediatric shock. *J Emerg Nurs.* 2015;41(2):113–118.

- If obstructive shock is present, it requires emergent recognition and treatment of the cause (e.g., tension pneumothorax or hemothorax, cardiac tamponade, CHD with the closure of the ductus arteriosus, or pulmonary embolism). If shock is caused by a cardiac arrhythmia, such as supraventricular tachycardia, then treatments to restore normal sinus rhythm are essential initial steps.

Venous Access in Children

Before fluid resuscitation can begin in children with suspected shock, venous access must be obtained. Sites for venous access in children include the following[8]:

- Percutaneous peripheral attempts (limited to two attempts)
- IO needle placement
- Saphenous vein cutdown
- Percutaneous placement in the femoral vein
- Percutaneous placement in the subclavian vein
- Percutaneous placement in the external jugular vein (this site should not be used if a cervical collar is in place)
- Percutaneous placement in the internal jugular vein

Hypovolemic Shock

Intravascular fluid losses from hemorrhage, vomiting, diarrhea, osmotic diuresis, or capillary leak are the principal elements of hypovolemic shock. The management of hypovolemic shock focuses on fluid replacement and preventing ongoing fluid loss. Vasoactive medications will not improve the child's perfusion status; the tank must be filled first. Administer 20 mL/kg normal saline or lactated Ringer's solution or blood transfusion for hypovolemic shock for most children and repeat as needed. Each bolus should be infused over 5–10 minutes. Rapid infusion of fluids should be performed with caution in children with severe malnutrition.[8,209,210,212]

For children who have not improved after receiving a total of 60 mL/kg over 30–60 minutes, consider the following[8,209,210,212]:

- The amount of fluid lost may be underestimated as with burn injuries or there may be significant ongoing fluid loss from hemorrhage secondary to blunt abdominal trauma or capillary leak syndrome associated with bowel obstruction.
- Other conditions may be causing or contributing to shock (i.e., a child with multiple traumas who has an SCI).
- It is not a first-line treatment, but colloids are an option for patients with hypoalbuminemia (albumin <3 g/dL) or hyperchloremic metabolic acidosis who have not improved after initial therapy with at least 60 mL/kg of crystalloid solutions.
- Patients with hemorrhagic shock who have not improved should receive blood and require definitive treatment for the cause of hemorrhage. Delaying fluid resuscitation for traumatic hemorrhagic in children is not recommended.
- Hypovolemic shock is uncommon in children with DKA. Patients in DKA whose perfusion does not improve with 10 mL/kg of isotonic fluid should be evaluated for other causes of shock.

Cardiogenic Shock

A history of heart disease, an abnormal cardiac examination, and worsening clinical status with fluid resuscitation are suggestive of cardiogenic shock. Additional findings suggestive of cardiogenic shock include a gallop rhythm, pulmonary rales, jugular venous distention, hepatomegaly, tachycardia out of proportion to fever or respiratory distress, cyanosis unresponsive to oxygen, and absent femoral pulses. If these signs are present, a smaller isotonic crystalloid fluid bolus of 5–10 mL/kg infused over 10–20 minutes will decrease the chances of exacerbating heart failure. If needed, an additional 5- to 10-mL/kg aliquots may be given if needed for improvement in physiologic indicators. Cardiogenic shock is less common than other forms of shock in children, and early consultation with a pediatric cardiologist is recommended.[8,209,210,212]

Cardiogenic shock management issues include the following[8,209,210,212]:

- Cardiogenic shock should be considered for any child without an easily identifiable cause for shock whose condition worsens with fluid therapy.
- Some children with poor cardiac function may also be volume-depleted. Fluid should be administered slowly and in boluses of 5–10 mL/kg and reassessed.
- Treatment with dobutamine or phosphodiesterase enzyme inhibitors such as milrinone can improve myocardial contractility and reduce SVR (afterload).
- Cardiac arrhythmias (e.g., supraventricular or ventricular tachycardia) should be addressed before fluid resuscitation.

Distributive Shock

Distributive shock is characteristic of a marked decrease in SVR. This form of shock does well with both fluid resuscitation and vasopressor infusions depending on the underlying etiology, septic shock, anaphylactic shock, or neurogenic shock. Septic shock management is recommended by the American Critical Care Medicine guidelines for neonates and children with septic shock and includes the following[8,209,210,212–216]:

- Treatment with 20-mL/kg crystalloid bolus over 5–10 minutes and repeat until perfusion improves or until the child develops rales or hepatomegaly.
- Correct hypoglycemia and hypocalcemia.
- Begin antibiotics after cultures are obtained.
- Septic shock may be classified as a cold or warm shock based on clinical findings. Children in cold septic shock exhibit cool extremities, delayed capillary refill, and poor pulses. They also have low CO and elevated SVR in an attempt to maintain perfusion pressure. Warm shock presents with vasodilation, low SVR, increased CO, clinical quick capillary refill, warm extremities, and bounding pulses. Traditionally, it was thought that septic shock was a cold shock, but recent data suggest community-acquired septic shock usually does not present as cold shock. Hospital-acquired or central line-associated septic shock frequently presents as warm shock.
- Fluid refractory shock will need inotropic support. To reverse cold shock start dopamine and titrate infusion; if resistant, initiate epinephrine infusion and titrate. To reverse warm shock, initiate and titrate a norepinephrine infusion.
- Catecholamine-resistant shock will need hydrocortisone started if a patient is at risk for adrenal insufficiency.
- Cold shock with normal blood pressure is managed by titrating fluids and epinephrine infusion; consider starting milrinone.
- Cold shock with low blood pressure requires titration of fluids and epinephrine; consider adding norepinephrine.
- Warm shock with low blood pressure is managed by titrating fluids and norepinephrine; consider adding vasopressin.
- Refractory septic shock not responding to fluid resuscitation and inotropes may need ECMO therapy.

When the child has a history of allergies and/or the presence of stridor, wheezing, urticaria, or facial edema, anaphylactic shock is suggested. Children with possible anaphylaxis should receive

IM epinephrine, IV or IM diphenhydramine, and steroids, in addition to rapid infusions of normal saline. Wheezing should be treated with nebulized albuterol. Patients with cardiovascular collapse or those who respond poorly to IM epinephrine may require epinephrine intravenously.[8,209–211,214–216]

Neurogenic shock refers to hypotension, usually associated with bradycardia, as a result of an interruption of the autonomic pathways in the spinal cord causing decreased vascular resistance. Patients with traumatic SCI may also suffer from hemodynamic shock related to blood loss and other complications. Adequate blood pressure is believed to be critical in maintaining adequate perfusion to the injured spinal cord, limiting secondary ischemic injury. Appropriate mean arterial pressure for age should be maintained using IV fluids, transfusion, and pharmacologic vasopressors as needed. Bradycardia caused by cervical spinal cord or high thoracic spinal cord disruption may require external pacing or administration of atropine.[8,209–211,214–216]

Obstructive shock causes include tension pneumothorax, cardiac tamponade, hemothorax, pulmonary embolism, or ductal-dependent congenital heart defects and require specific interventions to relieve the obstruction to blood flow.[8,209–211,214–216]

Damage Control Resuscitation

Trauma is the leading cause of death in children. Hemorrhage continues to be the leading cause of preventable traumatic deaths in children. Damage control resuscitation (DCR) is intended to improve patient outcomes through the alleviation of the lethal triad of acidosis, hypothermia, and coagulopathy. The ACS adopted both DCR and permissive hypotension in adults in the ATLS curriculum. DCR is designed to be used on patients with severe uncontrollable hemorrhage and requires large amounts of blood products. DCR is not intended for those who respond to initial fluids without further interventions. Children have physiologic differences compared with adults when presenting with hypovolemic shock, such as the ability to compensate for approximately 45% circulating blood loss before shock is reflected in the child's blood pressure. This physiologic response suggests that permissive hypotension may not be a good choice in children, especially if they have a head injury and adequate CPP is indicated. The goal of initial resuscitation in children is hemodynamic stability and restoration of adequate tissue perfusion with an endpoint of urine output greater than 1 mL/kg/hour. It is important to remember to prevent hypothermia during fluid resuscitation because hypothermia may result in vasoconstriction, acidosis, and consumptive coagulopathy. Along with preventative hypothermic measures, the prehospital provider should initiate fluid resuscitation starting with a 20 mL/kg fluid bolus of Ringer's lactate or isotonic sodium chloride solution. This may be given up to two times, and then the provider should consider blood components. In the prehospital environment, excessive volume replacement (over-resuscitation) with crystalloids in injured children increases the tendency for higher rates of multiorgan failure and mortality.[216,217]

Children with evidence of hemorrhagic shock who fail to respond to fluid resuscitation should begin receiving blood and blood products. Guidelines are not well established in pediatric trauma patients describing the best time to switch from crystalloid fluids to blood and blood products. Current data suggest early identification of coagulopathy and the need to treat patients with red blood cells, fresh frozen plasma, and platelets in a 1:1:1 unit ratio, limiting the use of crystalloid administration. This may

improve survival in pediatric patients with severe traumatic injury and life-threatening bleeding.[218,219]

Other Pediatric Medical and Trauma Conditions

Seizures

Status epilepticus (SE) is one of the most common pediatric neurologic emergencies. The mortality in children is up to 3%. Morbidities include cognitive and neurodevelopmental impairments, epilepsy, and recurrent SE. SE refractory to the initial antiepileptic medications is associated with poor outcomes. SE is defined as any continuous convulsive seizure activity or intermittent convulsive seizure activity lasting more than 30 minutes without regaining consciousness between the seizures. SE in children is the most common life-threatening neurologic emergency. Classification of SE falls into four categories. Acute symptomatic SE occurs because of a neurologic insult such as trauma, CNS infection, or metabolic disorders. Remote symptomatic SE includes patients with neurologic disorders, such as chronic encephalopathies, which predispose these children to seizures. Idiopathic seizures are those that occur in known epileptic patients who abruptly stop taking anticonvulsant medications. The febrile SE includes epileptic seizures associated with fever lasting more than 30 minutes without CNS infection.[220–222]

Children begin to suffer neurologic damage when seizures last 30 minutes or longer and can be complicated by focal neurologic deficits, cognitive impairment, behavior problems, airway compromise, or other adverse events. Seizures account for the second most common condition requiring EMS pediatric transport. Several studies in the pediatric prehospital literature compared administration routes of benzodiazepines for seizure patients and found similar results between the IV route and the IM, intranasal (IN), buccal, and rectal routes. The literature suggests alternative routes of administration (specifically IM, IN, and buccal) are equally effective and comparable to IV, with the same side effect profiles; therefore, they should be considered preferentially for children in the prehospital setting. EMS providers can administer benzodiazepine to a seizing child as quickly as possible and repeat if the seizure persists longer than 5–10 minutes. Avoid giving more than two doses of benzodiazepines because of an increased risk of respiratory depression. The most commonly seen adverse effect of benzodiazepines is respiratory depression. Hypoglycemia is an infrequent but important cause of pediatric seizures and can be easily and quickly identified via the use of a point-of-care glucometer.[220–222]

Concussive Head Injuries in Children

Concussions in children and adolescents account for 90% of all TBIs. It is estimated that one in five children will experience a concussion by the age of 10 years. Falls and sports-related activities are the most common causes of concussions. A concussion is a form of mild TBI that occurs as a result of a direct impact on the child's head or an impact on the body that transmits forces to the head. Common early symptoms include headaches, dizziness, vertigo or imbalance, lack of awareness of surroundings, brief loss of consciousness, and nausea and vomiting. Confusion is a hallmark sign of concussions and may include amnesia usually of the traumatic event and occasionally the preceding event.[223,224]

There is emerging evidence that repetitive concussions may cause persistent neurocognitive changes. Repetitive concussions have been a contributing factor to neurodegenerative conditions including chronic traumatic encephalopathy, post-traumatic stress disorder, substance abuse, anxiety, and depression.[223,224]

The prehospital provider will be transporting more concussive children because of the rising numbers of children actively engaging in sports-related activities. Another factor increasing concussion numbers is the media bringing concussions to the forefront and discussing professional athletes who are beginning to experience long-term deficits from concussions experienced years before.[223,224]

Pediatric Dog Bites and Attacks

Dog bites are common in the United States and can result in significant morbidity in pediatric patients. The injuries may range from superficial wounds to life-threatening head and neck injuries and fatalities. It is estimated that 4.5 million ED visits are for animal bites each year, with 85%–90% being dog bites, and 40% accounting for significant pediatric trauma involving pre-hospital emergency transport, with 10–20 animal-related pediatric fatalities every year. There is no single dog breed responsible for all animal bites. However, the Pitbull and Rottweiler breeds are responsible for the majority of human fatalities over the last 20 years. The majority of dog bite victims are children and they involve the head, neck, and face. Adolescents receive the majority of dog bites to their extremities. Psychologic trauma may result and manifest itself in fear and nightmares and is documented to harm the quality of life for both the child and parents. Dog bite injuries frequently affect the head, neck, and facial areas of children and are the most common reason for emergency transport. These injury areas are vascular, tissue damage could be extensive, and the child's airway may be affected. It is essential to clean these wounds effectively, and treatment is usually primary closure by a plastic surgeon to limit scarring morbidities and secondary infections in children. These children will require antibiotics, tetanus, and possibly rabies prophylaxis.[225–227]

Prehospital Pain Management in Children

Pain is commonly seen in prehospital care. The under-recognized and inadequate treatment of pain is associated with adverse physiologic and emotional effects such as slower healing, emotional trauma, and alterations in pain processing. Children whose pain is untreated can have lasting effects into adulthood, including fear of medical encounters, post-traumatic stress disorder, and misuse of medical care. Pain is an important part of the body's response to tissue injury, and the intensity is related to the extent, severity, and location of injury. Untreated pain can lead to shock from pain, making pain management one of the most important therapies needed in the patient after trauma, especially for children. Pain management in a child with an injury should include nonpharmacologic and pharmacologic interventions. Nonpharmacologic interventions include ice packs and immobilization of fractures. If these measures are ineffective in relieving pain, then pharmacologic methods are needed. Correctly providing pain management in the injured child after injury significantly affects the disease prognosis. The prehospital care provider needs to ensure that each child transported has their pain level assessed and documented in the chart and appropriate interventions should be provided.[228,229]

Children With Special Needs

It is estimated that there are more than 12 million children with special healthcare needs (CSHCNs) in the United States. CSHCNs are one of the fastest growing populations that use a significant proportion of healthcare resources within their communities. As medical technology and understanding of chronic conditions improve and surgical interventions such as repair of congenital heart defects, gastroschisis, omphalocele, and myelomeningocele continue to improve, these children are living longer and more fulfilling lives at home with their families. These children present daily challenges for their families, but they especially present a unique set of challenges for the prehospital provider. The prehospital provider is frequently unfamiliar with their medical issues and the medical technology that they need to sustain themselves at home.

CSHCNs are those who require additional long-term needs greater than 6 months that are more significant than the general population, and they are technology-dependent (i.e., ventilator dependent) or have significant behavioral or developmental disorders (i.e., autism). The need for emergency services in this population is not uncommon, and EMS prehospital providers are frequently responding to medical and traumatic emergencies involving children with severe cardiac, pulmonary, or neurologic conditions, or more advanced technologies such as mechanical ventilation, tracheostomies, gastrostomy or jejunostomy tubes, central venous lines, and ventriculoperitoneal CSF shunts.

In 1997, the EMS for Children program assembled a special task force designed to explore the growing emergency care needs of this population and to focus on ways to improve the quality of prehospital care delivered to children with complex medical health issues. The task force and local hospitals are working to help identify these patients in the community to help the prehospital provider be more prepared to care for the children in their area. Prehospital providers may require additional education to be able to provide the appropriate care and transport needs of these patients. The prehospital provider should remember to use the patient's family members or caregivers as a valuable resource of knowledge regarding the child's routine care because they manage most issues that occur with the child and have been trained in the maintenance and operation of the child's medical devices and technology. There is new information available with the addition of the emergency information form (EIF) to help provide additional information for the prehospital provider. Because of concerns that the family member may not be as knowledgeable regarding the child's care or a language barrier, both the American AAP and the ACEP recommend a copy of the EIF for the CSHCN be placed in the freezer of the child's home so that it can be located quickly and easily in the event of a medical emergency. The emergency transport of CSHCN for definitive medical care requires that the prehospital provider has adequate information in caring for the patient to be able to provide the highest level of care during transport. CSHCN children would be better cared for if the prehospital provider was able to transport them to a pediatric facility. Because this may not always be an option, once the child is stabilized, the interfacility transport of the child to a pediatric center may be done by a specialized pediatric transport team. Research has shown specialized pediatric transport teams improve overall care and outcomes in these children.[230,231]

Behavioral and Mental Health Issues

Prehospital EMS transports for nonemergent pediatric health issues are considerable and drastically rising. Transporting a pediatric psychiatric patient can be challenging; with a child acting out it is unclear if the child is reacting normally to stress in the environment, or if there is an imminent risk of harm to self or others, and parents may be anxious or apprehensive. It is estimated that one in five children aged 13–18, or over 21%, will experience a severe mental disorder at some point during their life, and for children aged 8–15 the estimate is 13%.[230–232]

The etiology of pediatric psychiatric diagnoses is extensive and influenced by a multitude of variables that may be internal or external to the patient. Many of these variables are not modifiable, such as genetic predisposition and personality, or a response to environmental factors, such as family dynamics. Factors that may affect a psychiatric illness in a child include intelligence, social abilities, and having some kind of talent, such as an athletic ability, which can minimize the negative effects of the illness. The patients who are substance abusers almost always seem to exacerbate the course of the psychiatric illness. A large number of pediatric psychiatric patients begin to show symptoms during early childhood and early recognition, intervention, and treatment may modify the effects or control the illness and hopefully prevent severe dysfunction as the child goes into young adulthood. See Table 18.21 for pediatric psychiatric disorders affecting children 5–12 years of age and see Table 18.22 for adolescent psychiatric disorders. The pediatric EMS prehospital provider will be transporting a great deal more of these children because of the significant rise in the number of pediatric and adolescent mental health psychiatric disorders and substance use being diagnosed. The prehospital EMS provider will be transporting either from an out-of-control behavioral outburst in the home or at school, a child who has inflicted injury to themselves such as cutting, or a teenager who has overdosed on medication or attempted to hang or shoot themselves in an attempt to commit suicide. The knowledge of these disorders may help the provider with a safe transport.[230–232]

TABLE 18.21 Pediatric Psychiatric Diagnoses With Age of Onset 5–12 Years

Intermittent Explosive Disorder (IED)	Reactive Attachment Disorder (RAD)	Pervasive Developmental Disorder (PDD)
Periods of aggression or violence followed by remorse, guilt, or anxiety	History of severe abuse, neglect, abandonment in infancy There is a persistent, prolonged disregard for the physical and emotional well-being of the child by caregivers	This disorder includes autism and Asperger's syndrome Symptoms may be noticed by parents in infancy but typically around 3 years, these children have impairments in social interaction and communication skills, many have difficulty with spoken language, and do not grasp social cues (i.e., humor, facial expressions or body language)
Precipitating event such as a restriction or limit set by others, but child reacts out of proportion to situation Unmanageable aggression or violence is reason for transport to emergency department	Child has difficulty with trust, empathy, establishing healthy relationships At younger ages exhibiting disturbing behaviors such as cruelty to animals and other children, lying, stealing, sexually acting out is common Impulsiveness, aggression, agitation, and unmanageable behaviors are reason they are transported	These children are hypersensitive to noise and lights, have ritualistic behaviors and a rigid adherence to routines These children have exaggerated emotional reactions Uncontrollable behavior is one of the reasons for transport or they truly have a medical illness
Key strategy for dealing with IED is to establish rapport with child to reduce anxiety and provide reassurance	Children with RAD develop other disorders during adolescence such as conduct disorder, oppositional defiance disorder, or borderline personality disorder	May need to ask parents for advice about the best methods to interact with the child

Data from Gilbert SB. Beyond acting out: managing pediatric psychiatric emergencies in the emergency department. *Adv Emerg Nurs J.* 2012;34(2):147–163.

TABLE 18.22 Adolescent Psychiatric Disorders With Age Onset of 13–17 Years

Major Depressive Disorder	Oppositional Defiant Disorder	Conduct Disorder	Borderline Personality Disorder
Adolescents are at high risk for depression and multiple stressors from home, school, and relationships They overwhelm the teenager's normal coping mechanisms	Disorder unique to children and adolescents characterized by behavioral problems at home and school Open defiance of rules, arguing with adults and peers, difficulty taking responsibility	Teenagers tend to have more severe behavioral problems than those with ODD Behaviors are more aggressive, threatening, and without concern for others	History of early childhood abuse, neglect, and abandonment, growing up without a sense of being protected or nurtured and developing poor coping skills

Continued

TABLE 18.22	Adolescent Psychiatric Disorders With Age Onset of 13–17 Years—cont'd			
Major Depressive Disorder	**Oppositional Defiant Disorder**	**Conduct Disorder**	**Borderline Personality Disorder**
Parental conflict, relationship breakups, and educational difficulties are the most common precipitating factors Others include being the victim of bullying, which increases depression and suicidal ideation Adolescents do not have perspective or understand the inevitable changes that occur over time, and many choose to end or attempt to end their lives Depression leads to a loss of rational, objective thinking Teenagers feel excessively guilty, isolated, and embarrassed They may be overly sensitive to criticism The parents of these children have no idea anything is wrong until the child attempts an overdose and requires emergent transport	In school, children with ODD have trouble making and keeping friends; they are difficult to redirect and need to be in control and have the last word whether it is with parents, peers, or other adults Etiology is unclear but has associations with history of neglect, family dysfunction, and abuse or chaotic home situation They present with anger and are resentful and uncooperative, which is the most common reason for transport They may easily be frustrated or irritated but typically they are not violent or aggressive unless provoked Teenagers with ODD are more likely to engage in risky behaviors, experiment with substances, and have minor legal issues	History of cruelty to animals or younger children, sexual deviancy with use of force, tendency to provoke physical fights Lack of respect for authority, complete disregard for rules Manipulative behaviors include lying and blaming others Truancy, running away, and substance abuse are common Ring leaders and encouraging others to break the rules or laws; lack of empathy, compassion, and concern for others, which allows them to engage in cruel acts without regret Treatment options are minimal but some behavioral modifications may result from early intensive interventions such as therapeutic residential treatment Long-term outcomes tend to be poor, and many of these adolescents develop antisocial and sociopathic personality disorders as adults	BPD traits emerge in adolescence and continue into adulthood These are characterized by dramatic attention-seeking behaviors, self-harming, suicidal gestures, anger, defensive, resistant to interventions from others, and blames parents rather than take responsibility for their behaviors Teens are often hypersensitive to criticism from adults, even under normal circumstances Quick to anger if directly confronted or challenged about their behaviors During transport they become more anxious and agitated if they sense disapproval Anxiety may be expressed as argumentativeness, resistance, or hostility Manipulative behaviors are a tactic to get their needs met or gain control of the situation

BPD, Borderline personality disorder; *ODD*, oppositional defiant disorder.
Data from Gilbert SB. Beyond acting out: managing pediatric psychiatric emergencies in the emergency department. *Adv Emerg Nurs J*, 2012;34(2):147–163.

References

1. PedsGuide. Version 1.32. Kansas City, MO. Children's Mercy Hospital; 2022.
2. Pediatric Emergency Guide. Version 3.1.1. Washington, DC: Protean, LLC; 2018.
3. Hobson MJ, Chima RS. Pediatric hypovolemic shock. *Open Pediatr Med J*. 2013;7(Suppl1:M3):10–15.
4. Leeper CM, McKenna C, Gaines BA. Too little too late: hypotension and blood transfusion in the trauma bay are independent predictors of death in injured children. *J Trauma Acute Care Surg*. 2018;85(4):674–678. doi: 10.1097/TA.0000000000001823
5. Valentine SL, et al. Consensus recommendations for RBC transfusion practice in critically ill children from the pediatric critical care transfusion and anemia expertise initiative. *Pediatr Crit Care Med*. 2018;19(9):884–898. doi: 10.1097/PCC.0000000000001613
6. Cornelius B, et al. Current practices in tranexamic acid administration for pediatric trauma patients in the United States. *J Trauma Nurs*. 2021;28(1):21–25. doi: 10.1097/JTN.0000000000000553
7. Patel MM, Hebbar KB, Dugan MC, Petrillo T. A survey assessing pediatric transport team composition and training. *Pediatr Emerg Care*. 2020;36(5):e263–e267. doi:10.1097/PEC.0000000000001655
8. ASTNA; Holleran RS, Wolfe AC, Frakes MA, eds. *Patient Transport*: Principles and Practice. 5th ed. St. Louis, MO: Mosby Elsevier; 2017.
9. Stroud MH, et al. Pediatric and neonatal interfacility transport: results from a national consensus conference. Pediatrics. 2013; 132(2):359–366.
10. Commission on Accreditation of Medical Transport Systems, ed. *Tenth Edition Accreditation Standards of The Commission on Accreditation of Medical Transport Systems*. 10th ed. Sandy Springs, SC: CAMTS; 2015.
11. Schmidt CD, et al. Pediatric transport-specific illness severity scores predict clinical deterioration of transported patients. *Pediatr Emerg Care*. 2022;38(8):e1449–e1453. doi: 10.1097/PEC.0000000000002789
12. Nagler J. Emergency airway management in children: unique pediatric considerations. UpToDate, June 2016. Available at: https://www.uptodate.com/contents/emergency-airway-management-in-children-unique-pediatric-considerations.
13. Mick NW. Airway management in patients with abnormal anatomy or challenging physiology. *Clin Pediatr Emerg Med*. 2015;16(3): 186–194.
14. Wing R, Armsby CC. Noninvasive ventilation in pediatric acute respiratory illness. *Clin Pediatr Emerg Med*. 2015;16(3):154–161.
15. de Caen AR, et al. Part 12: Pediatric advanced life support: 2015 American Heart Association guidelines update for cardiopulmonary resuscitation and emergency cardiovascular care. *Circulation*. 2015;132(18 Suppl 2):S526–S542.
16. Belanger J, Kossick M. Methods of identifying and managing the difficult airway in the pediatric population. *Am Assoc Nurse Anesth*. 2015;83(1):35–41.
17. Bailey P. Continuous oxygen delivery systems for infants, children, and adults. UpToDate, Aug 2016. Available at: http://www.uptodate.com/contents/continuous-oxygen-delivery-systems-for-infants-children-and-adults.
18. Milesi C, et al. High-flow nasal cannula: recommendations for daily practice in pediatrics. *Ann Intensive Care*. 2014;4:1–7.
19. Long E, Babl FE, Duke T. Is there a role for humidified heated high-flow nasal cannula therapy in paediatric emergency departments? *Emerg Med J*. 2016;33(6):386–389.
20. Fan G, Diao B, Zhang Y. Application of modified oropharyngeal airway in emergency care of patients with traumatic brain injury. *Int Med J*. 2014;21(2):163–165.

21. Emerson B, Shepherd M, Auerbach M. Technology-enhanced simulation training for pediatric intubation. *Clin Pediatr Emerg Med.* 2015;16(3):203–212.

22. Heyming T, et al. Accuracy of paramedic Broselow tape use in the prehospital setting. *Prehosp Emerg Care.* 2012;16(3):374–380.

23. McCans K, Varma S, Ramgopal S, Martin-Gill C, Owusu-Ansah S. Variation in prehospital protocols for pediatric respiratory distress management in the United States. *Pediatr Emerg Care.* 2022;38(7):e1355–e1361. doi: 10.1097/PEC.0000000000002620

24. Anders J, et al. Evidence and controversies in pediatric prehospital airway management. *Clin Pediatr Emerg Med.* 2014;15(1):28–37.

25. Hammer J. Acute respiratory failure in children. *Paediatr Respir Rev.* 2013;14(2):64–69.

26. Smith KA, et al. Risk factors for failed tracheal intubation in pediatric and neonatal critical care specialty transport. *Prehosp Emerg Care.* 2015;19(1):17–22.

27. Hansen M, et al. Out-of-hospital pediatric airway management in the United States. *Resuscitation.* 2015;90:104–110.

28. Piegeler T, et al. Advanced airway management in the anaesthesiologist-staffed helicopter emergency medical service (HEMS): a retrospective analysis of 1047 out-of-hospital intubations. *Resuscitation.* 2016;105:66–69.

29. Nadler I, et al. Time without ventilation during intubation in neonates as a patient-centered measure of performance. *Resuscitation.* 2016;105:41–44.

30. Eber E. Respiratory emergencies in children. *Paediatr Respir Rev.* 2013;14(2):62–63.

31. Pfleger A, Eber E. Management of acute severe upper airway obstruction in children. *Paediatr Respir Rev.* 2013;14(2):70–77.

32. Stansell C, Cherry B. A systematic approach to ventilator management for the pediatric patient during air medical transport. *Air Med J.* 2020;39(1):27-34. doi: 10.1016/j.amj.2019.09.011

33. Cheema B, Welzel T, Rossouw B. Noninvasive ventilation during pediatric and neonatal critical care transport: a systematic review. *Pediatr Crit Care Med.* 2019;20(1):9–18. doi: 10.1097/PCC.0000000000001781

34. American Academy of Pediatrics, et al. Equipment for ground ambulances. *Prehosp Emerg Care.* 2014;18(1):92–97.

35. Peters J, et al. Indications and results of emergency surgical airways performed by a physician-staffed helicopter emergency service. *Injury.* 2015;46(5):787–790.

36. Kline-Krammes S, Robinson S. Childhood asthma: a guide for pediatric emergency medicine providers. *Emerg Med Clin North Am.* 2013;31(3):705–732.

37. Ostermayer DC, Gausche-Hill M. Supraglottic airways: the history and current state of prehospital airway adjuncts. *Prehosp Emerg Care.* 2014;18(1):106–115.

38. Huang A, Jagannathan N. The role of supraglottic airways in pediatric emergency medicine. *Clin Pediatr Emerg Med.* 2015;16(3):162–171.

39. Mittiga MR, RInderknecht AS, Kerrey BT. A modern and practical review of rapid-sequence intubation in pediatric emergencies. *Clin Pediatr Emerg Med.* 2015; 16(3):172–185.

40. Kovacich NJ, et al. Incidence of bradycardia and the use of atropine in pediatric rapid sequence intubation in the emergency department. *Pediatr Emerg Care.* 2022;38(2):e540–e543.

41. Walls R, Murphy M, eds. *Manual of Emergency Airway Management.* 4th ed. Philadelphia, PA: Lippincott Williams & Wilkins; 2012.

42. McCormick T, et al. Atropine pretreatment and adverse events in emergency pediatric intubation. *Ann Emerg Med.* 2021;78(4):S157.

43. Sankaran D, et al. Non-invasive carbon dioxide monitoring in neonates: methods, benefits, and pitfalls. *J Perinatol.* 41(12):2698–2699. doi: 10.1038/s41372-021-01174-8

44. Jagannathan N, et al. An update on newer pediatric supraglottic airways with recommendations for clinical use. *Pediatr Anesth.* 2015; 25(4):334–345.

45. Freeman JF, et al. Use of capnographs to assess quality of pediatric ventilation with 3 different airway modalities. *Am J Emerg Med.* 2016;34(1):69–74.

46. World Allergy Organization. Treatment of asthma in children 5 years and under, based on different global guidelines. Available at: http://www.worldallergy.org/professional/allergic_diseases_center/ treatment_of_asthma_in_children/; 2015.

47. Bush A, Fleming L. Diagnosis and management of asthma in children. *Br Med J.* 2015;350:h996.

48. Navanadan N, et al. Defining treatment response for clinical trials of pediatric acute asthma. *J Allergy Clin Immunol Pract.* 2023;1:1–9. doi: 10.1016/j.jaip.2022.12.033

49. Chen L, Collado K, Rastagi D. Contribution of systemic and airway immune responses to pediatric obesity-related asthma. *Paediatr Respir Rev.* 2021;37:3–9. doi: 10.1016/j.prrv.2020.02.005

50. Koninckx M, Buysse C, de Hoog M. Management of status asthmaticus in children. *Paediatr Respir Rev.* 2013;14(2):78–85.

51. Sordillo JE, et al. Prenatal and infant exposure to acetaminophen and ibuprofen and the risk for wheeze and asthma in children. *J Allergy Clin Immunol.* 2015;135(2):441–448.

52. Hollenbach JP, Cloutier MM. Childhood asthma management and environmental triggers. *Pediatr Clin North Am.* 2015;62(5):1199-1214.

53. Akturk H, et al. Impact of respiratory viruses on pediatric asthma exacerbations. *J Pediatr Infect.* 2016;10(1):14-21.

54. Aniapravan R, et al. Question 5: Magnesium sulphate for acute asthma in children. *Pediatr Respir Rev.* 2020;36:112-117. doi: 10.1016/j.prrv.2020.05.005

55. Misra SM. The current evidence of integrative approaches to pediatric asthma. *Curr Probl Pediatr Adolesc Health Care.* 2016;46(6):190–194.

56. Long B, Rezaie SR. Evaluation and management of asthma and chronic obstructive pulmonary disease exacerbation in the emergency department. *Emerg Med Clin North Am.* 2022;40(3):539–563. doi: 10.1016/j.emc.2022.05.007

57. Doymaz S, Schneider J, Sagy M. Early administration of terbutaline in severe pediatric asthma may reduce incidence of acute respiratory failure. *Ann Allergy Asthma Immunol.* 2014;112(3):207–210.

58. Schwarz ES, Cohn BG. Is dexamethasone as effective as prednisone or prednisolone in the management of pediatric asthma exacerbations? *Ann Emerg Med.* 2015;65(1):81–82.

59. Ohn M, Jacobe S. Magnesium should be given to all children presenting to hospital with acute severe asthma. *Paediatr Respir Rev.* 2014;16(4):319–321.

60. Dionne A, Son MBF, Randolph AG. An update on multisystem inflammatory syndrome in children related to SARS-CoV-2. *Pediatr Infect Dis J.* 2022;41(1):e6–e9. doi: 10.1097/INF.0000000000003393

61. Kalyanaraman M, Anderson MR. COVID-19 in children. *Pediatr Clin North Am.* 2022;69(3):547–571. doi: 10.1016/j.pcl.2022.01.013

62. Blumenthal JA, Duvali MG. Invasive and noninvasive ventilation strategies for acute respiratory failure in children with coronavirus disease 2019. *Curr Opin Pediatr.* 2021;33:311–318. doi: 10.1097/ MOP.0000000000001021

63. Rimesnberger PC, et al. Caring for critically ill children with suspected or proven coronavirus disease 2019 infection: recommendations by the Scientific Sections' Collaborative of the European Society of Pediatric and Neonatal Intensive Care. *Pediatr Crit Care Med.* 2021;22(1):56-67. doi: 10.1097/pcc.0000000000002599

64. Gottlieb M, et al. Multisystem inflammatory syndrome in children with COVID-19. *Am J Emerg Med.* 2021;49:148–152. doi: 10.1016/ j.ajem.2021.05.076

65. Nierengarten MB. Diagnosis and management of croup in children. *Contemp Pediatr.* 2015;32(3):31–33.

66. Bagwell T, et al. Management of croup in the emergency department. *Pediatr Emerg Care.* 2020; 36(7):e387–e392. doi: 10.1097/ PEC.0000000000001276

67. Quraishi H, Lee DJ. Recurrent croup. *Pediatr Clin North Am.* 2022;69:319–328. doi: 10.1016/j.pcl.2021.12.004

68. Kathuria H. E-cigarette or vaping product use-associated lung injury (EVALI). UpToDate, Jan 2023. Available at: https://www.uptodate.com/ contents/e-cigarette-or-vaping-product-use-associated-lung-injury-evali.

69. Hamberger ES, Halpern-Felsher B. Vaping in adolescents: epidemiology and respiratory harm. *Curr Opin Pediatr.* 2020;32:378–383. doi: 10.1097/MOP.0000000000000896

70. Kaslow JA, Rosas-Salazar C, Moore PE. E-cigarette and vaping produce use-associated lung injury in the pediatric population: a critical review of the current literature. *Pediatr Pulmonol.* 2020;56:1857–1867. doi: 10.1002/ppul.25384

71. Centers for Disease Control and Prevention. Outbreak of lung injury associated with the use of e-cigarette, or vaping, products. CDC; February 25, 2020. Available at: https://cdc.gov/tobacco/basic_information/e-cigarettes/severe-lung-disease.html.

72. Thakrar PD, et al. E-cigarette, or vaping, product use-associated lung injury in adolescents: a review of imaging features. Pediatr Radiol. 2020;50:338–344. doi: 10.1007/s00247-019-04572-5

73. Helfgott D, et al. E-cigarette or vaping product use associated lung injury (EVALI) in the time of COVID-19: a clinical dilemma. *Pediatr Pulmonol.* 2022;57:623–630. doi: 10.1002/ppul.25804

74. Lowe DA, Vasquez R, Maniaci V. Foreign body aspiration in children. *Clin Pediatr Emerg Med.* 2015;16(3):140–148.

75. Cevik M, et al. The characteristics and outcomes of foreign body ingestion and aspiration in children due to lodged foreign body in the aerodigestive tract. *Pediatr Emerg Care.* 2013;29(1):53–57.

76. Chapman T, Sandstrom CK, Parnell SE. Pediatric emergencies of the upper and lower airway. *Appl Radiol.* 2012;41(4):10–17.

77. Adramerina A, et al. How parents' lack of awareness could be associated with foreign body aspiration in children. *Pediatr Emerg Care.* 2016;32(2):98–100.

78. Hegde SV, Hui PKT, Lee EY. Tracheobronchial foreign bodies in children: imaging assessment. *Semin Ultrasound CT MRI.* 2015;36(1):8–20.

79. Singh H, Parakh A. Tracheobronchial foreign body aspiration in children. *Clin Pediatr.* 2014;53(5):415–419.

80. Ettyreddy AR, et al. Button battery injuries in the pediatric aerodigestive tract. *Ear Nose Throat J.* 2015;94(12):486–493.

81. Gurevich Y, Sahn B, Weinstein T. Foreign body ingestion in pediatric patients. *Curr Opin Pediatr.* 2018;30:677–682. doi: 10.1097/MOP.0000000000000670

82. Liao W, Wen G, Zhang X. Button battery intake as foreign body in Chinese children. *Pediatr Emerg Care.* 2015;31(6):412–415.

83. Strickland M, Rosenfield D, Fecteau A. Magnetic foreign body injuries: a large pediatric hospital experience. *J Pediatr.* 2014;165(2):332–335.

84. Casey G. Bronchiolitis: a virus of infancy. *Nurs N Z.* 2015;21(7):20–24.

85. Gill PJ, Chanchlani N, Mahant S. Bronchiolitis. *CMAJ.* 2022;194:E216. doi: 10.1503/cmaj.211810

86. Kirolos A, et al. A systematic review of clinical practice guidelines for the diagnosis and management of bronchiolitis. *J Infect Dis.* 2019;222:S672-S679. doi: 10.1093/infdis/jiz240

87. Aziz N, Yousuf R, Gattoo I, Latief M. Clinical predictors of hospital admission in children aged 0–24 months with acute bronchiolitis. *Int J Pediatr.* 2015;3(2.1):75–79.

88. Teshome G, Gattu R, Brown R. Acute bronchiolitis. *Pediatr Clin North Am.* 2013;60(5):1019–1034.

89. Jain S, et al. Community-acquired pneumonia requiring hospitalization among U.S. children. *N Engl J Med.* 2015;372(22):2166–2168.

90. Elemraid MA, et al. Changing clinical practice: management of paediatric community-acquired pneumonia. *J Eval Clin Pract.* 2014;20(1):94–99.

91. Esposito S, Principi N. Unsolved problems in the approach to pediatric community-acquired pneumonia. *Curr Opin.* 2012;25(3):286–290.

92. Koppolu R, Simone S. Medical and surgical management of pediatric pneumonia. National Association of Pediatric Nurse Practitioners. Available at: https://www.napnap.org/sites/default/files/userfiles/education/2015SpeakerHO/213-%20Koppolu%20%26%20Simone.pdf.

93. Tam PI, Hanisch BR, O'Connell M. The impact of adherence to pediatric community-acquired pneumonia guidelines on clinical outcomes. *Clin Pediatr.* 2015;54(10):1006–1008.

94. Hoshina T, et al. The utility of biomarkers in differentiating bacterial from non-bacterial lower respiratory tract infection in hospitalized children: difference of the diagnostic performance between acute pneumonia and bronchitis. *J Infect Chemother.* 2014;20(10):616–620.

95. Esposito S, et al. Measurement of lipocalin-2 and syndecan-4 levels to differentiate bacterial from viral infection in children with community-acquired pneumonia. *BMC Pulmon Med.* 2016;16(1):1–8.

96. Neuman MI, et al. Emergency department management of childhood pneumonia in the United States prior to publication of national guidelines. *Acad Emerg Med.* 2013;20(3):240–246.

97. Chee E, et al. Systematic review of clinical practice guidelines on the management of community acquired pneumonia in children. *Paediatr Respir Rev.* 2022;42: 59–68. doi: 10.1016/j.prrv.2022.01.006

98. Wiser RK, et al. A pediatric high-flow nasal cannula protocol standardizes initial flow and expedites weaning. *Pediatr Pulmonol.* 2021;56:1189–1197. doi: 10.1002/ppul.25214

99. Centers for Disease Control and Prevention. Vaccines and preventable diseases: Pertussis: summary of vaccine recommendations. CDC; 2020. Available at: cdc.gov/vaccines/vpd/pertussis/recs-summary.html.

100. Staudt A, Mangla AT, Alamgir, H. Investigation of pertussis cases in a Texas county, 2008–2012. *South Med J.* 2015;108(7):452–457.

101. Pavic-Espinoza I, et al. High prevalence of *Bordetella pertussis* in children under 5 years old hospitalized with acute respiratory infections in Lima, Peru. *BMC Infect Dis.* 2015;15(1):1–7.

102. Cornia P, Lipsky BA. Pertussis infection: epidemiology, microbiology, and pathogenesis. UpToDate, Oct 2015. Available at: https://www.uptodate.com/contents/pertussis-infection-epidemiology-microbiology-and-pathogenesis.

103. Yeh S, Mink CM. Pertussis infection in infants and children: clinical features and diagnosis. UpToDate, Jan 2017. Available at: https://www.uptodate.com/contents/pertussis-infection-in-infants-and-children-clinical-features-and-diagnosis.

104. Cornia P, Lipsky BA. Pertussis infection in adolescents and adults: treatment and prevention. UpToDate, April 2017. Available at: https://www.uptodate.com/contents/pertussis-infection-in-adolescents-and-adults-treatment-and-prevention.

105. Sidhu N, et al. Evaluation of anaphylaxis management in a pediatric emergency department. *Pediatr Emerg Care.* 2016;32(8):508–512.

106. Tiyyagura GK, Arnold L, Cone DC, Langhan M. Pediatric anaphylaxis management in the prehospital setting. *Prehosp Emerg Care.* 2014;18(1):46–51.

107. Zilberstein J, McCurdy MT, Winters ME. Anaphylaxis. *J Emerg Med.* 2014;47(2):182–187.

108. Trainor JL, Pittsenbarger ZE, Joshi D, et al. Outcomes and factors associated with prehospital treatment of pediatric anaphylaxis. *Pediatr Emerg Care.* 2022;38(1):e69–e74.

109. Carrillo E, Hern HG, Barger J. Prehospital administration of epinephrine in pediatric anaphylaxis. *Prehosp Emerg Care.* 2016;20(2):239–244.

110. Kim SL, et al. Increase in epinephrine administration for food-induced anaphylaxis in pediatric emergency departments from 2007 to 2015. *J Allergy Clin Immunol Pract.* 2022;10(1):200–205.e1.

111. Kher K, Sharron M. Approach to the child with metabolic acidosis. UpToDate, July 2016 [updated Sep 2023]. Available at: https://www.uptodate.com/contents/approach-to-the-child-with-metabolic-acidosis.

112. Park E, Pearson NM, Pillow MT, Toledo A. Neonatal endocrine emergencies. *Emerg Med Clin North Am.* 2014;32(2):421–435.

113. Barker JM, Bajaj L. Hypo and hyper: common pediatric endocrine and metabolic emergencies. *Adv Pediatr.* 2015;62(1):257–282.

114. Hsia DS, Alimi A, Coss-Bu JA. Fluid management in pediatric patients with DKA and rates of suspected clinical cerebral edema. *Pediatr Diabetes.* 2015;16(5):338–344.

115. Bakes K, et al. Effect of volume of fluid resuscitation on metabolic normalization in children presenting in diabetic ketoacidosis: a randomized controlled trial. *J Emerg Med.* 2016;50(4):551–559.

116. Brink SJ. Paediatric and adolescent diabetic ketoacidosis. *Pract Diabetes*. 2014;31(8):342–347.

117. Olivieri L, Chasm R. Diabetic ketoacidosis in the pediatric emergency department. *Emerg Med Clin North Am*. 2013;31(3):755–773.

118. Glaser N. Diabetic ketoacidosis in children: treatment and complications. UpToDate. Available at: https://www.uptodate.com/contents/diabetic-ketoacidosis-in-children-treatment-and-complications.

119. Barata IA. Cardiac emergencies. *Emerg Med Clin North Am*. 2013;31(3):677–704.

120. Yates MC, Rao PS. Pediatric cardiac emergencies. *Emerg Med Open Access*. 2013;3(6):1–7.

121. Altman CA. Identifying newborns with critical congenital heart disease. UpToDate, June 2016. Available at: https://www.uptodate.com/contents/identifying-newborns-with-critical-congenital-heart-disease.

122. Oster M. Newborn screening for critical congenital heart disease using pulse oximetry. UpToDate, Mar 2017. Available at: https://www.uptodate.com/contents/newborn-screening-for-critical-congenital-heart-disease-using-pulse-oximetry.

123. American College of Surgeons. *Advanced Trauma Life Support for Doctors*: ATLS Student Course Manual. 9th ed. Chicago, IL: American College of Surgeons; 2013.

124. Stewart TC, et al. A comparison of injuries, crashes, and outcomes for pediatric rear occupants in traffic motor vehicle collisions. *J Trauma Acute Care Surg*. 2013;74(2):628–633.

125. Centers for Disease Control and Prevention. Childhood Injury Report. CDC; 2015. Available at: http://www.cdc.gov/safechild/child_injury_data.html.

126. McFadyen JG, Ramaiah R, Bhananker SM. Initial assessment and management of pediatric trauma patients. *Int J Crit Illn Inj Sci*. 2012;2(3):121–127.

127. Kelleher DC, et al. Factors associated with patient exposure and environmental control during pediatric trauma resuscitation. *J Trauma Acute Care Surg*. 2013;74(2):622–626.

128. Bullock JA, Haddow GD, Coppola DP. *Managing Children in Disasters: Planning for their Unique Needs*. Boca Raton, FL: Taylor and Francis Group; 2010.

129. Guzzetta C. Family presence during resuscitation and invasive procedures. *Crit Care Nurse*. 2016;36(1):e11–e14.

130. Joyce CN, Libertin R, Bigham MT. Family-centered care in pediatric critical care transport. *Air Med J*. 2015;34(1):32–36.

131. Forgey M, Bursch B. Assessment and management of pediatric iatrogenic medical trauma. *Curr Psychiatry Rep*. 2013;15(2):340.

132. Seid T, Ramaiah R, Grabinsky A. Pre-hospital care of pediatric patients with trauma. *Int J Crit Illn Inj Sci*. 2012;2(3):114–120.

133. Ballow SL, Kaups KL, Anderson S, Chang M. A standardized rapid sequence intubation protocol facilitates airway management in critically injured patients. *J Trauma Acute Care Surg*. 2012;73(6):1401–1405.

134. Tovar JA, Vasquez JJ. Management of chest trauma in children. *Paediatr Respir Rev*. 2013;14(2):86–91.

135. Air & Surface Transport Nurses Association. *Transport Professional Advanced Trauma Course*. 6th ed. Aurora, CO: Air & Surface Transport Nurses Association; 2015.

136. Snyder SR, Kivlehan SM, Collopy KT. Thoracic trauma: What you need to know. *EMS World*. 2012;41(7):60–66.

137. Lima M, ed. *Pediatric Thoracic Surgery*. Milan, Italy: Springer-Verlag Italia; 2013.

138. Ballouhey Q, Fesseau R, Benouaich V, Leobon B. Benefits of extracorporeal membrane oxygenation for the major blunt tracheobronchial trauma in the paediatric age group. *Eur J Cardio-Thoracic Surg*. 2013;43(4):864–865.

139. Okur MH, et al. Traumatic diaphragmatic rupture in children. *J Pediatr Surg*. 2014;49(3):420–423.

140. Ballouhey Q, et al. Management of blunt tracheobronchial trauma in the pediatric age group. *Eur J Trauma Emerg Surg*. 2013;39(2):167–171.

141. Kadish H. Chest wall injuries in children. UpToDate, March 2016. Available at: https://www.uptodate.com/contents/chest-wall-injuries-in-children.

142. Flaherty EG, Perez-Rossello J, Levine MA, Hennrikus WL. Evaluating children with fractures for child physical abuse. *Pediatrics*. 2014;133(2):e477–e489.

143. Hernandez DJ, Jatana KR, Hoff SR, Rastatter JC. Emergency airway management for pediatric blunt neck trauma. *Clin Pediatr Emerg Med*. 2014;15(3):261–268.

144. Chatterjee D, et al. Airway management in laryngotracheal injuries from blunt neck trauma in children. *Pediatr Anesth*. 2016;26(2):132–138.

145. Golden J, et al. Limiting chest computed tomography in the evaluation of pediatric thoracic trauma. *J Trauma Acute Care Surg*. 2016;81(2):271–277.

146. Puckett Y, et al. Imaging before transfer to designated pediatric trauma centers exposes children to excess radiation. *J Trauma Acute Care Surg*. 2016;81(2):229–235.

147. Swanson EW, et al. Application of the mandible injury severity score to pediatric mandibular fractures. *J Oral Maxillofac Surg*. 2015;73(7):1341–1349.

148. Al Shetawi AH, et al. Pediatric maxillofacial trauma: a review of 156 patients. *J Oral Maxillofac Surg*. 2016;74(7):1420.e1–1420.e4.

149. Flint PW, et al. *Cummings Otolaryngology-Head and Neck Surgery*. 6th ed. Philadelphia, PA: Elsevier Saunders; 2015.

150. Mendez DR. Overview of intrathoracic injuries in children. UpToDate, Feb 2016. Available at: http://www.uptodate.com.libproxy.usouthal.edu/contents/overview-of-intrathoracic-injuries-in-children.

151. Legome E, Kadish H. Cardiac injury from blunt trauma. UpToDate, Jan 2016. https://www.uptodate.com/contents/cardiac-injury-from-blunt-trauma. Accessed September 16, 2023.

152. Mendez DR. Initial evaluation and stabilization of children with thoracic trauma. UpToDate, May 2017. Available at: https://www.uptodate.com/contents/initial-evaluation-and-stabilization-of-children-with-thoracic-trauma.

153. Kamdar G, Santucci K, Emerson BL. Management of pediatric cardiac trauma in the ED. *Clin Pediatr Emerg Med*. 2011;12(4):323–332.

154. Maeda K, Ono S, Baba, K, Kawahara I. Management of blunt pancreatic trauma in children. *Pediatr Surg Int*. 2013;29(10):1019–1022.

155. Mendez DR. Overview of blunt abdominal trauma in children. UpToDate, April 2017. Available at: http://www.uptodate.com.libproxy.usouthal.edu/contents/overview-of-blunt-abdominal-trauma-in-children.

156. Holmes JF, et al. Identifying children at very low risk of clinically important blunt abdominal injuries. *Ann Emerg Med*. 2013;62(2):107–116.

157. Guyther JE. Advances in pediatric abdominal trauma: what's new in assessment and management. *Trauma Rep*. 2016;17(5):1–15.

158. Wesson DE. Liver, spleen, and pancreas injury in children with blunt abdominal trauma. UpToDate, Oct 2016. Available at: http://www.uptodate.com.libproxy.usouthal.edu/contents/liver-spleen-and-pancreas-injury-in-children-with-blunt-abdominal-trauma.

159. Tran S, Kabre R. Selective nonoperative management of pediatric penetrating abdominal trauma. *Pediatr Emerg Med*. 2014;15(3):219–222.

160. Paris C, Brindamour M, Ouimet A, St-Vil D. Predictive indicators for bowel injury in pediatric patients who present with a positive seat belt sign after motor vehicle collision. *J Pediatr Surg*. 2010;45(5):921–924.

161. Biswas S, Adileh M, Almogy G, Bala M. Abdominal injury patterns in patients with seatbelt signs requiring laparotomy. *J Emerg Trauma Shock*. 2014;7(4):295–300.

162. Borgialli DA, et al. Association between the seat belt sign and intra-abdominal injuries in children with blunt torso trauma in motor vehicle collisions. *Acad Emerg Med*. 2014;21(11):1240–1248.

163. Sheybani EF, et al. Pediatric nonaccidental abdominal trauma: what the radiologist should know. *Radiographs*. 2014;34(1):139–153.

164. Guzzo H, Middlesworth W. Hollow viscus blunt abdominal trauma in children. In: UpToDate, Oct 2016. Available at: http://www.uptodate.com.libproxy.usouthal.edu/contents/hollow-viscus-blunt-abdominal-trauma-in-children.

165. Dangle PP, et al. Evolving mechanisms of injury and management of pediatric blunt renal trauma – 20 years of experience. *Urology*. 2016;90:159–163.

166. Lee JN, et al. Predictive factors for conservative treatment failure in grade IV pediatric blunt renal failure. *J Pediatr Urol*. 2016;12(2):93.e1–e7.

167. Fiechtl J. Pelvic trauma: initial evaluation and management. UpToDate, Jan 2017. Available at: http://www.uptodate.com/contents/pelvic-trauma-initial-evaluation-and-management.

168. Delaney KM, et al. Risk factors associated with bladder and urethral injuries in female children with pelvic fractures: an analysis of the National Trauma Data Bank. *J Trauma Acute Care Surg*. 2016;80(2):472–476.

169. Shaath MK, et al. Associated injuries in skeletally immature children with pelvic fractures. *J Emerg Med*. 2016;51(3):246–251.

170. Ortega HW, et al. Patterns of injury and management of children with pelvic fractures at a non-trauma center. *J Emerg Med*. 2014;47(2):140–146.

171. Stone KP, White K. Femoral shaft fractures in children. UpToDate, March 2017. Available at: http://www.uptodate.com/contents/femoral-shaft-fractures-in-children.

172. Kliegman RM, Stanton B, St Geme J, et al., eds. *Nelson Textbooks of Pediatrics*. 19th ed. Philadelphia, PA: Elsevier Saunders; 2011.

173. Rowland SP, et al. Venous injuries in pediatric trauma: systematic review of injuries and management. *J Trauma Acute Care Surg*. 2014;77(2):356–363.

174. Wahlgren CM, Kragsterman B. Management and outcome of pediatric vascular injuries. *J Trauma Acute Care Surg*. 2015;79(4):563–567.

175. Hoffmann F, et al. Comparison of the AVPU scale and the pediatric GCS in prehospital setting. *Prehosp Emerg Care*. 2016;20(4):493–498.

176. Lumba-Brown A, Pineda J. Evidence-based assessment of severe pediatric traumatic brain injury and emergent neurocritical care. *Semin Pediatr Neurol*. 2014;21(4):275–283.

177. Youngblut JM, Caicedo C, Brooten D. Preschool children with head injury: comparing injury severity measures and clinical care. *Pediatr Nurs*. 2013;39(6):290–298.

178. Fuhrman BP, Zimmerman J, eds. *Pediatric Critical Care*. 4th ed. Philadelphia, PA: Elsevier Health Sciences; 2011.

179. GCS. The Glasgow Structured Approach to Assessment of the Glasgow Coma Scale. n.d. Available at: http://www.glasgowcomascale.org/.

180. Ducharme-Crevier L, Wainwright M. Acute management of children with traumatic brain injury. *Clin Pediatr Emerg Med*. 2015;16(1):48–54.

181. Burns ECM, et al. Scalp hematoma characteristics associated with intracranial injury in pediatric head injury. *Acad Emerg Med*. 2016;23(5):576–582.

182. Medscape. Classification and complications of traumatic brain injury. Available at: http://emedicine.medscape.com/article/326643-overview#a1.

183. Schutzman S. Minor head trauma in infants and children: evaluation. UpToDate, April 2017. Available at: http://www.uptodate.com/contents/minor-head-trauma-in-infants-and-children-evaluation.

184. Pitfield AF, Carroll AB, Kissoon N. Emergency management of increased intracranial pressure. *Pediatr Emerg Care*. 2012;28(2):200–204.

185. Agrawal D. Rapid sequence intubation (RSI) in children. UpToDate, May 2017. Available at: http://www.uptodate.com/contents/rapid-sequence-intubation-rsi-in-children.

186. Hansen G, Vallance JK. Ventilation monitoring for severe pediatric TBI during interfacility transport. *Int J Emerg Med*. 2015;8:41.

187. Allen BB, et al. Age-specific cerebral perfusion pressure thresholds and survival in children and adolescents with severe traumatic brain injury. *Pediatr Crit Care Med*. 2014;15(1):62–70.

188. Mangat HS, et al. Hypertonic saline reduces cumulative and daily intracranial pressure burdens after severe traumatic brain injury. *J Neurosurg*. 2015;122(1):202–210.

189. Taha AA, Westlake C, Badr L, Mathur M. Mannitol versus 3% NaCl for management of severe pediatric traumatic brain injury. *J Nurse Pract*. 2015;11(5):505–510.

190. Leonard JR, et al. Cervical spine injury patterns in children. *Pediatrics*. 2014;133(5):e1179–e1188.

191. Huisman TAGM, et al. Pediatric spinal trauma. *J Neuroimaging*. 2015;25(3):337–353.

192. Sun R, et al. A pediatric cervical spine clearance protocol to reduce radiation exposure in children. *J Surg Res*. 2013;183(1):341–346.

193. Mahajan P, et al. Spinal cord injury without radiologic abnormality in children imaged with magnetic resonance imaging. *J Trauma Acute Care Surg*. 2013;75(5):843–847.

194. Rosati SF, et al. Implementation of pediatric cervical spine clearance guidelines at a combined trauma center: twelve-month impact. *J Trauma Acute Care Surg*. 2015;78(6):1117–1121.

195. Tat ST, Mejia MJ, Freishtat RJ. Imaging, clearance, and controversies in pediatric cervical spine trauma. *Pediatr Emerg Care*. 2014;30(12):911–918.

196. McMahon PM, et al. Protocol to clear cervical spine injuries in pediatric trauma patients. *Radiol Manage*. 2015;37(5):42–48.

197. Leonard JC, et al. Factors associated with cervical spine injury in children after blunt trauma. *Ann Emerg Med*. 2011;58(2):145–155.

198. Leonard JC, Mao J, Jaffe DM. Potential adverse effects of spinal immobilization in children. *Prehosp Emerg Care*. 2012;16(4):513–518.

199. Clemency BM, et al. Patients immobilized with a long spine board rarely have unstable thoracolumbar injuries. *Prehosp Emerg Care*. 2016;20(2):266–272.

200. Collopy KT, Kivlehan SM, Snyder SR. Pediatric spinal cord injuries. *EMSWorld*; 2012. Available at: http://www.emsworld.com/article/10736962/pediatric-spinal-cord-injuries.

201. Kim EG, et al. Variability of prehospital spinal immobilization in children at risk for cervical spine injury. *Pediatr Emerg Care*. 2013;29(4):413–418.

202. White IV CC, Domeier RM, Millin MG. EMS spinal precautions and the use of the long backboard – resource document to the position statement of the National Association of EMS Physicians and the American College of Surgeons committee on trauma. *Prehosp Emerg Care*. 2014;18(2):306–314.

203. Corneli HM. Hypothermia in children: clinical manifestations and diagnosis. UpToDate, Aug 2016. Available at: https://www.uptodate.com/contents/hypothermia-in-children-clinical-manifestations-and-diagnosis.

204. Corneli JM. Hypothermia in children: management. UpToDate, Dec 2016. Available at: https://www.uptodate.com/contents/hypothermia-in-children-management.

205. Ishimine P. Heat stroke in children. UpToDate, Oct 2016. Available at: https://www.uptodate.com/contents/heat-stroke-in-children.

206. Semple-Hess J, Campwala R. Pediatric submersion injuries: emergency care and resuscitation. 2014. Available at: http://cdn7.slremeducation.org/wp-content/uploads/2015/02/Peds0614-Submersion-Injuries.pdf.

207. Paul AR, Adamo MA. Non-accidental trauma in pediatric patients: a review of epidemiology, pathophysiology, diagnosis and treatment. *Transl Pediatr*. 2014;3(3):195–207.

208. Bechtel K, Bennett BL. Evaluation of sexual abuse in children and adolescents. UpToDate, March 2017. Available at: https://www.uptodate.com/contents/evaluation-of-sexual-abuse-in-children-and-adolescents.

209. Friedman ML, Bone MF. Management of pediatric septic shock in the emergency department. *Clin Pediatr Emerg Med*. 2014;15(2):131–139.

210. Waltzman ML. Pediatric shock. *J Emerg Nurs*. 2015;41(2):113–118.

211. Waltzman M. Initial evaluation of shock in children. UpToDate, Feb 2017. Available at: https://www.uptodate.com/contents/initial-evaluation-of-shock-in-children.

212. Waltzman M. Initial management of shock in children. UpToDate, Aug 2016. Available at: https://www.uptodate.com/contents/initial-management-of-shock-in-children.

213. Waltzman M. Physiology and classification of shock in children. UpToDate, Feb 2017. Available at: https://www.uptodate.com/contents/initial-evaluation-of-shock-in-children.

214. Thompson GC, Macias CG. Recognition and management of sepsis in children: practice patterns in the emergency department. *J Emerg Med*. 2015;49(4):391–395.

215. Kim YA, Ha EJ, Jhang WK, Park SJ. Early blood lactate area as prognostic marker. *Intensive Care Med*. 2013;39(10):1818–1823.

216. Weiss SL, Pomerantz WJ. Septic shock: rapid recognition and initial resuscitation in children. UpToDate, May 2017. Available at: https://www.uptodate.com/contents/septic-shock-rapid-recognition-and-initial-resuscitation-in-children.

217. Marjanovic V, Budic I. Fluid resuscitation and massive transfusion protocol in pediatric trauma. *Acta Fac Med Naiss*. 2016;33(2):91–99.

218. Hughes NT, Burd RS, Teach ST. Damage control resuscitation: permissive hypotension and massive transfusion protocols. *Pediatr Emerg Care*. 2014;30(9):651–656.

219. American Heart Association. Highlights of the 2015 American Heart Association: Guidelines Update for CPR and ECC. AHA; 2015. Available at: https://www.uchealth.org/wp-content/uploads/2016/10/PROF-TC-2015-AHA-Guidelines-Highlights.pdf.

220. Carey JM, Shah MI. Pediatric prehospital seizure management. *Clin Pediatr Emerg Med*. 2014;15(1):59–66.

221. Fernandez IS, et al. Time from convulsive status epilepticus onset to anticonvulsant administration in children. *Neurology*. 2015;84(23):2304–2311.

222. Barzegar M, Mahdavi M, Behbehani AG, Tabrizi A. Refractory convulsive status epilepticus in children: etiology, associated risk factors and outcome. *Iran J Child Neurol*. 2015;9(4):24–31.

223. Browne GJ, Dimou S. Concussive head injury in children and adolescents. *Aust Fam Physician*. 2016;45(7):470–476.

224. Semple BD, et al. Repetitive concussions in adolescent athletes–translating clinical and experimental research into perspectives on rehabilitation strategies. *Front Neurol*. 2015;6:1–16.

225. Ellis R, Ellis C. Dog and cat bites. *Am Fam Physician*. 2014; 90(4):239–243.

226. O'Brien DC, et al. Dog bites of the head and neck: an evaluation of a common pediatric trauma and associated treatment. *Am J Otolaryngol*. 2015;36(1):32–38.

227. Garvey EM, Twitchell DK, Ragar R, Egan JC, Jamshidi R. Morbidity of pediatric dog bites: a case series at a level one pediatric trauma center. *J Pediatr Surg*. 2015;50(2):343–346.

228. Rutkowska A, Skotnicka-Klonowicz G. Prehospital pain management in children with traumatic injuries. *Pediatr Emerg Care*. 2015;31(5):317–320.

229. Browne LR, et al. Prehospital opioid administration in the emergency care of injured children. *Prehosp Emerg Care*. 2016;20(1): 59–65.

230. Gilbert SB. Beyond acting out: managing pediatric psychiatric emergencies in the emergency department. *Adv Emerg Nurs J*. 2012;34(2):147–163.

231. Knowlton AR, et al. Pediatric use of emergency medical services: the role of chronic illnesses and behavioral health problems. *Prehosp Emerg Care*. 2015;20(3):362–368.

232. National Alliance on Mental Illness. Mental Health by the Numbers. Available at: http://www.nami.org/Learn-More/Mental-Health-By-the-Numbers.

19

Care and Transport of the Geriatric Patient

P.S. MARTIN, KYLE HURST, EMILY A. OLLMANN, MICHAEL SHUKIS, FRANCESCA BARUFFI, JAMES SCHEIDLER, SANDRA NIXON, SAHIL DAYAL, JANNA BAKER-ROGERS, AND ALLISON TADROS

COMPETENCIES

1. Describe the norms for pathophysiology and vital signs for the geriatric populations.
2. State the effects of aging on bodily systems.
3. Describe the specific effects of injury on the aging population.
4. State the effects of classes of medication on the geriatric population.
5. Discuss the effects of Do Not Resuscitate directives on decisions in the transport environment.

Introduction

Geriatric medicine is a branch of medicine that focuses on the diseases and disabilities prevalent in older adults. The geriatric population is generally defined as those who are 65 years and older; however, starting at age 40 the mortality from severe trauma begins to increase, and for each year over the age of 65 mortality increases by about 6%.[1] Currently this demographic makes up 10% of the world population and is anticipated to increase to 16% by 2050. This geriatric population is one of the fastest growing in the United States and is not only increasing in size but also in age (Fig. 19.1).[2–5]

Human physiology changes with aging and leads to both geriatric-specific diseases and alteration of the body's response to medical conditions. These changes occur to all organ systems and the following are only a few of the major changes that affect caring for this population.

Changes to the cardiovascular system leads to blood vessel stiffening causing increased afterload and widening of the pulse pressure along with the decreased ability to buffer sudden hypovolemic states such as hemorrhage. This is further compounded by a decrease in cardiac beta-adrenergic responsiveness and pharmacologic effects of beta-blocking agents commonly used in the elderly that dampens the body's ability to increase cardiac output by increasing heart rate. Geriatric patients often have kyphotic spines and suffer decreased pulmonary elasticity, vital capacity, and alveolar surface area predisposing them to hypoxia and hypercapnia. Osteoporosis and decreased skin elasticity lead to fractures and lacerations from lower energy traumas compared to younger patients. Medical providers must keep changes in the geriatric patient's physiology in mind when reviewing vital signs and developing a treatment plan.

Geriatric patients utilize Emergency Medical Services (EMS) at four times the rate of younger patients and require more Advanced Life Support care and longer scene times.[6,7] This patient population is also generally sicker, with most older adults having at least one chronic medical condition and 53% of geriatric EMS calls that are transported to the hospital result in admission.[7,8]

Geriatric traumas have been increasing in incidence over the years making up 30% of total trauma patients and 46% of deaths.[9,10] It is also important to recognize that these patients have a higher mortality rate when sustaining a low-energy mechanism of injury when compared to a younger patient.[11] Geriatric patients are more likely to suffer from blunt traumatic injury (98.5%) than penetrating (1.5%).[10] The majority of geriatric trauma patients will present after falls (83%) or motor vehicle collisions (MVCs) (12.3%) (Fig. 19.2).[10] The injury severity score (ISS) is a primary determinant of mortality, however, there is increased mortality in the elderly when compared to the younger patient with the same ISS scores.[12] Pre-existing conditions such as cirrhosis, coagulopathy, chronic obstructive pulmonary disease (COPD), coronary artery disease (CAD), and/or diabetes mellitus (DM) put them at nearly two times the risk of dying when compared to those without these pre-existing conditions, and almost one out of four geriatric patients have a pre-existing condition.[12] The geriatric patient's advanced age and comorbidities put them at increased risk for poor outcomes in a trauma situation; however, these outcomes can be improved with appropriate treatment and monitoring.[9]

Initial Assessment of Elderly Patients – the ABCDEs

Airway

Assessment of the airway in the elderly patient requires special considerations given the development of anatomical and physiologic

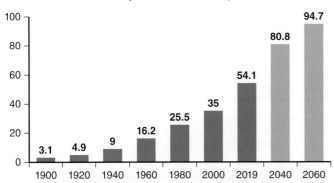

Number of persons age 65 and older, 1900–2060
(numbers in millions)

• **Fig. 19.1** Number of Persons Age 65 and Older, 1900–2060 (numbers in millions). Note: Increments in years are uneven. Lighter bars (2040 and 2060) indicate projections. (Source: U.S. Census Bureau, Popularion Estimates and Projections. From Administration of Aging; Administration for Community Living. (May 2021). 2020 Profile of Older Americans. US Department of Health and Human Services. Accessed February 22, 2023.)

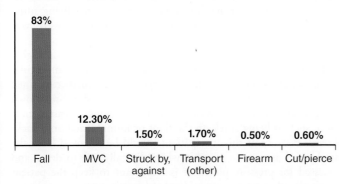

• **Fig. 19.2** Mechanism of Injury for Elderly Patients. (Data from American College of Surgeons. National Trauma Data Bank 2016 Annual Report. https://www.facs.org/media/ez1hpdcu/ntdb-annual-report-2016.pdf. Retrieved March 27, 2023.)

TABLE 19.1	Age-related Changes in Geriatric Airway Anatomy and Associated Management Strategies
Anatomic Changes	**Management Strategies**
• Decreased cervical spine range of motion • Decrease in tension of hyoepiglottic ligament • Edentulous ± presence of dentures; facial atrophy • Restricted mouth opening • Dry oral mucosa • Decreased esophageal sphincter tone	• Video laryngoscopy if intubating • Use Miller > Mac blade if intubating • Remove dentures if intubating; if BVM, ensure tight seal while bagging • Use of lubrication if need for oropharyngeal airway • Increased risk of aspiration; anticipate with suction and consider use of supraglottic device

BVM, Bag-valve-mask.

changes (Table 19.1). Elderly patients may have decreased range of motion of the neck, muscle, and bone wasting in the face, and are frequently edentulous or have dentures, which may complicate the use of a bag-valve-mask (BVM) or performing orotracheal intubation. Physiologically, these patients also have an increased risk of

peri-intubation arrest or hemodynamic instability given decreased physiologic reserve and an increase in the number of comorbidities. Patients are also at increased risk for aspiration due to dementia and reduced functionality of the esophageal sphincter, especially in the setting of ventilation with a BVM.[13,14]

If orotracheal interventions are deemed necessary in the field, the above considerations should be assessed prior to intervention. If the patient has a history or risk of aspiration, consider an laryngeal mask airway (LMA)-type device for ventilation over a typical BVM. If orotracheal intubation is required, the use of a Miller blade over a Mac blade may prove to be more successful due to decreased tensile strength of the hyoepiglottic ligament, causing similar problems with control of the epiglottis as in pediatric intubations.[15,16]

Breathing

Pulmonary reserve and compliance deteriorate over time in elderly patients. The first responder must consider that in the elderly patient there is commonly decreased pulmonary reserve due to multiple factors, including reduced chest wall expansion due to decreased compliance; as well as the progression of comorbidities such as COPD, pulmonary hypertension, and obstructive sleep apnea (OSA).[13,17] Approximately 16% of elderly patients over the age of 65 have increased hypoxemia during sleep or obtundation in combination with comorbidities and decreased pulmonary functional status.[18] The primary objectives of treatment are for respiratory support and reversal of any existing hypoxemia, hypercarbia, and acidosis. Noninvasive (NIV) respiratory adjuncts include a nasal cannula, simple nonrebreather mask, high-flow nasal cannula, continuous positive airway pressure (CPAP), and bilevel positive airway pressure (BiPAP) depending on the level of support needed for oxygenation and ventilation (Table 19.2).[19]

Circulation

Elderly patients have important considerations with regard to comorbidities when assessing the hemodynamic status and baseline reserve. Many studies have attempted to define or better identify shock in elderly patients. Complications such as a history of hypertension or the ubiquitous use of beta-blockers in this population may hide a hemodynamically unstable patient. For example, a patient who appears normotensive may be hypotensive from their baseline. Patients who regularly take beta-blockers may not exhibit a tachycardic response to shock given the beta-blockade which is masking this important marker.[20] This patient may indeed be "unstable" and therefore the clinical assessment of a patient and gestalt is equally as important as taking stock of vital signs.[15] In addition to beta-blockers, elderly patients are frequently known to have multiple prescriptions, known as "polypharmacy." These may be potential grounds for drug–drug interaction as well as cloud the hemodynamic response to injury and shock. These patients are also more likely to be anticoagulated; therefore, even minor trauma may be the cause for serious or precipitous hemodynamic instability due to bleeding.[20]

Suggested cutoff points to pinpoint shock and hemodynamic instability in the elderly vary in the literature. There is a growing consensus that cutoffs should attempt to be more sensitive or err on the side of conservative cutoff points to incorporate geriatric patients more broadly in shock. A systolic blood pressure of under 110 mmHg has been suggested as a cutoff measurement for shock in the elderly. This number is conservative, and would no doubt

TABLE 19.2	**Noninvasive Respiratory Support: Indications and Contraindications**	
Respiratory Adjunct	**Indications**	**Contraindications**
Nasal cannula	Deliver supplemental O_2 for SpO_2 <94% and not in severe respiratory distress Or as temporizing measure for noninvasive ventilation (NIV)	Nasal bone fracture Not a good choice for severe respiratory distress or acute respiratory failure as it does not provide ventilatory support
Nonrebreather	Deliver concentrated supplemental O_2 for hypoxemia	Vomiting
High-flow nasal cannula	Deliver supplemental O_2 for hypoxemia and provide some ventilatory support	Nasal trauma Pneumothorax Central apnea
CPAP/BiPAP	Deliver concentrated supplemental O_2 with moderate ventilatory support.	Vomiting Relative contraindication with altered mental status

BiPAP, Bilevel positive airway pressure; *CPAP*, continuous positive airway pressure.

incorporate several patients who are not hemodynamically unstable; however, in this population, the multiple comorbidities described above and the aging physiology of the geriatric patient have close clinical correlation with the patient in front of you.[21,22] Other metrics that have been offered as tools for the identification of shock in the elderly include an age-adjusted "shock index," which when greater than 50, should prompt concern for shock. The age-adjusted formula is as follows: (Heart rate / Systolic blood pressure) × Age.[15,16]

Disability

As in other parts of the prehospital assessment of geriatric patients, the assessment of disability may rely on family or primary caretaker sources. The evaluation of mental status is especially complicated given that dementia and other neurocognitive disorders are seen with increased prevalence in the elderly population.[23] Therefore, knowledge of a baseline mental status is extremely helpful in initial neuro assessment. The often-used Glasgow Coma Scale (GCS) is a useful adjunct in the field and communication with hospital providers, however, it was initially designed for traumatic brain injury and lacks sensitivity in mild traumatic brain injury or other medical causes for the change in mental status. It should therefore be used in context and the patient's baseline referenced when transporting.[15] In addition to the GCS, patients should be evaluated for orientation and potential cognitive impairment, whether acute or chronic, with simple questions pertaining to person, place, or time.[24]

Delirium, though traditionally thought to afflict hospitalized patients, can occur both in patients who reside in nursing homes and patients who reside at home. It can present as hyperactive, hypoactive, or mixed delirium. Delirium can be preceded by an inciting event such as infection, metabolic derangements, polypharmacy, or decreased sensorium brought on by poor hearing or vision.[24]

Substance use disorder must also be a consideration when considering etiologies for altered mental status; over 17% of adults 60 years and older have substance use disorder with alcohol, street drugs, or prescription drugs.[24]

Environment and Exposure

When initially assessing the patient in their home it is important to note factors in the environment that may make their home unsafe. This can include trip hazards such as rugs, poorly lit areas, and lack of handholds in high fall-risk areas of the home. More information on modifications to the patient's living situation can be referenced at the following website: https://www.healthinaging.org.[25]

While caring for elderly patients, note that they are at higher risk for developing hypothermia due to decreased thermoregulation, as well as musculoskeletal changes that are further outlined below. Additionally, patients are more prone to skin breakdown from relatively minor injuries, including prolonged immobilization, such as being stuck on the floor or immobilized on a backboard. Because of this, the patient should be removed from the backboard as soon as possible when clinically safe to do so and assessed for pressure ulcers. It is important to keep the patient covered and warm to prevent further hypothermia.

Effects of Aging

Significant physiologic changes are present in the elderly patient which have a great effect on prehospital management. These are briefly summarized in Table 19.3.

Cardiovascular

In part due to age and the accumulation over time of comorbidities such as hypertension, diabetes, and hyperlipidemia, in these patients there is decreased elasticity and compliance of arterial vessels.[13] Aging of the arteries alone begets multisystem dysfunction which can manifest in an acutely ill or injured geriatric patient. These patients may present with low circulatory reserves such as an increased risk of peri-intubation arrest, or intolerance of certain drugs which may predispose the elderly patient toward hypotension.

Pulmonary

Decreased vital capacity, as well as decreased lung airway compliance, can lead to increased airway resistance, resulting in end-stage organ diseases such as COPD and emphysema. In addition, patients can have decreased chemoreceptor response to pathophysiology such as hypercapnia and hypoxemia, which can cause decreased or rapid decline in respiratory drive. Additionally, the elderly patient may have worsened interstitial disease, which can

TABLE 19.3 Physiologic Effects of Aging	
Changes with Aging	**Clinical Consequences**
CNS	**CNS**
• Neuronal loss	• Increased risk of delirium
• Cochlear degeneration	• Presbyacusis/high-tone hearing loss
• Increased lens rigidity	• Presbyopia/abnormal near vision
• Lens opacification	• Cataract
• Anterior horn cell loss	• Muscle weakness and wasting
• Dorsal column loss	• Reduced position and vibration sense
• Slowed reaction times	• Increased risk of falls
Respiratory System	**Respiratory System**
• Reduced lung elasticity and alveolar support	• Reduced vital capacity and peak expiratory flow
• Increased chest wall rigidity	• Increased residual volume
• Increased V̇/Q̇ mismatch	• Reduced inspiratory reserve volume
• Reduced cough and ciliary action	• Reduced arterial oxygen saturation
	• Increased risk of infection
Cardiovascular System	**Cardiovascular System**
• Reduced maximum heart rate	• Reduced exercise tolerance
• Dilatation of aorta	• Widened aortic arch on x-ray
• Reduced elasticity of conduit/capacitance vessels	• Widened pulse pressure
• Reduced number of pacing myocytes in sinoatrial node	• Increased risk of postural hypotension
	• Increased risk or atrial fibrillation
Endocrine System	**Endocrine System**
• Deterioration in pancreatic β-cell function	• Increased risk of impaired glucose tolerance
Renal System	**Renal System**
• Loss of nephrons	• Impaired fluid balance
• Reduced glomerular filtration rate	• Increased risk of dehydration/overload
• Reduced tubular function	• Impaired drug metabolism and excretion
Gastrointestinal System	**Gastrointestinal System**
• Reduced motility	• Constipation
Bones	**Bones**
• Reduced bone mineral density	• Increased risk of osteoporosis

Data from Basicmedical Key. Ageing and disease. https://basicmedicalkey.com/ageing-and-disease-2/.

result in increased diffusion capacity. This poor exchange of gases can result in hypoxemia and hypercarbia.

COPD is a disease process which is multifactorial in etiology, particularly with a history of smoking or environmental/industrial exposure resulting in obstructive airway disease, poor oxygenation, and retention of CO_2 related to COPD. As with caring for the average adult, adjuncts for the management of these diseases should be readily available and appropriate for the disease process at hand. Both COPD and OSA can lead to hypercarbia. COPD exacerbation will present with acute respiratory distress. As the exacerbation progresses, the patient will become progressively more hypercapnic which can result in obtundation and acute respiratory failure.[26] Patients may present with wheezing, productive cough, altered mental status secondary to hypercapnia, and suprasternal and subcostal retractions. Patients even with slightly increased work of breathing are at risk of worsening and respiratory failure; therefore, care should be taken to appropriately manage COPD exacerbations during transport.

Nebulized treatments with albuterol and ipratropium act as bronchodilators to reduce the obstructive process of the disease. Early administration of systemic glucocorticoids should be given in the form of oral prednisone or intravenous (IV) glucocorticoids; take care that patients with hyperglycemia may have worsening of this condition due to steroid effects. Finally, IV magnesium may be given if the patient is refractory to breathing treatments. When administering oxygen, care should be taken to avoid excess oxygenation, as in a chronically hypercapnic or hypoxic patient this may result in decreased respiratory drive and precipitate acute respiratory failure. When administering oxygen, a target SpO_2 of 88%–92% is appropriate for COPD patients.[27–29]

Renal System

Elderly patients have a decrease in overall renal cell mass and decreased functional ability for the kidney to filter. This can cause complications such as decreased drug elimination of renally excreted medications. Elderly patients also have an overall decrease in thirst response, as well as a decrease in total body water. This can cause them to be at higher risk of dehydration and electrolyte abnormalities. The kidneys are also responsible for the hydroxylation of vitamin D, and decreased function puts the elderly at higher risk of hypercalcemia and osteopenia.

Musculoskeletal System

Elderly patients have atrophy of synovial fluid, and cartilaginous tissue, which can result in joint laxity, joint pain, and decreased mobility. In combination with this, elderly patients have decreased bone mass and muscle atrophy, which places them at higher risk for falls and fractures. Changes in muscle mass and adipose tissue can also change the pharmacokinetics of any medications that are administered.

Immune System

The elderly have an overall decreased immune response to infection. This places them at a higher risk for infection, and causes them to have a blunted response, making the diagnosis of infection more difficult. Up to 30% of patients with a serious infection can present with a blunted or absent fever response.[30] The elderly also have decreased cell-mediated immunity, which can place them at higher risk for reactivation of latent disease, as well as increased risk of neoplasm.

Metabolic and Endocrine

Metabolic effects and endocrine disorders may lead to the presenting illness or injury in the elderly patient. One of the most common chronic diseases in the geriatric population is diabetes mellitus (DM). Patients in these populations are at high risk of hypoglycemic events leading to falls, malaise, and altered mental status. Therefore, obtaining a blood glucose level is recommended. In part, this is due to frailty, as discussed below. Some medications used in the treatment of diabetes may also be prescribed inappropriately or difficult to regulate as in the case of insulin, by caregivers or patients themselves.[31] This may lead to overmedication or improper monitoring, which can result in hypoglycemia. In geriatric patients, it may be difficult to distinguish hypoglycemia from other chronic neurocognitive issues. Additionally, typical signs and symptoms of hypoglycemia in the average non-elderly adult may be missed in elderly patients due to potentially diminished end-organ response.

Geriatric patients often have several medications to manage multiple comorbidities accrued over time. These drugs may include those with narrow therapeutic windows, and given patients with multiorgan comorbidities, improper use or even proper use of these prescriptions may result in serious health consequences.[32] This is further complicated by a decrease in renal and/or hepatic metabolism. The American Geriatric Society (AGS) regularly updates a list of medications called The Beers Criteria, which identifies potential problem drugs related to geriatric-specific physiology. This list is extensively reviewed based on evidence-based medicine and provides a rationale for the cautious use of certain classes of drugs in the elderly.[33] In addition to the published list of Beers Criteria, the AGS also has a mobile application, iGeriatrics, available for use by clinicians and healthcare providers to regularly access the full list of recommendations.

Frailty and Deconditioning

The term "frailty" in geriatric patients has been described on a spectrum but has been defined as "age- and disease-related loss of adaptation, such that events of previously minor stress result in disproportionate biomedical and social consequences."[34] Frailty often results because of a decrease in physiologic reserve affecting all organ systems. This causes older patients to be less able to compensate for external stressors, and subsequently have a rapid decline. Common ways for frailty and deconditioning to present include decreased ability to accomplish activities of daily living, decreased bone density, and repeated falls.

Specific Effects of Injury in the Elderly

Brain and Spinal Injuries

Head injuries are the most common cause of mortality in geriatric trauma patients and the most common mechanism of these injuries are ground-level falls.[35,36] The lifetime prevalence of geriatric traumatic brain injury (TBI) is up to 40% in adults and is most common in elderly White females. Geriatric patients are more susceptible to TBI and spinal cord injury as the average life expectancy increases.[37] These patients are more prone to TBI and spinal injuries for multiple reasons.

The brain is prone to atrophy as we age, which results in decreased protection of brain tissue by the skull. There are veins in the subarachnoid space called "bridging veins" that stretch as the brain atrophies, resulting in increased tension on these veins causing them to tear more easily.[35] This causes an increased risk of subdural and intraparenchymal hematoma in the elderly population, that can occur even with low mechanism trauma and very minor head injury.[35,37] Some studies show that one out of every 50 elderly trauma patients who sustain a head injury require neurosurgical intervention.[36]

Another contributing factor to higher rates of significant head injuries in the elderly population is that many of these patients are on anticoagulation medications (i.e., warfarin, heparin, or direct oral anticoagulants [DOACs]), increasing their risk for intracranial bleeding. It is important to determine if the patient is on these medications, as the concern for intracranial bleed significantly increases. Geriatric patients with a head injury who are anticoagulated have an increased risk for late-onset severity, even if initial assessment only revealed a mild TBI, such as a small head contusion.[38]

Virtually all geriatric trauma patients with a head injury will undergo a computed tomography (CT) scan of their brain based on their increased risk of bleed, but this becomes significantly more important if they are on anticoagulation medications. If a patient is on these medications and a bleed is noted on a CT scan, reversal of these medications is important.[35] Lab values, specifically coagulation labs, should be monitored and corrected if possible. Whether a geriatric patient is on anticoagulation or not, they are three times more likely to undergo a CT scan of their brain and four times more likely to be admitted to a step-down or intensive care unit (ICU) than a younger patient with the same mechanism of injury and/or initial complaint.[37] The most common abnormal finding on a CT brain scan in an elderly trauma patient is a cerebral contusion, followed by subdural hematoma.[36]

When initially evaluating an elderly patient with even a slight potential for head trauma, it is important not to assume that altered mental status is secondary to dementia.[35] If you are able, attempt to obtain a clinical history from family members or others who know the patient well to establish a relative baseline mental status for the patient. The Glasgow Coma Scale (GCS) score is a helpful tool when assessing mental status, but it does not give the full picture, especially in elderly patients who may have a decreased GCS score at baseline.[37] Additionally, due to the increased space in the skull caused by brain atrophy with aging, initial GCS may not accurately reflect the severity of the TBI as the hematoma may have more time to expand before causing a decline in mental status.[37] The GAP score, defined as age divided by GCS, can be used in this population to help determine relative morbidity and mortality risk. A high GAP score is greater than 12, and studies revealed that a score over 12 correlated with a drastic increase in mortality and rehab/skilled nursing facility placement upon discharge.[39] Another reliable indication of morbidity or mortality for a head injury patient is the volume of intracranial blood and rate of expansion of hematoma.[35] Understandably so, elderly patients with significant comorbidities or poor health preceding a TBI had worse outcomes than those who were healthier prior to the event. It has been shown that many older adults with TBI do respond well to aggressive therapy and rehabilitation.[37]

Geriatric trauma patients are twice as likely to sustain a spinal injury from trauma than younger patients with a similar mechanism.[35] This is due to several factors including decreased mobility and osteoporosis. Decreased joint mobility often leads to spinal stenosis as we age, which causes an increase in vertebral injury and spinal cord damage.[36] Cervical spine fractures most commonly occur at levels C1–C3, and a type II odontoid fracture is the most common spinal fracture in elderly trauma patients. Thoracic and lumbar compression fractures resulting from trauma are also relatively common in these patients.[36] Based on the Canadian C-spine Rule, all patients over the age of 65 who sustain any trauma should have a C-collar placed. These patients should also undergo a CT scan of their cervical spine, even if the injury seems minor and the patient has no neck pain or neurologic findings on exam.[35] The use of a backboard in trauma patients is more controversial and falling out of favor, especially in regard to elderly trauma patients. These patients are prone to the rapid development of tissue necrosis or decubitus ulcers, so a backboard should be avoided if possible. If a backboard must be used, a padded backboard or at least a padding of all voids between the patient and the backboard is preferred.[35]

Thoracic Injuries

Elderly patients are more prone to sustaining a significant injury in the setting of blunt thoracic trauma and are less able to compensate when injury does occur.[35] Thoracic trauma has the second-highest mortality rate in the geriatric population, after head injury.[40] Injuries to the thorax include rib fractures, sternal fractures, lung injury, and injuries to vessels including the thoracic aorta.

As patients age, their cardiovascular reserve declines and the heart is unable to compensate as well for hypovolemia. In the setting of volume loss, these patients have a blunted physiologic response, which can lead to worse outcomes than the same injury in younger patients. Many of these patients are on cardiovascular medications such as beta-blockers, calcium channel blockers, or digoxin which can further blunt the cardiac response to trauma or blood loss as documented earlier. Geriatric patients also commonly have coronary artery disease, which can lead to an increase in demand for ischemia in the setting of hypovolemia.[36]

Rib Fractures

The most common abnormal findings after blunt thoracic trauma in the elderly are rib fractures and hemothorax.[41] Geriatric patients are more prone to rib fractures due to stiffening of the thoracic cage and loss of cortical bone mass that occurs with aging.[37] The most common mechanisms of isolated and multiple rib fractures in these patients are falls and MVCs. Studies have shown that elderly patients have twice the risk of morbidity and mortality than younger patients with the same fractures.[42] One study revealed that with each additional rib fracture in a geriatric trauma patient, mortality increased by 19% and risk of pneumonia increased by 27%.[35]

The most frequent concomitant injury in the setting of rib fracture(s) in the geriatric population is lung contusion, followed by pneumothorax then hemopneumothorax. There is a high association between pulmonary complications and overall mortality.[42] Longer-term complications of rib fractures in elderly patients include pneumonia, pleural effusion, and acute respiratory failure.[42] There is only a slightly increased risk of elderly patients developing lung failure in the setting of rib fractures, but mortality is significantly increased if lung failure does develop.[43] Pain control, especially in the setting of multiple rib fractures, is vital in this patient population to improve ventilation. These patients should be monitored with continuous pulse oximetry and capnometry, and the provider should have a low threshold to intubate early in the setting of severe chest trauma or if the respiratory rate is over 40 due to a high risk of decompensation.[35] They should also undergo strict blood glucose control and aggressive chest physiotherapy to aid in the recovery process.[42] Sternal fractures can also be indicative of underlying myocardial or pulmonary contusion and large vessel injury.

Pulmonary Injury

Respiratory muscles weaken with aging, lungs become less compliant, and bones are more brittle, which combine to result in a higher incidence of injury to the lungs in the setting of trauma.[36] These patients are prone to respiratory failure and a more difficult recovery than younger patients with similar injuries. Studies have shown that age greater than 60 years is an independent risk factor for the development of lung failure after thoracic trauma.[35] Our bodies increase our tidal volume and respiratory rate in order to compensate for hypoxia and hypercarbia, conditions commonly seen in pulmonary trauma. However, elderly patients have elevated respiratory rates and decreased tidal volume at baseline, so they have less ability to respond to injury and decompensate more quickly.[43] In-hospital morbidity and mortality and the number of patients who develop lung failure requiring intubation/ICU stays during hospitalization is higher than younger patients with thoracic injury as well.[43]

Abdominal Injury

There are multiple complications of blunt abdominal trauma that elderly patients are more prone to the physiologic changes that come with aging. The most commonly damaged organ is the spleen. While rare, a few other diagnoses to have a heightened concern for in older patients are aortic dissection, atheroembolic disease, and small intestinal perforation.[44] The abdominal physical exam in a geriatric patient is unreliable, as even a relatively minor blunt injury to the abdomen (i.e., fall from standing) can cause organ damage without significant suggestive signs or complaints of pain.[44] A Focused Assessment with Sonography for Trauma (FAST) exam to assess for free fluid is vital to triage patients for immediate surgical intervention.[35] Plain films of the chest and pelvis can assist with evaluating for internal abdominal injury, but if the patient is stable a CT scan is obtained for a more detailed assessment when the FAST is inconclusive. In the prehospital setting, it is important to have a low threshold for giving fluid or blood products in the setting of blunt abdominal trauma, especially if a patient has blood pressures on the low side of normal or complaint of any abdominal pain, as the abdomen can hold up to 5 liters of blood and significant hemorrhagic shock can result.

Pelvic and Hip Fractures

Hip fractures are the most common injury that leads to the hospitalization in elderly patients and has a very high mortality rate, up to 70% without surgical intervention.[35,45] Almost every patient with a hip or femur fracture, despite their age or comorbidities, will undergo surgical fixation because the mortality rate decreases to approximately 21% after surgery. Patients with hip fractures will most likely have a shortened and externally rotated lower extremity. It is important to immobilize the extremity in the prehospital setting and provide adequate pain control. Both pelvic and hip fractures can occur in very low energy mechanism traumas in elderly patients, such as a fall from standing, due to degenerative changes of bone and joints. However, younger patients require a relatively high mechanism of injury such as a high-speed MVC to sustain these same fractures.[35] Pubic ramus fracture is the most common type of pelvic fracture, and a lateral compression injury is the most common mechanism resulting in a pelvic fracture.[35]

Some of the more common unstable pelvic fractures are "open book" fractures, vertical shear fractures, and lateral compression fractures.[46] Open book fractures are unstable on both sides when bilateral pressure is applied to the iliac crests. A binder should be placed on confirmed open book fracture or unstable blunt trauma patients when the bleeding source has not been identified in the prehospital setting. Placement should be centered at the level of the greater trochanters on the hips as opposed to higher up around the abdomen. This helps to tamponade bleeding. Like the abdomen, the pelvis can hold a large amount of blood, so fluids and blood products should be given early in the setting of a suspected pelvic fracture. In the setting of pelvic fracture, elderly patients were shown to have a severe outcome in 73% of cases, as opposed to only 31% in the young adult group.[46] Early definitive treatment, supportive care, and pain control are all important.

Burn Injury

Burns are the fourth leading cause of unintentional mortality in patients over 65 years old and the second most common cause of geriatric traumatic death inside the home.[35,47] The most common type of burn sustained is a flame burn (50%), followed by scald burns at 19% and flammable liquid burns at 10%.[36] Cooking is a common cause of burn injury in "younger" elderly patients and bathing is a common cause of burn injury in "older" elderly patients.[47] The incidence of burn injury is higher in younger patients, but the morbidity and mortality rates in the setting of burn injury are much higher in the geriatric population.[36] The mortality rate in older patients who suffer burns is twice that of younger patients, and they have a greater incidence of long-term disability and loss of independence.[47] There are multiple reasons that geriatric patients have a much more difficult recovery in the setting of burn injury including thinner skin and decreased immunocompetency.[36] Burns in these patients are often deeper and more extensive because reaction time, mobility, and skin sensitivity all decrease with age thus causing difficulty quickly reaching safety.[36,46,48] When assessing burn patients, determining a rough estimate of the percentage of total body surface area (TBSA) burned is important regarding resuscitation.

Fluid resuscitation and pain control are the most important early interventions in burn patients. Early and adequate fluid resuscitation helps to prevent decreased perfusion, organ failure, sepsis, and overall mortality.[48] The Parkland Formula is used to determine the amount of fluid required for adequate fluid resuscitation based on the percentage of TBSA burned and the weight of the patient. The formula is (4 mL × body weight in kg × %TBSA) = total crystalloid fluids required in the first 24 hours after the burn. Half of this amount is given in the first 8 hours, and the other half is given in the last 16 hours. The gold standard for measuring adequate fluid resuscitation in a burn injury is urine output of 0.5–1.0 mL/kg/hr, but an average mean arterial pressure (MAP) of 70 can also be used for a rough estimate of good perfusion.[48] There is no difference in mortality when using the Parkland formula vs. goal-directed fluid resuscitation.[48]

It is also very important to examine the oropharynx and face to assess for inhalational burns, i.e., soot in or around the mouth, as patients with these burns can quickly lose their airway and require a low threshold for early intubation. Pain control is vital and is often inadequate in elderly patients due to concern for hemodynamic instability.[16] Continue to resuscitate the patient while simultaneously treating pain.

Elderly patients who survive a burn injury are shown to have significantly increased length of hospital stay, slower recovery time, and more complications. There is a higher risk of complications from burns including pulmonary edema, congestive heart failure, and pneumonia (especially with inhalational burns).[48] There is a concern with worsened heart failure and fluid overload in these patients due to their comorbidities, but fluid resuscitation in significant burn injury is more important during initial treatment.[35]

Medication Therapy in the Geriatric Patient

This section serves two main roles, the first being a quick reference/encyclopedia of worrisome drugs in their uses, drug interactions, side effects, and ramifications with over- or under-dosing. The second is to provide a basic understanding of why all these possible complications occur, establishing a larger knowledge base for both new and returning learners to explore.

Nomenclature

Drugs have a variety of names meaning the same thing. So, it is handy to know some of the more common names to interchange them or have a basis to look them up and confirm the medication with which you are working. Every drug has a (1) chemical, (2) generic, and (3) trade name. For example, ibuprofen[49]:

Chemical name: 2-(4-isobutylphenyl) propanoic acid

Generic name: ibuprofen

Trade names: Motrin, Advil

Motrin is manufactured by Johnson & Johnson, and Advil is manufactured by GlaxoSmithKline Pharmaceuticals.[49] They both have the same active ingredients.

Some drugs have different trade names because of how they are distributed while having the same generic name. For example, acetaminophen is called Tylenol in oral form, but Ofirmev when it is given intravenously.[49]

Mechanism of Action, Indications, and Side Effects

Drugs are often grouped by their mechanism of action (MOA). We refer to "beta-blockers" as the group of drugs that work on beta-1 and/or beta-2 (beta) antagonism rather than saying "propranolol, metoprolol, esmolol..." and so on.[50] While each drug is unique in its properties such as half-life and efficacy, knowing the groupings can help hone your patient care toward specific outcomes.

The "Medication Classes of Concern" section goes into these groupings in more detail to better explain *why* they have such indications and side effects. Table 19.4 provided below aims to be a quick reference and is not intended to impart the complete knowledge of geriatric pharmacology by itself.

Fig. 19.3 is a list of the most commonly prescribed medications (in descending order) for patients older than 65 years of age. This list is compiled from the popularly used EPCR EPIC and, as can be seen, it accounts for millions of prescriptions. As we progress through this section, think of all the potential complications to which these commonly prescribed medications can lead.

TABLE 19.4 Considerations for Medications Commonly Used in Geriatric Care

Generic Drug Name	Trade Names	Mechanism of Action	Uses	Side Effects	Overdose	Comments
Atorvastatin	Lipitor, Caduet	HMG-CoA reductase inhibitor	Mainly lowers LDL, also slightly raises HDL and lowers triglyceride levels	Increase in LFTs, myalgia, statin-associated myopathy (can manifest as rhabdomyolysis)	Myopathy/rhabdo risk increases with dose increase	Metabolized by CYP3A4 (CYP inhibitors can increase statin concentration)
Acetylsalicylic acid	Aspirin, Anacin, Ecotrin, Excedrin, Alka-Seltzer, Pamprin, Percodan	Irreversible COX-1 and COX-2 inhibitor	Antipyretic, anti-inflammatory, and analgesic; inhibits platelet aggregation at certain doses	GI ulcers, bleeding	Tinnitus, tachypnea, coma, seizures, pulmonary edema, AKI	Reye syndrome and aspirin-exacerbated respiratory disease
Lisinopril	Prinivil, Prinzide, Zestoretic, Zestril	ACEI	Treats HTN and scleroderma, nephroprotective, increased survivability in heart failure	Cough, angioedema, pemphigus vulgaris, teratogenicity, hypotension, hyperkalemia, increased creatinine, low GFR	Can cause AKI in those with pre-existing renal hypoperfusion, hyperkalemia	NSAIDs decrease antihypertension effectiveness, increases lithium levels, compound hypotensive effect with other antihypertensives
Albuterol	DuoNeb, AccuNeb, Combivent, Pro-Air, Proventil, Ventolin	Short-acting beta-2 agonist	Treats asthma, COPD, and hyperkalemia	Arrhythmias, vasoconstriction, angina, tremor, hyperglycemia	Hypokalemia	Onset should be within 5 minutes
Acetaminophen	Tylenol, Acephen, Alagesic, Bupap, Capacet, Excedrin, Fever-All, Goody's, Midol, Ofirmev, Percogesic	COX inhibitor	Antipyretic and analgesic	Minimal gastric side effects	Hepatotoxic, can cause acute liver failure	No anti-inflammatory effect, 4 g daily maximum dose (adults)
Levothyroxine	Levothroid, Levoxyl, Synthroid, Unithroid	Synthetic form of T4	Treats hypothyroidism and myxedema coma	Sweating, tachycardia, tremors, weight loss, osteoporosis, arrhythmias	Thyrotoxicosis, thyroid storm	Drug interactions with PPIs, calcium, iron supplements, glucocorticoids
Hydrocodone-acetaminophen	Vicodin, Norco, Lorcet, Hycet, Lortab, Anexsia, Xodol, Zamicet	Opiate agonist, COX inhibitor	Analgesic, antitussive, antipyretic	Respiratory depression, addiction	Same as "Oxycodone"; remember acetaminophen causes liver damage	This formulation has two different drugs in it, see "Oxycodone" or "Acetaminophen" for more

Continued

TABLE
19.4
Considerations for Medications Commonly Used in Geriatric Care—cont'd

Generic Drug Name	Trade Names	Mechanism of Action	Uses	Side Effects	Overdose	Comments
Metoprolol	Lopressor, Toprol XL	Beta-1 antagonist	Anti-arrhythmic, anti-ischemic and anti-remodeling in heart failure, treats HTN	Bradycardia, orthostatic hypotension, fatigue, seizures	Bradycardia, cardiogenic shock, hypoglycemia, wheezing	Withdrawal (missing doses with no taper) can cause reflexive tachycardia and/or HTN. Tapers should be used for increasing or decreasing dosage
Furosemide	Lasix	Loop diuretic	Treats HTN, renal failure, and hypercalcemia; used in forced diuresis (pulmonary edema treatment)	Gout, ototoxicity, hypokalemia, nephritis, dehydration, metabolic alkalosis	No specific effects, but can exacerbate other conditions (hypovolemic shock)	Sulfa drug; "laSIX lasts 6 hours"
Prednisone	Deltasone, Prednicot, Sterapred, Prapred, Millipred, Veripred	Glucocorticoid/steroid	Anti-inflammatory, immunosuppression, increases sodium and decreases potassium	Increases blood pressure, insulin resistance, gluconeogenesis, and appetite; and decreases fibroblast activity, immune response, and bone formation	Psychosis, HTN, Cushing's disease (long-term use)	Can cause adrenal crisis if not tapered off
Metformin	Metabet, Fortamet, Glumetza, Invokamet, Janumet, Jentadueto, Segluromet, Synjardy	Enhances insulin effect	Main treatment for DM2	Metformin-associated lactic acidosis, vitamin B_{12} deficiency, dysgeusia		Metformin and sulfonylureas together are associated with an increase in cardiovascular mortality
Losartan	Cozaar, Hyzaar	Angiotensin-receptor blocker	Same as "Lisinopril"	Angioedema, hyperkalemia, hypotension, teratogenicity, leukopenia, rash	Same as ACEIs (see "Lisinopril")	2nd-line treatment compared to ACEIs
Gabapentin	Neurontin, Gralise, Horizant	Decreases glutamate release via calcium channel inhibition	Treats neuropathic pain and peripheral neuropathy, 2nd-line treatment for focal seizures	Dry mouth, somnolence, nausea, ataxia	Respiratory depression	Morphine increases gabapentin concentrations
Omeprazole	Prilosec, Zegerid	PPI	Peptic ulcer disease, GERD, gastritis, *H. pylori*, gastrinoma, gastropathy	GI effects (nausea, vomiting, diarrhea, abdominal pain, flatulence), increases *C. difficile* infection risk, decreased absorption of iron, vitamin B_{12}, calcium, magnesium	No specific effects, but tons of drug interactions because of CYP2C19	Noteworthy interactions include decreased clopidogrel activation, decreased warfarin, diazepam, and nifedipine clearance, increased phenytion and carbamazepine clearance
Pantoprazole	Protonix	PPI, increases stomach pH	Same as "Omeprazole"	Same as "Omeprazole"	Same as "Omeprazole"	Same as "Omeprazole"; targets stomach more specifically

TABLE 19.4   Considerations for Medications Commonly Used in Geriatric Care—cont'd

Generic Drug Name	Trade Names	Mechanism of Action	Uses	Side Effects	Overdose	Comments
Fluticasone	Flonase, Advair, Diskus, Flovent	Glucocorticoid/steroid	Flonase for seasonal allergies, the rest for asthma and COPD	Same as "Prednisone"	Same as "Prednisone"	This steroid is more local acting, does not cause the systemic effects as easily
Tramadol	Conzip, Qdolo, Ultram, Ultracet, Zydol	Opiate agonist	Analgesic	Addiction, constipation, increased risk of serotonin syndrome and seizures	Same as "Oxycodone"	Same as "Oxycodone"; used often for moderate chronic pain
Tamsulosin	Flomax	Alpha-1 antagonist	Benign prostatic hyperplasia	Orthostatic hypotension, retrograde ejaculation, priapism	Hypotension	Half life of 9–15 hours depending on urine excretion
Hydrochlorothiazide	Microzide, Accuretic, Aldactazide, Avalide, Dyazide, Hyzaar, Maxzide, Prinzide, Tribenzor, Uniretic, Vaseretic, Zestoretic, Ziac	Thiazide diuretic	Treats HTN, edema, and nephrogenic diabetes insipidus; prevention of calcium kidney stones and osteoporosis	Hyperglycemia, hyperlipidemia, hyperuricemia, hypercalcemia, and hypokalemia	Same as "Furosemide"	Drug interactions can worsen metabolic interactions, such as steroids and hypokalemia, propranolol and hypoglycemia
Apixaban	Eliquis	Direct Factor Xa inhibitor	Anticoagulation (nonvalvular atrial fibrillation, DVT prophylaxis, post-operation)	Dose-dependent increase in bleeding	Bleeding; reversal agent: andexanet alfa	Certain antifungal medications double apixaban efficiency
Cephalexin	Keflex	Inhibits bacterial cell wall production	Antibiotic against Gram-positive organisms	Cross-reactivity with penicillin allergies, vitamin K deficiency, disulfiram-like reaction, seizures	No specific events	Nephrotoxic when combined with aminoglycosides; decreases metformin clearance
Oxycodone	Percocet, Endocet, Endodan, Oxaydo, Oxecta, Oxycontin, Primlev, Roxicet, Roxicodone	Opiate agonist	Analgesic	Addiction, constipation, hypogonadism in prolonged use	Respiratory depression, altered mental status, miosis, bradycardia, hypotension	Half-life is 3–5 hours; reversal agent: nalaxone
Rosuvastatin	Crestor, Ezallor	HMG-CoA reductase inhibitor	Same as "Atorvastatin"	Same as "Atorvastatin"	Same as "Atorvastatin"	Most potent of all statins; minimally metabolized by CYP
Polyethylene glycol	Miralax, Gavilax, Glycolax	Osmotic laxative	Constipation	Diarrhea, dehydration, flatulence, bloating	No specific effects, but can exacerbate other conditions (hypovolemic shock)	Chronic use can lead to hypokalemia and metabolic alkalosis
Potassium (oral)	Effer-K, Kaon-Cl, Kay Ciel, K-Lor, Klor-Con, Klotrix, K-Tab, Micro-K	Synthetic/natural potassium	Treats hypokalemia, adjunct in diet for HTN	Hyperkalemia, metabolic acidosis, GI lesions	Arrhythmia	Commonly prescribed along with K-wasting diuretics (Lasix)

ACEI, Angiotensin-converting enzyme inhibitor; *AKI*, acute kidney injury; *COPD*, chronic obstructive pulmonary disease; *COX*, cyclo-oxygenase; *CYP*, cytochrome P450; *DM2*, diabetes mellitus type 2; *DVT*, deep vein thrombosis; *GERD*, gastroesophageal reflux disease; *GFR*, glomerular filtration rate; *GI*, gastrointestinal; *HDL*, high-density lipoprotein; *HMG-CoA*, 3-hydroxy-3-methylglutaryl-coenzyme A; *HTN*, hypertension; *LDL*, low-density lipoprotein; *LFT*, liver function tests; *NSAID*, nonsteroidal anti-inflammatory drug; *PPI*, proton pump inhibitor; *T4*, thyroxine.

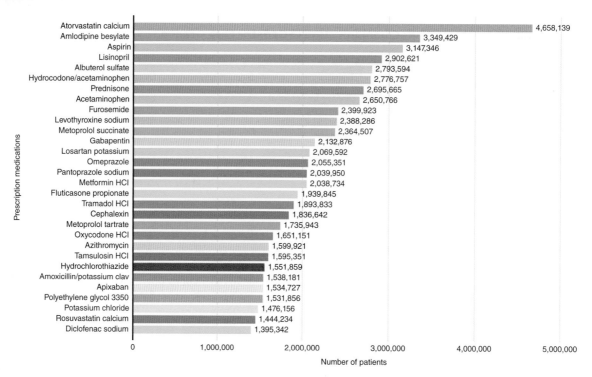

• **Fig. 19.3** Top 30 Prescription Medications for Patients 65 or Older from the Epic Cosmos Database. Between 1/1/2020 and 12/31/2022. This is a HIPAA limited data set of more than 183 million patients from 198 Epic customers. These are counting unique patients that have an active prescription for the medication during the report timeframe (1/1/2020 – 12/31/2022). (Data from Epic Cosmos Database. https://cosmos.epic.com/.)

Physiology and Pharmacology

Growing old has physiological changes for us all. As life progresses, medication, procedures, surgery, and treatments are a true possibility. Even with all that, medicine merely delays the inevitable as the body will reach a point where it cannot sustain the basic life support functions, such as oxygenation of the blood, and the patient dies. While grim, this is the reality all geriatric patients face in a much more consistent manner than anyone younger than 65 years of age. For example, their heart does not pump as well compared to 25,000 miles ago (or 25 years). To steer more toward medical jargon, their ability to resist stress and compliance is reduced, in multiple organ systems. The purpose of this section is to provide more insight into the effects of medication on the elderly compared to the younger population.

Basic Pharmacology

There is an adage for dosing in the elderly, "start low, go slow,"[51] (i.e., low-dose, slow titration compared to a younger and healthier adult). The rest of the section explains why this is the case, most of the time. First, there are some important concepts and terminology to understand:

Pharmacology: The science that studies substances that interact with living systems through chemical processes, especially by binding to regulatory molecules and activating or inhibiting normal body processes.[52]

Pharmacokinetics (PK): The branch of pharmacology concerned with the movement of drugs within the body. PK can be thought of as "what the body does to a drug."[52]

Pharmacodynamics (PD): The branch of pharmacology concerning the study of the biochemical and physiological effects of a drug and their mechanisms of action at the organ system/subcellular/macrocellular levels. PD can be thought of as "what the drug does to the body."[52]

Within pharmacology, pharmacokinetics is influenced by four main categories: **absorption**, **distribution**, **metabolism**, and **excretion** (ADME).[53] Some drugs need to be absorbed with food to work better. Some don't distribute to tissues that are not well vascularized. Others need to be metabolized by the liver or kidneys before they "turn on."[53] Finally, some drugs just don't leave the body if the kidneys, for example, don't work. As you can imagine, there are a variety of both normal and abnormal conditions the human body can be subject to that would change how these drugs would work. Pregnancy, shock, kidney disease, obesity, substance abuse, and dehydration just to name a few.[53] You will see these four categories being referenced as we proceed.

Pharmacodynamics, on the other hand, relates to what the drug does after it starts to work, i.e., the mechanism of action (MOA). Sometimes, the PD can affect the PK.[52] For example, terazosin is used to improve urinary flow. It also is eliminated 40% by urine.[49] This is useful, because as urinary flow improves, the drug is no longer needed. It has a *negative feedback loop*. Some drugs do the opposite. They stay in the body longer, thereby exerting their effect longer per newly synthesized/metabolized molecule. PD concepts will come up often as we begin to talk about geriatric physiology and drug–drug interactions.

Changes in Physiology

There is no absolute change in physiology for elderly adults. Every patient is unique. As an example, say we have an 81-year-old who walks 5 miles every day before 10 a.m. and a 76-year-old with chronic kidney disease due to possible longstanding diabetes.

One obviously cannot metabolize and excrete certain medications as well as the other. The healthier active person can likely metabolize drugs better than younger patients. That being said, there are some trends to be aware of from the current literature.

Effects of aging include stiffening of the arteries and calcification of valves (cardiovascular system), osteoporosis and increased risk of fracture (musculoskeletal system), decreased chest wall compliance and increased ventilation–perfusion mismatch (respiratory system), susceptibility to recurrent infections and malignancies (immune system), and decline in cognitive function and changes in sleep patterns (nervous system).[50,51,53–62]

To go through every physiological change in geriatric patients is beyond the scope of this chapter, but we can discuss the big ones that are related to pharmacology. Remember that all cells and all organ systems are subject to the natural processes of aging that ultimately lead to progressive functional decline.[50]

Aging Changes[50–62]

An increase in age increases the risk for presbyopia, presbycusis (reduced sense of smell and taste), reduced sensation such as touch and temperature (increased risk of ulcers, burns), decreased reflexes, and decreased balance and gait stability (hence increased fall risk and general psychomotor slowing). Although fluid intelligence decreases, crystallized intelligence increases. There is a general neuronal loss in the brain, leading to decreased cerebral blood flow and brain volume. Sleep patterns are also altered in the elderly, namely waking up earlier, sleeping later, and decreased REM sleep.

There is increased chest wall stiffness due to muscle weakness, kyphosis, and calcification. This leads to decreased chest wall compliance, which has a host of respiratory effects, including increased residual volume, decreased forced vital capacity (FVC), and decreased forced expiratory volume after one second (FEV_1). The heart, having (hopefully) never stopped since birth, becomes more hypertrophied and stiffened, mostly in the left ventricle. This increases wall size and decreases the cavity size. The mitral and aortic valves thicken and calcify, leading to their respective stenosis murmurs. The aorta, having been beat against consistently, increases in diameter with time. There is a general vascular sclerosis and stiffness, leading to increased blood pressure.

There is decreased lean body mass due to muscle atrophy and sarcopenia. The muscle weakness affects respiration, movement, and swallowing, leading to increased aspiration, falls, and hypoxia. There is decreased colonic motility, leading to increased constipation. The stomach loses its mucosal protection with time, increasing ulcer risk.

The immune system also becomes weaker, and the bone marrow decreases in mass as there is decreased hematopoiesis. This increases the risk of infection, decreases vaccination response, and increases the risk of inflammatory diseases.

For the genitourinary system, there is increased sclerosis of glomeruli, leading to decreased glomerular filtration rate (GFR). There is an increased prevalence of voiding dysfunction, also increasing urinary tract infection rates. Finally, there is decreased libido, typically more pronounced in women than in men.

While not a physiologic change, it is worth noting that age is a suicide risk in individuals with physical illness, mental illness (particularly depression), functional impairment, and stressful life events (e.g., loss of a partner).

In light of all these changes, age is a non-modifiable risk factor for multiple diseases, including cardiovascular disease, cancer, urinary incontinence, prostate hyperplasia, and several others.

Linking the Physiology to Pharmacology

How medication kinetics and dynamics are affected is complex. Drugs are made up of chemicals, and all chemicals and elements have an affinity or charge attraction: acidic, neutral, basic. This then relates to a drug's affinity to certain body stores, such as the gut, and being hydrophilic (charged ions like water more) or lipophilic (neutral carbon-based molecules like fats). Digoxin, for example, is hydrophilic, so as an elderly patient's muscle mass and total body water decrease, the ability for digoxin to accumulate and produce an effect decreases. Propofol is lipophilic, so as muscle is replaced by fat, less propofol is needed to produce the same effect in the elderly (all other variables ignored).[50–62] Decreased protein (albumin) decreases the binding of certain drugs, such as levothyroxine (Synthroid).[50–62]

Despite slow gastric emptying and an increase in gastric pH, however, absorption remains typically unaffected in older adults.[50–62]

Due to older adults often having multiple drug regimens, this group is particularly at risk for drug and food interactions. For example, cimetidine is a common over-the-counter acid reflux drug, but it is an inhibitor of liver enzymes (most important is cytochrome P450 3A4 or CYP3A4). If a patient who is taking warfarin, which is metabolized by the liver, starts taking cimetidine on their own initiative, the warfarin will not be metabolized (ADME) as well and therefore will have a smaller therapeutic effect. The warfarin dose needs to be increased to compensate for this change. There are lengthy lists of CYP inhibitors and stimulators. Milk and milk products decrease the absorption of oral bisphosphonates, which is why they are instructed to be taken on empty stomachs. Refer to Table 19.4 for some of the more prevalent drug interactions.

As mentioned in the physiology section, advanced age increases renal dysfunction. Approximately one-third of elderly patients have a normal glomerular filtration rate. Several drugs are excreted renally. If they are not being filtered out as effectively, they then circulate in the body for a longer time, increasing efficacy. The decreased hepatic mass and splanchnic blood flow also decreases the liver's metabolization of drugs. Consequently, lower therapeutic doses should be considered in elderly individuals. This can be achieved by decreasing the total daily dosage (100 mg daily to 75 mg daily) or changing the frequency (100 mg daily to 50 mg twice a day).[49,50,63–66]

Medication Classes of Concern

There are several classes of drugs represented by medications included in Table 19.4 and in Fig. 19.3.

Statins

These drugs were designed to lower low-density lipoprotein (LDL) cholesterol. Their main risk is statin-induced myopathy and hepatotoxicity. The literature does not mention any increased risk in the elderly, but it can be assumed that as liver function declines with age, these drugs can wreak more havoc and are more likely to cause worrisome side effects.[62]

NSAIDs

Nonsteroidal anti-inflammatory drugs (NSAIDs) are common, both over-the-counter and prescribed. The most common is aspirin (ASA), which acts like an "NSAID+" as it is anti-inflammatory at some doses and is also antiplatelet at others. It is common practice to prescribe 81 mg ASA dose after stroke, heart attack, and pre-eclampsia. Ibuprofen is commonly used as well for pain. NSAIDs are not perfect cure-alls, however; there is an increased risk of gastrointestinal bleeding or peptic ulcer disease. This risk is accrued over time and is also dose-related. There is also an increased risk of kidney injury. Older patients are at increased risk of peptic ulcers, and bleeding. Acetaminophen, while not technically an NSAID, does still cause liver damage, especially in acute toxic overdoses.[33,65,67–70]

Diuretics

Diuretics are used to treat hypertension commonly, as they help the patient decrease their total body water volume. As mentioned, older patients have a decreased water volume already, so they are at risk of dehydration and drastic decreases in blood pressure. Lisinopril does have similar effects on the elderly. It is used to treat hypertension, prevents kidney disease, and is part of standard heart failure treatment. Look out for hypotension, dizziness, syncope, fatigue, hyperkalemia, acute kidney injury, and cough. It is a bad recipe for falls in the elderly.[33,61,64]

Steroids and Hormonal Analogues

Prednisone and steroids are used for multiple ailments. Because of their lipophilic properties, steroids need to be tapered as they have long half-lives and thereby can have stacking effects if not dosed correctly. Levothyroxine is a thyroid hormone analog, which itself can cause tachycardia and other "turned up" symptoms such as hyperthermia and clonus. There are no specific indications for changes in steroids or hormones in older patient populations.[49,50]

Opioids and Analgesics

Pain, sleeping changes/disorders, and anxiety are the most common reasons for these kinds of drugs to be prescribed. These can be opioids, benzodiazepines, barbiturates, and more. Especially in the elderly, these drugs can cause respiratory depression to the point of apnea. This effect is multiplied when more than one class is prescribed (e.g., opioids and benzos). Overdose is a huge risk with these, as is addiction. Overdose deaths have been associated with tachycardia, respiratory failure, seizures, coma, and serotonin syndrome. With the increasing aged population, drug misuse and abuse are increasing in these patients. It has been reported that long-term use of opioids and benzos increases the risk of falls, hip fractures, and traffic accidents. Elderly patients have increased sensitivity and decreased metabolism of the long-acting agents in these classes.[33,49,50,59,65,69,71–78]

As an aside, there are changes to sedation and induction agent dosing for rapid sequence intubation (RSI) that are recommended in older adults. Etomidate can have a dose reduction between 20% and 50%. Propofol dosing can be reduced by 20%. A dose reduction of 33% is recommended for dexmedetomidine in the elderly. Rocuronium, a paralytic often used for RSI, has a longer elimination half-life in the elderly compared to younger controls by roughly 16 minutes. Thus, redosing intervals should be longer in the geriatric population.[33,49–51,59,65,69,71–78]

Beta-Blockers and Cardiac Drugs

If the cardiac disease is the leading cause of death in the world, then the prevalence of congestive heart failure (CHF) has to be high as well. Goal-directed medical therapy (GDMT) refers to a variety of drugs that all CHF patients should adhere to take as they progress through their disease process. Beta-blockers are a staple of this. They can cause hypotension, bradycardia, dizziness, fatigue, depressed mood, confusion, and erectile dysfunction, more so in older populations than younger patients. Like analgesics and benzos, there is an increased risk of falls, syncope, and orthostatic hypotension with concurrent rate-control drugs (calcium channel blockers and beta-blockers, or beta-blockers and benzos).[79–85]

Anticoagulants/Antithrombotic

Age is an independent risk factor for the development of atrial fibrillation (AF). Older patients represent the largest majority of those with AF. AF patients are often treated with rate-control drugs but also need to be anticoagulated because of their increased CHA_2DS_2-VASc risk score for thrombosis and clots. With increased fragility and fall risk in the elderly, there is some hesitance in anticoagulating these populations because of increased brain hemorrhage risk. Studies show a lack of anticoagulant prescribing for these patients when it is clinically indicated. The risk of falls should not be considered a contraindication to the use of anticoagulants. High bleeding risk should not be interpreted as a contraindication to the use of antithrombotics.[86] Important drug interactions are aspirin or NSAIDs along with blood thinners. Ginkgo biloba is a common herbal medicine that increases the risk of bleeding with antithrombotic drugs as well. Warfarin is CYP3A4 metabolized and has a slew of interactions with drugs and foods.[33,55,63,64,66,85,87–89]

Beers Criteria

As mentioned above, the Beers Criteria is a comprehensive resource to help guide pharmacy decisions to improve the care of patients 65 years of age and older. It comprises a consensus list of medicines considered to be inappropriate for long-term care facility residents for a variety of reasons.[33]

Physical and Mental Abuse of the Elderly

Eldercare Locator Hotline (1-800-677-1116) and website (https://eldercare.acl.gov) can help to find the appropriate agency for reporting older adult abuse.

The sad truth is that 16% of older adults experience abuse at some point, and this may be an underestimation. Older adult abuse is defined as any form of physical, sexual, psychological, or financial mistreatment or neglect of an older adult at the hands of a caregiver. Multiple circumstances can facilitate abuse, including dementia, social isolation, lack of support, and living in an assisted living facility. Individuals with greater physical limitations are more vulnerable to abuse. Elder abuse is perpetrated most commonly by someone close to the victim, frequently a male spouse or adult child. Resident-to-resident abuse may be more prevalent than staff-to-resident abuse at nursing facilities. In the United States, minority adults may be at higher risk for mistreatment and also are much less likely to report or seek assistance from available services. Black Americans experience three times as much financial exploitation and four times as much psychologic abuse as their White counterparts. Remember, some of these patients cannot make their own medical decisions or even daily decisions, much like some children. They could be completely unaware of the situation.[90–95]

For screening tools, there is the Detection of Elder Mistreatment Through Emergency Care Technicians (specific for EMS), the Elder Abuse Suspicion Index, Elder Assessment Instrument, ED Senior AID, Vulnerability to Abuse Screening Scale, Geriatric

Injury Documentation Tool (Geri-IDT), and Responding to Elder Abuse in GERiAtric Care – Provider questionnaire (REAGERA-P).[90–105] Some key features that can be gleaned during an interview include conflicting accounts of events/history, caregiver interrupts/answers for the older adult, older adult seems fearful of or hostile toward the caregiver, unengaged/inattentive in caring for the patient, caregiver seems frustrated, tired, angry, burdened, overwhelmed by the older adult, lack knowledge of the patient's care needs, and illicit substance use. Look out for reports of theft, unexplained injuries such as multiple bruises or burns, trauma, irregular alopecia, parallel injuries, the patterned shape of bruising, different healing stages of lesions, dehydration, malnutrition, unusual fractures, depression, and unusual or hostile behavior, especially if it is a marked change. If the patient has ulcers or other medical conditions that have been "ignored," it could be caregiver neglect, an often-missed form of abuse.[90–102] There are a variety of different warning signs of elder abuse, however no one sign is specific. It falls upon you to rely upon gut feeling and being aware of a nonconsistent story. Listen to the patient. Be their advocate.

Elder abuse, like any abuse, is thought to be grossly underreported. Medical providers have a legal and ethical obligation to report older adult abuse, even if the patient is consenting. Despite the obvious potential to increase detection and initiate intervention, the US Preventive Services Task Force found insufficient evidence that screening for elder abuse in clinical settings reduces harm. There is no association between abuse and earlier death. Despite the lack of evidence for harm reduction, the American Medical Association and other professional organizations still recommend assessing patients for elder abuse, citing an ethical responsibility to attempt to detect this life-threatening condition. There is protection from litigation if you report unfounded cases of abuse. Depending on the life-threatening danger to the patient and how imminent action must be taken, you can inform law enforcement, Adult Protective Services, and/or the Long-Term Care Ombudsman program (if the patient lives in a facility/nursing home). While this is the only studied intervention, using local resources to help control factors would be beneficial. Keep in mind also that some US states require reporting within a certain period of time, check your state or local protocols, policies, or procedures.[90,94,97,98,103,104]

Older adults who suffer from abuse have worse outcomes from preexisting health conditions and are more likely to be placed in a long-term care facility. All types of abuse increase the risk of depression and anxiety, and abuse victims may have an increased risk for thoughts of suicide compared with unexposed peers. Older people exposed to abuse are more likely to utilize EMS services, and the emergency department, and to require hospitalization.[92,96,99,100,105–107]

Cases Involving Hospice, Palliative Care, and Do Not Resuscitate Orders

Prehospital provider training is primarily focused on resuscitation and saving lives. Not uncommonly, however, they find themselves responding to calls for patients who are enrolled in hospice, are comfort measures only, or are receiving palliative care. While providing palliative care may not have been considered traditional expertise for prehospital providers, there is evidence that providing this type of care is becoming more accepted and integrated into their evolving professional identity.[106] The need for palliative

care skills is increasingly being recognized by EMS providers and additional experience and education with palliative care results in a greater appreciation for its importance.[107] At the same time, prehospital providers often report they do not feel adequately trained to care for patients in hospice or with comfort-focused treatment.[108–110] They are also faced with managing intense and complex emotions from family members.[111,112] Understanding the nature and goals of palliative care, and the issues that frequently arise in the out-of-hospital setting, can empower prehospital nurses to provide patient-centered care in challenging circumstances.

Overview

Palliative care is care focused on the quality of life in patients with serious illness.[113] When the medical care that a patient is receiving is exclusively focused on palliative measures, patients often elect to enroll in hospice care. The goal of hospice care is to keep patients with short life expectancies as comfortable as possible. In the US, hospice care is most often provided in the patient's home setting, be it a private residence or a nursing facility.[114] When considering health care at the end of life, emergency health care and terminal hospitalizations can be inappropriate due to ineffective resource utilization and inconsistency with goals of care.[115] To promote goal-concordant care, quality of life, and effective healthcare utilization, efforts have been ongoing to integrate palliative care earlier in patients' disease trajectories; however, despite this, most patients do not receive palliative care until a few weeks before death.[115]

Utilizing EMS for Palliative Care and Hospice Patients

Most EMS providers will interface with patients at the end of life. A US survey of EMS providers revealed that 84.1% had cared for at least one hospice patient in their career.[116] Canadian researchers have found that in the last 2 weeks of life, 40% of patients with goals focused on palliative care visit an emergency department, and over half of these visits involve emergency medical services.[106] Approximately one-third of EMS calls for patients enrolled in hospice or whose medical goals were comfort measures only were for patients in a nursing facility, and the remaining calls are from home according to one study. While prehospital providers recognize that transport of patients at the end of life to the hospital setting may not be optimal in all cases, an Australian study found that nearly 75% of these calls resulted in transport to the hospital.[106,117]

Some common themes identified by hospice providers as to why a patient in hospice or their family member seek hospital care include: not fully understanding hospice, lack of understanding about disease prognosis, desire to continue receiving care from nonhospice physicians and hospital, caregiver burden, difficulty managing symptoms, caregivers' reluctance to administer medications, 911's faster response time compared to hospice, and families' difficulty accepting patients' mortality.[118,119] A lack of understanding about the dying process, an abrupt change in the patient's status, or a change in the caregiver's ability to handle the clinical situation are also reasons for contacting EMS.[110,120] A review of EMS records for patients who are comfort measures only or enrolled in hospice cited respiratory complaints (96; 18.0%), altered mental status (96; 18.0%), weakness (58; 10.9%), and cardiac arrest (45; 8.4%) as the most common impressions.[119] Other clinical reasons for engaging emergency medical services include pain, massive bleeding episodes, and falls.[117,120] EMS may also be called for end-of-life or hospice patients residing in nursing homes. In a retrospective study conducted in the US, approximately one-third of EMS calls for hospice and comfort care patients originated from skilled nursing facilities.[119] There can be several reasons for this; crises in clinical care, dying-related turmoil, unfavorable staffing ratios, and organizational protocols were frequently perceived reasons that nursing home staff initiate emergency medical services contact.[121]

Contribution of EMS in Palliative Care and Collaboration

EMS can play an important role in providing palliative care, and the need and opportunities exist.[107] The provision of, and integration of, prehospital palliative care is important to provide "care across boundaries."[115] As in many situations, emergency medical services are often called upon to fill in the gap when an extensive outpatient palliative care system is lacking.[112] EMS providers can be integral in managing distressing symptoms, in addition to supporting patients and their caregivers by providing goal-concordant care in line with the wishes expressed in advanced directives.[115] In addition, when a patient experiences a clinical emergency that may be terminal, EMS might be the first point of contact with the healthcare system.[122] Decisions made in the prehospital setting can set the trajectory for further palliative care.[107] Additionally, there are situations in which utilization of emergency medical services may be the only way to transport patients from the inpatient setting back to home or a desired location closer to home, providing a critical link to facilitate patients in their end-of-life wishes.[107,115,120] By supporting patients in providing pre-hospital palliative care, EMS services are an important part of an ethical healthcare system that upholds patient autonomy, beneficence, non-maleficence, and human dignity.[107] Collaboration between emergency medical services and community-based palliative care organizations results in more goal-aligned care for palliative care patients when emergency medical situations arise.[123] Several innovative prehospital palliative care models have been developed to meet these needs. Some services have developed prehospital palliative care specialty teams or have identified a palliative care specialist or champion.[107] In some areas, mobile integrated hospice healthcare programs have been developed to fill this need.[124,125] Palliative homecare organizations have also forged collaborative relationships with EMS services, creating a "home urgent care" service for palliative care patients that they serve.[126] It is likely that additional service models will develop as the role of prehospital providers in palliative care becomes increasingly recognized and researched.

Barriers to the Provision of Prehospital Palliative Care

Despite the role of prehospital providers in palliative care and the alignment of providing this type of care with their professional identity, EMS personnel still experience many challenges and barriers when the need and opportunity for these services arise. Traditional views of EMS care as focused on the goal of hospitalization can still dominate.[107,127] Arriving on the scene in stressful

circumstances, EMS providers may have insufficient information about the patient, condition, and overall situation to make decisions about palliative or comfort care or to deviate from "normal" transport procedures.[107,127,128] Even when providers and patients recognize that avoiding hospitalization may be desirable, limited community availability or access to additional or alternative care support may constrain the ability of EMS providers to maintain the patient in the home.[127]

There may be insufficient system-level support for EMS services to provide palliative care. Lack of provider education in palliative care and limited research on the role of EMS and end-of-life and palliative care are two important barriers.[107,110,115] These are two factors contributing to the current lack of a defined role for prehospital personnel in palliative care.[110] Current protocols and guidelines may be inadequate to support prehospital palliative care.[107,110,115] In fact, a study published in 2002 indicated that only 5.8% of EMS agencies had palliative care protocols.[129] A lack of "treat and release" protocols may limit a provider's ability or confidence in avoiding hospital transport. Clinical situations, such as severe symptoms requiring palliative management, may not be adequately addressed in existing protocols. Lack of equipment, medications, or other resources may impede optimal palliation.[107,120]

The time needed to address patient and family concerns in prehospital palliative scenarios can also cause challenges. Providers who remain on-scene to provide palliative care for symptom management and avoid transport may be penalized by quality metrics that prioritize fast scene times.[110] Another important barrier to providing high-quality prehospital palliative care is the opportunity cost. Long scene-times to care for patients can limit the ability of the unit to respond to other calls in the community.[110] Transporting patients back to their homes at the end of life, or to hospice facilities for additional palliative treatment and support, may limit availability to respond to other EMS calls.[107] This can create a systems-level dilemma, as well as provider stress. Finally, unresolved legal considerations and concerns may affect protocol development, research, and clinical provision of palliative care.[107,115,130,131]

Identifying Goals of Care and Treatment Limitations

Determining a patient's wishes and treatment limitations can be challenging for a patient residing at home and for nursing home patients as well.[132] A POST, or Provider Orders for Scope of Treatment, is a form that is voluntarily completed by a patient to specify their preferences for medical care. A POST dictates a patient's wishes regarding medical interventions such as cardiopulmonary resuscitation (CPR), intubation, vasopressors, artificial nutrition, and IV fluids.[111] All 50 states in the US have some version of a POST form. Some states have online registries of medical orders for treatment limitations and advanced directives, such as medical power of attorney. This can be a reference for EMS personnel if time and opportunity allow. One study found that accessing these types of registries changed the care of the patient in 44% of cases; in 26% of cases, it changed the decision to transport the patient.[133] Studies suggest that prehospital providers feel comfortable interpreting a POST form, but at times find them confusing. Most paramedics feel confident in deciding when to start or withhold CPR on pulseless patients, but when a patient is still breathing and has a pulse, the forms can be harder to decipher.[133,134] At times, the forms may contain conflicting information.[119,131] Difficulty can also arise when a patient's family say they know the dying patient's wishes, but there is no documentation to support it, or there is documentation, but it is not available.[112,135–137]

Prehospital providers can experience pressure from family members, nursing home staff, and even colleagues to provide care or interventions that are against a patient's best interest or expressed wishes.[115] Conflict occurs when a family member claims that the patient has a DNR order but does not have the documentation, or when DNR documentation is present and the family member is asking the paramedic to provide care against the wishes of the patient.[112,122,134] Specific challenges may include situations in which the family revokes an existing Do Not Resuscitate order at the time of a terminal event, or when CPR has been initiated and a DNR order is subsequently located.[130] Disagreements can also occur between family members, or between the patient and their family members.[107,112] When accessing online information is not possible, or when conflict persists, the online medical direction can help support prehospital providers.[134]

Clinical Care and Communication

Some providers have the perception that providing life-sustaining treatment, such as mechanical ventilation, is the only way to relieve discomfort due to serious illness or the dying process; however, these interventions can be burdensome and prolong life.[110] When a patient has expressed their desire to limit these types of interventions, prehospital providers still have many options to provide support and treatment for uncomfortable or painful symptoms. Unfortunately, very few studies have been published that examine the economic implications of providing prehospital palliative care or investigated the implementation of clinical practice guidelines regarding providing end-of-life care by prehospital providers.[138]

Prehospital providers are uniquely positioned to arrive quickly on the scene of a patient or family in distress at the end of life and provide prompt relief of symptoms and suffering. Waldrop et al.

described a multifocal assessment that prehospital providers can provide when attending the end-of-life calls. This assessment includes assessing the patient, assessing the family, and assessing the environment.[112] On patient assessment, dyspnea may be present. Opioid medications can relieve the discomfort associated with respiratory distress at the end of life.[139–141] If dyspnea is not adequately controlled with opioid medication, especially if there is associated anxiety, a benzodiazepine medication can be useful.[142] The use and benefit of supplemental oxygen in patients experiencing breathlessness at the end of life are more controversial.[141,143] Opioid medication may also be required to control pain at the end of life and repeat doses may be necessary to produce an adequate response.[141,144,145]

Providers have noted that intense emotions from family members can be harder to manage than the care of the patient.[112] The field of palliative care recognizes several communication skills and strategies that could potentially be helpful in the prehospital setting.[146] These skills include techniques for empathetic communication, delivering bad news, and alignment with patient and family goals.

Future Directions

Prehospital providers should be given additional training and support for administering clinical palliative care and addressing related communication tasks. Protocols and medical oversight should be established to assist providers caring for those at the end of life. EMS personnel should have access to registries containing advanced care planning documents and be sufficiently trained to interpret such documents. Primary care and palliative providers should also encourage their patients to keep copies of POST forms and similar documents readily available for emergencies. Additional research in the area of prehospital palliative care can help further define the role of EMS, identify additional educational needs, and suggest system-level advancements to empower EMS providers to support their patients and community in palliative and end-of-life care.

Summary

The care and transport of geriatric patients are complicated by many factors from the effects of aging on essentially every organ system to the medications they are taking, their sensitivity to various therapies, comorbidities, and even a need to respect their autonomy when they have made end-of-life decisions. Such transports require the provider to have a strong grasp on these concepts, thus allowing them the opportunity to anticipate potential pitfalls they may encounter and respond appropriately.

References

1. American Medical Association. Geriatric medicine (FM). FREIDA: American Medical Association Residency & Fellowship Database. Available at: https://freida.ama-assn.org/specialty/geriatric-medicine-fm.

2. Aschkenasy MT, Rothenhaus TC. Trauma and falls in the elderly. *Emerg Med Clin North Am.* 2006;24(2):413–432. doi: 10.1016/j.emc.2006.01.005

3. United Nations Department of Economic and Social Affairs, Population Division. World Population Prospects 2022: Summary of Results. UN DESA/POP/2022/TR/NO February 22, 2023.

4. Administration for Community Living; US Department of Health and Human Services. Projected future growth of older population. [Last modified May 4, 2022.]

5. United States Census Bureau. Population 65 years and over in the United States. American Community Survey, 2022: ACS 1-Year Estimates Subject Tables, Table S0103. Available at: https://data.census.gov/table/ACSST1Y2022.S0103?q=s0103.

6. Dickinson ET, Verdile VP, Kostyun CT, Salluzzo RF. Geriatric use of emergency medical services. *Ann Emerg Med.* 1996;27:199–203. doi: 10.1016/S0196-0644(96)70323-2

7. Shah MN, Bazarian JJ, Lerner EB, et al. The epidemiology of emergency medical services use by older adults: an analysis of the National Hospital Ambulatory Medical Care Survey. *Acad Emerg Med.* 2007;14:441–447. doi.org/10.1111/j.1553-2712.2007.tb01804.x

8. Administration of Aging; Administration for Community Living. 2020 Profile of older Americans. US Department of Health and Human Services; 2021. Available at: https://acl.gov/sites/default/files/Profile%20of%20OA/2020ProfileOlderAmericans_RevisedFinal.pdf

9. Jiang L, Zheng Z, Zhang M. The incidence of geriatric trauma is increasing and comparison of different scoring tools for the prediction of in-hospital mortality in geriatric trauma patients. *World J Emerg Surg.* 2020;15:59. doi: 10.1186/s13017-020-00340-1

10. American College of Surgeons, Committee on Trauma, National Trauma Data Bank (NTDB). Graph and Table retrieved from http://www.facs.org/trauma/ntdb.

11. Wilson MS, Konda SR, Seymour RB, Karunakar MA; The Carolinas Trauma Network Research Group. Early predictors of mortality in geriatric patients with trauma. *J Orthopaedic Trauma.* 2016;30(9): e299–e304. doi: 10.1097/BOT.0000000000000615

12. Min L, Burruss S, Morley E, et al. A simple clinical risk nomogram to predict mortality associated geriatric complications in severely injured geriatric patients. *J Trauma Acute Care Surg.* 2013;74(4):1125–1132.

13. Bryan Y, Johnson K, Botros D, Groban L. Anatomic and physio-pathologic changes affecting the airway of the elderly patient: implications for geriatric-focused airway management. *Clin Interv Aging.* 2015;10:1925–1934. doi: 10.2147/cia.s93796

14. Panjiar P, Bhat K, Yousuf I, Kochhar A, Ralli T. Study comparing different airway assessment tests in predicting difficult laryngoscopy: a prospective study in geriatric patients. *Ind J Anaesth.* 2021;65(4):309. doi: 10.4103/ija.ija_1413_20

15. Eichinger M, Robb HDP, Scurr C, Tucker H, Heschl S, Peck G. Challenges in the PREHOSPITAL emergency management of geriatric trauma patients – a scoping review. *Scand J Trauma, Resusc Emerg Med.* 2021;29(1):100. doi: 10.1186/s13049-021-00922-1

16. Pandit V, Rhee P, Hashmi A, et al. Shock index predicts mortality in geriatric trauma patients. *J Trauma Acute Care Surg.* 2014;76(4):1111–1115. doi: 10.1097/ta.0000000000000160

17. Duvillard C, Lafaie L, de Magalhaes É, et al. Implementation of a systematic comprehensive geriatric assessment for elderly patients suspected of pulmonary hypertension. *Respir Med Res.* 2020;78: 100785. doi: 10.1016/j.resmer.2020.100785

18. Peruzza S, Sergi G, Vianello A, et al. Chronic obstructive pulmonary disease (COPD) in elderly subjects: impact on functional status and quality of life. *Respir Med.* 2003;97(6):612–617. doi: 10.1053/rmed.2003.1488

19. Stoller J. COPD Exacerbations: Management. UpToDate, Aug 8, 2022. Available at: https://www.uptodate.com/contents/copd-exacerbations-management.

20. Newgard CD, Lin A, Eckstrom E, et al. Comorbidities, anticoagulants, and geriatric-specific physiology for the field triage of injured older adults. *J Trauma Acute Care Surg.* 2019;86(5):829–837. doi: 10.1097/ta.0000000000002195

21. Brown JB, Gestring ML, Forsythe RM, et al. Systolic blood pressure criteria in the National Trauma Triage Protocol for geriatric trauma. *J Trauma Acute Care Surg.* 2015;78(2):352–359. doi: 10.1097/ta.0000000000000523

22. Alshibani A, Alharbi M, Conroy S. Under-triage of older trauma patients in prehospital care: a systematic review. *Eur Geriat Med.* 2021;12(5):903–919. doi: 10.1007/s41999-021-00512-5

23. Rosen P. *Rosen's Emergency Medicine: Concepts and Clinical Practice.* 6th ed, St. Louis, MO: Mosby; 2006.

24. Cone D, Brice JH, Delbridge TR, Myers JB. *Emergency Medical Services: Clinical Practice and Systems Oversight*, 2 Volume Set. Hoboken, NJ: John Wiley & Sons; 2015.

25. HealthinAging.org. Wellness & Prevention. Available at: https://www.healthinaging.org.

26. Cazzola M et al. *Acute Exacerbations in COPD (Therapeutic Strategies).* Fayetteville, NC: Clinical Publishing; 2009.

27. Abdo WF, Heunks LM. Oxygen-induced hypercapnia in COPD: myths and facts. *Crit Care.* 2012;16(5):323. doi: 10.1186/cc11475

28. O'Driscoll BR, Howard LS, Davison AG. BTS guideline for emergency oxygen use in adult patients. *Thorax.* 2008;16(Suppl 6):vi1–68.

29. Austin MA, Wills KE, Blizzard L, Walters EH, Wood-Baker R. Effect of high flow oxygen on mortality in chronic obstructive pulmonary disease patients in prehospital setting: randomised controlled trial. *BMJ.* 2010;16:c5462. doi: 10.1136/bmj.c5462

30. Norman D. Fever in the elderly. *Clin Infect Dis.* 200;31(1):148–151. doi: 10.1086/313869

31. Malabu U, Vangaveti V, Kennedy L. Disease burden evaluation of fall-related events in the elderly due to hypoglycemia and other diabetic complications: a clinical review. *Clin Epidemiol.* 2014;6: 287–294. doi: 10.2147/clep.s66821

32. Aggarwal P, Woolford SJ, Patel HP. Multi-morbidity and polypharmacy in older people: challenges and opportunities for clinical practice. *Geriatrics.* 2020;5(4):85. doi: 10.3390/geriatrics5040085

33. The 2019 American Geriatrics Society Beers Criteria Update Expert Panel. American Geriatrics Society 2019 Updated AGS Beers Criteria for Potentially Inappropriate Medication Use in Older Adults. *J Am Geriatr Soc.* 2019;67(4):674–694. doi: 10.1111/jgs.15767

34. Cifu DX. *Braddom's Physical Medicine and Rehabilitation.* Elsevier; 2020.

35. Tintinalli JE, Ma OJ, Yealy D, et al. *Tintinalli's Emergency Medicine: A Comprehensive Study Guide.* 9th ed. New York: McGraw Hill Professional; 2019:1677–1680.

36. Marx JA, Walls RM. *Rosen's Emergency Medicine: Concepts and Clinical Practice.* Vol 1. 6th ed. St. Louis, MO: Mosby Elsevier; 2006:344–349.

37. Gardner RC, Dams-O'Connor K, Morrissey MR, Manley GT. Geriatric traumatic brain injury: epidemiology, outcomes, knowledge gaps, and future directions. *J Neurotrauma.* 2018;35(7): 889–906. doi: 10.1089/neu.2017.5371

38. Suehiro E, Fujiyama Y, Kiyohira M, et al. Risk of deterioration of geriatric traumatic brain injury in patients treated with antithrombotic drugs. *World Neurosurg.* 2019;127:1221–1227. doi: 10.1016/j.wneu.2019.04.108

39. Khan M, O'Keeffe T, Jehan F, et al. The impact of Glasgow Coma Scale–age prognosis score on geriatric traumatic brain injury outcomes. *J Surg Res.* 2017;216:109–114. doi: 10.1016/j.jss.2017.04.026

40. Mentzer CJ, Walsh NJ, Talukder A, et al. Thoracic trauma in the oldest of the old: an analysis of the nationwide inpatient sample. *Am Surg.* 2017;83(5):491-494. doi: 10.1177/000313481708300524

41. González R, Fuentes A, Riquelme A, et al. Traumatismo torácico en el adulto mayor. *Revista Chilena de Cirugía.* 2020;72(3):224–230.

42. Elmistekawy E, Hammad AA. Isolated rib fractures in geriatric patients. *Ann Thorac Med.* 2007;2(4):166. doi: 10.4103/1817-1737.36552

43. Vollrath JT, Schindler CR, Marzi I, Lefering R, Störmann P. Lung failure after polytrauma with concomitant thoracic trauma in the elderly: an analysis from the TraumaRegister DGU. *World J Emerg Surg.* 2022;17(1):12. doi: 10.1186/s13017-022-00416-0

44. Schattner A, Mavor E, Adi M. Unsuspected serious abdominal trauma after falls among community-dwelling older adults. *QJM.* 2014;107(8):649–653. doi: 10.1093/qjmed/hcu050

45. Kanezaki S, Miyazaki M, Notani N, Tsumura H. Clinical presentation of geriatric polytrauma patients with severe pelvic fractures: comparison with younger adult patients. *Eur J Orthop Surg Traumatol.* 2016;26(8):885–890. doi: 10.1007/s00590-016-1822-7

46. Gage M, Dunbar RP, Lowe JA. Pelvic fractures. OrthoInfo. American Academy of Orthopedic Surgeons. [Last reviewed May 2023.] Available at: https://orthoinfo.aaos.org/en/diseases—conditions/pelvic-fractures/.

47. Rosen T, Mulcare MR, Stern ME, et al. 225 Geriatric burn injuries presenting to the emergency department of a major burn center: clinical characteristics and outcomes. *Ann Emerg Med.* 2014; 64(4):S81. doi: 10.1016/j.annemergmed.2014.07.252

48. Abu-Sittah GS, Chahine FM, Janom H. Management of burns in the elderly. *Ann Burns Fire Disasters.* 2016;29(4):249–254.

49. AHFS Drug Information. Essentials. AHFS Clinical Drug Information. Bethesda, MD: American Society of Health-System Pharmacists; Updated 2021.

50. Dashboard – AMBOSS. December 26, 2022. Available at: https://next.amboss.com/us.

51. Wastesson JW, Morin L, Tan ECK, Johnell K. An update on the clinical consequences of polypharmacy in older adults: a narrative review. *Expert Opin Drug Saf.* 2018;17(12):1185–1196. doi: 10.1080/14740338.2018.1546841

52. Andres TM, McGrane T, McEvoy MD, Allen BFS. Geriatric pharmacology. *Anesthesiol Clin.* 2019;37(3):475–492. doi: 10.1016/j.anclin.2019.04.007

53. Means KM, Kortebein PM, eds. *Geriatrics.* New York: Demos Medical; 2013.

54. Benson JM. Antimicrobial pharmacokinetics and pharmacodynamics in older adults. *Infect Dis Clin North Am.* 2017;31(4):609–617. doi: 10.1016/j.idc.2017.07.011

55. Gronich N, Stein N, Muszkat M. Association between use of pharmacokinetic-interacting drugs and effectiveness and safety of direct acting oral anticoagulants: nested case-control study. *Clin Pharmacol Ther.* 2021;110(6):1526–1536. doi: 10.1002/cpt.2369

56. Montecino-Rodriguez E, Berent-Maoz B, Dorshkind K. Causes, consequences, and reversal of immune system aging. *J Clin Invest.* 2013;123(3):958–965. doi: 10.1172/JCI64096

57. Yun M. Changes in regenerative capacity through lifespan. *Int J Mol Sci.* 2015;16(10):25392–25432. doi: 10.3390/ijms161025392

58. Sharma G, Goodwin J. Effect of aging on respiratory system physiology and immunology. *Clin Interv Aging.* 2006;1(3):253–260. doi: 10.2147/ciia.2006.1.3.253

59. Ailabouni NJ, Marcum ZA, Schmader KE, Gray SL. Medication use quality and safety in older adults: 2019 Update. *J Am Geriatr Soc.* 2021;69(2):336–341. doi: 10.1111/jgs.17018

60. Tarn DM, Barrientos M, Wang AY, Ramaprasad A, Fang MC, Schwartz JB. Prevalence and knowledge of potential interactions between over-the-counter products and apixaban. *J Am Geriatr Soc.* 2020;68(1):155–162. doi: 10.1111/jgs.16193

61. Denic A, Glassock RJ, Rule AD. Structural and functional changes with the aging kidney. *Adv Chron Kidney Dis.* 2016;23(1):19–28. doi: 10.1053/j.ackd.2015.08.004

62. Horodinschi RN, Stanescu AMA, Bratu OG, Pantea Stoian A, Radavoi DG, Diaconu CC. Treatment with statins in elderly patients. *Medicina (Mex).* 2019;55(11):721. doi: 10.3390/medicina55110721

63. Comans AL, Sennesael AL, Bihin B, Regnier M, Mullier F, de Saint-Hubert M. Inappropriate low dosing of direct oral anticoagulants in older patients with non-valvular atrial fibrillation: impact on plasma drug levels. *Thromb Res.* 2021;201:139–142. doi: 10.1016/j.thromres.2021.02.034

64. De Vincentis A, Gallo P, Finamore P, et al. Potentially inappropriate medications, drug–drug interactions, and anticholinergic burden in elderly hospitalized patients: does an association exist with post-discharge health outcomes? *Drugs Aging.* 2020;37(8):585–593. doi: 10.1007/s40266-020-00767-w

65. Gutiérrez-Valencia M, Izquierdo M, Cesari M, Casas-Herrero Á, Inzitari M, Martínez-Velilla N. The relationship between frailty and polypharmacy in older people: a systematic review. Frailty and polypharmacy: a systematic review. *Br J Clin Pharmacol.* 2018;84(7):1432–1444. doi: 10.1111/bcp.13590

66. Agbabiaka TB, Wider B, Watson LK, Goodman C. Concurrent use of prescription drugs and herbal medicinal products in older adults: a systematic review. *Drugs Aging.* 2017;34(12):891–905. doi: 10.1007/s40266-017-0501-7

67. Morin L, Laroche ML, Vetrano DL, Fastbom J, Johnell K. Adequate, questionable, and inadequate drug prescribing for older adults at the end of life: a European expert consensus. *Eur J Clin Pharmacol.* 2018;74(10):1333–1342. doi: 10.1007/s00228-018-2507-4

68. Cisewski DH. Pain in older adults. In: *Pain Management Guide: Evidence-Based Alternative Analgesia* (ch. 13). Emergency Medicine Residents' Association; 2020: ch. 13. Available at: http://www.emra.org/books/pain-management/geriatric-pain/.

69. van der Gaag WH, Roelofs PD, Enthoven WT, van Tulder MW, Koes BW. Non-steroidal anti-inflammatory drugs for acute low back pain. *Cochrane Database Syst Rev.* 2020;4(4):CD013581. doi: 10.1002/14651858.CD013581

70. Reginster JY, Beaudart C, Al-Daghri N, et al. Update on the ESCEO recommendation for the conduct of clinical trials for drugs aiming at the treatment of sarcopenia in older adults. *Aging Clin Exp Res.* 2021;33(1):3–17. doi: 10.1007/s40520-020-01663-4

71. Carpenter CR, Cameron A, Ganz DA, Liu S. Older adult falls in emergency medicine. *Clin Geriatr Med.* 2019;35(2):205–219. doi: 10.1016/j.cger.2019.01.009

72. Carpenter CR, Cameron A, Ganz DA, Liu S. Older adult falls in emergency medicine—a sentinel event. *Clin Geriatr Med.* 2018; 34(3):355–367. doi: 10.1016/j.cger.2018.04.002

73. Lee J, Negm A, Peters R, Wong EKC, Holbrook A. Deprescribing fall-risk increasing drugs (FRIDs) for the prevention of falls and fall-related complications: a systematic review and meta-analysis. *BMJ Open.* 2021;11(2):e035978. doi: 10.1136/bmjopen-2019-035978

74. Ryba N, Rainess R. Z-drugs and falls: a focused review of the literature. *Sr Care Pharm.* 2020;35(12):549–554. doi: 10.4140/TCP.n.2020.549

75. Seppala LJ, Petrovic M, Ryg J, et al. STOPPFall (Screening Tool of Older Persons Prescriptions in older adults with high fall risk): a Delphi study by the EuGMS Task and Finish Group on Fall-Risk-Increasing Drugs. *Age Ageing.* 2021;50(4):1189–1199. doi: 10.1093/ageing/afaa249

76. Rodrigues MCS, Oliveira C de. Drug–drug interactions and adverse drug reactions in polypharmacy among older adults: an integrative review. *Rev Lat Am Enfermagem.* 2016;24:e2800. doi: 10.1590/1518-8345.1316.2800

77. Kim J, Parish AL. Polypharmacy and medication management in older adults. *Nurs Clin North Am.* 2017;52(3):457–468. doi: 10.1016/j.cnur.2017.04.007

78. Mizokami F, Koide Y, Noro T, Furuta K. Polypharmacy with common diseases in hospitalized elderly patients. *Am J Geriatr Pharmacother.* 2012;10(2):123–128. doi: 10.1016/j.amjopharm.2012.02.003

79. Ates Bulut E, Isik AT. Abuse/misuse of prescription medications in older adults. *Clin Geriatr Med.* 2022;38(1):85–97. doi: 10.1016/j.cger.2021.07.004

80. Xu Y, Li W, Wan K, et al. Myocardial tissue reverse remodeling after guideline-directed medical therapy in idiopathic dilated cardiomyopathy. *Circ Heart Fail.* 2021;14(1):e007944. doi: 10.1161/CIRCHEARTFAILURE.120.007944

81. Adams J, Mosler C. Safety and efficacy considerations amongst the elderly population in the updated treatment of heart failure: a review. *Expert Rev Cardiovasc Ther.* 2022;20(7):529–541. doi: 10.1080/14779072.2022.2098118

82. Goyal P, Gorodeski EZ, Marcum ZA, Forman DE. Cardiac rehabilitation to optimize medication regimens in heart failure. *Clin Geriatr Med.* 2019;35(4):549–560. doi: 10.1016/j.cger.2019.06.001

83. Nassif ME, Windsor SL, Borlaug BA, et al. The SGLT2 inhibitor dapagliflozin in heart failure with preserved ejection fraction: a multicenter randomized trial. *Nat Med.* 2021;27(11):1954–1960. doi: 10.1038/s41591-021-01536-x

84. Orso F, Herbst A, Pratesi A, et al. New drugs for heart failure: what is the evidence in older patients? *J Card Fail.* 2022;28(2):316–329. doi: 10.1016/j.cardfail.2021.07.011

85. Steinman MA, Dimaano L, Peterson CA, et al. Reasons for not prescribing guideline-recommended medications to adults with heart failure. *Med Care.* 2013;51(10):901–907. doi: 10.1097/MLR.0b013e3182a3e525

86. Polidori MC, Alves M, Bahat G, et al. Atrial fibrillation: a geriatric perspective on the 2020 ESC guidelines. *Eur Geriatr Med.* 2022;13(1):5–18. doi: 10.1007/s41999-021-00537-w

87. Sukumar S, Orkaby AR, Schwartz JB, et al. Polypharmacy in older heart failure patients: a multidisciplinary approach. *Curr Heart Fail Rep.* 2022;19(5):290–302. doi: 10.1007/s11897-022-00559-w

88. Lachuer C, Benzengli H, Do B, Rwabihama JP, Leglise P. Oral anticoagulants: interventional pharmaceutical study with reminder of good practices, and iatrogenic impact. *Ann Pharm Fr.* 2021; 79(4):409–417. doi: 10.1016/j.pharma.2021.01.004

89. Stämpfli D, Boeni F, Gerber A, Bättig VAD, Hersberger KE, Lampert ML. Contribution of patient interviews as part of a comprehensive approach to the identification of drug-related problems on geriatric wards. *Drugs Aging.* 2018;35(7):665–675. doi: 10.1007/s40266-018-0557-z

90. American Bar Association Commission on Law and Aging. Adult Protective Services Reporting Chart [Current April 2022]. Available at: https://www.americanbar.org/content/dam/aba/administrative/law_aging/2020-elder-abuse-reporting-chart.pdf.

91. Centers for Disease Control and Prevention. Fast Facts: Preventing elder abuse. CDC; 2021. Available at: https://www.cdc.gov/violenceprevention/elderabuse/fastfact.html.

92. Cimino-Fiallos N, Rosen T. Elder abuse—a guide to diagnosis and management in the Emergency Department. *Emerg Med Clin North Am.* 2021;39(2):405–417. doi: 10.1016/j.emc.2021.01.00

93. Clarysse K, Kivlahan C, Beyer I, Gutermuth J. Signs of physical abuse and neglect in the mature patient. *Clin Dermatol.* 2018;36(2):264–270. doi: 10.1016/j.clindermatol.2017.10.018

94. Lachs MS, Pillemer K. Elder abuse. *Lancet.* 004;364(9441):1263–1272. doi: 10.1016/S0140-6736(04)17144-4

95. Nowak K, Ouellette L, Chassee T, Seamon JP, Jones J. Emergency services response to elder abuse and neglect – then and now. *Am J Emerg Med.* 2018;36(10):1916–1917. doi: 10.1016/j.ajem.2018.02.036

96. Rosen T, Bao Y, Zhang Y, et al. Identifying patterns of health care utilisation among physical elder abuse victims using Medicare data and legally adjudicated cases: protocol for case–control study using data linkage and machine learning. *BMJ Open.* 2021;11(2):e044768. doi: 10.1136/bmjopen-2020-044768

97. Huecker MR, King KC, Jordan GA, Smock W. Domestic violence. In: StatPearls [Internet]. Treasure Island, FL: StatPearls Publishing; 2022. Available at: http://www.ncbi.nlm.nih.gov/books/NBK499891/.

98. Statutes to Combat Elder Abuse in Nursing Homes. *Virtual Mentor.* 2014;16(5):359–364. doi: 10.1001/virtualmentor.2014.16.05.hlaw1-1405

99. Kayser J, Morrow-Howell N, Rosen TE, et al. Research priorities for elder abuse screening and intervention: a Geriatric Emergency Care Applied Research (GEAR) network scoping review and consensus statement. *J Elder Abuse Negl.* 2021;33(2):123–144. doi: 10.1080/08946566.2021.1904313

100. National Center on Elder Abuse. Intervention partners. Available at: https://ncea.acl.gov/What-We-Do/Practice/Intervention-Partners.aspx.

101. Simmons J, Wenemark M, Ludvigsson M. Development and validation of REAGERA-P, a new questionnaire to evaluate health care provider preparedness to identify and manage elder abuse. *BMC Health Serv Res.* 2021;21(1):473. doi: 10.1186/s12913-021-06469-2

102. Rosen T, Stern ME, Elman A, Mulcare MR. Identifying and initiating intervention for elder abuse and neglect in the Emergency Department. *Clin Geriatr Med.* 2018;34(3):435–451. doi: 10.1016/j.cger.2018.04.007

103. Kogan AC, Rosen T, Navarro A, Homeier D, Chennapan K, Mosqueda L. Developing the Geriatric Injury Documentation Tool (Geri-IDT) to improve documentation of physical findings in injured older adults. *J Gen Intern Med.* 2019;34(4):567–574. doi: 10.1007/s11606-019-04844-8

104. Hoover RM, et al. Detecting elder abuse and neglect: assessment and intervention. *Am Fam Phys.* 2014;89(6):453–460.

105. Richmond NL, Zimmerman S, Reeve BB, et al. Ability of older adults to report elder abuse: an emergency department–based cross-sectional study. *J Am Geriatr Soc.* 2020;68(1):170–175. doi: 10.1111/jgs.16211

106. Carter AJE, Harrison M, Goldstein J, et al. Providing palliative care at home aligns with the professional identity of paramedics: a qualitative study of paramedics and palliative health care providers. *Canad J Emerg Med.* 2022;24(7):751–759. doi: 10.1007/s43678-022-00369-y

107. Gage CH, Geduld H, Stassen W. South African paramedic perspectives on prehospital palliative care. *BMC Palliative Care.* 2020;19(1):1–11. doi: 10.1186/s12904-020-00663-5

108. Carron N, Dami F, Diawara F, Hurst S, Hugli S. Palliative care and prehospital emergency medicine: analysis of a case series. *Medicine (Baltimore).* 2014;(25):e128. doi: 10.1097/MD.0000000000000128

109. Donnelly C, Armstrong K, Perkins M, et al. Emergency medical services provider experiences of hospice care. *Prehosp Emerg Care.* 2018;22(2):237–243. doi: 10.1080/10903127.2017.1358781

110. Lord B, Récoché K, O'Connor M, Yates P, Service M. Paramedics' perceptions of their role in palliative care: analysis of focus group transcripts. *J Palliative Care.* 2012;28(1), 36–40. doi: 10.1177/082585971202800106

111. Murphy-Jones G, Timmons S. Paramedics' experiences of end-of-life care decision making with regard to nursing home residents: an exploration of influential issues and factors. *Emerg Med J.* 2016;33(10):722–726. doi: 10.1136/emermed-2015-205405

112. Waldrop DP, Clemency B, Lindstrom HA, Clemency Cordes C. "We are strangers walking into their life-changing event": How prehospital providers manage emergency calls at the end of life. *J Pain Symptom Manage.* 2015;50(3):328–334. doi: 10.1016/j.jpainsymman.2015.03.001

113. Connor SR. Development of hospice and palliative care in the United States. *Omega J Death Dying.* 2007;56(1):89–99. doi: 10.2190/OM.56.1.h

114. National Hospice and Palliative Care Organization. *NHPCO Facts and Figures 2022 Edition.* Available at: www.nhpco.org/wp-content/uploads/NHPCO-Facts-Figures-2022.pdf.

115. Peran D, Uhlir M, Pekara J, Kolouch P, Loucka M. Approaching the end of their lives under blue lights and sirens – Scoping Review. *J Pain Symptom Manage.* 2021;62(6):1308–1318. doi: 10.1016/j.jpainsymman.2021.04.023

116. Barnette Donnelly C, Armstrong KA, Perkins MM, Moulia D, Quest TE, Yancey AH. Emergency medical services provider experiences of hospice care. *Prehosp Emerg Care.* 2018;22(2):237–243. doi: 10.1080/10903127.2017.1358781

117. Lord B, Andrew E, Henderson A, Anderson D, Smith K, Bernard S. Palliative care in paramedic practice: a retrospective cohort study. *Palliat Med.* 2019;33(4):445–451. doi: 10.1177/0269216319828278

118. Phongtankuel V, Scherban B, Reid M, et al. Why do home hospice patients return to the hospital? A study of hospice provider perspectives. *J Palliat Med.* 2016;19(1):51–56. doi: 10.1089/jpm.2015.0178

119. Breyre AM, Bains G, Moore J, Siegel L, Sporer KA. Hospice and comfort care patient utilization of emergency medical services. *J Palliative Med.* 2022;25(2):259–264. doi: 10.1089/jpm.2021.0143

120. Ingleton C, Payne S, Sargeant A, Seymour J. Barriers to achieving care at home at the end of life: transferring patients between care settings using patient transport services. *Palliative Med.* 2009;23(8):723–730. doi: 10.1177/0269216309106893

121. Waldrop DP, McGinley JM, Clemency B. Mediating systems of care: emergency calls to long-term care facilities at life's end. *J Palliative Med.* 2018;21(7):987–991. doi: 10.1089/JPM.2017.0332

122. Lamba S, Schmidt TA, Chan GK, et al. Integrating palliative care in the out-of-hospital setting: four things to jump-start an EMS-palliative care initiative. *Prehosp Emerg Care.* 2013;17(4):511–520. doi: 10.3109/10903127.2013.811566

123. Burnod A, Lenclud G, Ricard-Hibon A, Juvin P, Mantz J, Duchateau FX. Collaboration between prehospital emergency medical teams and palliative care networks allows a better respect of a patient's will. *Eur J Emerg Med.* 2012;19(1):46–47. doi: 10.1097/MEJ.0b013e328347fa9c

124. Anastasio BM, Bruce JD, Mezo J. (2015). Mobile integrated healthcare Part 4: Integrating home care, hospice and EMS. *EMS World.* 2015;April.

125. Breyre A, Taigman M, Salvucci A, Sporer K. Effect of a mobile integrated hospice healthcare program on emergency medical services transport to the emergency department. *Prehosp Emerg Care.* 2022;26(3):364–369. doi: 10.1080/10903127.2021.1900474

126. Montgomery CL, Pooler C, Arsenault JE, et al. Innovative urgent care for the palliative patient at home. *Home Healthcare Now.* 2017;35(4):196–201. doi: 10.1097/NHH.0000000000000526

127. Hoare S, Kelly MP, Prothero L, Barclay S. Ambulance staff and end-of-life hospital admissions: a qualitative interview study. *Palliative Med.* 2018;32(9):1465–1473. doi: 10.1177/0269216318779238

128. Kirk A, Crompton P, Knighting K, et al. Paramedics and their role in end-of-life care: perceptions and confidence. *J Paramed Pract.* 2017;9:71–79.

129. Ausband SC, March JA, Brown LH. National prevalence of palliative care protocols in emergency medical services. *Prehosp Emerg Care.* 2002;6(1): 36–41. doi: 10.1080/10903120290938751

130. Waldrop DP, Waldrop MR, McGinley JM, Crowley CR, Clemency B. Prehospital providers' perspectives about online medical direction in emergency end-of-life decision-making. *Prehosp Emerg Care.* 2022;26(2):223–232. doi: 10.1080/10903127.2020.1863532

131. Wiese CHR, Bartels UE, Marczynska K, Ruppert D, Graf BM, Hanekop GG. Quality of out-of-hospital palliative emergency care depends on the expertise of the emergency medical team-a prospective multi-centre analysis. *Supportive Care Cancer.* 2009;17(12): 1499–1506. doi: 10.1007/s00520-009-0616-4

132. Murphy-Jones G, Timmons S. Paramedics' experiences of end-of-life care decision making with regard to nursing home residents: an exploration of influential issues and factors. *Emerg Med J.* 2016;33(10):722–726. doi: 10.1136/emermed-2015-205405

133. Schmidt TA, Olszewski EA, Zive D, Fromme EK, Tolle SW. The Oregon Physician Orders for Life-Sustaining Treatment Registry: a preliminary study of emergency medical services utilization. *J Emerg Med.* 2013;44(4):796–805. doi: 10.1016/j.jemermed.2012.07.081

134. Schmidt T, Hickman S, Tolle S, Brooks H. The Physician Orders for Life-Sustaining Treatment program: Oregon emergency medical technicians' practical experiences and attitudes. *J Am Geriatr Soc.* 2004;(9):1430–1434. doi: 10.1111/j.1532-5415.2004.52403.x

135. Breyre A, Sporer K, Davenport G, Isaacs E, Glomb N. Paramedic use of the Physician Order for Life-Sustaining Treatment (POLST) for medical intervention and transportation decisions. *BMC Emerg Med.* 2022;22(1):145. doi: 10.1186/s12873-022-00697-3

136. Wenger A, Potilechio M, Redinger K, Billian J, Aguilar J, Mastenbrook J. Care for a dying patient: EMS perspectives on caring for hospice patients. *J Pain Symptom Manage.* 2002:64(2):e71–e76. doi: 10.1016/j.jpainsymman.2022.04.175

137. Waldrop DP, McGinley JM, Dailey MW, Clemency B. Decision-making in the moments before death: challenges in prehospital care. *Prehosp Emerg Care.* 2019;23(3):356–363. doi: 10.1080/10903127.2018.1518504

138. Juhrmann M, Vandersman P, Butow B, Clayton J. Paramedics delivering palliative and end-of-life care in community-based settings: a systematic integrative review with thematic synthesis. *Palliative Med.* 2002;36(3):405–421. doi: 10.1177/02692163211059342

139. Benítez-Rosario M, Rosa-González I, González-Dávila E, Sanz E. Fentanyl treatment for end-of-life dyspnoea relief in advanced cancer patients. *Support Care Cancer.* 2019;(1):157–164. doi: 10.1007/s00520-018-4309-8

140. Clary P, Lawson P. Pharmacologic pearls for end-of-life care. *Am Fam Phys.* 2009;79(12):1059–1065.

141. Murakami M. (2019). Opioids for relief of dyspnea immediately before death in patients with noncancer disease: a case series study. *Am J Hosp Palliat Care.* 36(8):734–739. doi: 10.1177/1049909119832816

142. Slawnych M. Management of dyspnea at the end of life. *CMAJ.* 2020;192(20):E550. doi: 10.1503/cmaj.200488

143. Abernethy A, McDonald C, Frith P, Clark K, Herndon J, et al. Effect of palliative oxygen versus room air in relief of breathlessness in patients with refractory dyspnea: a double-blind, randomised controlled trial. *Lancet.* 2010;376(9743):784–793. doi: 10.1016/S0140-6736(10)61115-4

144. Clemens K, Quednau I, Klaschik E. Use of oxygen and opioids in the palliation of dyspnea in hypoxic and non-hypoxic palliative care patients: a prospective study. *Support Care Cancer.* 2008;17(4):367–77. doi: 10.1007/s00520-008-0479-0

145. Hunter Groninger H, Vijayan J. Pharmacologic management of pain at the end of life. *Am Fam Physician.* 2014;90(1):26–32.

146. Back AL, Arnold RM, Tulsky JA. *Mastering Communication with Seriously Ill Patients: Balancing Honesty with Empathy and Hope.* Cambridge: Cambridge University Press; 2009.

20

Care and Transport of the Bariatric Patient

MARION L. JONES, BRADLEY ARTHUR KUCH, AND FRANCIS GUYETTE

COMPETENCIES

1. Introduce and discuss the transport of bariatric patients.
2. Describe the general assessment and physiological differences in a bariatric patient.
3. Identify the significant cardiovascular and respiratory physiologic sequelae associated with obesity and its challenges when caring for patients in the transport environment.
4. Demonstrate effective decision-making when dispatching crew configuration and vehicle considerations for transporting bariatric patients.
5. Describe the clinical management of the bariatric patient in the transport environment.
6. Identify the fundamental concepts of patient integrity in the bariatric population.
7. Identify limitations and describe the ergonomic techniques regarding bariatric patient transfers.

Introduction

Greater than 40% of adults over the age of 20 in the United States are considered obese with a body mass index (BMI) >30.[1] The incidence of obesity has increased across all sociodemographic classes and age groups and is associated with poor dental care, diabetes, and hypertension.[1] Additionally, obesity-related conditions such as heart disease, stroke, type II diabetes, and certain cancers remain preventable causes of premature death.

Bariatric patients can present clinical challenges to healthcare professionals treating and caring for this patient population. Diabetes mellitus, cardiovascular disease, renal disease, respiratory disorders, and airway difficulties are comorbidities often requiring critical care intervention(s) that exceed resources available at community healthcare facilities. As a result, it is necessary to transport a subset of these patients to tertiary care facilities that can provide emergent diagnostics and treatment. This chapter presents logistical and clinical perspectives on the general assessment, physiological differences, comorbid illness, dispatching decisions, mission planning, clinical management, patient integrity, and ergonomic transfer techniques used when caring for bariatric patients during transport.

According to the CDC, a weight greater than what is considered healthy for a given height is considered overweight or obese. Data from the Centers for Disease Control (CDC) reflect an increasing prevalence in US adults self-reporting obesity (Fig. 20.1 and Table 20.1).[2–5] Body mass index (BMI) is the accepted albeit imperfect screening tool and measure for overweight and obesity

and is calculated the same way for adults and children. BMI is easily calculated by dividing a person's weight in kilograms by the square of height in meters.

$$\text{Formula kilograms and meters} : \frac{weight\ (kg)}{\left[height\ (m)\right]^2}$$

or

$$\text{Formula pounds and inches} : \frac{weight\ (lb)}{\left[height\ (in)\right]^2} \times 703$$

A high BMI is associated with high body fat concentrations. Advocated BMI classifications are defined as[6]:

BMI <18.5, underweight

BMI 18.5 to <25, healthy weight

BMI 25.0 to <30, overweight

BMI 30.0 or higher, obesity range

Obesity is frequently subdivided into three categories[6]:

Class 1: BMI of 30 to <35

Class 2: BMI of 35 to <40

Class 3: BMI of 40 or higher is categorized as "*severe*" obesity

The term "bariatrics" refers to the branch of medicine treating obesity and weight-related problems, where obesity is the state of having excess body fat.

BMI and Obesity Class may provide helpful information regarding the treatment and transport of bariatric patients. Still,

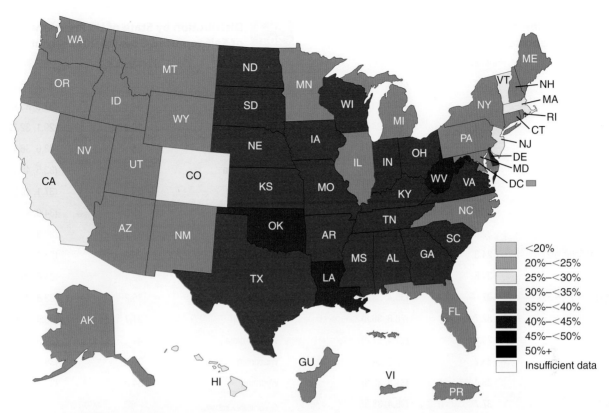

• **Fig. 20.1** United States adult self-reported obesity prevalence by state and territory. Data are from the Behavioral Risk Factor Surveillance System (BRFSS), 2022. The prevalence of obesity in the United States from 2020 to 2022 was over 30%.[3–5] (From Centers for Disease Control and Prevention (CDC). Adult obesity prevalence maps. https://www.cdc.gov/obesity/data/prevalence-maps.html.)

they should be one of many measures used to determine the operational needs for transport of this patient population. Clinical and operational research may draw on BMI, Predicted Body Weight (PBW), IDW Ideal Body Weight (IDW), and an individual's physical measurements to effectively assess, manage, and transfer patients. When critical care transport programs design an operational bariatric transport process, ample consideration must be given to the capabilities and size of the transport vehicles and patient stretchers utilized. BMI is reductive, while height and weight are necessary measurements. Determining the greatest straight-line width and abdominal height will directly affect whether a specific fixed-wing, rotor-wing, or ground ambulance can safely transport a bariatric patient.

General Bariatric Assessment

The primary aim of any transport system is the safe and timely transfer of patients to centers providing specialized care without an increased risk of morbidity and mortality. As a result, critical care teams are generally reserved for high-acuity patients. However, the bariatric population requires unique assessment skills, additional specialized equipment, and resources frequently found in specialty critical care transport systems. In addition, specialty transport programs can expedite transport of this patient population when other prehospital agencies cannot accommodate them due to limited resources or gaps in the requisite clinical training to care for this patient population.

The bariatric patient population is admitted to the critical care unit for three primary purposes. First, they may experience acute complications associated with restrictive gastric surgery. These include intraoperative complications related to comorbid illness or anesthesia. Postoperative complications include failed extubation, staple line rupture, anastomotic leak, stomal stenosis, dumping syndrome, surgical site perforation, infection, and pulmonary embolus.[7] Secondly, patients may experience problems related to their intercurrent illnesses that require intensive care monitoring and support. Various cardiac, vascular, respiratory, endocrine, and immunologic issues with multiple systems implications may mandate critical care admission. Thirdly, the obese patient may suffer a trauma requiring intensive care. Of note is that injuries may be missed as radiologic assessment may be compromised due to accessibility barriers related to weight restrictions of diagnostic equipment and limitations in image quality.[7] Many facilities may not have the resources to adequately care for this patient population, necessitating transport.

Upon arrival at the bedside, it is necessary to perform a complete assessment of the patient's clinical condition, physical environment, and transport resources (i.e., equipment, need for specialized vehicles, and people) available to move the patient.

Clinical Assessment

Always complete a primary assessment and perform initial intervention(s) necessary to stabilize the patient. With the bariatric patient, obtaining accurate vitals via physical assessment, cardiac monitoring, automatic noninvasive blood pressures, and pulse oximetry can be complicated and less accurate due to placement challenges resulting from excessive amount of adipose tissue.

TABLE 20.1 Distribution by State of US Prevalence of Self-reported Obesity, 2022		
State	Prevalence	95% CI
Alabama	38.3	(36.3, 40.3)
Alaska	32.1	(30.4, 33.9)
Arizona	33.2	(31.6, 34.9)
Arkansas	37.4	(35.6, 39.2)
California	28.1	(26.8, 29.4)
Colorado	25	(23.9, 26.2)
Connecticut	30.6	(29.1, 32.1)
Delaware	37.9	(35.6, 40.2)
District of Columbia	24.3	(22.2, 26.5)
Florida	31.6	(29.9, 33.4)
Georgia	37	(35.4, 38.7)
Guam	32.7	(28.8, 36.8)
Hawaii	25.9	(24.4, 27.4)
Idaho	33.2	(31.7, 34.7)
Illinois	33.4	(31.5, 35.3)
Indiana	37.7	(36.4, 38.9)
Iowa	37.4	(36.0, 38.8)
Kansas	35.7	(34.4, 37.0)
Kentucky	37.7	(35.6, 39.9)
Louisiana	40.1	(38.3, 41.9)
Maine	33.1	(31.8, 34.5)
Maryland	33.2	(31.9, 34.4)
Massachusetts	27.2	(26.0, 28.5)
Michigan	34.5	(33.2, 35.8)
Minnesota	33.6	(32.6, 34.7)
Mississippi	39.5	(37.5, 41.4)
Missouri	36.4	(34.9, 38.0)
Montana	30.5	(29.1, 32.0)
Nebraska	35.3	(33.7, 36.9)
Nevada	33.5	(31.0, 36.2)
New Hampshire	30.2	(28.6, 32.0)
New Jersey	29.1	(27.6, 30.7)
New Mexico	32.4	(30.5, 34.4)
New York	30.1	(29.1, 31.2)
North Carolina	34.1	(32.1, 36.1)
North Dakota	35.4	(33.6, 37.3)
Ohio	38.1	(37.0, 39.3)
Oklahoma	40	(38.4, 41.6)
Oregon	30.9	(29.4, 32.4)

TABLE 20.1 Distribution by State of US Prevalence of Self-reported Obesity, 2022—cont'd		
State	Prevalence	95% CI
Pennsylvania	33.4	(31.2, 35.5)
Puerto Rico	34.1	(32.3, 35.9)
Rhode Island	30.8	(29.1, 32.7)
South Carolina	35	(33.6, 36.4)
South Dakota	36.8	(33.5, 40.1)
Tennessee	38.9	(37.1, 40.8)
Texas	35.5	(34.0, 37.1)
Utah	31.1	(29.9, 32.4)
Vermont	26.8	(25.4, 28.3)
Virgin Islands	32.1	(25.4, 39.6)
Virginia	35.2	(33.8, 36.6)
Washington	31.7	(30.9, 32.5)
West Virginia	41	(39.3, 42.8)
Wisconsin	37.7	(36.4, 39.0)
Wyoming	34.3	(32.3, 36.2)

CI, Confidence interval.

Data from the Behavioral Risk Factor Surveillance System (BRFSS). (From Centers for Disease Control and Prevention (CDC). Adult obesity prevalence maps. https://www.cdc.gov/obesity/php/data-research/adult-obesity-prevalence-maps.html

Utilizing monitor-specific pacer or defibrillation pads for ECG tracing, thigh cuffs for blood pressure monitoring, or an appropriately sized bariatric cuff, and pulse oximetry via an ear probe can improve the ability to monitor and obtain accurate vital signs. Invasive monitoring of blood pressure may be necessary when titrating vasoactive medications. Establishing vascular access may also be difficult due to the absence of traditional landmarks and increased soft tissue thickness. Therefore, access should be anticipated and performed in a controlled environment before transport.

Primary Assessment

The initial or primary assessment should be conducted in the same fashion as all other patient groups and includes an evaluation of the patient's airway, breathing, circulation, neurological disability, and exposure(s) (ABCDE). During this assessment, patient problems are identified, and interventions are initiated. Habitus of this patient population introduces unique challenges and needs to be addressed with a focused assessment. All challenges should be communicated and documented for consideration of ongoing care at the receiving institution.

Airway

Compared with non-bariatric patients, bariatric patients have an increased tongue size, a smaller pharyngeal area, redundant pharyngeal tissue, an increased neck circumference, and increased chest girth.[8] The bariatric patient population tends to have higher rates of respiratory failure and subsequent intubation. Studies on obesity as a risk factor for airway problems indicate that obesity is a statistically significant but weak predictor of difficult intubation.[8] In an emergent situation, however, obesity may contribute to complex airway management and require additional resources.[8]

Assessment should include evaluation of airway patency, level of consciousness, skin appearance (i.e., ashen pale, grey, cyanotic, or poor perfusion), preferred posture to maintain airway, and audible sounds of obstruction. If airway compromise or difficulty is identified, stabilizing intervention should occur as soon as practicable and prior to transport. Preferred posture is an essential consideration in the high BMI population.

Breathing

Alterations in breathing patterns may include increased respiratory rates, greater oxygen consumption from metabolic requirements of excess tissue, increased work of breathing, and decreased tidal volume. These changes can lead to reduced time to desaturation, greater oxygen requirements, and hypoventilation with supine spontaneous ventilation.[8]

Bariatric patients may have an increased work of breathing due to abnormal chest elasticity, abnormal diaphragm position, chest wall compliance, and upper airway resistance. Work of breathing may increase by as much as 60% in the obese bariatric patient and 250% in the morbidly obese bariatric patient.[9] Persons with obesity-related pulmonary dysfunction will desaturate more quickly due to decreased functional residual capacity (FRC). Avoid supine positioning (including lithotomy and Trendelenburg) as these are associated with significant declines in lung volumes.[9]

Assessment of breathing begins from the door, identifying whether the patient has adequate respiration and the presence of respiratory distress. Immediate intervention is indicated if the patient is apneic or in severe respiratory distress. The breathing assessment should include an evaluation of the rate and depth of respiration, presence of cyanosis, work of breathing, use of accessory muscles, position of the trachea, breath sounds, and oxygen saturation.

Respiratory rate (RR) should be measured by counting breaths for 1 minute. Electric respiratory impedance technology used by the monitors can be inaccurate, visual measures of respiratory rate may be more precise. Physical assessment, including auscultation of breath sounds, can be complex in patients with higher BMI or increased chest adipose tissue. Breath sounds may sound distant or "diminished." Additionally, pulse oximetry values may be obscured by adipose tissue; ensure proper placement and readings. Correlate all measurements with the cardiac monitor to ensure accuracy.

Abnormal respiratory assessment findings that may require physician consult include:

- Increase/decrease in respiratory rate
- Change in respiratory pattern
- Change in level of consciousness or orientation
- Decrease in pulse oximetry <90% for 5 min
- Increase in end-tidal CO_2 or change in PCO_2 from baseline
- Nasal flaring or use of accessory muscles to breathe

Circulation

Assessment of cardiovascular function presents unique challenges as typical symptoms of heart failure are potentially unreliable. Excess adipose tissue makes auscultation of heart sounds challenging. Signs of cardiac failure, such as jugular venous distention, hepatomegaly, and peripheral edema, may be masked by body habitus and chronic peripheral edema. Circulatory assessment includes evaluation of pulse rate and quality, skin color (i.e., perfusion), peripheral pulse strength, skin temperature, level of consciousness (LOC), urine output, blood pressure (BP), and cardiac monitoring. Auscultate heart sounds, ensuring minimalization of extraneous noise. It may be necessary to displace tissue, placing the stethoscope on the chest wall. When placing monitor leads, ensure the waveform is reliable.

BP measures are critical in the high BMI patient, as chronic hypertension is cofounding comorbidity. When evaluating noninvasive BP, the cuff should exceed the circumference of the extremity by 20%, the cuff width should be greater than or equal to 40% of the arm circumference, and the same extremity should be used for repeated measures. If the BP cuff size is the barrier, consider using the forearm. Leblanc et al. reported less difference between the intra-arterial and forearm methods than the upper-arm methods.[10] The decreased difference was found in the systolic and diastolic blood pressures.[10]

Disability: Neurologic Evaluation

Concise assessment of neurologic function provides insight into the patient's current clinical state. An altered level of consciousness may result from an intracranial process (i.e., cerebral vascular accident), respiratory failures, or toxic ingestion, such as alcohol or other drugs. The simplest assessment method is the AVPU mnemonic, as defined:

A – Alert
V – Responds to verbal stimuli
P – Responds to painful stimuli
U – Unresponsive

The Glasgow Coma Scale (GCS) is more detailed and is associated with morbidity and mortality. A thorough assessment of the neurologic status and monitoring for changes will aid in defining the subsequent interventional escalation in care.

Key Physiological Considerations

Understanding the physiological differences in the bariatric patient provides the ability to properly prepare, treat, and manage patients safely and effectively during transport.[11] We describe obesity-related physiological differences (see Table 20.3) and the need for awareness and preparedness related to clinical interventions and the safe transport of high BMI patients.

Pulmonary Considerations

Bariatric and Respiratory Symptomology

Overweight patients are more likely to experience respiratory symptoms compared to patients with normal BMI, despite the absence of lung disease (Table 20.2).[12] Some theorized that this is related to increased respiratory workload and oxygen demand.[13] This, coupled with coexisting medical conditions, cofound the development of respiratory symptomology. The transport environment may also induce anxiety and uncertainty, contributing to the feeling of dyspnea.

Respiratory Physiology

The effects of obesity on the respiratory system are often underappreciated. Safe and effective transport of these patients requires a firm understanding of these effects, which includes alterations in lung mechanics, adipose tissue-induced systemic inflammation, central and obstructive apneas, chronic obstructive pulmonary disease (COPD), and uni- and bilateral heart failure resulting in

TABLE 20.2 Transport Environment–Related Comorbidities Associated with Obesity

Organ System	Confounding Dysfunction/Comorbidity
Cardiovascular	Hypertension Ischemic heart disease Cor pulmonale (right-sided heart failure) Cardiomyopathy Cerebrovascular disease Peripheral disease Deep vein thrombosis Pulmonary embolism
Respiratory/Pulmonary	Obesity hypoventilation syndrome Obstructive sleep apnea Asthma *See* Table 20.4 for additional detail
Endocrine/Metabolic	Diabetes mellitus Metabolic syndrome Hypothyroidism Cushing syndrome (abnormally high levels of cortisol)
Gastrointestinal	Fatty liver Liver disease Gallbladder disease
Malignancies	Colorectal Pancreatic
Musculoskeletal	Osteoarthritis of weight-bearing joints Lower back pain
Dermatologic	Cellulitis Pressure ulcers
Neuropsychiatric	Anxiety Depression Idiopathic intracranial hypertension Intracranial processes (i.e., stroke)

Modified from Catenacci VA, Hill JO, Wyatt HR. The obesity epidemic. *Clin Chest Med.* 2009;30:423.

TABLE 20.3 Anatomic and Physiologic Changes Associated with Obese Patients Secondary to Increased Adipose Tissue

Anatomic Location	Physiologic Effect
Large tongue, excessive upper airway tissue, and reduced pharyngeal dilator muscle function	Increased risk of upper airway obstruction Obstructive sleep apnea (OSA)
Pharyngeal structure	Decreased airway lumen Difficult superlaryngeal mask seat/seal
Face	Difficult bag-valve-mask (BVM) ventilation Difficult noninvasive ventilation (NIV) mask fitting
Neck	Difficult surgical airway access
Chest/thorax	Reduction in chest wall compliance Reduced functional residual capacity (FRC)
Abdomen	Reduced diaphragmatic excursion Micro-atelectasis in the supine position

TABLE 20.4 Respiratory Physiologic Adaptations Associated with Obesity

Respiratory Physiologic Measure	Physiologic Adaptions
Ventilation	Increased respiratory rate Decreased tidal volume
Oxygenation	Wide alveolar–arterial (A–a) gradient Hypoxemia Increased oxygen consumption
Lung volumes	Decreased expiratory reserve volume (ERV) Decreased FRC Reduced residual volume (RV) FRC approaches RV (risk of atelectasis) Closing capacity may be >FRC in the range of tidal volume
Compliance	Decreased chest wall compliance Decreased lung compliance
Airway resistance	Increased airway resistance: Reduced lung volume Small airway closure Airway remodeling (pro-inflammatory adipokines)

pulmonary edema and hypoxemia (see Table 20.3).[12] Clinical presentation and management of these underlying pathologies are related to the compliance and resistance of the respiratory system or a combination of both (see Table 20.3, Table 20.4).

Dynamic compliance, defined as the change in lung volume per unit change in transmural pressure gradient (i.e., between alveolus and pleural space) or the lung's ability to stretch and expand, is a property of the structural properties of the tissues. Compliance can be further grouped into its contribution to the chest wall, lung elastance, and abdominal components. Lung compliance decreases with increasing BMI and is not fully understood.[14] Contributing factors include increased thoracic blood volume, mediastinal fat compressing the lung, and premature closure of dependent airways resulting in chronic atelectasis and increased alveolar surface tension.[15] Decreased compliance decreases lung volume and increases respiratory muscle workload resulting in chronic respiratory insufficiency and increased use of noninvasive respiratory support. These factors will present additional challenges and should be considered when providing respiratory support (see Table 20.4).

Resistance is defined as the pressure difference between the oral opening and alveoli, divided by airflow, with the primary location of airway resistance being the medium-sized bronchi. It has been well documented that airway resistance increases with increasing BMI.[16–19] Increased resistance in the bariatric population is located in the smaller airways, which is different from the lower BMI cohort and is related to reduced lung volume.[17] Bariatric patients may benefit from bronchodilators when clinically indicated by physical assessment. Therefore, transport team members should remain cognizant of potential increased airway resistance, assessing breath sounds across all lung fields (see Table 20.4).

Asthma

Several reports associate obesity with asthma, with one account demonstrating a 38% higher incidence of asthma in overweight patients and 92% higher in obese patients (see Table 20.2).[19] Although it is unclear whether asthma symptoms are related to airway inflammation or increased BMI, emerging evidence suggests asthma symptoms are primarily due to ventilatory mechanics (i.e., decreased compliance, reduction in airway size and tone) rather than inflammatory ones (see Table 20.4).[12] Despite the etiology, reduction in airway lumen size increases the risk of gas trapping, wheezing, and dynamic hyperinflation, all hallmarks of an asthma exacerbation, most notably during respiratory tract infections.

Bariatric patients diagnosed with asthma are known to have more severe exacerbations, increased use of asthma medications, and more frequent emergency room visits than non-bariatric patients with asthma.[21] For this reason, the transport professional should not ignore asthma symptoms in a bariatric patient. Proper assessment and treatment within the accepted protocols should occur with particular attention to underlying medical conditions contributing to dyspnea and wheezing. Congestive heart failure and signs of fluid overload should be evaluated during the primary assessment, including past medical history and current treatment modalities.

Chronic Obstructive Pulmonary Disease (COPD)

The prevalence of obesity is higher in COPD patients than in non-COPD patient subjects; therefore, it should be considered when evaluating a high BMI patient for transport.[22] In a narrative review, Zewari et al. reported an obesity prevalence between 18% and 54% in patients with COPD.[22] Obesity and COPD have similarities that potentially exacerbate each condition. Each is associated with decreased lung function, mild systemic inflammation, and hypoxia, increasing morbidity and mortality risk. This clinical presentation, combined with an increased incidence of obesity hypoventilation syndrome (OHS) and obstructive sleep apnea, result in chronic hypoxia, decreased pulmonary reserve, and right-heart dysfunction, potentially complicating the transfer and care of the patient (see Table 20.2). Obesity complicates airway and respiratory management and high BMI patients may have either acute or chronic respiratory insufficiency.

Comparison of Acute vs. Chronic Respiratory Insufficiency

High BMI patients are at significant risk of developing acute on chronic respiratory failure secondary to OHS, disorders in lung mechanics, ventilatory drive, and infectious processes.[23] OHS is defined as the presence of obesity (BMI >30 kg/m^2) and arterial hypercarbia ($PaCO_2$ >45 mmHg) during waking hours.[23] Patients with OHS may have arterial blood gas (ABG) values demonstrating mild hypoxia with compensated respiratory acidosis (normal pH and elevated bicarbonate). Masa et al. reported the clinical features of 757 patients with OHS from 15 studies – illustrating mean ABG values of pH 7.38, PaO_2 53 mmHg, $PaCO_2$ 56 mmHg, and serum bicarbonate of 32.[24] The crew needs to identify the presence of acute on chronic respiratory failure, as obese patients with chronic respiratory insufficiency can rapidly deteriorate into acute respiratory failure (ARF). The presence of any of the following may be considered an acute respiratory failure.[23]

- Acute acidemia pH <7.30
- Decreased level of consciousness or coma
- Hemodynamic instability
- Refractory hypoxemia
- Intolerance to positive airway pressure (PAP) therapy (i.e., continuous PAP, bilevel PAP)

The presence of one or more of these indicators requires intervention prior to transport and may benefit from Medical Direction consultation.

Airway

Increasing BMI is associated with greater anatomic and physiologic challenges related to oxygenation and airway management. Anatomic changes result primarily from excess adipose tissue in the pharyngeal structures, face, neck, and thorax (see Table 20.3).[8] Increased adipose tissue deposition in the pharyngeal structure, most commonly in the lateral pharyngeal walls, results in the narrowing of the airway lumen, most notably on inspiration.[25] Coupled with a large tongue and dysfunction of the pharyngeal dilator muscles, obese patients have a greater risk of obstructive sleep apnea (see Table 20.2). This triad of upper airway physiologic changes poses an increased risk of airway obstruction and decompensation during induction and should be considered before advanced airway maneuvers.

In addition to upper airway obstruction, the clinician must also consider the negative effect of excess fatty tissue on the face, neck, chest, thorax, and abdomen, which possess significant challenges related to patient positioning, neck extension, bag-valve-mask ventilation, oxygenation, and intubation. An extensive review of complications of airway management found a four-fold increased risk of severe complications in obese patients compared with non-obese patients with 25% of patients suffering brain damage or death.[9] For this reason, the air medical crew must understand the risks and interventions to limit secondary complications (hypoxia, hypotension, and hypercarbia) during advanced airway management (see Tables 20.2–20.4).

Airway Assessment (Prediction)

Rapid assessment and identification of a potentially difficult airway is the first aspect of a stepwise approach to successful intubation. Multiple assessment tools and scores have been developed and evaluated for use in the prehospital setting, an environment with space, time, and provider limitations – vastly different than the operating room. As a result, an airway assessment tool chosen for the transport setting should be designed for and validated in the prehospital environment. Even when using a validated airway assessment tool, the air medical crew should be cognizant of physical and situational conditions increasing the risk of difficult intubations.

Physical Findings

Several investigations in the intra- and prehospital settings have identified physical attributes associated with difficult intubation. These physical findings include but are not limited to the following:

- BMI >30 kg/m^2 [26]
- Mallampati score ≥3[26]
- Short neck[26]
- Mouth opening <3 cm /limited mouth opening[26,27]
- Large tongue[27]
- Poor neck flexibility[27]

Environmental Factors

In addition to the patient's physical findings, environmental risk factors should also be considered. These factors pose a significant challenge to the resource-limited environment and include the following:

- Confined or restricted space[27]
- Vomitus, blood, or secretions in the airway[27]
- Intubation in an ambulance or helicopter[27]
- Cervical spine immobilization[26,27]

Pre-intubation Support

Positioning

The most critical aspect of pre-intubation management is creating the optimal position for the bariatric patient prior to induction. Proper positioning will allow the patient to maintain their natural airway, decrease right heart workload, allow for effective pre-oxygenation techniques, and promote patient comfort thus reducing oxygen consumption. The transport environment is challenged with space and patient positioning limitations. For this reason, the best option is the head-up position. The head-up position is defined as placing the patient in a position with their head at 25 degrees. A randomized controlled trial found that pre-oxygenating the patient in the "head-up" position resulted in 23% higher arterial oxygen tension than in the supine position and an increase in the duration of apnea before desaturation.[28] Head-up position also improves laryngeal visualization during direct laryngoscopy.[29] Improved visualization is created with the horizontal alignment of the sternal notch with the external auditory canal in a "ramped" position with the patient ear parallel to the top of the chest wall.[8] Achieving this alignment is quickly done by placing multiple folded blankets under the upper body, shoulders, and head or raising the head of the stretcher.[8] Using the readily available resources to create proper alignment will facilitate the next steps in management and pre-oxygenation.

Management and Oxygenation

Regardless of the method, agent selection, and technique, induction is a high-risk period beginning with effective pre-oxygenation. Patients with increased BMI have pulmonary physiologic changes that include decreased spontaneous tidal volume, prone to upper airway obstruction, wide arterial to alveolar gradient (A–a gradient), decreased functional residual capacity (FRC), and reduced residual volume, all of which result in a shorter duration of apnea and profound hypoxemia (see Table 20.4). These physiologic changes decrease the time available for the induction period and stress the importance of effective pre-oxygenation.

Sufficient pre-oxygenation arterial saturation (SpO_2) level in obese patients is considered >90% in the skilled provider.[30] That said, the highest SpO_2 achievable is recommended given the clinical circumstance. Several techniques have been advocated. Spontaneous 3-minute breathing through a "well-sealed" face-mask is standard practice.[8] When using a nonrebreather mask, the clinician must ensure the bag remains fully inflated and does not entirely deflate during deflation. In addition to high-concentration oxygen delivery, supplemental nasopharyngeal oxygen insufflation provides added gas flow resulting in decreased room air entrainment and anatomic dead space carbon dioxide clearance. High-flow nasal oxygen may provide a longer duration of apnea without hypoxemia and hypercarbia. Other adjunctive techniques include semi-recumbent positioning, continuous positive airway pressure (CPAP), positive end-expiratory pressure (PEEP), and pressure-support ventilation before induction.[8] A single-center study demonstrated that 94% (16/17) of obese patients undergoing pre-oxygenation followed by nasopharyngeal insufflation in a recumbent position (25-degree head-up position) maintained a SpO_2 at 100% during an apnea period of 4 minutes compared to controls of only pre-oxygenation, showing SpO_2 decrease after 27-seconds.[31] Supplementing pre-oxygenation with nasopharyngeal insufflation in a recumbent position may help prevent hypoxia during induction.

A high-flow nasal cannula (HFNC) is an emerging oxygen delivery modality in adults. The therapeutic effect is similar to pharyngeal insufflation, only differing by the set liter flow. The conditioning (warmed and humidified) of inspired gas allows for a higher flow rate resulting in the filling of the bronchial-tracheal tree – increasing FiO_2 delivery while decreasing rebreathed CO_2; these characteristics potentially benefit the bariatric population. Although the use of HFNC requires more research, its use has been reported to reduce CO_2 and increase FRC and oxygen reserves.[32,33]

Bag-Valve-Mask Ventilation

High BMI has been demonstrated to be a strong predictor of difficult bag-valve-mask (BVM) ventilation.[34] A large prospective study found that a BMI >26 kg/m^2 is an independent predictor of difficult BVM.[34] This was later validated by a study that demonstrated a BMI >30 mg/m^2 to be a predictor of difficult BVM and, ultimately, intubation.[35] Other factors associated with difficult BVM include radiotherapy to the neck, male sex, presence of a beard, and Mallampati scores of 3 to 4. Therefore, in clinical situations where one or more of these risk factors are identified, the clinician should anticipate difficult BVM and have additional support (respiratory therapist, skilled intubator) and a readily available supraglottic airway.

Advanced Airway Management and Intubation

Supraglottic Airway Devices

Supraglottic airway (SGA) devices are important adjuncts in complex airway management pathways and are validated in pre- and interhospital transport environments. Historically, laryngeal mask airways (LMA) with an inflatable mask have been the device of choice. However, airway seal pressure remained a limitation leading to the "unseating of the device." Natalini et al. report that the inflatable cuff LMA required greater pressure to create an airway seal than gel cuff devices in high BMI patients.[36] Development of gel masks with an integrated gastric tube channel has improved airway seal and provided a means for decompressing the stomach during temporary ventilation.

An SGA should be readily available when a potential for a difficult airway is identified or expected. Equipment gathered during preparation for advance airway placement should include a correctly sized and one-size-smaller SGA. It is essential to ensure all crew are aware of the proper sizing considerations in the bariatric patient, as actual weight may overestimate the correct size. In the case of a bariatric patient, some reference should be made specific to the SGA device when discerning whether ideal or actual body weight should be used.

Once the SGA is in place, confirm by utilizing ETCO$_2$, bilateral breath sound assessment, presence of chest rise, and improvement of arterial saturation. If the SGA is ineffective in achieving the ventilation goals the medical crew should be well trained in troubleshooting the device and continue working through their difficult airway algorithm. The transport environment is dynamic and always presents the risk of airway dislodgment. The secured SGA should be evaluated with visual inspection and ETCO$_2$ following each patient movement.

Intubation

Visualization and successful placement of an advanced airway may be difficult using direct laryngoscopy because of positioning and anatomic changes found in bariatric patients (see Table 20.3). Juvin et al. found a higher rate of difficult intubation in a bariatric patient than lean subjects (15% vs. 2%).[37] Video laryngoscope technology continues to improve. It has become the gold standard in the transport environment. These devices have been advocated in the bariatric patient population, as their use is associated with a high success rate, shortened intubation times, and decreased risk of arterial desaturation in high-risk patients.[38–41] Transport teams should consider additional airway management support from the referring institution, including direct video laryngoscopy or awake fiberoptic intubation.

Keys to an uncomplicated, successful placement of an advanced airway in any patient population begins with identifying a potentially difficult airway, preparation, and proper intubation technique. Sequencing these previously discussed pre-intubation steps include the following (Box 20.1):
- Airway assessment – prediction of difficult airway
  - Physical findings
- Environmental factor consideration

• BOX 20.1   Intubation Preparation

Patient Preparation
- Pulse oximeter and ECG monitor
- Functional IV with fluids attached/running
- Appropriate RSI medications
- Pre-oxygenation sitting patient up if possible
  - NRB, BVM, noninvasive positive airway pressure therapy (i.e., CPAP or BiPAP)

Procedural Equipment
- BVM on oxygen source #1
- Nasal cannula on oxygen source #2
- End-tidal carbon dioxide either in-line or detector available
- Suction on and functioning
- Video laryngoscope on and functioning
- Two (2) endotracheal tubes with intact balloon (i.e., correct size and one-size smaller)
- 10-mL syringe
- Bougie
- Stylet
- Stethoscope
- Commercial tube holder
- Wrist restraints

Back-Up Plan
- Back-up handle, blade(s), tube(s), stylet
- Supraglottic device(s)
- Secondary support provider (i.e., anesthesia)
- Surgical airway

BiPAP, Bilevel positive airway pressure; *BVM,* bag-valve-mask; *CPAP,* continuous positive airway pressure; *ECG,* electrocardiogram; *IV,* intravenous; *NRB,* nonrebreather; *RSI,* rapid sequence induction.

- Equipment gathering
  - Suction
  - ETCO$_2$
  - Endotracheal tubes (one predicted size and one size smaller)
  - Securing device
- Pharmacological adjuncts
- Pre-intubation support
  - Positioning
  - Pre-intubation oxygenation – tracheal insufflation via nasal cannula may be considered
  - Noninvasive positive pressure therapy
  - Bag-valve-mask ventilation
- Back-up adjuncts
  - Supraglottic airway devices
  - Potential need for back-up support (i.e., anesthesia, awake fiberoptic intubation)
  - Surgical airway
- Communication of the process with the care team
- Technique and visualization

Before an advanced airway attempt, resuscitate the patient appropriately to decrease the risk of further clinical decompensation. Resuscitation may include volume challenge, inotropic support, and increased ventilatory support. High BMI patients are at risk of low cardiopulmonary reserve and right-sided heart failure, which may make them less responsive to fluid challenges and increase the risk of cardiovascular decompensation during induction and airway placement. The medical crew should plan accordingly, engaging additional resources, following their clinical protocols, and consulting medical command if decompensation is suspected during intubation.

Elastic bougies can facilitate intubation in difficult airway patients. Driver et al. performed a randomized trial evaluating the first-attempt success rate in patients with difficult airways undergoing emergency intubation, comparing the bougie to the endotracheal tube with a stylet in the emergency department.[42] They reported a higher first-attempt success rate in the bougie group compared to the endotracheal with a stylet subject (96% vs. 82%; $P < 0.001$).[42] Jabre and colleagues reported a 75% intubation success rate in patients with a difficult airway and a 94% success rate in subjects without factors of a difficult airway.[43] Given these data, using a bougie may be a valuable adjunct for advanced airway management of bariatric patients.

Mechanical Ventilation

Obesity, as previously mentioned, results in altered respiratory anatomy and physiology and requires additional considerations when providing invasive and noninvasive mechanical ventilation. These considerations become critical during the acute stabilization phase of respiratory support. The initiation and management of respiratory support will facilitate ventilatory and oxygenation stabilization.

The increased chest and abdominal mass will affect respiratory mechanics and impair gas exchange.[44] Impaired gas exchange may require higher mean airway pressures, changes in positioning or increased PEEP. Other impairments include cranial displacement of the diaphragm in the supine position and loss of FRC, which is exacerbated by the loss of muscle tone.[44] A decrease in FRC results in airway closure, atelectasis, and increased intrapulmonary dead space in the dorsal aspect of the lung.[44] Recruitment and PEEP may mitigate the effects of a decreased FRC. More detailed lists of these anatomical and physiological changes are indicated in Tables 20.3 and 20.4.

Noninvasive Ventilation

Noninvasive ventilation (NIV) modalities include both CPAP (one level of airway pressure) and BiPAP (two levels of airway pressure) support using an interface that may consist of masks or nasal pillows. Use for management of ARF continues to be recommended as it has been associated with a decreased need for intubation and reduction in mortality/morbidity compared to standard oxygen therapy.[45,46] The increase in FRC associated with NIV may be advantageous in reversing hypoxia, as set PEEP potentially increases total lung volume and alveolar recruitment.[44]

Hypercarbic ARF may be a marker of the clinical progression of OHS, cardiogenic pulmonary edema, pneumonia, asthma, and exacerbation of COPD.[44] BiPAP adds two levels of airway pressure, end-expiratory level – PEEP – and inspiratory level – pressure support (PS) to mitigate central hypoventilation and facilitate CO_2 removal. PEEP's goals are to increase end-expiratory volume, thus increasing FRC, reversing atelectasis, and decreasing FiO_2 requirements. Set the inspiratory level to increase tidal volume (Vt), minute ventilation, and decrease CO_2 levels.[47]

Managing ARF with or without hypercarbia begins with stabilizing the underlying cause and initiating NIV via a three-step process.[47] The following approach has been recommended by Lauria et al.[47]:
1. Optimize respiratory mechanics:
   a. Initiate CPAP (EPAP) at 6–8 cmH_2O
   b. Titrate CPAP (EPAP) up by 2 cmH_2O till the work of breathing and oxygenation improves
2. Optimize oxygenation:
   a. Initiate FiO_2 at 1.0 or 100%
   b. After respiratory mechanics are optimized, FiO_2 can be decreased as tolerated to maintain SpO_2
3. Optimize ventilation:
   a. Initiate inspiratory level (IPAP) at 10–12 cmH_2O (PS above CPAP of 4–6 cmH_2O)
   b. Increase IPAP (PS above CPAP) by 2–4 cmH_2O to increase Vt, correct hypercarbia, and achieve a pH > 7.35
   c. Some bariatric patients may require PS as high as 30 cmH_2O

Other considerations should include proper mask selection and tolerance. Caution should be taken to decrease the risk of tissue injury while maintaining proper mask fit with a manageable leak. Modern ventilatory devices can compensate for a 60 L/min mask leak. However, not all leaks are bad. Some level of mask leak will facilitate CO_2 elimination and increase patient tolerance. Additionally, the mask should be sufficiently tightened to create a seal. The soft mask flange is designed to expand with positive pressure, creating an enhanced seal with decreased tissue pressure on the chin and bridge of the nose.

If the patient is not tolerating the NIV mask and therapy, HFNC may be considered. Stephan et al. reported in a secondary analysis of 272 bariatric patients that NIV lacked superiority regarding treatment failure compared to HFNC, 15% vs. 13%, respectively.[48] Given the physiologic alteration previously stated, NIV may be considered a first-line therapy in bariatric patients with ARF. However, if the patient is not tolerating NIV, HFNC is a potentially effective second-line approach for hypoxemic respiratory failure.[49] That said, caution should be taken, as HFNC may be less effective in primary ventilatory failure.

Regardless of the respiratory support provided, the patient's vital signs, mental status, work of breathing, respiratory pattern, tidal volume, SpO_2, and blood gas values should be monitored. In the absence of clinical improvement on optimized device settings, the presence of physiological deterioration, or the patient not tolerating NIV, intubation with mechanical ventilation should be considered.

Invasive Mechanical Ventilation

Following successful intubation, the goals of effective mechanical ventilation focus on targeting appropriate Vt, identifying optimal PEEP, achieving blood gas hemostasis via adequate minute ventilation, and decreasing the risk of ventilator-induced lung injury (VILI).[47] Tidal volume should be set to limit VILI and progressive inflammation in more compliant ventilation-dependent areas.[46] An accepted Vt target is 6–8 mL/kg ideal body weight (IBW).[47] Using the patient's actual body weight may overestimate the Vt resulting in lung injury, and should be avoided.

Positioning is an important consideration during mechanical ventilation, as placing the patient in either a ramped or reverse Trendelenburg position will unload the abdomen's weight off the diaphragm. Removing the excess weight results in better Vt distribution, oxygenation, and lower pressures necessary for effective ventilation.[47] Early return of spontaneous respiration can also preserve the diaphragmatic tone and redistribute ventilation to dependent regions of the lung.[47]

As mentioned, bariatric patients have decreased functional residual volume compared to normal-weight patient populations and will benefit from higher PEEP levels. Initial PEEP levels ranging between 8 and 10 cmH_2O were reported. PEEP helps keep the alveolar pressure greater than the closing pressure, thus maintaining end-expiratory lung volume or functional residual volume. PEEP will not necessarily recruit alveolar units but rather prevent derecruitment.[50] The added weight of chest adipose tissue results in higher closing pressures in the obese patient. That said, this does not result in higher PEEP pressures.[50] "Best PEEP" strategies should be used for PEEP titration, targeting oxygenation and improvement in lung mechanics.

Set respiratory rate should be done to achieve targeted minute ventilation goals and blood gas values. Management should focus on correcting the respiratory component of the pH and not correcting the PCO_2 which may be elevated as part of normal compensatory mechanisms. Rate settings do not vary from the standard adult patient population. The crew should maintain adequate time for lung emptying by maintaining an inspiratory:expiratory ratio of at least 1:2. In some clinical situations, the ratio may need to be augmented to meet oxygenation or prolonged expiratory times. In these cases, the medical crew should consult with medical direction. When indicated, ventilation information reported to the command physician should include all pertinent ventilator information. In addition, information should consist of the setting upon arrival, blood gas measures, and current ventilator settings. This information will help discern the next steps in the medical direction.

Pharmacology

Depending on the size of the bariatric patient, the medical crew responsible for administering medications should discuss and review all medication orders with a command physician. The absorption, metabolism, and primarily the distribution and excretion of drugs can be altered due to the size and body composition of the bariatric patient being transported.[51] Changes in distribution may require a smaller or larger dose. A drug that distributes well into fatty tissue will be dosed using the patient's total body weight (TBW). A drug with a low affinity for adipose tissue is restricted to the blood and other tissues. Such a drug would require a calculated ideal body weight (IBW) or a dosing weight (DW). An IBW reflects a person's "lean" body weight and incorporates gender and height in its calculation.[51]

Changes in excretion may require a shorter or longer dosing frequency. Renal elimination has been found to increase in obese patients taking several drugs and is often attributed to greater kidney mass.[51] Differences in the proportion of adipose and lean muscle tissue and fluid status can significantly affect the pharmacokinetics, absorption, distribution, metabolism, and excretion of drugs.[52] The size of the bariatric patient can increase total blood volume and cardiac output and cause alterations in plasma protein binding. Hepatic clearance is usually normal or even increased in obese patients, and renal clearance can increase because of increased kidney weight, renal blood flow, and glomerular filtration rate. The volume of distribution in bariatric patients can be dramatically different from that in normal-weight patients, and the extent of change is based on the intrinsic characteristics of a medication.[52] Hospitals should promote collaboration between staff and transport teams to ensure the safe transfer; active involvement of clinical pharmacologists in the dosing of medications is highly recommended. Necessary actions include using the appropriate weight-based calculations, educating the medical crew, and establishing protocols for medications used in emergent situations for the bariatric population of critical care transport.

Diagnostics

Radiology departments face increasing challenges in performing imaging studies with acceptable diagnostic quality in bariatric patients.[53] Because of thick layers of adipose tissue, computed tomography, magnetic resonance imaging, ultrasound, radiography, and nuclear medicine studies often yield distorted images with limited diagnostic value.[53] These factors can delay or limit the value of studies, placing the healthcare staff in a diagnostic predicament, to which most referring facilities will seek a transfer to a tertiary care center that may have the capabilities to perform the necessary diagnostic tests for the bariatric patient.

The scanners commonly used for computed tomography and magnetic resonance imaging have gantry aperture diameter (chest and abdominal girth) restrictions and table load limits. Patients must be able to freely move in and out of the machine's opening during the procedure. In addition, size restrictions exist to prevent structural damage to the equipment and subsequent injury to the patient. However, devices are now available that accommodate patients weighing up to 650 lb (292 kg), but the patient must meet the aperture diameter standards.[53] Knowledge of the girth and weight restrictions and capabilities of the receiving facilities' diagnostic equipment should be determined if the patient is being transported for diagnostics that were unable to be completed at the referring facility due to the patient's size.

Transport Operations

Critical care transport programs must determine thresholds based on the capabilities of each mode of transport and the types of transport vehicles offered by their program. Standard dispatch and response of resources may need to be adapted into a predetermined and educated communication process to effectively and safely transport bariatric patients.

A thorough understanding of the capabilities and limitations of the aircraft, including ambulance and aircraft stretchers and whether adaptions can be made to accommodate the bariatric patient, needs to be evaluated. Next, measurements of the vehicle's interior, where the patient is loaded and unloaded, and the weight capacity of the stretchers and mounts utilized are necessary to determine if transporting a bariatric patient is possible. This data should be known to crews and the dispatch center to facilitate mission planning. Finally, once a vehicle is determined to be capable of safe transport of the bariatric patient, synthesis of this data is necessary to coordinate whether the service's available vehicles can safely accommodate the patient or whether an alternate mode of transportation is necessary.

The following information is essential to ensure the correct asset is sent for transport:
- Patient weight
- Height of patient
- The straight-line width of the patient's widest part
- Height of the abdomen at the tallest part

The referring facility may request immediate assistance due to the bariatric patient's acuity. Failure to obtain information regarding weight, height, straight line width, and abdominal height to determine the appropriate asset to respond to the request may lead to further delays throughout the transport related to a lack of initial information gathering and inadequate preparation. With rotor-wing transport, determining the time frame of the closest asset and if the referring facility has a remote landing zone is essential. Remote landing zones may require multiple transfers and specialty vehicles negating the time benefit of a rotorcraft. There may be cases where it is reasonable to send a clinical team by rotor wing for immediate care, followed with a different aviation vehicle or a ground vehicle to complete the transport.

Following dispatch, the communication center should call the referring and receiving facilities and request appropriate resources to facilitate the transfer of the patient at both locations. Considerations include:
- Adequate personnel to assist in moving the patient to the referring/receiving unit and loading/unloading the patient at the aircraft. The National Institute for Occupational Safety and Health has a voluntary guideline suggesting that each individual on the lifting team lift no more than 51 pounds.[54]
- A hydraulic hospital stretcher or bariatric bed may be needed at the helipad. If a nonhydraulic bed is used, access to power will be needed at the helipad.
- Bariatric bed at the receiving hospital unit.
- Transfer slide board or specialized lifting sheet.
- If using a remote landing zone, a bariatric ambulance must be coordinated to take the patient to or from the remote landing zone, with EMS or fire personnel available to assist in transferring the patient to or from the aircraft.

Crew

Once the bariatric patient transport is relayed to the crew staffing the aircraft, the preparation and planning will depend on the synthesis of information relayed by the communication center.

Aviation will determine the weight and balance needs, fuel quantity, and weather-related issues. In addition, the pilots will reconfigure the aircraft to accommodate the specific stretcher configuration communicated. The medical crew will determine the necessary equipment and remove unnecessary bags and items irrelevant to the transport. In addition, the team will assist with reconfiguring the aircraft and determine if specific bariatric equipment is necessary to assist in the transport. All team members will be educated on the reconfiguration procedures, stretcher use and placement, equipment bag needs, placement and securing, and types of bariatric transfer devices the service utilizes.

Sample Bariatric Equipment Bag
- Stretcher belt extenders
- Air mattress system (inflatable mattress, blower, batteries)
- Back-up inflatable mattress
- Large bariatric tarp with handles
- Heavy duty Bucher mounts × 2
- Extra foils and mega mover

Bedside Priorities

Upon arrival at the bedside, transport teams should assess the clinical, environmental, and transport needs. Clinical concerns are identified, and initial interventions needed to stabilize the patient are completed. Before transferring the patient onto the cardiac transport monitor, intravenous infusion pumps, and any oxygen delivery devices, clarify the patient's physical and cognitive needs.

If the patient is alert and oriented, communicate the plan on how the transfer will occur. Open communication will provide the crew with information on how the patient can assist and will ease the patient as they will have concerns, which may include the risk of crew injury or them falling on the floor. Depending on patient size and weight, transfer may require additional assistance.

Proceed by placing any movement-assist devices (i.e., sliders, inflatable movers, and handled movers) by rolling the patient with assistance then placing the device under the patient. Ensure all handles are visible or have an extension added for access.

Based on the size of the patient and the configuration of the aircraft, determine if the patient can be transported on the aircraft stretcher, a bariatric hydraulic stretcher, or the bariatric bed to the aircraft. Ensure the weight limit is checked prior to utilizing the hospital's hydraulic stretcher. Pay attention to the head of the hydraulic stretcher or the bariatric bed. Consider whether the frame will permit sliding the patient from the head into an aircraft. A stretcher may have to be reversed if the head of the stretcher precludes the transfer into an aircraft. An assessment of the stretcher and an understanding of the operational components is necessary to avoid complications when you get to the aircraft with the patient.

In addition, review the route taken through the referring facility to ensure ease of movement through halls and into and out of elevators, and that these will accommodate the crew, necessary devices, and the type of stretcher/bed the patient is transported on. Measurement of doorways, elevators, etc., should be completed before transferring the patient onto a transport stretcher.

After all the patient's monitoring devices, intravenous infusions, and other equipment (i.e., ventilator and assist devices) have been transferred, ensure adequate slack of the wires and tubing before transferring the patient onto the transport stretcher.

Once the patient is on the transport stretcher, ensure placement of each device to allow ease of access. Leaving an intravenous access point available is imperative for continuous assessment of the infusions being administered and accessibility for additional medication administration. Most bariatric patients are unable to lay flat for more than a few minutes; ensure all safety precautions when elevating the head by having extra assistance supporting the bottom of the transport stretcher with extra assistance at the top to elevate the head of the stretcher as the weight distribution will change and can cause a tip. Ensure the patient is secured through all phases of trans-

port. Stretcher belt extenders may be necessary to secure the patient adequately.

Preparing to Depart Bedside

Before departing the bedside with a bariatric patient, complete your routine assessment and checks before heading to the aircraft. The oxygen demand in this patient population needs careful consideration and calculation, as transport time from the bedside to the aircraft will be prolonged. Anticipate the need for additional oxygen cylinders and a plan for cylinder exchange during the transfer to the aircraft. Similarly, ensuring an adequate volume of intravenous medications for transport is necessary to ensure no gaps in medication administration. The transport stretcher or bed needs to be set to the level of the aircraft floor before departing. Knowing the floor height for the type of vehicle you are utilizing is a crucial measurement to obtain before a bariatric transport. If the stretcher is in the aircraft or ambulance and you are transferring the patient from a portable stretcher into the aircraft containing a stretcher, this height will need to be accounted for in addition to the height of the vehicle's floor. Finally, review the plan with the staff that will be assisting you. Delegate responsibilities before departing bedside. Ensure all team members verbalize understanding and provide time to address any questions or concerns the staff may have. If the patient is alert and oriented, ensure comfort, communicate the plan, and provide dignity throughout all transitions during the transport to the aircraft and into the aircraft.

As a final check, before departing the bedside:
- Ensure you have adequate personnel available for each patient transition to the aircraft (at the bedside and aircraft).
- Ensure the path to the helipad includes pathways, hallways, and elevators that can accommodate the stretcher or bed used.
- Obtain a transfer slide board and bring it to the aircraft.

Loading the Patient in the Transport Vehicle

Ensure adequate personnel is available to load the patient into the aircraft or ambulance. The personnel inside the vehicle should monitor advanced airways and equipment while guiding the patient into the correct position. Personnel should be positioned outside the aircraft to move the patient into the aircraft. The hydraulic stretcher or bed should be positioned at the back of the vehicle and level with the back of the aircraft but above the level of the stationary stretcher placed in the aircraft. This will prevent the mattresses from rolling underneath the patient. The plastic slide board can be utilized as a bridge if necessary. Move the patient into the aircraft with as much assistance as possible to the crew. It is critical to minimize the amount of time the patient is lying flat.

Off-Loading the Patient from the Transport Vehicle

The same careful preparation involved in moving the patient out of the hospital and into the transport vehicle are needed at the receiving end, but in reverse. Advance notice and preparation from the Communications Center will aid in marshalling the resources needed.

Personal and Environmental Bias

Caring for the bariatric patient must address the bias associated with caring for, treating, and transporting this specialized population.

These patients have failed many attempts to lose weight and are sensitive to how they are addressed publicly. They know they have care challenges and specialized needs. A successful program addresses the social needs of patients and their families. Patients' perceptions of being stigmatized by healthcare providers can lead to feelings of shame, marginalization, and anxiety. For these reasons among others, the priority is to provide the highest quality of care while ensuring dignity, demonstrating compassion and empathy during transport.

Bariatric Sensitivity

The Respect Model discusses that the key to providing quality, patient-centered, sensitive care to the bariatric patient is RESPECT.[55]

R – Rapport is an interpersonal relationship of connection, empathy, and understanding.

- *Tips to achieve rapport*: Use common courtesy, introduce yourself, listen attentively, maintain eye contact, and do not make assumptions about the person based on their weight: "See the person, not the pounds."

E – Environment/Equipment: the environment in which we care for the bariatric patient can convey concern for their unique physical comfort and safety needs or it cannot.

- *Tips to demonstrate a bariatric-friendly environment*: Provide and use appropriate size equipment; remember, "one size does not fit all," and know the weight limit of the equipment you use.

S – Safety: body weight and weight distribution in the bariatric patient may present a safety challenge when attempting to turn, lift or ambulate. Patients often fear falling or hurting the patient care staff when transferring. The goal is to build a safety culture for the patient and the medical crew.

- *Tips to achieve a safe environment*: Use bariatric equipment and assistive devices as indicated, know the weight limit of

your equipment, obtain the appropriate number of staff members to safely transfer the patient, and use proper body mechanics.

P – Privacy: to build and maintain trust with the bariatric patient, it is critical to safeguard their privacy, protect the confidentiality of patient information, and always preserve their dignity.

- *Tips to demonstrate attention to the privacy needs of the bariatric patient*: Keep the patient covered with the appropriate size gown/robe and discuss with the patient's family/friends only if the patient permits.

E – Encouragement: many bariatric patients have made multiple attempts to lose weight in the past without success. Motivation and attitude can play a significant role in the success of treatments and improve the quality of life for the bariatric patient.

- *Tips to encourage*: Provide positive feedback and recognize even the most minor successes during transport.

C – Caring/Compassion: caring is based on concern or interest in actions that contribute to the good, worth, dignity, or comfort of another human being. Caring is the connectedness and mutual respect between the patient and the patient care team members.

- *Tips to demonstrate caring and compassion:* Anticipate the patient's needs; plan when possible; recognize your personal biases and judgments about obesity; do not communicate your opinions about obesity to the bariatric patient and avoid blaming the patient; not all medical conditions are "caused" by obesity.

T – Tact is the ability to speak or act without offending another person.

- *Tips to demonstrate tact*: be aware of nonverbal signals, facial expressions, and body language, and avoid offensive terms when talking about or to the patient.

Summary

Bariatric transport is an emerging area of transport medicine. This trend is expected to continue to grow as obesity rates have increased across all sociodemographic classes and age groups. Care and transport of this specialized patient population poses unique challenges across all phases of the transport continuum. For this reason, transport of bariatric patients requires a firm understanding of the operational, clinical, and emotional needs of each patient to achieve the best possible outcomes.

Timely and safe transport of this population begins at the time of referral, requiring collaboration among the referring facility, local EMS, the transport service, and receiving center. Collaboration is ensured via concise communication, accurate measurements (i.e., *weight, height, straight-line of patient's widest part*, and *height of the abdomen at the tallest point*) and organized asset management using information gathering and identification of

environmental and vehicle limitations. Identifying all potential challenges and concerns among the transport stakeholders will help navigate potential delays and minimize risk and decrease crew workload. Situational awareness and good resource management are critical tools in ensuring success of these specialized transports.

Medical crews should understand the physiologic differences, common comorbidities, and challenges these patients create in the dynamic environment that is transport. Pre-planning and communication with goal-oriented care plans will further facilitate their safe transport. It is critical to limit bias and provide emotional support for the patient and their family. Developing operational and clinical processes for each of the aforementioned areas will help ensure safe and effective transport, while creating value for not only the patient and family, but also the community as well.

References

1. Hales CM, Carroll MD, Fryar CD, Ogden CL. Prevalence of obesity and severe obesity among adults: United States, 2017–2018. NCHS Data Brief, no. 360. Hyattsville, MD: National Center for Health Statistics; 2020.
2. Centers for Disease Control and Prevention (CDC). Overweight and Obesity. Obesity Factsheet 2010. Available at: https://tinyurl.com/bdefperj.
3. Centers for Disease Control and Prevention (CDC). Overweight and Obesity. Adult obesity prevalence maps. Available at: https://www.cdc.gov/obesity/data/prevalence-maps.html.
4. Centers for Disease Control and Prevention (CDC). Overweight & Obesity: Surveillance Systems. July 22, 2022. Available at: https://www.cdc.gov/obesity/data/surveillance.html#NPAO.
5. Stierman B, Afful J, Carroll MD, et al. National Health and Nutrition Examination Survey 2017–March 2020 prepandemic data files: development of files and prevalence estimates for selected health

outcomes. National Health Statistics Reports, no. 158. Hyattsville, MD: National Center for Health Statistics; 2021.

6. Centers for Disease Control and Prevention (CDC). Overweight and Obesity. Defining adult overweight and obesity. June 3, 2022. Available at: https://tinyurl.com/2jstz2es.

7. Hurst S, Blanco K, Boyle D, et al. Bariatric implications of critical care nursing. *Dimens Crit Care Nurs*. 2004;23(2):76–83.

8. Murphy C, Wong DT. Airway management and oxygenation in obese patients. *Can J Anesth*. 2013;60:929–945.

9. Cook TM, Woodall N, Frerk C; Fourth National Audit Project. Major complications of airway management in the UK: results of the Fourth National Audit Project of the Royal College of Anaesthetists and the Difficult Airway Society. Part 1: Anaesthesia. *Br J Anaesth*. 2011;106 617–631.

10. Leblanc M, Croteau S, Ferland A, et al. Blood pressure assessment in severe obesity: validation of a forearm approach. *Obesity*. 2013; 21(12):E533–E541.

11. Catenacci VA, Hill, JO, Wyatt HR. The obesity epidemic. *Clin Chest Med*. 2009;30:415–444.

12. Zammit C, Liddicoat H, Moonsie I, Makker H. Obesity and respiratory disease. *Int J Gen Med*. 2010;3:335–343.

13. Kress JP, Pohlman AS, Alverdy J, Hall JB. The impact of morbid obesity on the oxygen cost of breathing at rest. *Am J Resp Crit Care Med*. 1999;160:883–886.

14. Hegewald MJ. Impact of obesity on pulmonary function: current understanding and knowledge gaps. *Curr Opin Pulm Med*. 2021;27(2): 132–140.

15. Salome CM, King GG, Berend N. Physiology of obesity and effects on lung function. *J Appl Physiol 1985*. 2010;108:206–211.

16. Rubinstein I, Zamel N, DuBarry L, Hoffstein V. Airflow limitation in morbidly obese, nonsmoking men. *Ann Intern Med*. 1990;112:828–832.

17. Zerah F, Harf A, Perlemuter L, et al. Effects of obesity on respiratory resistance. *Chest*, 1993;103:1470–1476.

18. Ferretti A, Giampiccolo P, Cavalli A, et al. Expiratory flow limitation and orthopnea in massively obese subjects. *Chest*; 2001;119: 1401–1408.

19. Torchio R, Gobbi A, Gulotta C, et al. Mechanical effects of obesity on airway responsiveness in otherwise healthy humans. *J Appl Physiol 1985*. 2009;107:408–416.

20. Beuther DA, Sutherland ER. Overweight, obesity and incident asthma: a meta-analysis of prospective epidemiologic studies. *Am J Respir Crit Care Med*. 2007;175:661–666.

21. Rodrigo GJ, Plaza V. Body mass index and response to emergency department treatment in adults with severe asthma exacerbations: a Prospective Cohort Study. *Chest*. 2007;132:1513–1519.

22. Zewari S, Vos P, vanden Elshout F, et al. Obesity in COPD: revealed and unrevealed issues. *COPD J Chron Obstruct Pulm Dis*. 2017;14(6): 663–673.

23. BaHamman A. Acute ventilatory failure complicating obesity hypoventilation: update on a "critical care syndrome". *Curr Opin Pulm Med* 2010;16:543–551.

24. Masa JF, Pepi JL, Borel JC, et al. Obsity hypoventilation syndrome. *Eur Respir Rev*. 2019;28:180097.

25. Horner RL, Mohiaddin RH, Lowell DG, et al. Sites and sizes of fat deposits around the pharynx in obese patients with obstructive sleep apnoea and weight matched controls. *Eur Respir J* .1989;2:613–622.

26. Breckwoldt J, Klemstein S, Brunne B, et al. Difficult prehospital endotracheal intubation – predisposing factors in a physician based EMS. *Resuscitation*. 2011;82:1519–1524.

27. Wang HE, Kupas DF, Greenwood MJ, et al. An algorithmic approach to prehospital airway management. *Prehosp Emerg Care*. 2005;9:145–155.

28. Dixon BJ, Dixon JB, Carden JR, et al. Preoxygenation is more effective in the 25 degrees head-up position than in the supine position in severely obese patients: a randomized controlled study. *Anesthesiology*. 2005;102:1110–1115; discussion 5A.

29. Levitan RM, Mechem CC, Ochroch EA, Shofer FS, Hollander JE. Head-elevated laryngoscopy position: improving laryngeal exposure during laryngoscopy by increasing head elevation. *Ann Emerg Med*. 2003;41:322–330.

30. Tanoubi I, Drolet P, Donati F. Optimizing preoxygenation in adults. *Can J Anesth*. 2009;56:449–466.

31. Baraka AS, Taha SK, Siddik-Sayyid SM, et al. Supplementation of pre-oxygenation in morbidly obese patients using nasopharyngeal oxygen insufflation. *Anaesthesia*. 2007;62:769–773.

32. Ricottilli F, Ickx B, Van Obbergh L. High-flow nasal cannula pre-oxygenation in obese patients undergoing general anaesthesia: a randomized controlled trial. *Br J Anaesth*. 2019;123(3):E443–444.

33. Vourch M, Baud G, Feuillet F, et al. High-flow nasal cannulae versus non-invasive ventilation for preoxygenation of obese patients: the PREOPTIPOP randomized trial. *EClin Med*. 2019;13:112–119.

34. Langeron O, Masso E, Huraux C, et al. Prediction of difficult mask ventilation. *Anesthesiology*. 2000;92:1229–1236.

35. Kheterpal S, Han R, Tremper KK, et al. Incidence and predictors of difficult and impossible mask ventilation. *Anesthesiology*. 2006;105: 885–891.

36. Natalini G, Franceschetti ME, Pantelidi MT, et al, Comparison of the standard laryngeal mask airway and the ProSeal laryngeal mask airway in obese patients. *Br J Anaesth*. 2003;90:323–326.

37. Juvin P, Lavaut E, Dupont H, et al. Difficult tracheal intubation is more common in obese than in lean patients. *Anesth Analg*. 2003; 97:595–600.

38. Ndok SK, Amathieu R, Tual L, et al. Tracheal intubation of the morbidly obese patients: a randomized trial comparing the performance of the Macintosh and Airtraq laryngoscope. *Br J Anaesth*. 2008;100:263–268.

39. Anderson LH, Rovsing L, Olsen KS, et al. Glidescope videolaryngoscope vs. Macintosh direct laryngoscope for intubation of morbidly obese patients: a randomized trial. *Anesthesiol Scand*. 2011;55: 1090–1097.

40. Marrel J, Blanc C, Frascarolo P, et al. Videolaryngoscopy improves intubation conditions in morbidly obese patients. *Eur J Anaesthesiol*. 2007;24:1045–1049.

41. Moore AR, Schricker T, Court O. Awake videolaryngoscopy-assisted tracheal intubation of the morbidly obese. *Anaesthesia*. 2012;67: 232–235.

42. Driver BE, Prekker ME, Klein LR, et al. Effect of use of a bougie vs. endotracheal tube and stylet on first-attempt intubation success among patients with difficult airways undergoing emergency intubation: a randomized clinical trial. *JAMA*. 2018;319(21):2179–2189.

43. Jabre P, Combes X, Leroux B. Use of gum elastic bougie for prehospital difficult intubation. *Am J Emerg Med*. 2005;23:552–555.

44. De Jong A, Wrigge H, Hedenstierna G, et al. How to ventilate obese patients in the ICU. *Intens Care Med*. 2020;46:2423–2435.

45. Rochwerg B, Brochard L, Elliott MW, et al. Official ERS/ATS clinical practice guidelines: noninvasive ventilation for acute respiratory failure. *Eur Respir*. 2017;50(2):1602426.

46. Jaber S, Lescot T, Futier E, et al. Effect of noninvasive ventilation on tracheal reintubation among patients with hypoxic respiratory failure following abdominal surgery: a randomized clinical trial. *JAMA*. 2016;315:1345–1353.

47. Lauria MJ, Root CW, Gottula AL, Braude DA. Management of respiratory distress and failure in morbidity and super obese patients during critical care transport. *Air Med J*. 2022;41:133–140.

48. Stephan F, Berand L, Rezaiguia-Delclaux S, Amaru P. High-flow nasal cannula therapy versus intermittent noninvasive ventilation in obess subjects after cardiothoracic surgery. *Respir Care*. 2017;62: 1193–1202.

49. Drake MG. High-flow nasal cannula oxygen in adults: an evidence-based assessment. *Ann Am Thorac Soc*. 2018;15(2):145–155.

50. De Jong A, Chanques G, Jaber S. Mechanical ventilation in obese ICU patients: from intubation to extubation. *Crit Care*. 2017;21:63.

51. Davidson JE, Kruse MW, Cox DH, Duncan R. Critical care of the morbidly obese. *Crit Care Nurs Q.* 2003;26(2):105–116.

52. Berrios LA. The ABCDs of managing morbidly obese patients in intensive care units. *Crit Care Nurs.* 2016;36(5):17–26.

53. Phillips J. Care of the bariatric patient in acute care. *J Radiol Nurs.* 2013;32(1):21–31.

54. Waters TR, Putz-Anderson V, Garg A. *Applications Manual for the Revised NIOSH Lifting Equation.* Cincinnati, OH: U.S. Department of Health and Human Services, Centers for Disease Control and Prevention, National Institute for Occupational Safety and Health, DHHS Publication; no. (NIOSH) 94-110 (Revised 9/2021). Available at: https://stacks.cdc.gov/view/cdc/110725.

55. Bejciy-Spring SM. R-E-S-P-E-C-T: a model for the sensitive treatment of the bariatric patient. *Bariatr Nurs Surg Patient Care.* 2008; 3:47–56.

Index